The Microbiome in Rheumatic Diseases and Infection

Gaafar Ragab • T. Prescott Atkinson
Matthew L. Stoll
Editors

The Microbiome in Rheumatic Diseases and Infection

Springer

Editors
Gaafar Ragab
Faculty of Medicine
Cairo University
Cairo
Egypt

T. Prescott Atkinson
University of Alabama
Birmingham, AL
USA

Matthew L. Stoll
University of Alabama
Birmingham, AL
USA

ISBN 978-3-030-07708-2 ISBN 978-3-319-79026-8 (eBook)
https://doi.org/10.1007/978-3-319-79026-8

Printed on acid-free paper

This Springer imprint is published by the registered company Springer International Publishing AG part of Springer Nature.
The registered company address is: Gewerbestrasse 11, 6330 Cham, Switzerland

It has long been an axiom of mine that the little things are infinitely the most important

—Sherlock Holmes in A Case of Identity by Sir Arthur Conan Doyle.

This book is dedicated to our wives: Samia, Miriam, and Janice.

Foreword

It is fitting to now have a book dedicated entirely to the role of the microbiome in our rheumatic diseases. After all, the study of the infectious origins of rheumatoid arthritis alone is an exercise in exploration of the modern bestiary. From 30,000 feet I would like to draw attention to observations that may help to open our minds on this topic before entering this valuable new addition to the literature which bridges the fields of rheumatic and immunologic diseases and microbiology.

First, while I am genuinely excited at the exploration of the interface of rheumatic disease etiology, pathogenesis, and natural history and the human microbiome, I am more basically left in wonder by how our microbiome shapes our relationships not just with diseases but with our sum total of experiences with the natural world. Recognize that we are not humans at all but exist as superorganisms or holobionts who have been imprinted with a remarkable spectrum of microbial entities whose own interests may not coincide with ours at any given time. Furthermore and even more remarkable is that our DNA is about 8–10% of viral origin (i.e., endogenous retroviral elements) that has created a host-parasite co-evolutionary dynamic affecting everything from our integrated host defenses to our behavior. Based on this remarkable fact alone it is imperative that we increasingly dedicate our precious resources to furthering our understanding of these relationships and how they contribute to enhancing health and causing disease.

Second, I would like to remind us that the study of the microbiome and its relationship to health and diseases is a long road and that reductionist aspirations to find a microbial culprit that causes a given disease or to therapeutically manipulate the microbiome through microbial supplements or dietary change are likely to be unrewarding, at least for now. Study of the microbiome in many ways, including the massive global efforts to categorize it such as the Human Microbiome Project and the Earth Microbiome Project, remind me in many ways of the excitement and effort poured into the Human Genome Project which in the end taught us relatively little about specific human diseases but opened up a Pandora's box of ever new questions to be addressed. While we hope that some clarion concepts may arise from such reductionist approaches to the microbiome, we may find ourselves in the same situation, facing an ever increasing and complex set of questions to address if we are to move forward. To do so I urge us all to think expansively and consider how our microbiome interacts with other networks such as our food supply, our environment, and our society.

So with these humbling caveats which hopefully remind us of our small vantage point in our complex world I welcome you to *The Microbiome in Rheumatic Diseases and Infection.*

Leonard H. Calabrese
Department of Rheumatic and Immunologic Diseases
College of Medicine of Case Western Reserve University
Cleveland, OH
USA

Contents

List of Contributors

Daniel M. Altmann Department of Medicine, Hammersmith Hospital, Imperial College London, London, UK

Miika Arvonen Department of Pediatrics, Kuopio University Hospital, Kuopio, Finland

John W. Baddley Department of Medicine, Division of Infectious Diseases, University of Alabama at Birmingham, Birmingham, AL, USA

Medical Service, Birmingham VA Medical Center, Birmingham, AL, USA

Thomas Bardin INSERM U1132, Rheumatology Department, Hôpital Lariboisière, University Paris Diderot, Paris, France

Anne Barton Division of Musculoskeletal and Dermatological Sciences, The University of Manchester, Manchester, UK

Meriem Belheouane Max-Planck-Institute for Evolutionary Biology, Plön, Germany

Institute for Experimental Medicine, Christian-Albrechts-University of Kiel, Kiel, Germany

Dimitrios P. Bogdanos Department of Rheumatology and Clinical Immunology, Faculty of Medicine, School of Health Sciences, University of Thessaly, Larissa, Greece

Rosemary J. Boyton Department of Medicine, Hammersmith Hospital, Imperial College London, London, UK

Giorgio Bozzi Infectious Diseases Unit, University of Milan, L. Sacco Hospital, Milan, Italy

Paul A. Bryant Department of Medicine, Division of Infectious Diseases, University of Alabama at Birmingham, Birmingham, AL, USA

Patrice Cacoub Sorbonne Universités, UPMC Univ Paris 06, UMR 7211, and Inflammation-Immunopathology-Biotherapy Department (DHU i2B), Paris, France

INSERM, UMR_S 959, Paris, France

CNRS, FRE3632, Paris, France

AP-HP, Groupe Hospitalier Pitié-Salpêtrière, Department of Internal Medicine and Clinical Immunology, Referral Center for Rare Autoimmune Systemic Disorders, Paris, France

Sara Zandonella Callegher Rheumatology Clinic, Academic Hospital Santa Maria della Misericordia, Udine, Department of Medical and Biological Sciences, Udine, Italy

Luca Cantarini Research Center of Systemic Autoinflammatory Diseases, Behçet's Disease and Rheumatology-Ophthalmology Collaborative Uveitis Center, Department of Medical Sciences Surgery and Neurosciences, University of Siena, Siena, Italy

Madhura Castelino Department of Rheumatology, NIHR Manchester Musculoskeletal Biomedical Research Unit, The University of Manchester, Manchester, UK

Cloe Comarmond Sorbonne Universités, UPMC Univ Paris 06, UMR 7211, and Inflammation-Immunopathology-Biotherapy Department (DHU i2B), Paris, France

INSERM, UMR_S 959, Paris, France

CNRS, FRE3632, Paris, France

AP-HP, Groupe Hospitalier Pitié-Salpêtrière, Department of Internal Medicine and Clinical Immunology, Referral Center for Rare Autoimmune Systemic Disorders, Paris, France

Randy Q. Cron University of Alabama at Birmingham, Birmingham, AL, USA

Heleen Cypers Department of Rheumatology, Ghent University Hospital, Ghent, Belgium

Mario M. D'Elios University of Florence, Florence, Italy

Maria I. Danila University of Alabama at Birmingham, Division of Clinical Immunology and Rheumatology, Birmingham, AL, USA

Carina Dehner Department of Immunobiology, Yale School of Medicine, New Haven, CT, USA

Anne Claire Desbois Sorbonne Universités, UPMC Univ Paris 06, UMR 7211, and Inflammation-Immunopathology-Biotherapy Department (DHU i2B), Paris, France

INSERM, UMR_S 959, Paris, France

CNRS, FRE3632, Paris, France

AP-HP, Groupe Hospitalier Pitié-Salpêtrière, Department of Internal Medicine and Clinical Immunology, Referral Center for Rare Autoimmune Systemic Disorders, Paris, France

Salvatore De Vita Rheumatology Clinic, Academic Hospital Santa Maria della Misericordia, Udine, Department of Medical and Biological Sciences, Udine, Italy

Dirk Elewaut Department of Rheumatology, Ghent University Hospital, Ghent, Belgium

Unit for Molecular Immunology and Inflammation, VIB Inflammation Research Center, Ghent University, Ghent, Belgium

Esraa M. Eloseily Assuit University Children's Hospital, Assiut, Egypt

Jean-François Emile EA4340 and Pathology Department, Versailles University and Ambroise Paré Hospital, Boulogne, France

Guliz Erdem Nationwide Children's Hospital Medical Center, The Ohio State University, Infectious Diseases Section, Columbus, OH, USA

Steve Eyre Division of Musculoskeletal and Dermatological Sciences, The University of Manchester, Manchester, UK

Polly J. Ferguson University of Iowa Carver College of Medicine, Iowa City, IA, USA

Massimo Galli Infectious Diseases Unit, University of Milan, L. Sacco Hospital, Milan, Italy

Saviana Gandolfo Rheumatology Clinic, Academic Hospital Santa Maria della Misericordia, Udine, Department of Medical and Biological Sciences, Udine, Italy

Andrea Giacomelli Infectious Diseases Unit, University of Milan, L. Sacco Hospital, Milan, Italy

Hadi Goubran College of Medicine, University of Saskatchewan, Saskatoon, SK, Canada

Saskatoon Cancer Centre, Saskatoon, SK, Canada

Loïc Guillevin Department of Internal Medicine, Hôpital Cochin, Assistance Publique–Hôpitaux de Paris, Université Paris Descartes, Paris, France

Ahmet Gül Istanbul University, Istanbul Faculty of Medicine, Department of Internal Medicine, Division of Rheumatology, Istanbul, Turkey

Hazem Hamza Virology Laboratory, National Research Centre, Cairo, Egypt

Department of Immunology, Interfaculty Institute of Cell Biology, Eberhard Karls University Tübingen, Tübingen, Germany

Julien Haroche Department of Internal Medicine, French Reference Center for Rare Auto-immune and Systemic Diseases, Institut E3M, AP-HP, Pitié-Salpêtrière Hospital, Paris, France

Université Pierre et Marie Curie, University Paris 6, Paris, France

Saleh Ibrahim Lübeck Institute of Experimental Dermatology, University of Lübeck, Lübeck, Germany

College of Medicine and Sharjah Institute for Medical Research, University of Sharjah, Sharjah, United Arab Emirates

Ana Izcue Institute of Molecular Medicine, RWTH Aachen University, Aachen, Germany

Traci Jester Department of Pediatrics, Division of Gastroenterology, University of Alabama at Birmingham, Birmingham, AL, USA

Maria Kaparakis-Liaskos La Trobe University, Melbourne, VIC, Australia

Edward L. Kaplan University of Minnesota Medical School, Department of Pediatrics, Minneapolis, MN, USA

Martin Kriegel Department of Immunobiology, Yale School of Medicine, New Haven, CT, USA

Axel Künstner Max Planck Institute for Evolutionary Biology, Plön, Germany

Group for Medical Systems Biology, Lübeck Institute of Experimental Dermatology (LIED), University of Lübeck, Lübeck, Germany

S. Louis Bridges Jr. Division of Clinical Immunology and Rheumatology, Comprehensive Arthritis, Musculoskeletal, Bone and Autoimmunity Center, University of Alabama at Birmingham, Birmingham, AL, USA

Philip M. Murphy Laboratory of Molecular Immunology, National Institute of Allergy and Infectious Diseases, National Institutes of Health, Bethesda, MD, USA

Anoma Nellore Department of Medicine, Division of Infectious Diseases, University of Alabama at Birmingham, Birmingham, AL, USA

Derek Pearson College of Medicine, University of Saskatchewan, Saskatoon, SK, Canada

Saskatoon Cancer Centre, Saskatoon, SK, Canada

T. Prescott Atkinson Division of Pediatric Allergy, Asthma and Immunology, University of Alabama at Birmingham, Birmingham, AL, USA

Luca Quartuccio Rheumatology Clinic, Academic Hospital Santa Maria della Misericordia, Udine, Department of Medical and Biological Sciences, Udine, Italy

Gaafar Ragab Rheumatology and Clinical Immunology Unit, Department of Internal Medicine, Faculty of Medicine, Cairo University, Cairo, Egypt

Philipp Rausch Max Planck Institute for Evolutionary Biology, Plön, Germany

Institute for Experimental Medicine, Christian-Albrechts-University of Kiel, Kiel, Germany

Catherine J. Reynolds Department of Medicine, Hammersmith Hospital, Imperial College London, London, UK

Donato Rigante Institute of Pediatrics, Università Cattolica Sacro Cuore, Fondazione Policlinico Universitario "A. Gemelli", Rome, Italy

Hussien Rizk Department of Cardiology, Faculty of Medicine, Cairo University, Cairo, Egypt

Rossana Rocco Nephrology Unit, University Hospital, Parma, Italy

Ester Roffe Departamento de Bioquímica e Imunologia, Universidade Federal de Minas Gerais, Belo Horizonte, MG, Brazil

William Ruff Department of Immunobiology, Yale University School of Medicine, New Haven, CT, USA

David Saadoun Sorbonne Universités, UPMC Univ Paris 06, UMR 7211, and Inflammation-Immunopathology-Biotherapy Department (DHU i2B), Paris, France

INSERM, UMR_S 959, Paris, France

CNRS, FRE3632, Paris, France

AP-HP, Groupe Hospitalier Pitié-Salpêtrière, Department of Internal Medicine and Clinical Immunology, Referral Center for Rare Autoimmune Systemic Disorders, Paris, France

Lazaros I. Sakkas Department of Rheumatology and Clinical Immunology, Faculty of Medicine, School of Health Sciences, University of Thessaly, Larissa, Greece

Julia Spierings Department of Rheumatology and Clinical Immunology, University Medical Centre Utrecht, Utrecht, The Netherlands

Matthew L. Stoll Department of Pediatrics, Division of Rheumatology, University of Alabama at Birmingham, Birmingham, AL, USA

Konstantinos Thomas Joint Rheumatology Program, Clinical Immunology-Rheumatology Unit, 2nd Department of Medicine and Laboratory, National and Kapodistrian University of Athens, School of Medicine, Hippokration General Hospital, Athens, Greece

Augusto Vaglio Nephrology Unit, University Hospital, Parma, Italy

Jacob M. van Laar Department of Rheumatology and Clinical Immunology, University Medical Centre Utrecht, Utrecht, The Netherlands

Femke C. van Rhijn-Brouwer Department of Rheumatology and Clinical Immunology, University Medical Centre Utrecht, Utrecht, The Netherlands

Department of Nephrology and Hypertension, University Medical Centre Utrecht, Utrecht, The Netherlands

Dimitrios Vassilopoulos Joint Rheumatology Program, Clinical Immunology-Rheumatology Unit, 2nd Department of Medicine and Laboratory, National and Kapodistrian University of Athens, School of Medicine, Hippokration General Hospital, Athens, Greece

Antonio Vitale Research Center of Systemic Autoinflammatory Diseases, Behçet's Disease and Rheumatology-Ophthalmology Collaborative

Uveitis Center, Department of Medical Sciences Surgery and Neurosciences, University of Siena, Siena, Italy

David R. Webb The Department of Integrated Structural and Computational Biology, The Scripps Research Institute, La Jolla, CA, USA

Arthur Weinstein MedStar Washington Hospital Center, Washington, DC, USA

Georgetown University, Washington, DC, USA

Exagen Diagnostics, Vista, CA, USA

W. Winn Chatham University of Alabama at Birmingham (UAB), Division of Clinical Immunology and Rheumatology, Birmingham, AL, USA

Wayne Young Food Nutrition and Health Team, AgResearch, Palmerston North, New Zealand

Riddet Institute, Massey University, Palmerston North, New Zealand

High-Value Nutrition, National Science Challenge, Auckland, New Zealand

About the Editors

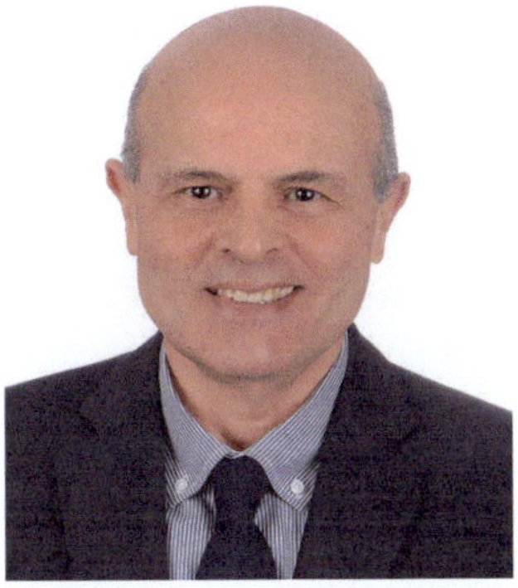

Gaafar Ragab graduated from the Faculty of Medicine, Cairo University, 1976, where he got his degrees in Internal Medicine: MSc, 1980, and PhD, 1985. He served his faculty as a Resident, Assistant Lecturer (1980), Lecturer (1985), Assistant Professor (1990), and Professor (1995) till now. He spent a sabbatical year 1989 at the UAB, USA, in the Department of Clinical Immunology and Rheumatology. He headed the Clinical Immunology and Rheumatology Unit affiliated to the Internal Medicine Department (2010–2015). He was Chief of the Internal Medicine Department's Research Committee (1995–2013). He is Fellow of the American College of Rheumatology (ACR) since 1989. He is a Co-founder of the Egyptian Society of Immunology and Rheumatology (EGYSIR) which he headed as its President from 2010 to 2013. He was chosen as President of the Egyptian League Against Rheumatism (ELAR) annual meeting in Alexandria, 2013. He is a member of the Advisory Board of the Egyptian Society of Internal Medicine (ESIM) and its journal and served as President of ESIM annual meeting, Cairo, 2014. He is the associate editor of the *Journal of Advanced Research* (JARE), the interdisciplinary publication of Cairo University, in charge of its medical branch. He won the prize of honor, Cairo University, for the great efforts in international publications, for the year 2008. He is a member of the Egyptian National Committee for the management of Hepatitis C Virus (the extrahepatic manifestation) as well as the International Study Group of Extrahepatic Manifestations Related to Hepatitis C Virus infection (ISGEHCV). He is also a member of the Geographical Variation in Rheumatoid Arthritis Group (GEO RA).

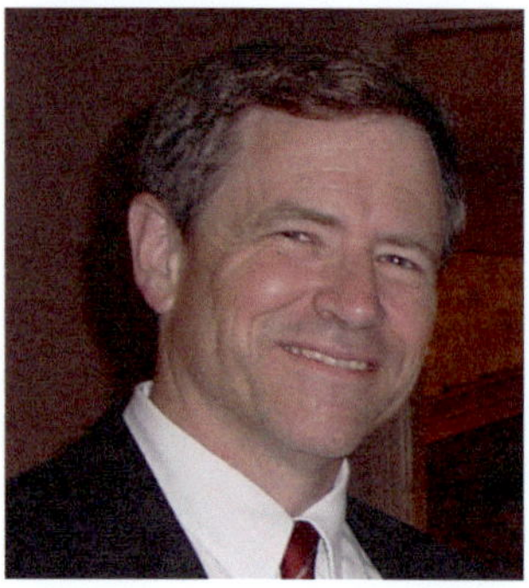

T. Prescott Atkinson is a native of Alabama, USA, born and raised in Montgomery. He attended Tulane University (1971–1975) in New Orleans, Louisiana, and then completed 6 years of active duty in the U.S. Navy. After his military tour of duty, he entered the Medical Scientist Training Program (MD-PhD) at Emory University (1981–1987). It was during his PhD work at Emory University that he became interested in immunologic cell signaling, and he carried this area of interest in immunology into Fellowship training at the National Institutes of Health as an NIAID Clinical Fellow in Allergy/Immunology (1987–1992). After moving to the University of Alabama at Birmingham in 1992 as an Assistant Professor of Pediatrics, he began seeing pediatric rheumatology and primary immunodeficiency patients in clinic, and benefited immensely from weekly review conferences/patient discussions with Dr. Max Cooper, one of the giants in the field of immunology. This is an area in which he still maintains an active clinical interest, and over the years, principally in collaboration with groups at the NIH, he has continued to pursue studies on the molecular etiology and clinical characteristics of this extraordinarily diverse group of disorders. He has also become interested in the role of chronic infection, particularly with mycoplasmas, in chronic diseases such as asthma and arthritis, particularly in patients with primary immunodeficiencies and rheumatic disorders. He is a former member and Chair of the American Board of Allergy and Immunology. Currently he is Professor and Director of the Division of Pediatric Allergy, Asthma, and Immunology at UAB.

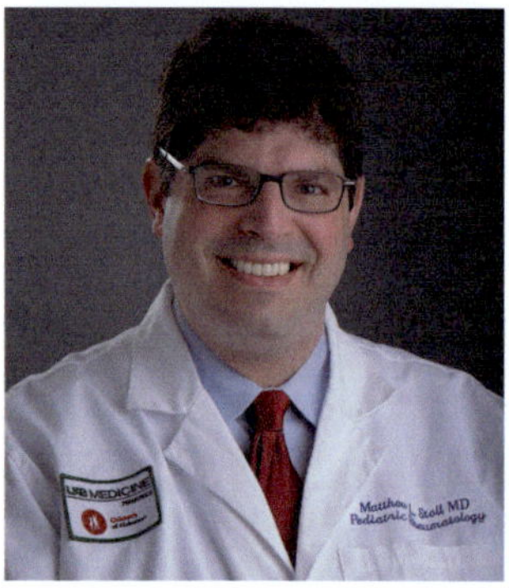

Matthew L. Stoll is a pediatric rheumatologist who earned his MD and PhD at Upstate Medical University (Syracuse, NY) in 2001, followed by completion of residency in pediatrics at the Long Island Jewish Medical Center in 2004 and fellowship in pediatric rheumatology at the Children's Hospital Boston in 2007. At the completion of his fellowship, he took a staff position at the University of Texas at Southwestern Medical Center (Dallas, TX), where he earned an MSCS degree. In 2011, he moved to the University of Alabama at Birmingham, where he remains. During his fellowship, Dr. Stoll developed an interest in the clinical epidemiology of spondyloarthritis, publishing on age-based subgroups of juvenile psoriatic arthritis as well as risk factors for sacroiliitis in patients with pediatric spondyloarthritis. He subsequently turned his attention to the links between spondyloarthritis and inflammatory bowel disease and reported on the use of fecal calprotectin as well as intestinal MRI to identify subclinical intestinal inflammation in children with spondyloarthritis. His current work focuses on the role of the intestinal microbiota in the pathogenesis of pediatric spondyloarthritis.

Part I

Introductory Chapters

1 The Microbiome: Past, Present, and Future

Matthew L. Stoll

Abbreviations

AS	Ankylosing spondylitis
EEN	Exclusive enteral nutrition
IBD	Inflammatory bowel disease
JIA	Juvenile idiopathic arthritis
RA	Rheumatoid arthritis

Past: Surprising Insights into Today's Microbial World

> All disease starts in the gut.—Attributed to Hippocrates

In the 1670s, Antony van Leeuwenhoek was the first to describe the presence of bacteria, which he described as "animalcules of the most minute size which moved themselves about very energetically [1]." Very little progress was made toward identifying or characterizing bacteria over the next two centuries. Infectious agents had not, it appears, captured the attention of the scientific community until Louis Pasteur promoted the concept that germs can cause transmissible disease, and Pasteur as well as Robert Koch further contributed to the field by developing techniques to culture bacteria [2]. As reviewed in 1911 [1], in the 1870s, two independent groups detected the presence of bacteria in stool. However, much of the work at the time, quite understandably, was focused on isolation of specific organisms associated with devastating diseases. Along those lines, there were some major discoveries at the time, including discovery of the bacteria causing anthrax in the blood of a dead animal accompanied by the demonstration that the disease could be transmitted through injection of the blood into a healthy animal as well as isolation and identification of the bacteria causing such diseases as tuberculosis, bacterial dysentery, and cholera [1]. Of note, the investigator who discovered both *Mycobacterium tuberculosis* in 1882 and *Vibrio cholerae* in 1884, Robert Koch, is still known today for his work proving pathogenicity of these bacteria.

Interest in the intestinal microbiota as a whole did not emerge until early in the twentieth century. Elie Metchnikoff had a rather dismal view of the microbiota, fearing that it released toxins into the systemic circulation that produced senility, and he therefore advocated altering the colonic microbiota [3]. An extreme method of doing so, which gained some attraction in the early twentieth century, was colectomy. There were some adherents to this belief, including Dr. Arbuthnot Lane, who performed colectomy or colonic bypass for a variety of

M. L. Stoll
Department of Pediatrics/Division of Rheumatology, University of Alabama at Birmingham, Birmingham, AL, USA
e-mail: mstoll@peds.uab.edu

G. Ragab et al. (eds.), *The Microbiome in Rheumatic Diseases and Infection*,
https://doi.org/10.1007/978-3-319-79026-8_1

indications [4]. By the 1920s, this procedure had fallen out of favor [3].

A more nuanced view of the intestinal microbiota was offered by Arthur Kendall, who hypothesized that they were typically benign, unless the host is colonized with specific pathogenic agents [1]. That the intestinal microbiota was essential for the health of the host was initially demonstrated in 1915, through studies on germ-free chicks, which showed poor development of the germ-free animals starting at 10 days of life [5]. These observations resulted in the conclusion that "man has a bacterial population in his intestinal tract; that under normal conditions the organisms in the intestinal tract are fairly characteristic and constant; normally they are harmless; [and] *they may be protective* [5]."

In addition to work in germ-free animals, several further lines of current research into the microbiota had their start 100 years ago. One of them is the functional capacity of intestinal bacteria, which today is studied through such tools as shotgun sequencing of microbial DNA and mass spectroscopy of fecal and plasma metabolites. Ford initially noted that bacteria differ in their ability to metabolize carbohydrates and proteins, characterizing bacteria into two categories: fermenters (carbohydrates metabolizers) and putrifiers (protein metabolizers) [6]. Kendall extended these findings, observing that "Food largely determines the type of intestinal bacteria [1]." Specifically, diets rich in carbohydrates resulted in the generation of bacteria with increased capacity to metabolize carbohydrates. Today, it is well recognized that fiber-rich diets result in increased abundance of bacteria capable of metabolizing complex carbohydrates [7]. While carbohydrate and protein metabolism were the focus of attention in the first two decades of the twentieth century, by mid-century, the microbial effects on multiple other endogenous substances were studied, including B-complex vitamins [8–10], vitamin C [11], and cholesterol [12].

Another area of active interest today that had its roots 100 years ago is interest in treating disease through alterations in the intestinal microbiota. While today's efforts, as will be seen throughout this textbook, focus on the treatment of chronic inflammatory diseases, interest in the pre-antibiotic era was in the management of infectious diseases. As discussed above, colectomy was an extreme method of altering the intestinal microbiota, but not the only one. Diet has long been recognized as a very effective means of doing so, beginning with observations from 1911 that bottle-fed and breast-fed infants had substantially different microbial populations, with these studies even showing increased "homogeneity" of the intestinal microbiota in bottle-fed infants [1]. These observations are a precursor to recent findings showing decreased alpha diversity in bottle-fed compared to nursed infants [13]. Torrey as well noted that diet strongly influenced the contents of the microbiota, writing "It has been my experience that the intestinal flora of dogs reacts very promptly and with great uniformity to changes in diet [14]." Kendall proposed using simple sugars to alter the microbiota as a therapeutic tool for bacterial dysentery, thus in effect introducing the first instance of a therapeutic prebiotic [1]. Lane followed therapeutic colectomies in the first decades of the twentieth century with introduction of pure cultures of bacteria, first *Lactobacillus bulgaricus* and later *Lactobacillus acidophilus*, an early use of probiotics [3]. In perhaps the first published fecal microbial transplant, Dalton transplanted *Escherichia coli* from a healthy subject to a child undergoing antibiotic therapy for meningitis, reporting that rectal but not oral administration of the organism resulted in successful uptake and may have contributed to resolution of the illness [15]. In 1955, Winkelstein evaluated *Lactobacillus acidophilus* as a therapeutic agent in 53 subjects with a variety of intestinal disorders, including ulcerative colitis, reporting mixed results [16]. For the most part, however, interest in probiotics remained low until the 1990s [3].

Loss of interest in probiotic therapy as a tool to alter the microbiota may have been due to the development of antibiotics, with penicillin introduced in 1928 and many others to follow. Improved public health measures in developed nations, including vaccinations and improved hygiene, likely also dampened enthusiasm in research into microbial-based therapy of intestinal infections. In any event, the widespread use of antibiotics spurred interest in the 1940s and 1950s on the effect of these therapies on the contents of the intestinal microbiota [17–20] and subsequently on the development of antibiotic resistance [21]. Another line of research in that era that pertained to antibiotics, which at the time was largely of interest to the agricultural field, were the effects of antibiotic therapy on the growth of livestock. Several studies demonstrated that young animals fed antibiotics demonstrated increased growth [22–24]. Observations that these growth-promoting effects of antibiotics did not occur in germ-free animals [25] and were associated with increased efficiency of absorption of dietary fatty acids [26] resulted in the conclusion that changes in the fecal microbiota mediated the increased weight gain of young animals treated with antibiotics [26]. Although this practice has fallen in disfavor due to concerns of transmission of antibiotic-resistant bacterial pathogens to humans, interest in the effects of antibiotics on growth remains, with a recent study showing that early exposure to antibiotics may be associated with an increased risk of childhood obesity [27].

One final theme that emerged in the 1950s and is germane to this textbook is the association of the intestinal microbiota with autoimmune diseases, including those not intrinsic to the gastrointestinal tract. Perhaps the first such study was published by Seneca, who reported increased total and coliform bacteria in the feces of 15 patients with UC as compared to four healthy controls [28]. Studies in the 1950s evaluated the intestinal microbiota in pediatric celiac disease [29] and acne [30]. Subsequent early studies on the intestinal microbiota were published in Crohn disease in 1969 [31], rheumatoid arthritis (RA) in 1966 [32], and ankylosing spondylitis (AS) in 1978 [33].

Ultimately, all of these efforts were limited by technology. For 100 years following the resurgence of interest in the intestinal microbiota, the only tool available to characterize them was culture, which we know today to be a highly inefficient means to characterize bacteria. It is often cited that only 20% of intestinal bacteria can be cultured [34]. Although this number may be higher [35], many of these bacteria require specialized media, and anaerobic culture is also technically demanding. In 1977, Carl Woese introduced the concept of identifying bacteria according to their ribosomal 16S DNA sequence [36], and 10 years later he published an immense database of bacterial 16S sequences [37]. This permitted use of DNA probes to characterize bacterial communities, and this technology was used in studies of RA [38] and AS [39] to name but two. However, the real explosion in microbial DNA technology had yet to come.

Present: "Democratization of Metagenomics"

> The intestinal tract is a wonderfully perfect incubator and culture medium combined… It must be evident that the direction that this flora takes will not be without influence upon the host.—Arthur Kendall (1911)

The last 10 years has witnessed an explosion of research into the microbiota. A PubMed search of microbiome or microbiota identified nearly 40,000 publications, the vast majority of which are under 10–15 years old. This research has been enabled by advances not only in sequencing technology but primarily in computing power; indeed, a typical smartphone contains more than 100,000 times the computing power of those that launched the lunar mission in 1969. More recently, even the initial sequencing of the Human Genome Project costs over $3 billion and took approximately 13 years, whereas today, the estimated cost of whole human exome sequencing is under $1000 http://www.genome.gov/sequencingcosts/ (accessed December 18, 2017). Due to the lower costs, investigators around the world are able to contribute to the field, a capacity that Jeff Gordon dubbed the "democratization of metagenomics [40]." These efforts around the world have been tremendously supported by massive centralized efforts to catalog the microbiota: the Human Microbiome Project in the United States [41] and Euro-HIT in Europe [42]. Thanks in no small part to these efforts, reference databases contain over

1.4 million bacteria and 53 thousand archaea [43] as of the end of 2016.

Much of the human work involving the microbiome consists of identifying differences in the microbiota between patient groups, e.g., those with versus without a particular disease. Such work is open to criticism that these differences are associative, but do not necessarily reflect a causal relationship. That is, the inflammatory milieu associated with a particular disease, or even its treatments, may result in alterations in the microbiota that are challenging to control for using comparison groups of healthy individuals. However, important work in animals and even in humans to some extent has shown the power of the microbiota to shape the disease, as well as the therapeutic potential of alterations of the microbiota.

Multiple animal models of inflammatory disease are attenuated or in some cases accelerated when the animals are raised in a germ-free setting, either in a true gnotobiotic facility or through treatment with broad-spectrum antibiotics. These include models of RA [44], ulcerative colitis [45], and chronic noninfectious osteomyelitis [46]. In each of these models, disease was highly attenuated in the germ-free state, and, furthermore, Koch's postulates of disease causation were partially established by recurrence of the disease when the microbiota were reintroduced into the animals.

A striking example of mediation of disease through the microbiota is the transfer of the obesity phenotype. Turnbaugh et al. studied mice that were genetically programmed to develop obesity based upon mutations in the gene coding for the satiety signal leptin [47]. Obese mice had increased *Firmicutes* in their intestines, findings typical in the obese state. Impressively, transfer of the fecal microbiota to germ-free mice resulted in increased weight gain among mice that received microbiota from obese as compared to lean mice. There were no differences in chow consumption, so this difference reflected increased energy harvest.

Another example is the HLA-B27 transgenic rat model of spondyloarthritis. Typically, transgenic rats develop a spontaneous arthritis, orchitis, and colitis. When raised in a sterile environment, the rats are protected against arthritis and colitis [48]; however, disease recurs when the animals are exposed to a cocktail of bacteria that includes *Bacteroides vulgatus* [49].

Human studies as well demonstrate that the microbiota can impact inflammatory diseases. One interesting illustration of this came from research in infants at risk for type I diabetes mellitus based upon HLA types [50]. The investigators obtained serial fecal specimens from 33 at-risk children from birth through age 3 years, finding that changes in the contents of the fecal microbiota preceded development of clinical disease.

Similarly, a study of adults with newly diagnosed RA showed an expansion of a single organism, *Prevotella copri*, in 75% of newly diagnosed subjects, that was not seen in healthy controls or established patients [51]. The pathogenic nature of this species was further demonstrated by oral gavage of mice, which resulted in colitis.

Finally, the impact of the microbiota on human disease is illustrated by therapeutic responses to treatment, possibilities that are still in their infancy. While antibiotic [52] and probiotic [53] therapy have long been a mainstay of treatment of inflammatory bowel disease, there has been increasing interest in the potential role of fecal microbial transplantation [54]. Additionally, it is clear that dietary manipulation through the use of exclusive enteral nutrition (EEN) can induce remission of inflammatory bowel disease (IBD) as effectively as can corticosteroids [55, 56], and EEN has also been reported to be beneficial in children with juvenile idiopathic arthritis [57]. Although dietary changes can induce rapid shifts in the microbiome [58], it is not clear whether the beneficial effects of dietary changes are mediated through the microbiome or some other mechanism. It remains to be seen whether microbial manipulation will have similar effects in other diseases.

It is not at all surprising that alterations in the microbiota can impact inflammatory diseases. The microbiota is required for normal development of the immune system [59], and the intestinal microbiota in particular represents the largest mass of microbial antigen and adjuvant that is encountered in life, thus setting the stage for marked effects on systemic and mucosal immune systems [60]. Indeed, antibodies directed against commensal microbial components are present and potentially pathogenic in a variety of autoimmune diseases, including IBD [61], spondyloarthritis [62], and RA [63].

Finally, it bears mentioning that certain microbiota may also be beneficial. Not only are certain bacteria generally considered protective (e.g., *Faecalibacterium prausnitzii* in IBD (Chap. 19)), but there is a body of literature that an entire class of organisms, helminth parasites, may also be protective against allergic or autoimmune diseases. The data in mice were summarized in a recent review [64]. Evidence that parasitic infection may be protective against allergy or autoimmunity is as follows: (a) A meta-analysis determined that current infection with an intestinal parasite was associated with reduced risk of allergic sensitization [65]; (b) worldwide rates of multiple sclerosis and parasitic infestation show an inverse correlation [66]; and (c) in an area endemic for filarial parasites, patients with RA were significantly less likely to be infected as compared to healthy controls [67]; an observational study of multiple sclerosis patients demonstrated that helminth infection was associated with reduced disease progression [68]. It does bear mention, however, that some studies have shown contradictory data with respect to helminth infection and atopic diseases [69–71], and consequently not all investigators have been convinced by the epidemiologic data [72]. Additionally, interventional studies of live parasites in a variety of human autoimmune disorders have generally shown mixed results (Table 1.1).

Table 1.1 Therapeutic trials of parasitic worms

Study	Patient population	Study design	Parasite	Outcome
Allergic rhinitis				
[79]	100 adults	RCT	*Trichuris suis*	No improvement in symptoms
[80]	100 adults	RCT	*Trichuris suis*	No changes in allergic reactivity
Asthma				
[81]	30 adults	RCT	*Necator americanus* larvae	No improvement in airway hyperreactivity
[82]	32 adults	RCT	*Necator americanus* larvae	No improvement in airway hyperreactivity
Inflammatory bowel disease				
[83]	4 adults with CD and 3 with UC	OL, uncontrolled	*Trichuris suis*	6/7 achieved remission for at least part of the study period
[84]	29 adults with CD	OL, uncontrolled	*Trichuris suis*	At week 24, 21/29 (72%) responded; 23/29 (79%) met criteria for remission
[85]	54 adults with UC	RCT	*Trichuris suis*	Favorable response seen in 13/30 (43%) in the treatment group versus 4/24 (15%) controls ($p = 0.04$). Remission occurred in ≤10% in both groups
[86]	36 adults with CD	RCT	*Trichuris suis*	Improvements in symptoms seen in placebo and treatment groups; no comparisons performed
Multiple sclerosis				
[87]	5 treatment-naïve adults	OL, uncontrolled	*Trichuris suis*	Decrease in number of new MRI lesions from 6.6 to 2; no change in self-reported symptoms
[88]	10 adults	OL, uncontrolled	*Trichuris suis*	Increase in number of new MRI lesions from 6 to 21
[89]	16 treatment-naïve adults	OL, uncontrolled	*Trichuris suis*	Nonsignificant improvement in MRI lesions; self-reported improvement in symptoms in 12/16

CD Crohn disease, *MRI* magnetic resonance imaging, *OL* open-label, *RCT* randomized controlled trial, *UC* ulcerative colitis

It is of particular interest that we have come full circle in our understanding that some of the chronic rheumatic diseases may have microbial causes. Over a century ago, C. Fred Bailey proposed that RA was likely caused by toxins elaborated by microorganisms, which potentially resided in the joints, nasopharynx, or gastrointestinal tract [73]. Sulfasalazine was developed as a therapeutic agent on the basis of this assumption that RA is an infectious disease [74]. Indeed, as discussed in the RA chapter (Chap. 15), there have been multiple successful trials of antibiotics in RA, yet by the late twentieth century, the notion that this was an infectious illness was abandoned, and the effectiveness of antibiotics was attributed to intrinsic anti-inflammatory effects of these agents [75]. Yet now, as shall be discussed as well in the RA chapter (Chap. 15), there is substantial evidence that specific microbes and their associated inflammatory properties underlie the disease.

Future: Microbiota-Based Therapeutics or Prevention

> A lack of knowledge of the normal intestinal bacteria and their relations will be a serious handicap in recognizing the abnormal bacteria and their relations… Arthur Kendall (1911)

Much work lies ahead to understand not only the contributory role of the microbiota to the disease but also the extent to which microbial manipulation may have therapeutic potential. As with any medication, this will require well-designed randomized studies to assess safety and efficacy. Many rheumatologists are familiar with the concept of a "window of opportunity" to treat an inflammatory disease. We are also familiar with the idea that the disease process begins long before the first symptom emerges, as illustrated by lupus-associated antibodies being formed years before the clinical onset of disease [76]. For diseases mediated by the microbiota, the window may be long before even the first disease manifestation. We will learn in the juvenile idiopathic arthritis (JIA) chapter (Chap. 17) of evidence that elevated fecal *Bacteroides* in JIA may reflect not intrinsic pathogenicity of this genus but altered immune development on account of it. We are also learning that early childhood events affecting the gut microbiota may influence the risk not only of pediatric autoimmune disease but possibly even adult disease as well. Gordon proposed the concept of microbial prevention, such as administering probiotics to infants immediately after birth, or even to their mothers just before delivery [40]. Probiotic studies involving infants have shown benefit in reducing the risk of type I diabetes [77] and atopy [78]. Thus, the future of microbiota-based therapeutics may prove to be as much of a public health measure as therapeutic measures for individual diseases.

References

1. Kendall AI. Certain fundamental principles relating to the activity of Bacteria in the intestinal tract. Their relation to therapeutics. J Med Res. 1911;25(1):117–87.
2. Smith KA. Louis pasteur, the father of immunology? Front Immunol. 2012;3:68.
3. Podolsky SH. Metchnikoff and the microbiome. Lancet. 2012;380(9856):1810–1.
4. Smith JL. Sir Arbuthnot lane, chronic intestinal stasis, and autointoxication. Ann Intern Med. 1982;96(3):365–9.
5. Kendall AI. The Bacteria of the intestinal tract of man. Science. 1915;42(1076):209–12.
6. Ford WW. Classification of intestinal bacteria: (preliminary note). J Med Res. 1901;6(1):211–9.
7. Heinritz SN, Weiss E, Eklund M, Aumiller T, Louis S, Rings A, et al. Intestinal microbiota and microbial metabolites are changed in a pig model fed a high-fat/low-fiber or a low-fat/high-fiber diet. PLoS One. 2016;11(4):e0154329.
8. Jimenez Diaz C, Ales JM, Vivanco F. Symbiotic action of intestinal microbial flora; studies on nicotinic acid, pyridoxine, folic acid, and vitamin B12 synthesis by microbial flora in the enteric tract. Bull Inst Med Res Univ Madr. 1953;6(2–3):105–28.
9. Abdel-Salaam A, Leong PC. Synthesis of vitamin B(1) by intestinal bacteria of the rat. Biochem J. 1938;32(6):958–63.
10. Ellinger P, Abdel Kader MM. The nicotinamide-saving action of tryptophan and the biosynthesis of nicotinamide by the intestinal flora of the rat. Biochem J. 1949;44(3):285–94.
11. Esselen WB, Fuller JE. The oxidation of ascorbic acid as influenced by intestinal bacteria. J Bacteriol. 1939;37(5):501–21.
12. Wainfan E, Henkin G, Rittenberg SC, Marx W. Metabolism of cholesterol by intestinal bacteria in vitro. J Biol Chem. 1954;207(2):843–9.

13. Azad MB, Konya T, Persaud RR, Guttman DS, Chari RS, Field CJ, et al. Impact of maternal intrapartum antibiotics, method of birth and breastfeeding on gut microbiota during the first year of life: a prospective cohort study. BJOG. 2015;123(6):983–93.
14. Torrey JC. The regulation of the intestinal flora of dogs through diet. J Med Res. 1919;39(3):415–47.
15. Dalton HW. Implantation of B. coli into the human intestine. Ir J Med Sci. 1951;308:384–6.
16. Winkelstein A. Lactobacillus acidophilus tablets in the therapy of various intestinal disorders: a preliminary report. Am Pract Dig Treat. 1955;6(7):1022–5.
17. Campos JV, Hoenen W, Costa A, Trabulsi L, Pontes JF. Changes in intestinal flora under tetracycline. Gastroenterology. 1958;34(4):625–35.
18. Anderson GW, Cunningham JD, Slinger SJ. Effect of terramycin and certain phenylarsonic acid derivatives on the growth and intestinal flora of Turkey poults. J Nutr. 1952;48(4):539–52.
19. Lipman MO, Coss JA Jr, Boots RH. Changes in the bacterial flora of the throat and intestinal tract during prolonged oral administration of penicillin. Am J Med. 1948;4(5):702–9.
20. Thomas AR, Levine M. Some effects of penicillin on intestinal bacteria. J Bacteriol. 1945;49(6):623–7.
21. Goldberg HS, Goodman RN, Lanning B. Low-level, long-term feeding of chlortetracycline and the emergence of antibiotic-resistant enteric bacteria. Antibiot Annu. 1958;6:930–4.
22. Stern JR, Mc GJ. Antibiotics and early growth of rats fed a soybean oil meal diet. Arch Biochem. 1950;28(3):364–70.
23. Berg LR, Bearse GE, Mc GJ, Miller VL. The effect of removing supplemental aureomycin from the ration on the subsequent growth of chicks. Arch Biochem. 1950;29(2):404–7.
24. Sieburth JM, Gutierrez J, Mc GJ, Stern JR, Schneider BH. Effect of antibiotics on intestinal microflora and on growth of turkeys and pigs. Proc Soc Exp Biol Med. 1951;76(1):15–8.
25. Forbes M, Park JT. Growth of germ-free and conventional chicks: effect of diet, dietary penicillin and bacterial environment. J Nutr. 1959;67(1):69–84.
26. Eyssen H, de Somer P. The mode of action of antibiotics in stimulating growth of chicks. J Exp Med. 1963;117(1):127–38.
27. Saari A, Virta LJ, Sankilampi U, Dunkel L, Saxen H. Antibiotic exposure in infancy and risk of being overweight in the first 24 months of life. Pediatrics. 2015;135(4):617–26.
28. Seneca H, Henderson E. Normal intestinal bacteria in ulcerative colitis. Gastroenterology. 1950; 15(1):34–9.
29. Anderson CM, Langford RF. Bacterial content of small intestine of children in health, in coeliac disease, and in fibrocystic disease of pancreas. Br Med J. 1958;1(5074):803–6.
30. Loveman DE, Noojin RO, Winkler CH Jr. Comparative studies of enteric bacterial flora in acne vulgaris. J Invest Dermatol. 1955;25(3):135–7.
31. Drasar BS, Shiner M. Studies on the intestinal flora. II. Bacterial flora of the small intestine in patients with gastrointestinal disorders. Gut. 1969;10(10):812–9.
32. Mansson I, Olhagen B. Intestinal Clostridium perfringens in rheumatoid arthritis and other connective tissue disorders. Studies of fecal flora, serum antitoxin levels and skin hypersensitivity. Acta Rheumatol Scand. 1966;12(3):167–74.
33. Ebringer RW, Cawdell DR, Cowling P, Ebringer A. Sequential studies in ankylosing spondylitis. Association of Klebsiella pneumoniae with active disease. Ann Rheum Dis. 1978;37(2):146–51.
34. Eckburg PB, Bik EM, Bernstein CN, Purdom E, Dethlefsen L, Sargent M, et al. Diversity of the human intestinal microbial flora. Science. 2005;308(5728):1635–8.
35. Goodman AL, Kallstrom G, Faith JJ, Reyes A, Moore A, Dantas G, et al. Extensive personal human gut microbiota culture collections characterized and manipulated in gnotobiotic mice. Proc Natl Acad Sci U S A. 2011;108(15):6252–7.
36. Woese CR, Fox GE. Phylogenetic structure of the prokaryotic domain: the primary kingdoms. Proc Natl Acad Sci U S A. 1977;74(11):5088–90.
37. Woese CR. Bacterial evolution. Microbiol Rev. 1987;51(2):221–71.
38. Vaahtovuo J, Munukka E, Korkeamaki M, Luukkainen R, Toivanen P. Fecal microbiota in early rheumatoid arthritis. J Rheumatol. 2008;35(8):1500–5.
39. Stebbings S, Munro K, Simon MA, Tannock G, Highton J, Harmsen H, et al. Comparison of the faecal microflora of patients with ankylosing spondylitis and controls using molecular methods of analysis. Rheumatology (Oxford). 2002;41(12):1395–401.
40. Gordon JI. Honor thy gut symbionts redux. Science. 2012;336(6086):1251–3.
41. Human Microbiome Project Consortium. Structure, function and diversity of the healthy human microbiome. Nature. 2012;486(7402):207–14.
42. Qin J, Li R, Raes J, Arumugam M, Burgdorf KS, Manichanh C, et al. A human gut microbial gene catalogue established by metagenomic sequencing. Nature. 2010;464(7285):59–65.
43. Schloss PD, Girard RA, Martin T, Edwards J, Thrash JC. Status of the archaeal and bacterial census: an update. MBio. 2016;7(3):e00201–16.
44. Wu HJ, Ivanov II, Darce J, Hattori K, Shima T, Umesaki Y, et al. Gut-residing segmented filamentous bacteria drive autoimmune arthritis via T helper 17 cells. Immunity. 2010;32(6):815–27.
45. Garrett WS, Lord GM, Punit S, Lugo-Villarino G, Mazmanian SK, Ito S, et al. Communicable ulcerative colitis induced by T-bet deficiency in the innate immune system. Cell. 2007;131(1):33–45.
46. Hubbard TD, Murray IA, Perdew GH. Indole and tryptophan metabolism: endogenous and dietary routes to Ah receptor activation. Drug Metab Dispos. 2015;43(10):1522–35.
47. Turnbaugh PJ, Ley RE, Mahowald MA, Magrini V, Mardis ER, Gordon JI. An obesity-associated gut

microbiome with increased capacity for energy harvest. Nature. 2006;444(7122):1027–31.
48. Taurog JD, Richardson JA, Croft JT, Simmons WA, Zhou M, Fernandez-Sueiro JL, et al. The germfree state prevents development of gut and joint inflammatory disease in HLA-B27 transgenic rats. J Exp Med. 1994;180(6):2359–64.
49. Dieleman LA, Goerres MS, Arends A, Sprengers D, Torrice C, Hoentjen F, et al. Lactobacillus GG prevents recurrence of colitis in HLA-B27 transgenic rats after antibiotic treatment. Gut. 2003;52(3):370–6.
50. Lahoti TS, John K, Hughes JM, Kusnadi A, Murray IA, Krishnegowda G, et al. Aryl hydrocarbon receptor antagonism mitigates cytokine-mediated inflammatory signalling in primary human fibroblast-like synoviocytes. Ann Rheum Dis. 2013;72(10):1708–16.
51. Scher JU, Sczesnak A, Longman RS, Segata N, Ubeda C, Bielski C, et al. Expansion of intestinal Prevotella copri correlates with enhanced susceptibility to arthritis. Elife. 2013;2:e01202.
52. Wilson L, Arabshahi A, Simons B, Prasain JK, Barnes S. Improved high sensitivity analysis of polyphenols and their metabolites by nano-liquid chromatography-mass spectrometry. Arch Biochem Biophys. 2014;559:3–11.
53. Li S, Pozhitkov A, Ryan RA, Manning CS, Brown-Peterson N, Brouwer M. Constructing a fish metabolic network model. Genome Biol. 2010;11(11):R115.
54. Castagnini C, Luceri C, Toti S, Bigagli E, Caderni G, Femia AP, et al. Reduction of colonic inflammation in HLA-B27 transgenic rats by feeding Marie Menard apples, rich in polyphenols. Br J Nutr. 2009;102(11):1620–8.
55. Sigall-Boneh R, Pfeffer-Gik T, Segal I, Zangen T, Boaz M, Levine A. Partial enteral nutrition with a Crohn's disease exclusion diet is effective for induction of remission in children and young adults with Crohn's disease. Inflamm Bowel Dis. 2014;20(8):1353–60.
56. Soo J, Malik BA, Turner JM, Persad R, Wine E, Siminoski K, et al. Use of exclusive enteral nutrition is just as effective as corticosteroids in newly diagnosed pediatric Crohn's disease. Dig Dis Sci. 2013;58(12):3584–91.
57. Berntson L, Hedlund-Treutiger I, Alving K. Anti-inflammatory effect of exclusive enteral nutrition in patients with juvenile idiopathic arthritis. Clin Exp Rheumatol. 2016;34(5):941–5.
58. Wu GD, Chen J, Hoffmann C, Bittinger K, Chen YY, Keilbaugh SA, et al. Linking long-term dietary patterns with gut microbial enterotypes. Science. 2011;334(6052):105–8.
59. Abramowicz S, Susarla HK, Kim S, Kaban LB. Physical findings associated with active temporomandibular joint inflammation in children with juvenile idiopathic arthritis. J Oral Maxillofac Surg. 2013;71(10):1683–7.
60. Saleh M, Elson CO. Experimental inflammatory bowel disease: insights into the host-microbiota dialog. Immunity. 2011;34(3):293–302.
61. Targan SR, Landers CJ, Yang H, Lodes MJ, Cong Y, Papadakis KA, et al. Antibodies to CBir1 flagellin define a unique response that is associated independently with complicated Crohn's disease. Gastroenterology. 2005;128(7):2020–8.
62. Mundwiler ML, Mei L, Landers CJ, Reveille JD, Targan S, Weisman MH. Inflammatory bowel disease serologies in ankylosing spondylitis patients: a pilot study. Arthritis Res Ther. 2009;11(6):R177.
63. Pianta A, Arvikar S, Strle K, Drouin EE, Wang Q, Costello CE, et al. Evidence for immune relevance of Prevotella copri, a gut microbe, in patients with rheumatoid arthritis. Arthritis Rheumatol. 2016;69(5):964–75.
64. Wu Z, Wang L, Tang Y, Sun X. Parasite-derived proteins for the treatment of allergies and autoimmune diseases. Front Microbiol. 2017;8:2164.
65. Feary J, Britton J, Leonardi-Bee J. Atopy and current intestinal parasite infection: a systematic review and meta-analysis. Allergy. 2011;66(4):569–78.
66. Fleming JO, Cook TD. Multiple sclerosis and the hygiene hypothesis. Neurology. 2006;67(11):2085–6.
67. Panda AK, Ravindran B, Das BK. Rheumatoid arthritis patients are free of filarial infection in an area where filariasis is endemic: comment on the article by Pineda et al. Arthritis Rheum. 2013;65(5):1402–3.
68. Correale J, Farez M. Association between parasite infection and immune responses in multiple sclerosis. Ann Neurol. 2007;61(2):97–108.
69. Cooper PJ, Chico ME, Platts-Mills TA, Rodrigues LC, Strachan DP, Barreto ML. Cohort profile: the Ecuador life (ECUAVIDA) study in Esmeraldas Province, Ecuador. Int J Epidemiol. 2015;44(5):1517–27.
70. Lynch NR, Palenque M, Hagel I, DiPrisco MC. Clinical improvement of asthma after anthelminthic treatment in a tropical situation. Am J Respir Crit Care Med. 1997;156(1):50–4.
71. Webb EL, Nampijja M, Kaweesa J, Kizindo R, Namutebi M, Nakazibwe E, et al. Helminths are positively associated with atopy and wheeze in Ugandan fishing communities: results from a cross-sectional survey. Allergy. 2016;71(8):1156–69.
72. Briggs N, Weatherhead J, Sastry KJ, Hotez PJ. The hygiene hypothesis and its inconvenient truths about Helminth infections. PLoS Negl Trop Dis. 2016;10(9):e0004944.
73. Bailey CF. The treatment of chronic rheumatic and rheumatoid arthritis by radiant heat and cataphoresis. Br Med J. 1909;1(2505):13–5.
74. Mayberry J. The history of 5-ASA compounds and their use in ulcerative colitis – trailblazing discoveries in gastroenterology. J Gastrointest Liver Dis. 2013;22(4):375–7.
75. O'Dell JR, Elliott JR, Mallek JA, Mikuls TR, Weaver CA, Glickstein S, et al. Treatment of early seropositive rheumatoid arthritis: doxycycline plus methotrexate versus methotrexate alone. Arthritis Rheum. 2006;54(2):621–7.
76. Arbuckle MR, McClain MT, Rubertone MV, Scofield RH, Dennis GJ, James JA, et al. Development

of autoantibodies before the clinical onset of systemic lupus erythematosus. N Engl J Med. 2003;349(16):1526–33.
77. Uusitalo U, Liu X, Yang J, Aronsson CA, Hummel S, Butterworth M, et al. Association of early exposure of probiotics and islet autoimmunity in the TEDDY study. JAMA Pediatr. 2016;170(1):20–8.
78. Zhang GQ, Hu HJ, Liu CY, Zhang Q, Shakya S, Li ZY. Probiotics for prevention of atopy and food hypersensitivity in early childhood: a PRISMA-compliant systematic review and meta-analysis of randomized controlled trials. Medicine (Baltimore). 2016;95(8):e2562.
79. Bager P, Arnved J, Ronborg S, Wohlfahrt J, Poulsen LK, Westergaard T, et al. Trichuris suis ova therapy for allergic rhinitis: a randomized, double-blind, placebo-controlled clinical trial. J Allergy Clin Immunol. 2010;125(1):123–30 e1–3.
80. Bourke CD, Mutapi F, Nausch N, Photiou DM, Poulsen LK, Kristensen B, et al. Trichuris suis ova therapy for allergic rhinitis does not affect allergen-specific cytokine responses despite a parasite-specific cytokine response. Clin Exp Allergy. 2012;42(11):1582–95.
81. Feary J, Venn A, Brown A, Hooi D, Falcone FH, Mortimer K, et al. Safety of hookworm infection in individuals with measurable airway responsiveness: a randomized placebo-controlled feasibility study. Clin Exp Allergy. 2009;39(7):1060–8.
82. Feary JR, Venn AJ, Mortimer K, Brown AP, Hooi D, Falcone FH, et al. Experimental hookworm infection: a randomized placebo-controlled trial in asthma. Clin Exp Allergy. 2010;40(2):299–306.
83. Summers RW, Elliott DE, Qadir K, Urban JF Jr, Thompson R, Weinstock JV. Trichuris suis seems to be safe and possibly effective in the treatment of inflammatory bowel disease. Am J Gastroenterol. 2003;98(9):2034–41.
84. Summers RW, Elliott DE, Urban JF Jr, Thompson R, Weinstock JV. Trichuris suis therapy in Crohn's disease. Gut. 2005;54(1):87–90.
85. Summers RW, Elliott DE, Urban JF Jr, Thompson RA, Weinstock JV. Trichuris suis therapy for active ulcerative colitis: a randomized controlled trial. Gastroenterology. 2005;128(4):825–32.
86. Sandborn WJ, Elliott DE, Weinstock J, Summers RW, Landry-Wheeler A, Silver N, et al. Randomised clinical trial: the safety and tolerability of Trichuris suis ova in patients with Crohn's disease. Aliment Pharmacol Ther. 2013;38(3):255–63.
87. Fleming JO, Isaak A, Lee JE, Luzzio CC, Carrithers MD, Cook TD, et al. Probiotic helminth administration in relapsing-remitting multiple sclerosis: a phase 1 study. Mult Scler. 2011;17(6):743–54.
88. Voldsgaard A, Bager P, Garde E, Akeson P, Leffers AM, Madsen CG, et al. Trichuris suis ova therapy in relapsing multiple sclerosis is safe but without signals of beneficial effect. Mult Scler. 2015;21(13):1723–9.
89. Fleming J, Hernandez G, Hartman L, Maksimovic J, Nace S, Lawler B, et al. Safety and efficacy of helminth treatment in relapsing-remitting multiple sclerosis: results of the HINT 2 clinical trial. Mult Scler. 2017. https://doi.org/10.1177/1352458517736377.

2 Methods for Microbiota Analysis: Sample Collection and Laboratory Methods

Saleh Ibrahim and Meriem Belheouane

Abbreviations

CD	*Clostridium difficile*
CD	Crohn's disease
CDI	*Clostridium difficile* infection
DGGE	Denaturing gradient gel electrophoresis
FACS	Flow cytometry (FCM) fluorescence-activated cell sorting (FACS)
FISH	Fluorescence in situ hybridization
GC-MS	Gas chromatography-mass spectrometry
MAR	Microautoradiography
OTU	Operational taxonomic unit
RTF	Reduced transport fluid
SIMS	Secondary ion mass spectrometry
SIP	Isotope-labeled substrates
TGGE	Temperature gradient gel electrophoresis
T-RFLP	Terminal restriction fragment length polymorphism

S. Ibrahim
Lübeck Institute of Experimental Dermatology, University of Lübeck, Lübeck, Germany

College of Medicine and Sharjah Institute for Medical Research, University of Sharjah, Sharjah, United Arab Emirates

M. Belheouane (✉)
Max-Planck-Institute for Evolutionary Biology, Plön, Germany

Institute for Experimental Medicine, Christian-Albrechts-University of Kiel, Kiel, Germany
e-mail: belheouane@evolbio.mpg.de

Introduction

We live in a world dominated by microbes [1]. In fact, various environments, including multicellular organisms, are inhabited by a myriad of complex and diversified microbial assemblages. The complete set of microorganisms that resides in a given habitat is referred to as "microbiota" and combines diverse microbial species such as bacteria, viruses, and fungi. Through this chapter, we will be mainly focusing on the bacterial communities that are associated with several human body sites.

Microbiota Research: From Culture- to Molecular-Based Methods

Until early in the twenty-first century, studies of microbiota were traditionally addressed using culture-dependent methods. Culture of pure microbial colonies using selective and diverse culture media (solid, semisolid, and liquid), which take advantage of the distinctive metabolic properties of the microorganisms, has enabled isolation, identification, and characterization of several microbial species, ultimately defining treatments against many pathogenic microbes [2, 3]. Nowadays, culture methods continue to be an approach in exploring microbial diversity [4–7] and are central for identifying pathogenic organisms from clinical specimens. However, numerous microbial species show fastidious growth

G. Ragab et al. (eds.), *The Microbiome in Rheumatic Diseases and Infection*,
https://doi.org/10.1007/978-3-319-79026-8_2

requirements which render their isolation and identification extremely challenging. In fact, culturable bacteria in laboratory conditions represent solely a tiny fraction of the entire bacterial diversity, and the unculturable species play essential roles in community functioning such as synthesizing and degrading key components [8]. Besides missing the unculturable members of the community, differences in growth requirements across different species potentially lead to biases in describing the relative abundances of the taxa within a mixed community. Indeed, bacteria with less fastidious growth requirements likely overcompete the more challenging species, thus providing an inaccurate estimation of the real relative abundances of the species within a community. Fortunately, over the last decades, methods of microbiota investigation have tremendously improved, allowing deep, detailed, and complete characterization of the microbial components in a given environment (Table 2.1). Specifically, with the introduction of the bacterial 16S rRNA genes described by Pace et al. [9] that harbor hypervariable and much conserved regions which permit the identification and reconstruction of the bacterial phylotypes phylogeny, the strong advancement of molecular-based approaches, and sequencing technologies, the field of microbiome research has massively expanded and host-microbiota interactions became a central interdisciplinary area of research in health and disease.

High-Throughput Sequencing of 16S rRNA Genes and Whole Community Profiling

With the aim to identify and quantify the relative abundances of microbial species, the 16S rRNA genes are amplified, commonly using primers that target one or two hypervariable regions such as V1–V2, V3–V4, or V6 regions. The primers for each sample contain a unique barcode sequence which allows merging several samples together in one sequencing run. Substantially, PCR products are pooled together at identical concentration and sequenced using high-throughput sequencing technology such as the Illumina platform [10, 11]. Of note, primer choice is crucial and might impact the detection of certain microbial species and thus impact the downstream analyses. Indeed, the ability to discriminate between diverse species is essential in clinical investigations. In this line, previous studies reported that the choice of the V1–V3 region is valuable in discriminating between common skin resident bacteria especially the *Staphylococcus* species [12, 13]. Deep sequencing of 16S rRNA genes offers phylogenetic and quantitative data, including for unknown species; however, phylogenetic definition depends on available databases, and the technique suffers from PCR biases and remains relatively expensive and laborious.

Whole community approaches or the so-called "omics" are advancing the characterization of microbial assemblages by addressing several community aspects. The Human Microbiome Project Consortium [14] employed metagenomics approach, which is based on the massive and parallel sequencing of the entire genomes of microbial communities associated with several human body sites. This technique takes advantage on genomics, sequencing tools, as well as bioinformatics analyses to define the genetic content of all community members and infer their functions [15]. The study reported higher stability among individuals at the level of bacterial metabolic pathways, whereas the structural disparities assessed via sequencing the 16S rRNA genes were substantial. Similarly, Oh et al. [16] applied metagenomics technique to the skin microbiota and reported that the microbial functional diversity varied along the different skin sites.

While metagenomics reveal the potential functions of the complete collection of microbes, it does not define the actual physiological or metabolic status of the community members. Metatranscriptomics provide further information about the current activity state. In fact, this method which requires RNA isolation identifies the relative expression of genes in a community, without characterizing the actual or direct enzymatic activity. Recently, Maurice et al. [17] defined the active part of gut-associated microbial communities in human using metatranscriptomics and revealed that the gut harbors a distinctive set of

Table 2.1 Description of various methods employed in microbiota research

Method	Description	Data provided
Culture	Isolation of bacteria on selective culture media and growth conditions	Identification and characterization of metabolic properties of the bacteria
Direct and high-throughput sequencing of 16S rRNA	Amplification of a hypervariable region of the 16S rRNA and massive parallel sequencing of the amplicons	Phylogenetic identification and quantification of bacteria of also unknown sequences
qPCR	Amplification of 16S rRNA with fluorescence labeled, primers or probes	Phylogenetic identification and quantification of species of known sequences
Cloning of the 16S rRNA	Amplification of full-length 16S rRNA gene using broad primers, cloning, and Sanger sequencing	Phylogenetic identification of bacteria
Microbiota array	Amplification of full-length 16S rRNA gene with degenerate primers; amplicons hybridize to an array that contains a set of specific probes	Phylogenetic identification and quantification of bacteria species of known sequences
Gram staining	Staining of bacteria cells based on the composition of the cell wall	Detection, localization, visualization, and sorting of bacteria species
Immunofluorescence	Binding of an antibody, linked to a fluorophore, and a specific bacterial antigen, e.g., lipopolysaccharide which generates fluorescence signal	Detection, localization, identification, and visualization of bacterial structure for bacteria of known sequences
Fluorescence in situ hybridization (FISH)	Fluorescence-labeled probes target the 16S rRNA genes of total and specific bacteria taxa	Phylogenetic identification, localization, visualization, and quantification of microbial presence and activity of known sequences
Microautoradiography (MAR)	Substrate absorption is quantified using radioactive-labeled substrates	Determination of the physiological status of a single cell
Temperature gradient gel electrophoresis (TGGE) and denaturing gradient gel electrophoresis (DGGE)	Gel separation of 16S rRNA PCR products using temperature or chemical denaturation	Comparative and quantitative assessment of bacterial profiles
Terminal restriction fragment length polymorphism T/RELP	16S RNA is amplified using fluorescence-labeled primers; amplicons are digested with restriction enzymes and separated by gel electrophoresis	Quantitative assessment of bacterial profiles
Flow cytometry (FCM) fluorescence-activated cell sorting (FACS)	Cell sorting based on cell properties including metabolic activity, cell damage, growth rate, gene content, and transcription levels	Definition of cell categories within a community based on the chosen sorting criteria, e.g., highly active vs. dormant cells
Mass spectrometry	Stable isotope labels of bacterial components such as peptides	Quantifies the actual metabolic activity within a single cell
Whole community profiling "omics"	Massive parallel sequencing of whole genome, transcriptome within a community	Phylogenetic identification, quantification, and reconstitution of functions, activity, and metabolic properties of the collection of microbes within a community
Single-cell omics	Whole genome, transcriptome, or proteome sequencing of a single cell, e.g., single-cell RNA sequencing (scRNA-seq)	Definition of gene content, function, activity and metabolic status of a single microbial cell

active species compared to the present species defined on the DNA level. Ultimately, metaproteomics provide information about the actual enzymatic functions that are expressed in a community [18]. Erickson et al. [19] took advantage of the improvements in protein isolation and preparation techniques reviewed by Xiong et al. [20] and combined shotgun metagenomics and metaproteomics methods to characterize and identify potential functional signatures of human gut microbiota in the context of Crohn's disease. This pioneering study reported novel differences in microbial communities between healthy and diseased individuals that include several genes, proteins, and pathways. An additional technique includes metabolomics, which focuses on the metabolome, i.e., the entire collection of metabolites such as hormones, and signaling molecules which belong to a given sample (e.g., cell, organism, and community). This method aims to define the metabolic profile by identifying, characterizing, and quantifying the metabolites of interest, as well as describing the biochemical pathways of metabolites. Antharam et al. [21] investigated the contribution of specific gut microbes to fecal metabolites in *Clostridium difficile*-associated gut microbiome. The researchers employed gas chromatography-mass spectrometry (GC-MS) and 16S rRNA deep sequencing, to analyze the metabolome and microbiome of fecal samples of patients suffering from *C. difficile* infection and from healthy controls. This study identified 63 human gut microbes with cholesterol-reducing activities, thus supporting a potential role of microbial components in host lipid metabolism. Overall, mass spectrometry quantifies the actual metabolic activity. This technique combines stable isotope labels and Raman microspectroscopy or secondary ion mass spectrometry (SIMS) [22, 23]. In addition, nuclear magnetic resonance spectroscopy technology is also employed to characterize the metabolic profile of the microbial communities. Mass spectrometry methods are powerful in terms of coverage, sensitivity, and quantification to characterize the metabolic properties of the cells including uncultured microorganisms and associate the structure and function in complex microbial assemblages. To date, these techniques remain fairly expensive.

In short, whole community approaches are focusing on a global characterization of the microbial species within a community; nonetheless, these techniques remain relatively costly, while the process of data analyses is laborious and time costly. Of note, annotations of the various databases (e.g., reference genomes, transcripts) continue to expand, to improve the accuracy of study's conclusions [24].

Beyond the 16S rRNA High-Throughput Sequencing

While sequencing of the 16S rRNA phylogenetic marker revolutionized the field of microbiome research, this approach provides a subset of information on the microbial assemblages, and additional techniques are valuable in providing supplementary pieces of information on several community aspects.

Quantitative PCR

Real-time PCR is frequently employed to identify and quantify microbial taxa, while quantification is based on the measure of fluorescent signals from primers or probes; identification is based on the use of specific primers that are commonly designed for the 16S rRNA gene [25, 26]. The specific primers target various taxonomical levels such as genus or species. Real-time PCR is sensitive and accurate, yet it is subject to PCR biases and targets solely taxa of known sequences. It is frequently used to confirm findings obtained through deep sequencing of the 16S rRNA gene.

Cloning of the 16S rRNA Genes

In this technique, 16S rRNA genes are amplified using broad-range primers; then PCR products are purified and cloned. A high number of colonies are randomly picked and processed for Sanger sequencing, and phylogenetic identification is performed using a classification database tool [27, 28]. This method provides phylogenetic data based on the full length of the 16S rRNA gene; however, it suffers from PCR and cloning biases and remains laborious and relatively expensive.

Microbiota Array

The microbiota array requires the amplification of full-length 16S rRNA gene with degenerate primers. PCR products hybridize to an array that comprises a set of specific probes whereby the specificity of the probes allows the identification of the taxa, while quantification of the bacterial taxa is achieved through the assessment of fluorescence signal [29, 30]. Nevertheless, cross hybridization is likely to occur, and unknown and very low abundant microbes are challenging to detect.

Staining-, Histology-, and Microscopy-Based Methods

Spatial localization of microbes is critical in the characterization of microbial assemblages. Accordingly, Nakatsuji et al. [31] investigated whether microbial species localize in deep sections of the skin and combined several staining techniques. Gram staining was employed to visualize and localize the bacterial structure across various skin layers. This technique discriminates bacteria based on the chemical and physical properties of their cell walls through detection of peptidoglycan, a structure present in Gram-positive bacteria [32]. Moreover, immunofluorescence was used to target particular bacterial structures. This technique is based on the specificity of an antibody to its antigen, e.g., lipopolysaccharide, whereby the specific binding triggers fluorescent signal that permits the visualization of the target species [33]. These techniques allow the detection, localization, and visualization of bacterial components and demonstrated that commensal bacteria are also localized in deep layers of the skin. Similarly, fluorescence in situ hybridization (FISH), which requires RNA isolation and labeled probes with fluorescent dyes such as cyanine 3 (Cy3) and/or cyanine 5 (Cy5), aims to define, localize, and quantify the 16S rRNA gene content. Broad and specific probes are employed separately or in combination to assess total and specific microbial abundance. Namely, the Eub338 targets the 16S rRNA of most but not all bacteria and defines the total bacterial abundance [34], while probes for specific taxa, for instance, Alf968 for α-proteobacteria [35] and Bet42a for β-proteobacteria [36], allow the detection of uniquely these taxa. Cottrell and Kirchman [37] quantified the relative abundances of major bacterial species inhabiting an estuary, while Earle et al. [33] quantified taxa abundances in different sections of the mouse gut. Both studies combined FISH and high-resolution microscopy. Of note, high-resolution microscopy and image analysis permit the description of relevant cell properties such as volume and size.

In addition to identifying, localizing, and quantifying the relative abundances of distinct taxa within a mixed community, FISH can be combined with microautoradiography (MAR), a technique employed to define the physiological state of a single cell. MAR is based on quantifying substrate absorption using radioactive-labeled substrates; for example, it can identify cells specifically uptaking radiolabeled leucine. Thus, MAR defines the metabolic state of the cell [38], while FISH provides phylogenetic data, and the two procedures can be used in tandem to identify which bacteria are metabolizing a specific compound of interest. Overall, these techniques are sensitive and accurate, though they do not define unknown species.

Electrophoresis-Based Methods

Methods that apply electrophoresis include the terminal restriction fragment length polymorphism (T-RFLP), which is based on fluorescently labeled primers that amplify 16S rRNA genes, whereby restriction enzymes digest the amplicons and the fragments are separated by gel electrophoresis. Sizes of every sample's terminal fragments are defined via sequencing and fluorescence intensity [39]. Similarly, temperature gradient gel electrophoresis (TGGE) and denaturing gradient gel electrophoresis (DGGE) use either a temperature or chemical gradient, respectively, to denature the sample during the migration process on an acrylamide gel. At last, sample specific profiles are generated during migration [40]. Zoetendal et al. [41] compared the composition of the active and present bacteria in human fecal samples by applying temperature gradient gel electrophoresis of 16S rRNA genes. Terminal restriction fragment length polymorphism and gradient gel electrophoresis provide only quantitative data, and henceforth are outdated methods.

Flow Cytometry (FCM)

Flow cytometry is a great tool that permits fast and simultaneous analysis of millions of cells. The microbial cells are held in suspension and exposed to a strong source of light, so that fluorescence signals for every single cell are collected and recorded [42]. Flow cytometry sorts cells based on different characteristics such as size, shape, intracellular content, or membrane integrity [17]. For example, cell damage, or whether a cell is deceased, can be investigated by examining the membrane integrity using exclusion dyes (PI, EtBr, TOPRO dyes). Furthermore, the enzymatic activity is assessed via quantifying the esterase activity, while nucleic acid content, to define cell activity levels, is measured using nucleic acid dyes such as SYBR Green or SYTO 13. An additional example includes substrate usage, which is quantified through isotope-labeled substrates (SIP). Recently, Peris-Bondia et al. [43] investigated the active fraction of human gut microbiota by measuring the nucleic acid content using Pyronin-Y, a fluorescent dye for total RNA, to sort the cells into categories based on the activity levels. A recently developed technique involves sorting intestinal bacteria based upon adhesion to mucosal IgA, with IgA^+ bacteria demonstrating greater ability to mediate colitis [44]. Flow cytometry performs high-throughput analysis, yet it does not define the phylogeny or the localization of the microbial cells.

Single-Cell Approaches

Single-cell approaches are valuable for characterizing various properties of the cell within a mixed microbial community. Based on cell sorting, these methods deeply describe intra- and intercellular variations of several properties including metabolic activity, cell damage, growth rate, gene content, and transcripts levels.

Several approaches of single-cell analyses have been developed and applied on microbial assemblages. These methods, which include whole-genome sequencing, transcriptomics, proteomics, and metabolomics, do not require prior culture and thus potentially reveal new genomes of unculturable species [45, 46]. Single-cell analysis was applied on an unculturable bacterium inhabiting the human oral cavity which belongs to the TM7 phylum, through which the whole-genome amplification and sequencing permitted the identification of thousands of genes and disclosed several microbial functional pathways. Ultimately, the collected genetic information likely contributes to understanding the culture requirements of this bacterium [47]. In the future, these methods will continue to improve to achieve deeper cell phenotyping, particularly when combinations of these analyses are performed within a single cell (e.g., genome sequencing, transcriptomics) [48–51].

Combination of Various Methods in Microbiota Studies

While using one method is common in investigating the microbiota, the approach of integrating several methods is also frequently employed. Indeed, combination of various methods is advantageous and allows the definition of complementary pieces of information on diverse community aspects and/or confirms each method outcome. Shankar et al. [52] characterized the gut microbiota of human patients suffering from *C. difficile* infection (CDI) by combining microbiota array, high-throughput Illumina sequencing of the 16S rRNA genes, and fluorescence in situ hybridization (FISH). Precisely, the microbiota array provides data on the phylogeny and abundances of microbial taxa, while the FISH localizes and also identifies the present taxa. Xu et al. [53] combined RNA sequencing and metabolomics to identify the pathogens in a clinical specimen in the context of esophageal squamous cell carcinoma, while Yu et al. [54] combined 16S rRNA sequencing and metabolomics to characterize association between gut microbial phenotypes and depression. On the other hand, previous studies have combined culture-dependent and culture-independent methods to investigate microbial assemblages. Molecular approaches successfully bring valuable insights on several features of a microbial community and overcome the inability to culture some microorganisms. However, comprehensive characterization of the physiology of microbial species and their interactions with their environments necessitates their culture in the laboratory. Fortunately, microbial growing techniques are improving, in particular when various techniques are combined, to increase the fraction of culturable bacteria. These methods include co-culture with other bacteria, restoring the "natural" environments in laboratory conditions, and microculture technology [8]. Lau et al. [55] employed a combination of culture and 16S rRNA gene sequencing, referred to as culture-enriched molecular profiling, whereby numerous culture media were used along with a large number of culture conditions. Following that, PCR amplification of the V3 region of the 16S rRNA gene was performed, and amplicons were processed for sequencing. Furthermore, the operational taxonomic units (OTUs) recovered by sequencing of the cultures were compared to those obtained from the uncultured community. Interestingly, the study revealed that a large number of species were successfully cultured. Similarly, Stearns et al. [56] and Sibley et al. [57] applied the same approach to the airway microbiome, to investigate shifts in community composition associated with age and cystic fibrosis. Likewise, Browne et al. [58] described a new approach that combines culture, whole-genome sequencing, phylogenetic analysis, and modeling on human fecal microbiota. Overall, these studies emphasize the advantage to combine several methods in order to boost the culturable fraction of the microbiome.

Sample Collection and Sampling Strategies in Microbiota Studies

Sample Collection

Any microbiota study starts with sample collection. This crucial step is performed according to the site of interest, the addressed question, and the planned downstream analyses. Globally, we distinguish three different sampling methods of the microbial material including swab, scrape, and punch biopsy (Fig. 2.1). First, the swab technique, which consists of vigorously swiping the

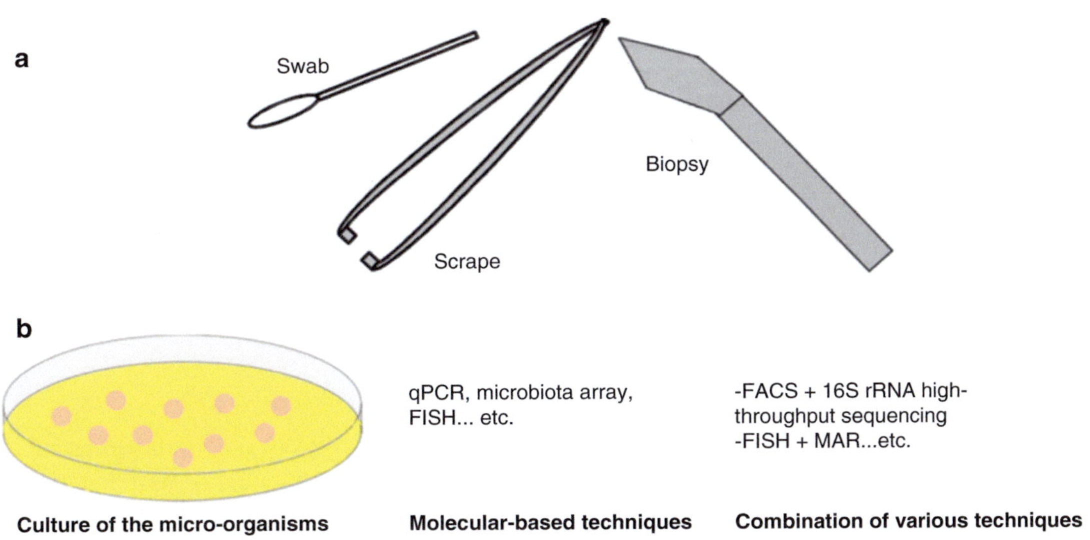

Fig. 2.1 Sampling methods and profiling approaches of the microbiota. (**a**) Sampling techniques of the microbial material. (**b**) Diversity of microbiota profiling techniques. *FISH* fluorescence in situ hybridization, *MAR* microautoradiography, *FACS* fluorescence-activated cell sorting

area to be sampled, is widely used to collect microbial material from the skin, oral and nasal cavities, vagina, and gastrointestinal tract. Studies of the skin microbiota have mainly employed swabs [59–62]. These investigations used a sterile Catch-All swab which consists of a cotton pledget that is usually pre-humidified with a lysis solution, and the body region of interest is energetically rubbed for about 30 s. After that, the swabs are either frozen in the lysis buffer or a homogenization buffer (i.e., the first solution to be used from the nucleic acids isolation kit). Likewise, The Catch-All swab is employed to collect material from the oral and nasal cavities where the interior mucosal surfaces are gently rubbed, and then the swabs are stored in the extraction kit buffer until the extraction process. Similarly, the vaginal cavity is sampled by swirling the Catch-All swab five times, withdrawing it, and transferring the specimen into a collection tube with a buffer from the nucleic acid isolation kit [63]. Recently, Budding et al. [64] investigated the properties and applicability of rectal swabs in a clinical routine setting with the purpose of profiling the gut microbiota in patients with different gastrointestinal diseases. Moreover, the researchers assessed the effect of storage and processing of rectal swabs by employing two storing protocols: the rectal swabs were snap frozen (i.e., dry swabs) or swabs were kept in reduced transport fluid (RTF) buffer prior to storage at −20 °C. Comparison of the two sampling approaches yielded highly similar microbiota profiles, and overall the rectal swabs seem to be a suitable approach for profiling the gut microbiota.

The punch biopsy has been applied on the skin commonly using, for example, 4 or 6 mm punch biopsy forceps [60, 65]. Likewise, in the gastrointestinal tract, mucosa, or epithelium tissues, sections are incised usually during medical examination such as gastroscopy [66, 67]. The scrapping technique has been employed on the skin where superficial scrapings were obtained from a 4 cm^2 area with two soft regular strokes of a sterile blade [68], while in the intestine, the mucosa was scraped off with slides for the examination of mucosal-associated microbiota [69].

Besides the choice of the sampling technique, sample collection and processing should include crucial steps: negative control or blank samples which consist of sampling the environment, e.g., ambient air, and/or keeping a collection tube with all extraction reagents except for the microbial material. These negative controls are necessary to assess the noise signal in the collected microbial material and thus define the accuracy of the data. Such inspection is particularly relevant for low biomass organs such as the skin [70]. In Fig. 2.2, we present an example of the proportion of contaminant estimates in mouse skin samples using the SourceTracker tool [71]. We assessed the similarity percentage between the core microbiota community and the extraction negative controls from which PCR products were detectable. We performed this analysis distinctively on the bacte-

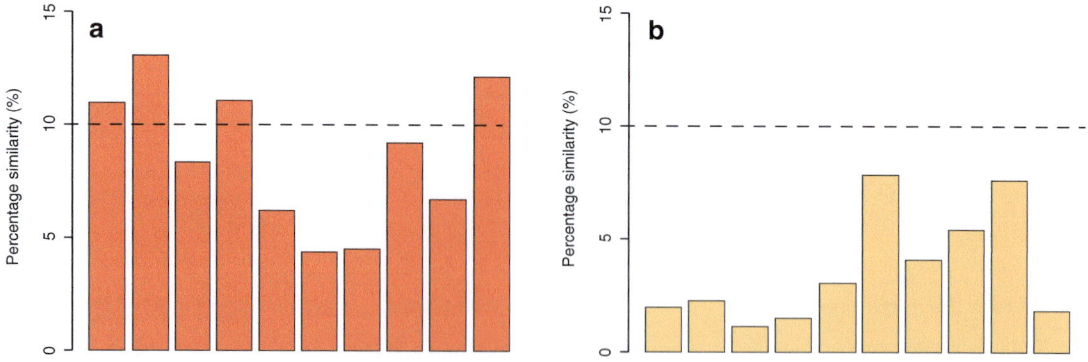

Fig. 2.2 Analysis of environmental contamination in ten mouse skin samples. (**a**) DNA, (**b**) RNA. Y-axis represents percentage similarity of the community (genus-level) between skin samples and extractions negative controls

rial genomic DNA and RNA reverse transcribed into complementary DNA (cDNA). We observe lower levels of contamination in the transcripts compared to genomic DNA, suggesting environmental noise is higher in the DNA [72]. This approach allows setting a threshold (e.g., 10%) beyond which the sample is considered contaminated and discarded from downstream analyses.

Choice and Consequences of the Sampling Method on a Microbiota Study

Previous microbiota investigations reported that the outcomes of a microbiota study are affected by the sampling method. Stearns et al. [73] collected biopsy samples from human healthy individuals along different sections of the gastrointestinal tract including the stomach, duodenum, and colon. Sample collection was achieved during a routine colonoscopy and gastroscopy performed in the context of inquiry of symptoms or screening for colorectal cancer, where a tissue was incised, placed in sterile solution of D-PBS, and frozen. Along with the biopsy tissue, stool samples were also collected and frozen at −20 °C. Profiling of the microbiota composition was performed in tissue and feces samples. The results revealed that composition of several biopsy sites was overall distinct from that in the stool. Moreover, noticeable representation of bacterial taxa in samples from the colon was not apparent in the stool. This observation suggests that the bacterial profiles derived from stool samples do not capture the complete diversity of the microbial species. Similarly, Gevers et al. [74] investigated the microbiome in a large human cohort of Crohn's disease (CD) and collected various biopsy tissues from different sections of the gastrointestinal tract along with stool samples. The researchers revealed that mucosal-associated dysbiosis in microbiota composition is slightly reflected in stool samples, while for evaluating the power of microbiome composition in diagnosing CD, the biopsy-associated microbiome performed well, whereas the stool samples yielded less accurate estimation. These results indicate that the biopsy technique is a preferable approach in characterizing the gut microbiota in health and disease contexts. For the most part, however, biopsy samples are limited by the requirement for the washout, which can affect the contents of the microbiota [75].

Similarly, Grice et al. [68] sampled human skin using three different methods that span distinct depths and layers of the skin, namely, swab, scrape, and punch biopsy. The swab catches the superficial layer of the skin, while the scrape reaches deeper level in the epidermis, and the biopsy incised all several layers. Of note, the investigators found that the three methods of swab, scrape, and punch biopsy captured similar core microbiome. On the other hand, Nakatsuji et al. [31] showed that microbial components are also located in the deep dermis, a skin layer which is missed when sampling is performed via swab or scrape. Furthermore, Kim et al. [76] investigated the vaginal microbiota using both swab and scrape and revealed that community compositions based on swab and scrape significantly differed, with scrape samples harboring higher microbial diversity. This disparity reflects differences in the sampling method and/or physiological changes at the sampling area during the collection process. While invasive methods seem to be preferable in characterizing the microbial assemblages, this approach is not always feasible, especially for healthy controls, and noninvasive techniques continue to be standard approaches in microbiota research. Altogether, these results emphasize that study conclusions may differ based on the chosen sampling method.

Additional Sources of Variability and Sampling Design

Earlier studies revealed precious insights on the composition, diversity, and distribution of the microbial assemblages across body sites. Specifically, investigations reported that within a given body site such as the skin and the gut, distinct parts of the organ harbor distinguishable distribution and composition of microbial species leading to "biogeography pattern" [73, 77].

Furthermore, temporal variability in community composition occurs in the diverse body sites. This baseline is critical to understand the normal microbiota variability and thus define meaningful shifts in community composition in disease state [78, 79]. Consequently, in a comparative investigation of microbiota between healthy and diseased individuals, the choice of the area to sample is crucial in the outcome, interpretation, and conclusions of a study. Indeed, the biogeographic pattern needs to be accounted for in the sampling strategy to avoid confounding the disparities in community composition which are caused by the disease state and those due to the biogeographic pattern. For a patient, the lesional area is sampled using one of the previously described methods (swab, scrape, biopsy), and the identical area should be sampled in the healthy controls. This comparison allows evaluating the extent of alterations in community aspects (e.g., composition, diversity) caused by disease characteristics. Likewise, a non-lesional area should also be sampled in patients and the matching region in the healthy controls. Contrasting community aspects between the lesional and non-lesional areas within a given patient determines the potential systemic changes caused by diseased state and whether the biogeographic pattern of microbial distribution can be recovered, while comparing the non-lesional sites between patients and healthy controls will further describe the extent of any effect of the disease on the microbiota composition (Fig. 2.3). Moreover, the sample sizes of patients and controls should be large and similar to detect any subtle disease effect on the microbiota. Ideally, the matched controls harbor similar characteristics of age, gender, and diet, to ensure accurate assessment of shifts in the microbiota between health and disease states, and draw clinically meaningful conclusions. Further, a

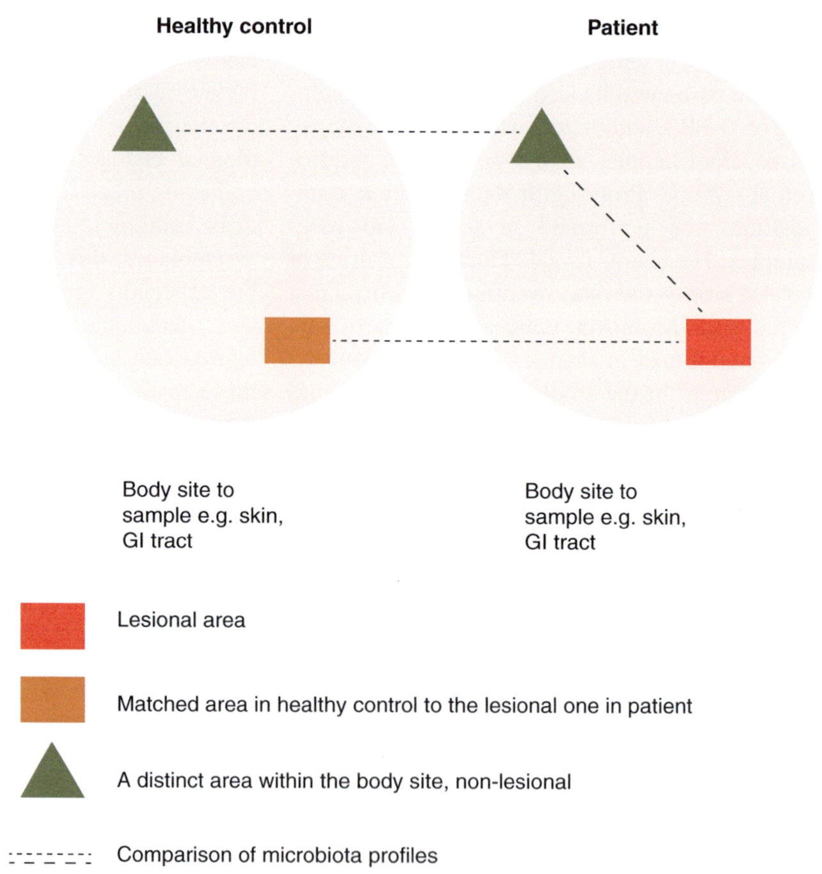

Fig. 2.3 Sampling strategies for microbiota profiling in health and disease states. *GI* Gastrointestinal tract

thorough description through a detailed questionnaire of patients and healthy controls is critical in a microbiome study. Alternatively, these potential confounding factors must be taken into account in the downstream analyses. Besides, for a powerful design, sampling and phenotyping of the microbiota over time is valuable as it likely disentangles the normal temporal and disease-driven variation in microbiota composition, thus allowing an accurate understating of the disease-triggered changes in the community. In summary, aspects of sampling strategies, sample collection,

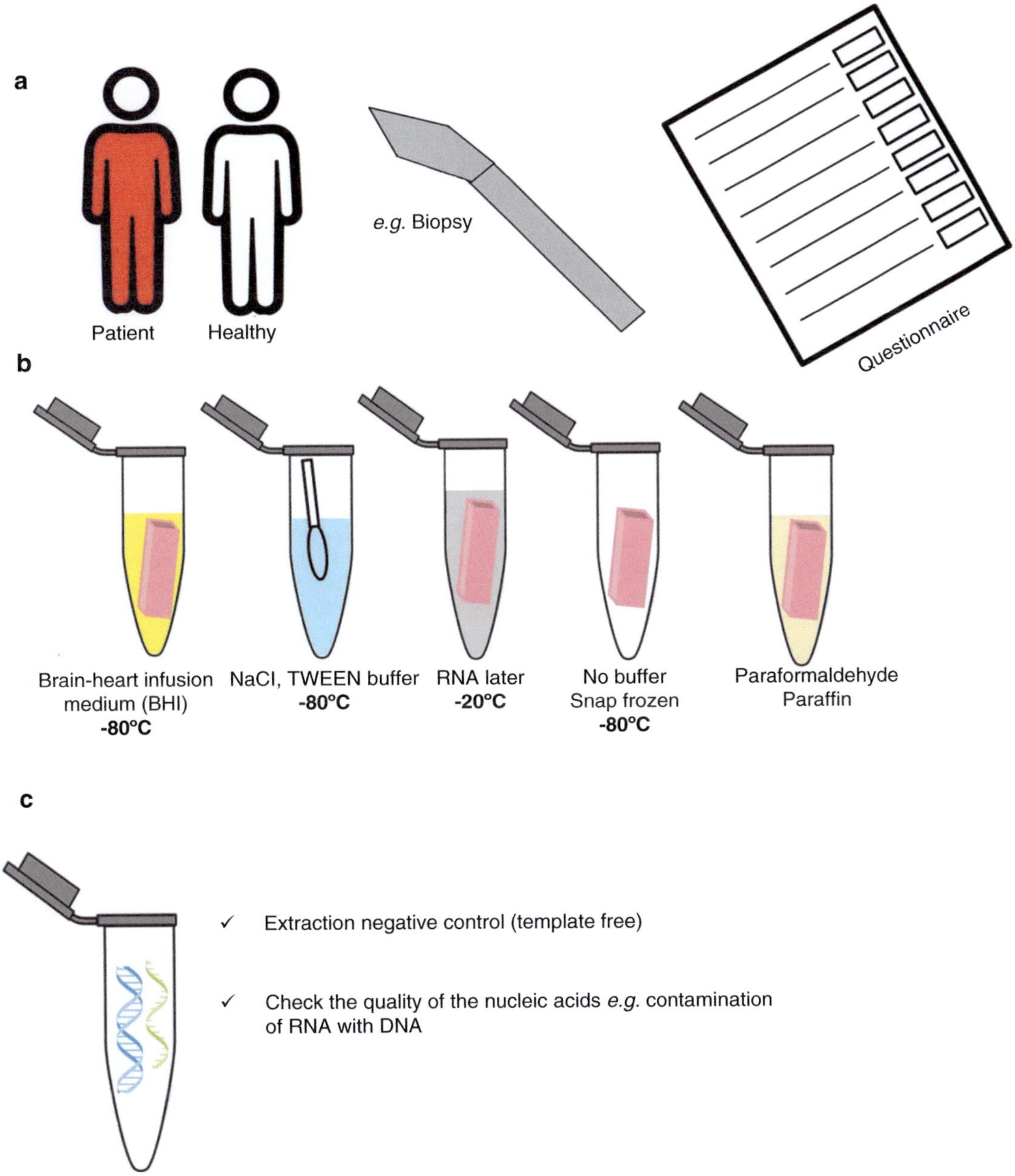

Fig. 2.4 Summary of critical steps in a microbiota study. (**a**) Study design which includes recruitment of patient and healthy controls, collection of microbial material, and collection of metadata. (**b**) Storage of microbial material in various laboratory investigation techniques. (**c**) Extraction of nucleic acids from hosts and microbiota

and storage and data generation influence the results of a microbiota study (Fig. 2.4). Furthermore, a robust study design should include consistent metadata collection, together with consideration of any possible confounding factors, standardized collection and storage of the samples, and the value of addition of negative blank and positive controls such as mock community cannot be overemphasized [70, 80].

Conclusion

Across the decades, methods to investigate the microbial assemblages have continued to improve. Nowadays, researchers have at their disposal a diversified panel of techniques that capture different and relevant pieces of information on the microbial communities, while various approaches can be combined to yield detailed description of the microbial communities. In the future, our understanding of host-microbiota interactions will continue to increase, hopefully allowing us to delineate the microbial disease associations and apply appropriate therapeutics.

References

1. McFall-Ngai MJ. Giving microbes their due – animal life in a microbially dominant world. J Exp Biol. 2015;218(Pt 12):1968–73.
2. Old DC, Duguid JP. Selective outgrowth of fimbriate bacteria in static liquid medium. J Bacteriol. 1970;103(2):447–56.
3. Lockman HA, Curtiss R 3rd. Isolation and characterization of conditional adherent and non-type 1 fimbriated Salmonella typhimurium mutants. Mol Microbiol. 1992;6(7):933–45.
4. Goodman AL, Kallstrom G, Faith JJ, Reyes A, Moore A, Dantas G, Gordon JI. Extensive personal human gut microbiota culture collections characterized and manipulated in gnotobiotic mice. PNAS. 2011;108(15):6252–7.
5. Lagier J-C, Edouard S, Pagnier I, Mediannikov O, Drancourt M, Raoult D. Current and past strategies for bacterial culture in clinical microbiology. Clin Microbiol Rev. 2015;28(1):208–36.
6. Myles IA, Reckhow JD, Williams KW, Sastalla I, Frank KM, Datta SK. A method for culturing gram-negative skin microbiota. BMC Microbiol. 2016;16:60.
7. Cosseaua C, Romano-Bertrandb S, Dupland H, Lucasa O, Ingrassiaa I, Pigassea C, Roquesa C, Jumas-Bilakb E. Proteobacteria from the human skin microbiota: species-level diversity and hypotheses. One Health. 2016;2:33–41.
8. Stewart EJ. Growing unculturable bacteria. J Bacteriol. 2012;194(16):4151–60.
9. Lane DJ, Pace B, Olsen GJ, Stahl DA, Sogin ML, Pace NR. Rapid determination of 16S ribosomal RNA sequences for phylogenetic analyses. Proc Natl Acad Sci U S A. 1985;82(20):6955–9.
10. Janda JM, Abbott SL. 16S rRNA gene sequencing for bacterial identification in the diagnostic laboratory: pluses, perils, and pitfalls. Clin Microbiol. 2007;45(9):2761–4.
11. Yang B, Wang Y, Yuan P. Sensitivity and correlation of hypervariable regions in 16S rRNA genes in phylogenetic analysis. BMC Bioinformatics. 2016;17:135.
12. Chakravorty S, Helb D, Burday M, Connell N, Alland D. A detailed analysis of 16S ribosomal RNA gene segments for the diagnosis of pathogenic bacteria. J Microbiol Methods. 2007;69(2):330–9.
13. Conlan S, Kong HH, Segre JA. Species-level analysis of DNA sequence data from the NIH human microbiome project. PLoS One. 2012;7(10):e47075.
14. Human Microbiome Project Consortium. Structure, function and diversity of the healthy human microbiome. Nature. 2012;486(7402):207–14.
15. Thomas T, Gilbert J, Meyer F. Metagenomics – a guide from sampling to data analysis. Microb Inform Exp. 2012;2:3.
16. Oh J, Byrd AL, Deming C, Conlan S, NISC Comparative Sequencing Program, Kong HH, Segre JA. Biogeography and individuality shape function in the human skin metagenome. Nature. 2014;514(7520):59–64.
17. Maurice CF, Turnbaugh PJ. Quantifying the metabolic activities of human-associated microbial communities across multiple ecological scales. FEMS Microbiol Rev. 2013;37:830–48.
18. Wilmes P, Bond PL. The application of two-dimensional polyacrylamide gel electrophoresis and downstream analyses to a mixed community of prokaryotic microorganisms. Environ Microbiol. 2004;6:911–20.
19. Erickson AR, Cantarel BL, Lamendella R, Darzi Y, Mongodin EF, Pan C, Shah M, Halfvarson J, Tysk C, Henrissat B, Raes J, Verberkmoes NC, Fraser CM, Hettich RL, Jansson JK. Integrated metagenomics/metaproteomics reveals human host-microbiota signatures of Crohn's disease. PLoS One. 2012;7:e49138.
20. Xiong W, Abraham PE, Li Z, Pan C, Hettich RL. Microbial metaproteomics for characterizing the range of metabolic functions and activities of human gut microbiota. Proteomics. 2015;15(20):3424–38.
21. Antharam VC, McEwen DC, Garrett TJ, Dossey AT, Li EC, Kozlov AN, Mesbah Z, Wang GP. An integrated Metabolomic and microbiome analysis identified specific gut microbiota associated with fecal cholesterol and coprostanol in clostridium difficile infection. PLoS One. 2016;11(2):e0148824.
22. Wagner M. Single-cell ecophysiology of microbes as revealed by Raman microspectroscopy or secondary

ion mass spectrometry imaging. Annu Rev Microbiol. 2009;63:411–29.
23. Musat N, Foster R, Vagner T, Adam B, Kuypers MM. Detecting metabolic activities in single cells, with emphasis on nanoSIMS. FEMS Microbiol Rev. 2012;36:486–511.
24. Kong HH. Details matter: designing skin microbiome studies. J Invest Dermatol. 2016;136(5):900–2.
25. Rinttilä T, Kassinen A, Malinen E, Krogius L, Palva A. Development of an extensive set of 16S rDNA-targeted primers for quantification of pathogenic and indigenous bacteria in faecal samples by real-time PCR. J Appl Microbiol. 2004;97(6):1166–77.
26. Haarman M, Knol J. Quantitative real-time PCR assays to identify and quantify Fecal Bifidobacterium species in infants receiving a prebiotic infant formula. Appl Environ Microbiol. 2005;71(5):2318–24.
27. Wang Y, Hoenig JD, Malin KJ, Qamar S, Petrof EO, Sun J, Antonopoulos DA, Chang EB, Claud EC. 16S rRNA gene-based analysis of fecal microbiota from preterm infants with and without necrotizing enterocolitis. ISME J. 2009;3:944–54.
28. Hayashi H, Sakamoto M, Benno Y. Phylogenetic analysis of the human gut microbiota using 16S rDNA clone libraries and strictly anaerobic culture-based methods. Microbiol Immunol. 2002;46(8):535–48.
29. Paliy O, Kenche H, Abernathy F, Michail S. High-throughput quantitative analysis of the human intestinal microbiota with a phylogenetic microarray. Appl Environ Microbiol. 2009;75:3572–9.
30. Rigsbee L, Agans R, Foy BD, Paliy O. Optimizing the analysis of human intestinal microbiota with phylogenetic microarray. FEMS Microbiol Ecol. 2011;75:332–42.
31. Nakatsuji T, Chiang HI, Jiang SB, Nagarajan H, Zengler K, Gallo RL. The microbiome extends to subepidermal compartments of normal skin. Nat Commun. 2013;4:1431.
32. Holt JG, Krieg N, Sneath PHA, Staley JT, Williams ST. Bergey's manual of determinative bacteriology. 9th ed. Philadelphia: Lippincott Williams & Wilkins; 1994. p. 11.
33. Earle KA, Billings G, Sigal M, Lichtman JS, Hansson GC, Elias JE, Amieva MR, Huang KC, Sonnenburg JL. Quantitative imaging of gut microbiota spatial organization. Cell Host Microbe. 2015;18(4):478–88.
34. Amann RI, Binder BJ, Olson RJ, Chisholm SW, Devereux R, Stahl DA. Combination of 16S ribosomal-RNA- targeted oligonucleotide probes with flow-cytometry for analyzing mixed microbial populations. Appl Environ Microbiol. 1990;56:1919–25.
35. Glöckner FO, Fuchs BM, Amann R. Bacterioplankton compositions of lakes and oceans: a first comparison based on fluorescence in situ hybridization. Appl Environ Microbiol. 1999;65:3721–6.
36. Manz W, Amann R, Ludwig W, Wagner M, Schleifer KH. Phylogenetic oligodeoxynucleotide probes for the major subclasses of proteobacteria – problems and solutions. Syst Appl Microbiol. 1992;15:593–600.
37. Cottrell MT, Kirchman DL. Single-cell analysis of bacterial growth, cell size, and community structure in the Delaware estuary. AME. 2004;34:139–49.
38. Nielsen JL, Nielsen PH. Advances in microscopy: microautoradiography of single cells. Methods Enzymol. 2005;397:237–56.
39. Liu W, Marsh T, Cheng H, Forney L. Characterization of microbial diversity by determining terminal restriction fragment length polymorphisms of genes encoding 16S rRNA. Appl Environ Microbiol. 1997;63(11):4516–22.
40. Fischer SG, Lerman LS. DNA fragments differing by single base-pair substitutions are separated in denaturing gradient gels: correspondence with melting theory. Proc Natl Acad Sci U S A. 1983;80:1579–83.
41. Zoetendal EG, Akkermans AD, De Vos WM. Temperature gradient gel electrophoresis analysis of 16S rRNA from human Fecal samples reveals stable and host-specific communities of active Bacteria. Appl Environ Microbiol. 1998;64(10):3854–9.
42. Shapiro HM. Pratical flow cytometry. New York: Wiley; 1995.
43. Peris-Bondia F, Latorre A, Artacho A, Moya A, D'Auria G. The active human gut microbiota differs from the total microbiota. PLoS One. 2013;6(7):e22448.
44. Palm NW, de ZoeteThomas MR, Cullen W, Barry NA, Stefanowski J, Hao L, Degnan PH, Hu J, Peter I, Zhang W, Ruggiero E, Cho JH, Goodman AL, Flavell RA. Immunoglobulin A coating identifies colitogenic bacteria in inflammatory bowel disease. Cell. 2014;158(5):1000–10.
45. Kalisky T, Blainey P, Quake SR. Genomic analysis at the single-cell level. Annu Rev Genet. 2011;45:431–45.
46. Lasken RS, McLean JS. Recent advances in genomic DNA sequencing of microbial species from single cells. Nat Rev Genet. 2014;15(9):577–84.
47. Marcy Y, Ouverney C, Bik EM, Lösekann T, Ivanova N, Martin HG, Szeto E, Platt D, Hugenholtz P, Relman DA, Quake SR. Dissecting biological "dark matter" with single-cell genetic analysis of rare and uncultivated TM7 microbes from the human mouth. Proc Natl Acad Sci U S A. 2007;104:11889–94.
48. Satija R, Farrell JA, Gennert D, Schier AF, Regev A. Spatial reconstruction of single-cell gene expression data. Nat Biotechnol. 2015;33:495–502.
49. Kimmerling RJ, Szeto GL, Li JW, Genshaft AS, Kazer SW, Payer KR, de Riba Borrajo J, Blainey PC, Irvine DJ, Shalek AK, Manalisb SR. A microfluidic platform enabling single-cell RNA-seq of multigenerational lineages. Nat Commun. 2016;7:10220.
50. Angermueller C, Clark SJ, Lee HJ, Macaulay IC, Teng MJ, Hu TX, Krueger F, Smallwood SA, Ponting CP, Voet T, Kelsey G, Stegle O, Reik W. Parallel single-cell sequencing links transcriptional and epigenetic heterogeneity. Nat Methods. 2016;13:229–32.
51. Welch JD, Williams LA, DiSalvo M, Brandt AT, Marayati R, Sims CE, Allbritton NL, Prins JF, Yeh JJ, Jones CD. Selective single cell isolation for

genomics using microraft arrays. Nucleic Acids Res. 2016;44(17):8292–301.
52. Shankar V, Hamilton MJ, Khoruts A, Kilburn A, Unno T, Paliy O, Sadowsky MJ. Species and genus level resolution analysis of gut microbiota in Clostridium difficile patients following fecal microbiota transplantation. Microbiome. 2014;2:13.
53. Xu J, Chen Y, Zhang R, He J, Song Y, Wang J, Wang H, Wang L, Zhan Q, Abliza Z. Global metabolomics reveals potential urinary biomarkers of esophageal squamous cell carcinoma for diagnosis and staging. Sci Rep. 2016;6:35010.
54. Yu M, Jia H, Zhou C, Yang Y, Zhao Y, Yang M, Zou Z. Variations in gut microbiota and fecal metabolic phenotype associated with depression by 16S rRNA gene sequencing and LC/MS-based metabolomics. J Pharm Biomed Anal. 2017;138:231–9.
55. Lau JT, Whelan FJ, Herath I, Lee CH, Collins SM, Bercik P, Surette MG. Capturing the diversity of the human gut microbiota through culture-enriched molecular profiling. Genome Med. 2016;8:72.
56. Stearns JC, Davidson CJ, McKeon S, Whelan FJ, Fontes ME, Schryvers AB, Bowdish DME, Kellner JD, Surette MG. Culture and molecular-based profiles show shifts in bacterial communities of the upper respiratory tract that occur with age. ISME J. 2015;9:1246–59.
57. Sibley CD, Grinwis ME, Field TR, Eshaghurshan CS, Faria MM, Dowd SE, Parkins MD, Rabin HR, Surette MG. Culture enriched molecular profiling of the cystic fibrosis airway microbiome. PLoS One. 2011;6(7):e22702.
58. Browne HP, Forster SC, Anonye BO, Kumar N, Neville BA, Stares MD, Goulding D, Lawley TD. Culturing of 'unculturable' human microbiota reveals novel taxa and extensive sporulation. Nature. 2016;533:543–6.
59. Gao Z, Tseng CH, Strober BE, Pei Z, Blaser MJ. Substantial alterations of the cutaneous bacterial biota in psoriatic lesions. PLoS One. 2008;3(7):e2719.
60. Zeeuwen PL, Boekhorst J, van den Bogaard EH, de Koning HD, van de Kerkhof PM, Saulnier DM, van Swam II, van Hijum SA, Kleerebezem M, Schalkwijk J, Timmerman HM. Microbiome dynamics of human epidermis following skin barrier disruption. Genome Biol. 2012;13(11):R101.
61. Alekseyenko AV, Perez-Perez GI, De Souza A, Strober B, Gao Z, Bihan M, Li K, Methé BA, Blaser MJ. Community differentiation of the cutaneous microbiota in psoriasis. Microbiome. 2013;1(1):31.
62. Horton JM, Gao Z, Sullivan DM, Shopsin B, Perez-Perez GI, Blaser MJ. The cutaneous microbiome in outpatients presenting with acute skin abscesses. J Infect Dis. 2015;211(12):1895–904.
63. Aagaard K, Petrosino J, Keitel W, Watson M, Katancik J, Garcia N, Patel S, Cutting M, Madden T, Hamilton H, Harris E, Gevers D, Simone G, McInnes P, Versalovic J. The human microbiome project strategy for comprehensive sampling of the human microbiome and why it matters. FASEB J. 2013;27(3):1012–22.
64. Budding AE, Grasman ME, Eck A, Bogaards JA, Vandenbroucke-Grauls CMJE, van Bodegraven AA, Savelkoul PHM. Rectal swabs for analysis of the intestinal microbiota. PLoS One. 2014;9(7):e101344.
65. van Rensburg JJ, Lin H, Gao X, Toh E, Fortney KR, Ellinger S, Zwickl B, Janowicz DM, Katz BP, Nelson DE, Dong Q, Spinola SM. The human skin microbiome associates with the outcome of and is influenced by bacterial infection. MBio. 2015;6(5):e01315.
66. Vujkovic-Cvijin I, Dunham RM, wai SI, Maher MC, Albright RG, Broadhurst MJ, Hernandez RD, Lederman MM, Huang Y, Somsouk M, Deeks SG, Hunt PW, Lynch SV, McCune JM. Dysbiosis of the gut microbiota is associated with HIV disease progression and tryptophan catabolism. Sci Transl Med. 2013;5(193):193ra91.
67. Jiang W, Wu N, Wang X, Chi Y, Zhang Y, Qiu X, Hu Y, Li J, Liu Y. Dysbiosis gut microbiota associated with inflammation and impaired mucosal immune function in intestine of humans with non-alcoholic fatty liver disease. Sci Rep. 2015;5:8096.
68. Grice EA, Kong HH, Renaud G, Young AC, NISC Comparative Sequencing Program, Bouffard GG, Blakesley RW, Wolfsberg TG, Turner ML, Segre JA. A diversity profile of the human skin microbiota. Genome Res. 2008;18(7):1043–50.
69. Liou AP, Paziuk M, Luevano J-M Jr, Machineni S, Turnbaugh PJ, Kaplan LM. Conserved shifts in the gut microbiota due to gastric bypass reduce host weight and adiposity. Sci Transl Med. 2013;5(178):178ra41.
70. Kong HH, Andersson B, Clavel T, Common JE, Jackson SA, Olson ND, Segre JA, Traidl-Hoffmann C. Performing skin microbiome research: a method to the madness. J Invest Dermatol. 2017;137:561–8.
71. Knights D, Kuczynski J, Charlson ES, Zaneveld J, Mozer MC, Collman RG, Bushman FD, Knight R, Kelley ST. Bayesian community-wide culture- independent microbial source tracking. Nat Methods. 2011;8(9):761–3.
72. Belheouane M, Gupta Y, Künzel S, Ibrahim S, Baines JF. Improved detection of gene-microbe interactions in the mouse skin microbiota using high-resolution QTL mapping of 16S rRNA transcripts. Microbiome. 2017;5(1):59.
73. Stearns JC, Lynch MDJ, Senadheera DB, Tenenbaum HC, Goldberg MB, Cvitko-vitch DG, Croitoru K, Moreno-Hagelsieb G, Neufeld JD. Bacterial biogeography of the human digestive tract. Sci Rep. 2011;1:170.
74. Gevers D, Kugathasan S, Denson LA, Vázquez-Baeza Y, Van Treuren W, Ren B, Schwager E, Knights D, Song SJ, Yassour M, Morgan XC, Kostic AD, Luo C, González A, McDonald D, Haberman Y, Walters T, Baker S, Rosh J, Stephens M, Heyman M, Markowitz J, Baldassano R, Griffiths A, Sylvester F, Mack D, Kim S, Crandall

W, Hyams J, Huttenhower C, Knight R, Xavier RJ. The treatment-naive microbiome in new-onset Crohn's disease. Cell Host Microbe. 2014;15(3):382–92.
75. Shobar RM, Velineni S, Keshavarzian A, Swanson G, DeMeo MT, Melson JE, Losurdo J, Engen PA, Sun Y, Koenig L, Mutlu EA. The effects of bowel preparation on microbiota-related metrics differ in health and in inflammatory bowel disease and for the mucosal and luminal microbiota compartments. Clin Transl Gastroenterol. 2016;7(2):e143.
76. Kim TK, Thomas SM, Ho M, Sharma S, Reich CI, Frank JA, Yeater KM, Biggs DR, Nakamura N, Stumpf R, Leigh SR, Tapping RI, Blanke SR, Slauch JM, Gaskins HR, Weisbaum JS, Olsen GJ, Hoyer LL, Wilson BA. Heterogeneity of vaginal microbial communities within individuals. J Clin Microbiol. 2009;47(4):1181–9.
77. Kong HH. Skin microbiome: genomics-based insights into the diversity and role of skin microbes. Trends Mol Med. 2011;17:320–8.
78. Grice EA, Segre JA. The skin microbiome. Nat Rev Microbiol. 2011;9(4):244–53.
79. Caporaso JG, Lauber CL, Costello EK, Berg-Lyons D, Gonzalez A, Stombaugh J, Knights D, Gajer P, Ravel J, Fierer N, Gordon JI, Knight R. Moving pictures of the human microbiome. Genome Biol. 2011;12(5):R50.
80. Goodrich JK, Di Rienzi SC, Poole AC, Koren O, Walters WA, Caporaso JG, Knight R, Ley RE. Conducting a microbiome study. Cell. 2014;158(2):250–62.

Analytic Methods in Microbiome Studies

3

Philipp Rausch and Axel Künstner

Abbreviations

AL	Average linkage
ANOSIM	Analysis of similarity
BLAST	Basic Local Alignment Search Tool
CCA	Canonical correspondence analysis
CL	Complete linkage
COI	Cytochrome c oxidase subunit I
DA	Differentially abundant
dbRDA	Distance-based redundancy analysis
DGE	Differential gene expression
ITS	Internal transcribed spacer
MDS	Multidimensional scaling
NAST	Nearest alignment space termination
NMDS	Nonmetric multidimensional scaling
OTU	Operational taxonomic unit
PAM	Partitioning around medoids
PCR	Polymerase chain reaction
PD	Phylogenetic diversity
PERMANOVA	Permutational multivariate analysis of variance
RA	Rheumatoid arthritis
RDA	Redundancy analysis
RDP	Ribosomal Database Project
rRNA	Ribosomal ribonucleic acid
SL	Single linkage
UniFrac	Unique fraction metric
UPGMA	Unweighted pair group method with arithmetic mean
ZIG	Zero-inflated Gaussian

P. Rausch
Max Planck Institute for Evolutionary Biology, Plön, Germany

Institute for Experimental Medicine, Christian-Albrechts-University of Kiel, Kiel, Germany

A. Künstner (✉)
Group for Medical Systems Biology, Lübeck Institute of Experimental Dermatology (LIED), University of Lübeck, Lübeck, Germany

Max Planck Institute for Evolutionary Biology, Plön, Germany
e-mail: axel.kuenstner@uni-luebeck.de

Universal Marker

In the past, anatomical and morphological differences were employed to structure the domains of life. For characterization of bacterial species, morphological, biochemical, or metabolic properties are important but require cultures. Unfortunately, cultivation in the laboratory is limited as many species and whole phyla are (still) not cultivable, or the efforts for cultivation are enormous [2–4]. However, it has been recognized that genetic information is a much richer

G. Ragab et al. (eds.), *The Microbiome in Rheumatic Diseases and Infection*,
https://doi.org/10.1007/978-3-319-79026-8_3

pool of characters for the inference of evolutionary ancestry and classification. Early on, universal markers were favored to allow for systematic comparison among organisms and led to a new way of ordering the biological world and the discovery of the domain archaea [5]. A universal marker has to fulfill certain requirements: (1) it has to occur among all species and (2) it has to accumulate enough variability to distinguish species and (3) still be stable enough to allow for comparisons among far diverged taxa. As one such marker, ribosomal RNAs (*rRNA*), central parts of the translational machinery, have been established [6]. Their secondary structure and central role in the cellular machinery prevent the sequences from accumulating too much diversity, while hypervariable regions allow for genetic variation even between different species [7].

A commonly used marker for bacterial and archaea classification is the *16S rRNA* gene [7]. The gene is about 1300 bp long and comprises nine hypervariable regions (V1–V9) of different informational content [8]. Traditional Sanger sequencing is able to capture the full sequence information of the gene. However, with recent advances in shotgun sequencing (next generation sequencing), short sequence technology became the most dominant technology, which allows for short reads up to 300 bp using Illumina technology [9] or 800 bp using Roche 454 technology [10]. Other technologies like Ion Torrent [11] and PacBio [12] allow for even longer read lengths with higher error rates compared to the two other methods. Due to the different information content of the V-regions, it is not necessary to sequence the full-length *16S rRNA*. The most representative regions are V1–V2 and V3–V4 [13, 14], and in combination with Illumina sequencing, these are the most widely used markers for classification. For eukaryotes the main marker genes became *18S rRNA*, *ITS* (internal transcribed spacer), and the *cytochrome c oxidase subunit I* (*COI*; universal barcode for eukaryotes [15]) and have been established as phylogenetic and taxonomic markers.

Note that even universal markers may have biases because variations in the conserved sequences make it difficult to capture all species with the same likelihood [8, 16, 17]. This even led to the underappreciation of whole phyla in marker gene analyses, as recently discovered for genetically unusual candidate phyla [17–19].

Sequence Preprocessing and OTU Binning

A typical workflow from bacterial DNA isolation to analyzing the data is shown in Fig. 3.1 and described below.

Merging and Trimming

Sequencing errors can blur taxonomic classification of sequences. Therefore, it is necessary to apply strict filtering steps to minimize sequencing errors [20]. Compared to single-end sequencing, paired-end sequencing has the inherent benefit that a large proportion of the sequence can be read twice and can also reach longer read lengths through partial merging. Basically, forward and backward reads of paired-end sequencing overhangs are trimmed, the remaining reads aligned and merged under consideration of the respective base quality [13, 21, 22]. That is, with paired reads, there is often overlap between the forward and reverse reads. As the two reads should be identical in their area of overlap, this overlap in essence constitutes double-checking the sequence. Furthermore, if there is disagreement between the forward and reverse read at a particular base pair, then the read with the higher quality score counts, or both reads are discarded depending on the stringency of the protocol.

Chimera Detection and Denoising

During library preparation, sequences are amplified using several PCR cycles. Although error-correcting polymerases are used, the resulting products are not free of errors. The typical per base error rate is in the range of 10^{-7} to 10^{-5}, depending on the polymerase used [23], and it further increases with the number of cycles [24].

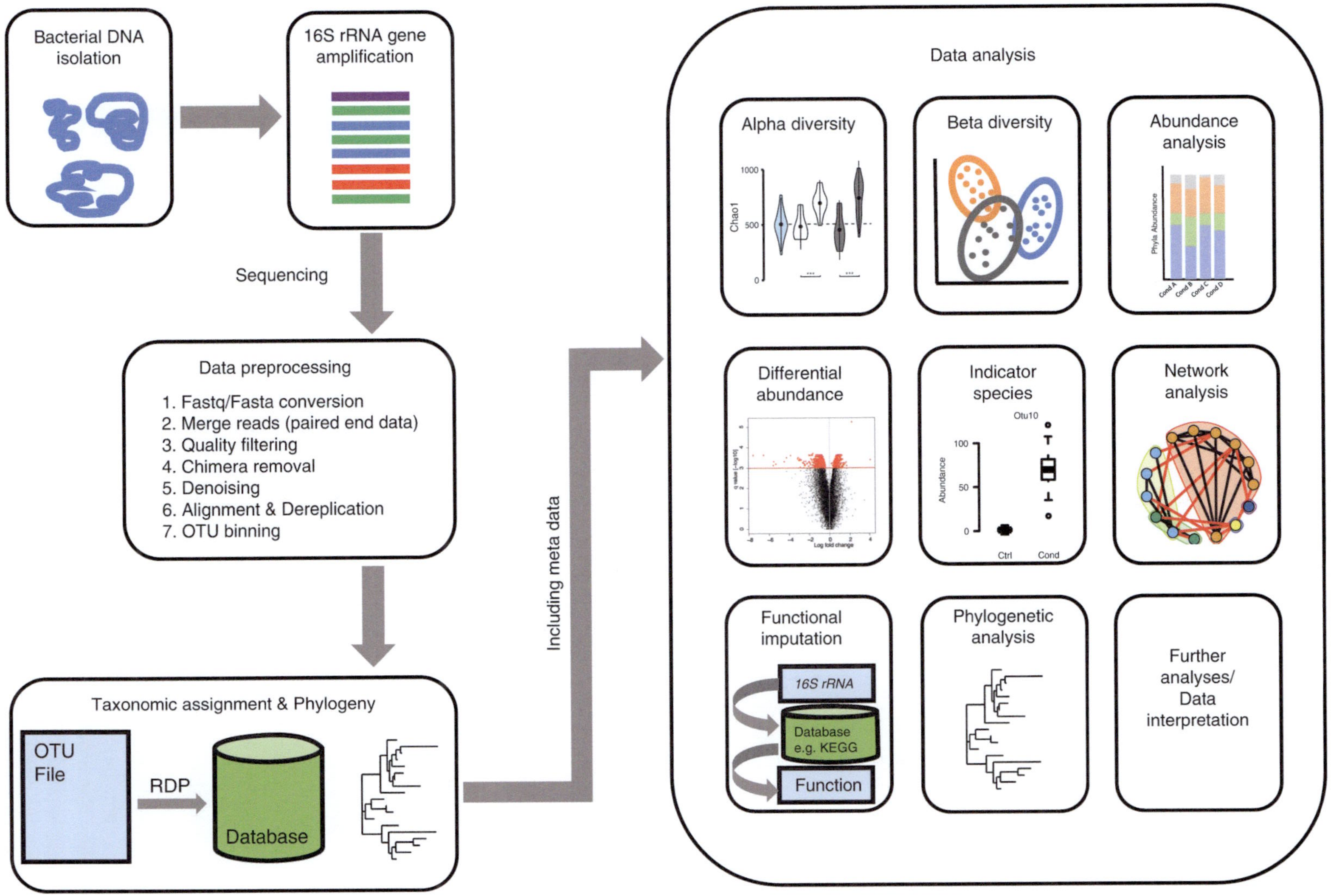

Fig. 3.1 Schematic overview about a typical *16S rRNA* workflow from bacterial DNA isolation to data analysis. The box “Data analysis” is not all encompassing and can be extended or reduced to fit the needs of specific studies or questions

When only short sequence fragments are used, sequencing errors can lead to misclassifications and in consequence lead to more diversity within and between samples. To reduce the impact of these uncertainties, different denoising strategies are applied, e.g., via clustering [13, 22, 25]. Additionally, abundance analysis can be applied to filter out uninformative variation [21].

Self-priming of PCR products leads to chimeric sequences, without biological relevance [26–28]. Database-driven approaches match sequences against a curated database to identify sequence fragments with multiple ancestry and potential breakpoints within the sequences, as implemented in ChimeraSlayer [26] or UCHIME [27, 29]. In addition to the alignment strategy, de novo approaches use the given dataset to construct a database and calculate the abundance distribution of sequences and exploit the characteristic abundance distribution of chimeric sequences [27]. Compared to database-driven methods, this is computationally more demanding.

OTU Binning

Many analytic protocols involve binning similar sequences into operational taxonomic units (OTUs), which constitute artificial species clusters of highly similar sequences. Before the clustering step is performed, it might be necessary to align them depending on the strategy used for clustering and classification. Different strategies for this have been developed and are mainly based on large and well-curated seed alignments (RDP core set, Silva core set). The nearest alignment space termination (NAST) algorithm [30–32] is the most common and most reliable alignment strategy, based on a primary search and subsequent alignment to the best database entry [33]. As a side note, lane masks which cover extremely variable sites in the NAST seed alignment (e.g., Greengenes) should be avoided [34].

OTUs are based on sequence similarity thresholds. Traditionally a similarity threshold of 97% is applied to delineate bacterial species. However, this threshold can be adjusted depending on the aspects of community assembly under investigation (e.g., Moeller et al. 2012, threshold of 99%) [35]. Basically, three approaches are available to bin sequences into OTUs: closed-reference clustering (e.g., as implemented in QIIME [36]), de novo clustering (as implemented in QIIME, mothur [37] or VSEARCH [38]), and open-reference clustering (e.g., implemented in QIIME). In closed-reference OTU picking, each sequence is aligned with an operator-selected database; those that do not align with the database are usually discarded. De novo OTU picking, in contrast, does not make any use of a query database. Instead, sequences are aligned and clustered only with each other. Open-reference OTU picking constitutes a hybrid approach, in which sequences are initially aligned to a database, while those that do not align to the database subsequently undergo de novo OTU picking. Due to the variety of approaches, it is important to know the benefits, weaknesses, and potential biases of the methods on the OTU assignments [39, 40].

The effectiveness of closed-reference clustering depends on an appropriate reference database on which sequences are aligned. The validity of the obtained OTUs highly depends on the order and diversity of the query, as well as on the quality of the reference database [39]. The advantages are that the approach scales linearly with the number of sequences and is easily parallelizable and its results are comparable between studies. The drawback is that species not represented in the database cannot be clustered into OTUs (the same applies to sequences too diverged). Additional problems occur if sequences match to two or more database entries leading to inconsistent assignments [39]. Closed-reference OTU picking works better for habitats that have been widely studied, such as human fecal specimens, as it is more likely to find relatives of those bacteria in the database.

De novo clustering of OTUs is based solely on the sequences within the respective dataset. Generally, two methods exist to perform this: distance-based and heuristic approaches. The traditional distance-based clustering relies on the hierarchical ordering of a distance matrix via different algorithms such as complete linkage

(CL; furthest neighbor), single linkage (SL; nearest neighbor), and average linkage (AL; unweighted pair group method with arithmetic mean) [41]. The CL method assigns a sequence (or group of sequences) to a cluster if it is similar to all members of the cluster. SL bins a sequence into an existing cluster if it is similar to any of the sequences in the cluster. AL links a sequence to a cluster if it is similar to the arithmetic average of the cluster and recalculates the average distance between the members of the cluster. AL is the preferred method as it represents a compromise between SL and CL leading to neither under- nor overestimation of OTU numbers and provides a high consistency of OTU assignments [39]. However, AL is computationally the most demanding method (scales quadratic with number of sequences). Heuristic methods are most similar to CL clustering as they are mainly based on greedy clustering, which tend to find local optimal solutions in reasonable time, but are not guaranteed to find the global optimal differentiation between OTUs, resulting in split OTUs or inconsistent sequence affiliations. Different methods are implemented, e.g., optimal global alignments (e.g., VSEARCH), heuristic seed with extend aligner (e.g., USEARCH [42]), or word length similarity (e.g., CD-HIT [43]). Heuristic methods are usually faster than distance methods but are not guaranteed to find the best clustering and tend to split OTUs and inflate diversity.

Classification, Taxonomic Assignment, and Phylogenetic Inference

Classification of sequences is another important step to investigate the composition of a community by placing sequences/OTUs in the context of a known taxonomy or phylogeny.

In the case of closed-reference clustering, taxonomic classification is already known for each OTU, while de novo clustering needs a posterior assignment to taxonomic groups. OTU sequences can be matched against several databases to obtain a consensus classification for each OTU. The most commonly used databases for *16S rRNA* gene sequences are Greengenes [44], the Ribosomal Database Project (RDP) [45, 46], and Silva [47, 48]. They share a common core of sequences but differ in their curation strategy (length, quality, chimeras) and in their taxonomic backbone. The Greengenes database was last updated in 2013, whereas the two others are updated more regularly. The Greengenes database has the advantage of carrying species level assignments, whereas the two latter ones contain information only to genus level. However, OTUs cannot always be classified to the lowest possible level (species or genus) due to missing information in either database or query sequence. In addition, classification by a majority vote instead of distance-based representative sequence usually provides better results [49]. That is, OTUs will constitute sequences that have similar but not identical taxonomies. One approach to assign taxonomy is to pick a "representative" sequence from each OTU, assess its taxonomy, and apply it to the rest of the OTU. The "majority vote" approach assigns taxonomy to each sequence within the OTU and selects the most common to apply to the entire OTU.

Classification has been the subject of many investigations regarding the algorithms and databases. The most widely used and validated method for amplicon-based analyses is the naïve Bayesian classifier developed by the RDP team [50]. This technique can be used for other marker genes as well with the appropriate training datasets (e.g., *ITS*, *18S rRNA*) [51] and is available as a stand-alone program or re-implementation in mothur. It derives support values via a bootstrap heuristic, for which empirical evidence suggests cutoff values ≥80%. As for every other classifier, it is only as good as the underlying database; thus decoy sequences to root the classification (e.g., human, plant sequences), as well as the option to adjust the database with additional sequences, can improve classifications [52, 53].

Recent developments also provide good alternatives based on *k*-mer similarity scores as implemented in UTAX/SINTAX [54] which reduces overclassification. Also the widely used Basic Local Alignment Search Tool (BLAST) [55] and variations thereof [25] can be used to classify short amplicon reads, although with certain shortcomings [56]. Furthermore, placement of sequences on a guide tree was developed for classification as well but may not be well suited for automated taxonomic assignments [56].

Phylogenetic Inferences

Phylogenetic inferences on highly conserved, slowly evolving genes like the *16S rRNA* gene are less reliable than multigene or whole genome inferences but have the power to delineate deep relationships among taxa [5], while the number of sequences and their heterogeneous divergence can be challenging to existing inference methods. FastTree has been specifically developed to accommodate short-read data using sophisticated evolutionary models [57, 58]. Alternative approaches which map sequences to curated guide trees as implemented in ARB [59] are also available [60]. Fast but less sophisticated tree building methods (e.g., neighbor-joining approaches) via clearcut (also part of mothur) [61, 62], however, may not represent the most accurate depiction of species relationships. Phylogenetic trees can later be examined and edited in dedicated programs (e.g., Dendroscope [63]) or incorporated into measures of alpha and beta diversity such as UniFrac (see below "Alpha and Beta Diversity").

Diversity Analysis

Alpha and Beta Diversity

A commonly used concept to compare ecological samples is that of the diversity within a given community (alpha diversity) or among communities (beta diversity). The two concepts were conceived by [64, 65]. Alpha diversity describes the local species pool in a sample or community and can be seen as a summary statistic, whereas beta diversity describes the total species diversity or (dis-) similarity between communities. Table 3.1 summarizes the categories of diversity indices.

Regardless of whether alpha or beta diversity is being used, all measurements can be distinguished broadly into two categories. First, some measurements use only the presence/absence of taxa (qualitative data; richness of samples), while others take into account the abundance (quantitative data; evenness of samples) of each taxon. Second, some measures treat all taxa equally in relation to each other (species-based), while others incorporate the relatedness (phylogeny) of the taxa (divergence-based). That is, with measures that incorporate phylogenetic information, extra weight is given for two OTUs that are distantly related (e.g., different phyla), compared to two that are from the same family or genus. Generally, methods with the same properties give quite similar results, but one or the other measurement is more suitable for a specific question (Table 3.1).

Table 3.1 Diversity measurements according to their category (qualitative vs quantitative and species vs divergence)

Category		Measurement of diversity	
		Alpha	Beta
Qualitative	Species	Chao1	Sörensen index
		ACE	Jaccard index
		Rarefaction	
	Divergence	Phylogenetic distance	UniFrac
Quantitative	Species	Shannon index	Bray-Curtis
		Simpson index	Morisita-Horn measure
	Divergence	θ	Weighted UniFrac

Alpha diversity is important to understand the complexity of different communities. For instance, we can compare the gut microbiota of patients and healthy controls with respect to species richness and/or evenness and ask about a general effect of the disease. Qualitative measurements like species richness and quantitative measurements like Shannon index [66] and Simpson index [67] as well as their more generalized versions [68, 69] have been successfully applied to summarize datasets. In contrast to these more traditional estimators, Faith's phylogenetic diversity (PD) [70] has been widely used to incorporate the phylogenetic relationship between species (or taxa) into the analysis of alpha diversity. Considering the divergence within and between the respective community members provides an insight into the history of community development and can even give proxies for functional differentiation among them [70, 71]. Alpha diversity indices implicitly assume that the total diversity in a community has been sampled, an assumption that is not always accurate if sequencing depth is low. To overcome this limitation, techniques like rarefication curves can be used to predict the coverage and total diversity by curve-fitting methods, or even approximated diversities like Chao1 [72] or ACE [73, 74] can be applied (Table 3.1). Put simply, given a particular sample, the more unique sequences that are present, the more diverse the sample will appear, everything else being equal.

Beta diversity is used to evaluate how the composition and structure of the microbiota differ between sample groups [75]. Commonly, Jaccard index/distance [76] and Bray-Curtis dissimilarity [77] are used to analyze the community data in a qualitative or quantitative way (shared presence, shared abundance), respectively (Table 3.1). Divergence can be incorporated into the analysis as well via the unique fraction metric (UniFrac) [78, 79] as a qualitative measurement. It assumes that phylogenetically similar communities (e.g., separated by a short branch) have only recently diverged, which would also imply functional similarities. The UniFrac metric was further extended to account for changes in (relative) abundances of species or lineages between samples, the weighted UniFrac measurement [79], which was further generalized in different ways [80, 81]. Note that phylogenetically informed alpha and beta diversity measures depend on the quality/type of the phylogenetic community trees [79, 83–85]. In simple terms, the smaller the overlap of bacterial species between two samples is, the larger will be their community distance and thus their beta diversity.

Keep in mind that especially quantitative data might be affected by biases introduced during DNA extraction and PCR amplification [85, 86]. Additionally, different copy numbers of the *16S rRNA* gene between bacteria introduce further biases [87, 88]. These biases are less pronounced in qualitative measurements compared to quantitative measurements. Other problematic issues are contamination [89] and samples with source bias or low biomass (e.g., skin samples) [90], which can affect qualitative and quantitative measurements.

Comparing Samples Using Diversity Estimates

Alpha diversity is a rather descriptive measure. Distribution of the data can be shown using, for instance, boxplots/violin plots or density plots to visually explore differences within and between groups. Samples or groups can be compared using statistical testing (e.g., Mann-Whitney *U* test, Kruskal-Wallis test). Additionally, confounding factors can be identified and quantified using more complex statistics like linear models and mixed effects models.

Beta diversity can be visualized using clustering algorithms, like neighbor-joining (NJ), UPGMA, or partitioning around medoids (PAM). The resulting dendrograms show the relatedness of the samples with respect to the chosen distance measurement and clustering algorithm.

Other commonly used exploratory tools are unconstrained and constrained ordination methods (indirect, direct gradient analysis). The former category comprises multidimensional scaling (MDS, e.g., principal coordinate analysis/PCoA) and nonmetric multidimensional scaling (NMDS). Constrained ordination methods include canonical correspondence analysis (CCA), redundancy analysis (RDA), and distance-based redundancy analysis (dbRDA) [92–94]. Generally, it is possible to correct for (partial out) confounding factors using constrained ordination methods before the constraints are applied (partial redundancy analysis), but this can also be addressed by appropriate permutation regimes. Besides these exploratory methods, hypothesis testing methods can be applied on beta diversity. Most commonly, permutational multivariate analysis of variance (PERMANOVA) [94] and analysis of similarity (ANOSIM) [95] are applied to determine if the microbial composition differs according to specific variables such as disease status or treatment.

Correlating Species with Habitats

As described above, microbiota data can be summarized and compared between conditions (e.g., disease phenotype and healthy controls) using diversity indices (alpha or beta diversity) or differences in total taxonomic abundance (e.g., on phylum or genus level). To gain more insights into differences between experimental conditions, the more relevant questions are which species (or OTUs) are indicators for a certain condition and which are differentially abundant (DA) between conditions? Clearly, this analysis is not restricted to the species level and can be performed on any taxonomic level (e.g., family or genera). Note, microbiota data are usually very sparse count data (most OTUs have zero counts) and are highly overdispersed (variance of the data is higher than variance expected by the model). These characteristics should be taken into account to build appropriate models to identify indicator species.

Indicator Species Analysis

Identifying indicator species to describe differences between habitats is a common concept in ecology [96]. Due to their niche preferences, indicator species can be used to describe and distinguish habitats also among bacterial communities. One of the most commonly used methods to detect indicator species is the method introduced by Dufrêne and Legendre [97] and its extensions by De Cáceres [98, 99]. The method estimates an indicator value to measure the association between a species and a habitat while accounting for both abundance and frequency of species and can be expanded to combinations of species. Statistical significance is tested using permutation tests, which do not explicitly account for overdispersion or zero-inflated data.

Supervised classification is an alternative method of classifying microbiome samples and identifying indicator microbes. For instance RandomForest classification became a popular method to test clustering of samples and also to perform regression analysis in microbial community analysis [100, 101]. A RandomForest classifier can be tuned by *k*-fold cross-validation (variable selection, optimization) and provides information about the importance of each feature (e.g., OTU) to discriminate the respective groups and can be used to identify indicator species.

Differential Abundance (DA) Analysis Based on Count Data

The problem of identifying DA taxa is quite similar to the problem of differential gene expression (DGE) analysis, namely, the issue of taking into account multiple comparisons. Therefore, McMurdie and Holmes [102] proposed to use methods that are commonly used in DGE analysis like edgeR [103], DESeq2 [104] or baySeq [105] to identify DA taxa. However, methods developed for DGE analysis may not perform well on microbiome data because they do not account for sparsity in the data (zero-inflated data) [106]. An approach more related to microbial marker surveys is implemented in metagenomeSeq [107]. It exploits cumulative sum scaling to normalize the data and a zero-inflated Gaussian model (ZIG model) that accounts for undersampling. Fernandes et al. proposed another approach (ALDEx2) that emphasizes the compositional nature of sequencing data and uses Monte Carlo sampling of Dirichlet distributions and averages *P*-values across resamples [108]. However, so far no general recommendation can be given about which approach to use for DA analysis because of the very nature of each dataset [109].

Network Analysis of Co-occurrence/ Co-abundance Relationships

Typically, ecological communities are not an assembly of independent entities that simply differ in number and abundance and develop accordingly in a neutral fashion but highly structured and intricate networks connected by various mechanisms (e.g., predator-prey, syntrophy). Thus, an analysis of interaction networks, or thereof their approximations, can increase our understanding of community assembly and dynamics, as well enable us to identify important species with central positions in those communities. However, microbial communities rarely allow the observation of clear biological interactions (e.g., via fluorescent in situ hybridization) due to their complexity and turnover. Thus, most analyses rely on abundance relationships and co-occurrences that only represent statistical interactions. Several techniques exist to calculate those statistical relationships, aside from the commonly used but biased conventional correlation routines [110, 111]. The main problems for the inference of interactions are the large number of tests, spurious signals by indirect correlations (false positives), compositionality of the data (relative counts), data sparsity, and a multitude of linear and nonlinear interaction types [112]. For example SparCC (also implemented in mothur) and CoNet (Cytoscape) were designed to handle the compositionality of metagenomic data by different techniques and generate empirical *P*-values through permutation and bootstrapping [110, 113, 114]. More detailed evaluations and selection criteria as for, e.g., time courses of networks (local similarity analysis [115]) can be found elsewhere [111, 116]. The resulting correlation matrices should be culled by an appropriate *P*-value threshold to reduce false positives and indirect interactions and analyzed with dedicated software packages (e.g., Cytoscape). The resulting networks denote bacteria as "nodes" and their correlation as "edges" (weighted/unweighted), for which indices and statistics can be derived, as well as for the network as a whole [118–120]. Measures to evaluate the positions of nodes and edges within a network can be employed to find important network members [121–124], from which degree centrality is the simplest (number of direct connections). Within a network one can employ permutation tests, network simulations, or null models (e.g., random Erdös-Renyi graphs) to analyze network properties or to specify the type of network (e.g., scale-free, small-world). Furthermore communities, cliques, and hierarchical structures can be inferred by various algorithms (e.g., walktrap algorithm [124]), to investigate the super structure of the network and identify interesting subpopulations.

Functional Imputation of Amplicon Data

As described above, amplicon data only give us information about the taxonomic composition of communities. However the ever-growing genomic databases and more sophisticated algorithms allow for an indirect approach to approximate the functional repertoire of communities. By matching amplicon reads to a database of well analyzed bacteria, it can be assumed that the functional content is present in the community in the abundance signified by the abundance of amplicons corrected by copy number and relatedness. First developed by Okuda et al. in 2012 [125] but popularized and molded into the software suite PICRUSt by Langille et al. [126], it became an interesting addition to taxonomic analyses with new applications being continuously developed [128–130]. PICRUSt in particular is available through QIIME, as a stand-alone version, and through a mothur-based workflow, mainly based on matching OTUs to the Greengenes taxonomy backbone in combination with the Galaxy PICRUSt pipeline (https://huttenhower.sph.harvard.edu/galaxy/) [44, 130]. The results, consisting of validity measures and functional category abundances, can be analyzed on their own or fed into pipelines like HumanN for additional inferences [131]. Results, however, have to be taken with caution, as these can only be seen as approximations of the metabolic capacities due to intrinsic problems (plastic bacterial genomes, incompleteness, accuracy). Although efforts to show their validity have been made [132], these techniques are not infallible and should be investigated for potential flaws (e.g., weighted Nearest Sequenced Taxon Index >0.15 for PICRUSt). Thus, shotgun DNA- or RNA-based metagenomic analysis is the only reliable method to derive functional information from microbial communities but requires larger financial and computational investments of the researcher.

Conclusion

In general marker gene analyses of complex communities are the first line of investigation and provide great first insights and hypotheses. They combine low costs with fairly well-established protocols and databases. However, as we have outlined, this type of analysis has its flaws (e.g., misrepresentation) which have to be taken into account to interpret results obtained.

References

1. Okada Y, Wu D, Trynka G, Raj T, Terao C, Ikari K, et al. Genetics of rheumatoid arthritis contributes to biology and drug discovery. Nature. 2014;506(7488):376–81.
2. He X, McLean JS, Edlund A, Yooseph S, Hall AP, Liu S-Y, et al. Cultivation of a human-associated TM7 phylotype reveals a reduced genome and epibiotic parasitic lifestyle. Proc Natl Acad Sci U S A. 2015;112(1):244–9.
3. Vartoukian SR, Adamowska A, Lawlor M, Moazzez R, Dewhirst FE, Wade WG. In vitro cultivation of ‘unculturable’ oral bacteria, facilitated by community culture and media supplementation with siderophores. PLoS One. 2016;11(1):e0146926.
4. Solden L, Lloyd K, Wrighton K. The bright side of microbial dark matter: lessons learned from the uncultivated majority. Curr Opin Microbiol. 2016;31:217–26.
5. Woese CR, Kandler O, Wheelis ML. Towards a natural system of organisms: proposal for the domains Archaea, Bacteria, and Eucarya. Proc Natl Acad Sci U S A. 1990;87(12):4576–9.
6. Woese CR, Fox GE. Phylogenetic structure of the prokaryotic domain: the primary kingdoms. Proc Natl Acad Sci U S A. 1977;74(11):5088–90.
7. Lane DJ, Pace B, Olsen GJ, Stahl DA, Sogin ML, Pace NR. Rapid determination of 16S ribosomal RNA sequences for phylogenetic analyses. Proc Natl Acad Sci U S A. 1985;82(20):6955–9.
8. Yarza P, Yilmaz P, Pruesse E, Glockner FO, Ludwig W, Schleifer K-H, et al. Uniting the classification of cultured and uncultured bacteria and archaea using 16S rRNA gene sequences. Nat Rev Microbiol. 2014;12(9):635–45.
9. Bentley DR, Balasubramanian S, Swerdlow HP, Smith GP, Milton J, Brown CG, et al. Accurate whole human genome sequencing using reversible terminator chemistry. Nature. 2008;456(7218):53–9.
10. Margulies M, Egholm M, Altman WE, Attiya S, Bader JS, Bemben LA, et al. Genome sequencing in microfabricated high-density picolitre reactors. Nature. 2005;437(7057):376–80.
11. Rothberg JM, Hinz W, Rearick TM, Schultz J, Mileski W, Davey M, et al. An integrated semiconductor device enabling non-optical genome sequencing. Nature. 2011;475(7356):348–52.
12. Eid J, Fehr A, Gray J, Luong K, Lyle J, Otto G, et al. Real-time DNA sequencing from single polymerase molecules. Science. 2009;323(5910):133–8.
13. Schloss PD. The effects of alignment quality, distance calculation method, sequence filtering, and region on the analysis of 16S rRNA gene-based studies. PLoS Comput Biol. 2010;6(7):e1000844.
14. Huttenhower C, Gevers D, Knight R, Abubucker S, Badger JH, Chinwalla AT. Structure, function and diversity of the healthy human microbiome. Nature. 2012;486:207.
15. Hebert PDN, Cywinska A, Ball SL, deWaard JR. Biological identifications through DNA barcodes. Proc R Soc Lond Ser B Biol Sci. 2003;270(1512):313–21.
16. Klindworth A, Pruesse E, Schweer T, Peplies J, Quast C, Horn M, et al. Evaluation of general 16S ribosomal RNA gene PCR primers for classical and next-generation sequencing-based diversity studies. Nucleic Acids Res. 2013;41(1):e1.
17. Eloe-Fadrosh EA, Ivanova NN, Woyke T, Kyrpides NC. Metagenomics uncovers gaps in amplicon-based

detection of microbial diversity. Nat Microbiol. 2016;1:15032.
18. Brown CT, Hug LA, Thomas BC, Sharon I, Castelle CJ, Singh A, et al. Unusual biology across a group comprising more than 15% of domain Bacteria. Nature. 2015;523(7559):208–11.
19. Rinke C, Schwientek P, Sczyrba A, Ivanova NN, Anderson IJ, Cheng J-F, et al. Insights into the phylogeny and coding potential of microbial dark matter. Nature. 2013;499(7459):431–7.
20. Bokulich NA, Subramanian S, Faith JJ, Gevers D, Gordon JI, Knight R, et al. Quality-filtering vastly improves diversity estimates from Illumina amplicon sequencing. Nat Methods. 2013;10(1):57–9.
21. Edgar RC, Flyvbjerg H. Error filtering, pair assembly, and error correction for next-generation sequencing reads. Bioinformatics. 2015;31(21):3476–82.
22. Kozich JJ, Westcott SL, Baxter NT, Highlander SK, Schloss PD. Development of a dual-index sequencing strategy and curation pipeline for analyzing amplicon sequence data on the MiSeq Illumina sequencing platform. Appl Environ Microbiol. 2013;79(17):5112–20.
23. McInerney P, Adams P, Hadi MZ. Error rate comparison during polymerase chain reaction by DNA polymerase. Mol Biol Int. 2014;2014:8.
24. Gohl DM, Vangay P, Garbe J, MacLean A, Hauge A, Becker A, et al. Systematic improvement of amplicon marker gene methods for increased accuracy in microbiome studies. Nat Biotechnol. 2016;34(9):942–9.
25. Huse SM, Dethlefsen L, Huber JA, Welch DM, Relman DA, Sogin ML. Exploring microbial diversity and taxonomy using SSU rRNA Hypervariable tag sequencing. PLoS Genet. 2008;4(11):e1000255.
26. Haas BJ, Gevers D, Earl AM, Feldgarden M, Ward DV, Giannoukos G, et al. Chimeric 16S rRNA sequence formation and detection in sanger and 454-pyrosequenced PCR amplicons. Genome Res. 2011;21(3):494–504.
27. Edgar RC, Haas BJ, Clemente JC, Quince C, Knight R. UCHIME improves sensitivity and speed of chimera detection. Bioinformatics. 2011;27(16):2194–200.
28. Ashelford KE, Chuzhanova NA, Fry JC, Jones AJ, Weightman AJ. New screening software shows that most recent large 16S rRNA gene clone libraries contain chimeras. Appl Environ Microbiol. 2006;72(9):5734–41.
29. Edgar R. UCHIME2: improved chimera prediction for amplicon sequencing. bioRxiv. 2016.
30. DeSantis TZ, Hugenholtz P, Keller K, Brodie EL, Larsen N, Piceno YM, et al. NAST: a multiple sequence alignment server for comparative analysis of 16S rRNA genes. Nucleic Acids Res. 2006;34(suppl 2):W394–W9.
31. Caporaso JG, Bittinger K, Bushman FD, DeSantis TZ, Andersen GL, Knight R. PyNAST: a flexible tool for aligning sequences to a template alignment. Bioinformatics. 2010;26(2):266–7.
32. Schloss PD. A high-throughput DNA sequence aligner for microbial ecology studies. PLoS One. 2009;4(12):e8230.
33. Schloss PD. Secondary structure improves OTU assignments of 16S rRNA gene sequences. ISME J. 2013;7(3):457–60.
34. White J, Navlakha S, Nagarajan N, Ghodsi M-R, Kingsford C, Pop M. Alignment and clustering of phylogenetic markers – implications for microbial diversity studies. BMC Bioinformatics. 2010;11(1):152.
35. Moeller AH, Degnan PH, Pusey AE, Wilson ML, Hahn BH, Ochman H. Chimpanzees and humans harbour compositionally similar gut enterotypes. Nat Commun. 2012;3:1179.
36. Caporaso JG, Kuczynski J, Stombaugh J, Bittinger K, Bushman FD, Costello EK, et al. QIIME allows analysis of high-throughput community sequencing data. Nat Methods. 2010;7(5):335–6.
37. Schloss PD, Westcott SL, Ryabin T, Hall JR, Hartmann M, Hollister EB, et al. Introducing mothur: open source, platform-independent, community-supported software for describing and comparing microbial communities. Appl Environ Microbiol. 2009;75(23):7537–41.
38. Rognes T, Flouri T, Nichols B, Quince C, Mahé F. VSEARCH: a versatile open source tool for metagenomics. PeerJ. 2016;4:e2584.
39. Westcott SL, Schloss PD. De novo clustering methods outperform reference-based methods for assigning 16S rRNA gene sequences to operational taxonomic units. PeerJ. 2015;3:e1487.
40. Schmidt TSB, Matias Rodrigues JF, von Mering C. Limits to robustness and reproducibility in the demarcation of operational taxonomic units. Environ Microbiol. 2015;17(5):1689–706.
41. Schloss P, Handelsman J. Introducing DOTUR, a computer program for defining operational taxonomic units and estimating species richness. Appl Environ Microbiol. 2005;71(3):1501–6.
42. Edgar RC, Search and clustering orders of magnitude faster than BLAST, Bioinformatics (2010);26(19):2460–1. doi: 10.1093/bioinformatics/btq461.
43. Li W, Jaroszewski L, Godzik A. Clustering of highly homologous sequences to reduce the size of large protein databases. Bioinformatics. 2001;17(3):282–3.
44. DeSantis TZ, Hugenholtz P, Larsen N, Rojas M, Brodie EL, Keller K, et al. Greengenes, a chimera-checked 16S rRNA gene database and workbench compatible with ARB. Appl Environ Microbiol. 2006;72(7):5069–72.
45. Cole JR, Wang Q, Cardenas E, Fish J, Chai B, Farris RJ, et al. The ribosomal database project: improved alignments and new tools for rRNA analysis. Nucleic Acids Res. 2009;37(suppl_1):D141–5.
46. Cole JR, Chai B, Marsh TL, Farris RJ, Wang Q, Kulam SA, et al. The ribosomal database project (RDP-II): previewing a new autoaligner that allows regular updates and the new prokaryotic taxonomy. Nucleic Acids Res. 2003;31(1):442–3.

47. Pruesse E, Quast C, Knittel K, Fuchs BM, Ludwig W, Peplies J, et al. SILVA: a comprehensive online resource for quality checked and aligned ribosomal RNA sequence data compatible with ARB. Nucleic Acids Res. 2007;35(21):7188–96.
48. Quast C, Pruesse E, Yilmaz P, Gerken J, Schweer T, Yarza P, et al. The SILVA ribosomal RNA gene database project: improved data processing and web-based tools. Nucleic Acids Res. 2013;41(D1):D590–6.
49. Schloss PD, Westcott SL. Assessing and improving methods used in operational taxonomic unit-based approaches for 16S rRNA gene sequence analysis. Appl Environ Microbiol. 2011;77(10):3219–26.
50. Wang Q, Garrity GM, Tiedje JM, Cole JR. Naive Bayesian classifier for rapid assignment of rRNA sequences into the new bacterial taxonomy. Appl Environ Microbiol. 2007;73(16):5261–7.
51. Liu K-L, Porras-Alfaro A, Kuske CR, Eichorst SA, Xie G. Accurate, rapid taxonomic classification of fungal large subunit rRNA genes. Appl Environ Microbiol. 2011;78(5):1523–33.
52. Newton I, Roeselers G. The effect of training set on the classification of honey bee gut microbiota using the naive Bayesian classifier. BMC Microbiol. 2012;12(1):221.
53. Werner JJ, Koren O, Hugenholtz P, DeSantis TZ, Walters WA, Caporaso JG, et al. Impact of training sets on classification of high-throughput bacterial 16s rRNA gene surveys. ISME J. 2012;6(1):94–103.
54. Edgar R. SINTAX: a simple non-Bayesian taxonomy classifier for 16S and ITS sequences. bioRxiv. 2016.
55. Altschul SF, Gish W, Miller W, Myers EW, Lipman DJ. Basic local alignment search tool. J Mol Biol. 1990;215(3):403–10.
56. Liu Z, DeSantis TZ, Andersen GL, Knight R. Accurate taxonomy assignments from 16S rRNA sequences produced by highly parallel pyrosequencers. Nucleic Acids Res. 2008;36(18):e120.
57. Price MN, Dehal PS, Arkin AP. FastTree: computing large minimum evolution trees with profiles instead of a distance matrix. Mol Biol Evol. 2009;26(7):1641–50.
58. Price MN, Dehal PS, Arkin AP. FastTree 2 – approximately maximum-likelihood trees for large alignments. PLoS One. 2010;5(3):e9490.
59. Ludwig W, Strunk O, Westram R, Richter L, Meier H, Yadhukumar, et al. ARB: a software environment for sequence data. Nucleic Acids Res. 2004;32(4):1363–71.
60. Matsen FA, Kodner RB, Armbrust EV. pplacer: linear time maximum-likelihood and Bayesian phylogenetic placement of sequences onto a fixed reference tree. BMC Bioinformatics. 2010;11(1):538.
61. Evans J, Sheneman L, Foster J. Relaxed neighbor joining: a fast distance-based phylogenetic tree construction method. J Mol Evol. 2006;62(6):785–92.
62. Sheneman L, Evans J, Foster JA. Clearcut: a fast implementation of relaxed neighbor joining. Bioinformatics. 2006;22(22):2823–4.
63. Huson DH, Richter DC, Rausch C, Dezulian T, Franz M, Rupp R. Dendroscope: an interactive viewer for large phylogenetic trees. BMC Bioinformatics. 2007;8(1):460.
64. Whittaker RH. Evolution and measurement of species diversity. Taxon. 1972;21(2/3):213–51.
65. Whittaker RH. Vegetation of the Siskiyou mountains, Oregon and California. Ecol Monogr. 1960;30(3):279–338.
66. Shannon CE. A mathematical theory of communication. Bell Syst Tech J. 1948;27:623–56.
67. Simpson EH. Measurement of diversity. Nature. 1949;163(4148):688.
68. Jost L. Entropy and diversity. Oikos. 2006;113(2):363–75.
69. Jost L. Partitioning diversity into independent alpha and beta components. Ecology. 2007;88(10):2427–39.
70. Faith DP. Conservation evaluation and phylogenetic diversity. Biol Conserv. 1992;61(1):1–10.
71. Cavender-Bares J, Kozak KH, Fine PVA, Kembel SW. The merging of community ecology and phylogenetic biology. Ecol Lett. 2009;12:693–715.
72. Chao A. Nonparametric-estimation of the number of classes in a population. Scand J Stat. 1984;11(4):265–70.
73. Chazdon RL, Colwell RK, Denslow JS, Guariguata MR. Statistical methods for estimating species richness of woody regeneration in primary and secondary rain forests of Northeastern Costa Rica; 1998. p. 285–309.
74. Chiu C-H, Wang Y-T, Walther BA, Chao A. An improved nonparametric lower bound of species richness via a modified good–turing frequency formula. Biometrics. 2014;70(3):671–82.
75. Koleff P, Gaston KJ, Lennon JJ. Measuring beta diversity for presence–absence data. J Anim Ecol. 2003;72(3):367–82.
76. Jaccard P. Étude comparative de la distribution florale dans une portion des Alpes et des Jura. Bull Soc Vaud Sci Nat. 1901;37:547–79.
77. Bray JR, Curtis JT. An ordination of the upland forest communities of southern Wisconsin. Ecol Monogr. 1957;27(4):326–49.
78. Lozupone C, Knight R. UniFrac: a new phylogenetic method for comparing microbial communities. Appl Environ Microbiol. 2005;71(12):8228–35.
79. Lozupone CA, Hamady M, Kelley ST, Knight R. Quantitative and qualitative beta diversity measures lead to different insights into factors that structure microbial communities. Appl Environ Microbiol. 2007;73(5):1576–85.
80. Chang Q, Luan Y, Sun F. Variance adjusted weighted UniFrac: a powerful beta diversity measure for comparing communities based on phylogeny. BMC Bioinformatics. 2011;12(1):118.
81. Chen J, Bittinger K, Charlson ES, Hoffmann C, Lewis J, Wu GD, et al. Associating microbiome composition with environmental covariates using generalized UniFrac distances. Bioinformatics. 2012;28(16):2106–13.

82. Swenson NG. Phylogenetic resolution and quantifying the phylogenetic diversity and dispersion of communities. PLoS One. 2009;4(2):e4390.
83. Davies TJ, Kraft NJB, Salamin N, Wolkovich EM. Incompletely resolved phylogenetic trees inflate estimates of phylogenetic conservatism. Ecology. 2011;93(2):242–7.
84. Vellend M, Drummond EBM, Tomimatsu H. Measuring phylogenetic biodiversity. In: Magurran AE, McGill BJ, editors. Biological diversity: frontiers in measurement and assessment. Oxford: Oxford University Press; 2011. p. 193–206.
85. Kanagawa T. Bias and artifacts in multitemplate polymerase chain reactions (PCR). J Biosci Bioeng. 2003;96(4):317–23.
86. von Wintzingerode F, Göbel UB, Stackebrandt E. Determination of microbial diversity in environmental samples: pitfalls of PCR-based rRNA analysis. FEMS Microbiol Rev. 1997;21(3):213–29.
87. Weider LJ, Elser JJ, Crease TJ, Mateos M, Cotner JB, Markow TA. The functional significance of ribosomal (r)DNA variation: impacts on the evolutionary ecology of organisms. Annu Rev Ecol Evol Syst. 2005;36:219–42.
88. Kembel SW, Wu M, Eisen JA, Green JL. Incorporating 16S gene copy number information improves estimates of microbial diversity and abundance. PLoS Comput Biol. 2012;8(10):e1002743.
89. Salter SJ, Cox MJ, Turek EM, Calus ST, Cookson WO, Moffatt MF, et al. Reagent and laboratory contamination can critically impact sequence-based microbiome analyses. BMC Biol. 2014;12:12.
90. Weiss S, Amir A, Hyde ER, Metcalf JL, Song SJ, Knight R. Tracking down the sources of experimental contamination in microbiome studies. Genome Biol. 2014;15(12):564.
91. Anderson MJ. A new method for non-parametric multivariate analysis of variance. Austral Ecol. 2001;26(1):32–46.
92. Legendre P, Anderson MJ. Distance-based redundancy analysis: testing multispecies responses in multifactorial ecological experiments. Ecol Monogr. 1999;69(1):1–24.
93. ter Braak CJF. Canonical correspondence analysis: a new eigenvector technique for multivariate direct gradient analysis. Ecology. 1986;67(5):1167–79.
94. Anderson MJ. Permutation tests for univariate or multivariate analysis of variance and regression. Can J Fish Aquat Sci. 2001;58(3):626–39.
95. Clarke KR. Non-parametric multivariate analyses of changes in community structure. Aust J Ecol. 1993;18(1):117–43.
96. Carignan V, Villard M-A. Selecting indicator species to monitor ecological integrity: a review. Environ Monit Assess. 2002;78(1):45–61.
97. Dufrene M, Legendre P. Species assemblages and indicator species: the need for a flexible asymmetrical approach. Ecol Monogr. 1997;67(3):345–66.
98. De Cáceres M, Legendre P. Associations between species and groups of sites: indices and statistical inference. Ecology. 2009;90(12):3566–74.
99. De Cáceres M, Legendre P, Moretti M. Improving indicator species analysis by combining groups of sites. Oikos. 2010;119(10):1674–84.
100. Knights D, Costello EK, Knight R. Supervised classification of human microbiota. FEMS Microbiol Rev. 2011;35(2):343–59.
101. Breiman L. Random forests. Mach Learn. 2001;45(1):5–32.
102. McMurdie PJ, Holmes S. Waste not, want not: why rarefying microbiome data is inadmissible. PLoS Comput Biol. 2014;10(4):e1003531.
103. Robinson MD, McCarthy DJ, Smyth GK. edgeR: a bioconductor package for differential expression analysis of digital gene expression data. Bioinformatics. 2010;26(1):139–40.
104. Love MI, Huber W, Anders S. Moderated estimation of fold change and dispersion for RNA-seq data with DESeq2. Genome Biol. 2014;15(12):550.
105. Hardcastle TJ, Kelly KA. baySeq: empirical Bayesian methods for identifying differential expression in sequence count data. BMC Bioinformatics. 2010;11(1):422.
106. Xu L, Paterson AD, Turpin W, Xu W. Assessment and selection of competing models for zero-inflated microbiome data. PLoS One. 2015;10(7):e0129606.
107. Paulson JN, Stine OC, Bravo HC, Pop M. Differential abundance analysis for microbial marker-gene surveys. Nat Methods. 2013;10(12):1200–2.
108. Fernandes A, Reid J, Macklaim J, McMurrough T, Edgell D, Gloor G. Unifying the analysis of high-throughput sequencing datasets: characterizing RNA-seq, 16S rRNA gene sequencing and selective growth experiments by compositional data analysis. Microbiome. 2014;2(1):15.
109. Thorsen J, Brejnrod A, Mortensen M, Rasmussen MA, Stokholm J, Al-Soud WA, et al. Large-scale benchmarking reveals false discoveries and count transformation sensitivity in 16S rRNA gene amplicon data analysis methods used in microbiome studies. Microbiome. 2016;4(1):62.
110. Faust K, Sathirapongsasuti JF, Izard J, Segata N, Gevers D, Raes J, et al. Microbial co-occurrence relationships in the human microbiome. PLoS Comput Biol. 2012;8(7):e1002606.
111. Weiss S, Van Treuren W, Lozupone C, Faust K, Friedman J, Deng Y, et al. Correlation detection strategies in microbial data sets vary widely in sensitivity and precision. ISME J. 2016;10(7):1669–81.
112. Reshef DN, Reshef YA, Finucane HK, Grossman SR, McVean G, Turnbaugh PJ, et al. Detecting novel associations in large data sets. Science. 2011;334(6062):1518–24.
113. Friedman J, Alm EJ. Inferring correlation networks from genomic survey data. PLoS Comput Biol. 2012;8(9):e1002687.

114. Faust K, Raes J. CoNet app: inference of biological association networks using Cytoscape. F1000Res. 2016;5:1519.
115. Ruan Q, Dutta D, Schwalbach MS, Steele JA, Fuhrman JA, Sun F. Local similarity analysis reveals unique associations among marine bacterioplankton species and environmental factors. Bioinformatics. 2006;22(20):2532–8.
116. Berry D, Widder S. Deciphering microbial interactions and detecting keystone species with co-occurrence networks. Front Microbiol. 2014;5(219):219.
117. Butts CT. Social network analysis with sna. J Stat Softw. 2008;24(6):1–51.
118. Csardi G, Nepusz T. The igraph software package for complex network research. InterJournal Complex Syst. 2006;1695:1–9.
119. Shannon P, Markiel A, Ozier O, Baliga NS, Wang JT, Ramage D, et al. Cytoscape: a software environment for integrated models of biomolecular interaction networks. Genome Res. 2003;13(11):2498–504.
120. Freeman LC. A set of measures of centrality based on betweenness. Sociometry. 1977;40(1):35–41.
121. Freeman LC. Centrality in social networks conceptual clarification. Soc Netw. 1979;1(3):215–39.
122. Bavelas A. Communication patterns in task-oriented groups. J Acoust Soc Am. 1950;22(6):723–30.
123. Allesina S, Pascual M. Googling food webs: can an eigenvector measure Species' importance for Coextinctions? PLoS Comput Biol. 2009;5(9):e1000494.
124. Newman MEJ, Girvan M. Finding and evaluating community structure in networks. Phys Rev E Stat Nonlin Soft Matter Phys. 2004;69(2):026113.
125. Okuda S, Tsuchiya Y, Kiriyama C, Itoh M, Morisaki H. Virtual metagenome reconstruction from 16S rRNA gene sequences. Nat Commun. 2012;3:1203.
126. Langille MGI, Zaneveld J, Caporaso JG, McDonald D, Knights D, Reyes JA, et al. Predictive functional profiling of microbial communities using 16S rRNA marker gene sequences. Nat Biotechnol. 2013;31(9):814–21.
127. Aßhauer KP, Wemheuer B, Daniel R, Meinicke P. Tax4Fun: predicting functional profiles from metagenomic 16S rRNA data. Bioinformatics. 2015;31(17):2882–4.
128. Iwai S, Weinmaier T, Schmidt BL, Albertson DG, Poloso NJ, Dabbagh K, et al. Piphillin: improved prediction of metagenomic content by direct inference from human microbiomes. PLoS One. 2016;11(11):e0166104.
129. Jing G, Sun Z, Wang H, Gong Y, Huang S, Ning K, et al. Parallel-META 3: comprehensive taxonomical and functional analysis platform for efficient comparison of microbial communities. Sci Rep. 2017;7:40371.
130. McDonald D, Price MN, Goodrich J, Nawrocki EP, DeSantis TZ, Probst A, et al. An improved Greengenes taxonomy with explicit ranks for ecological and evolutionary analyses of bacteria and archaea. ISME J. 2012;6(3):610–8.
131. Abubucker S, Segata N, Goll J, Schubert AM, Izard J, Cantarel BL, et al. Metabolic reconstruction for metagenomic data and its application to the human microbiome. PLoS Comput Biol. 2012;8(6):e1002358.
132. Xu Z, Malmer D, Langille MGI, Way SF, Knight R. Which is more important for classifying microbial communities: who's there or what they can do? ISME J. 2014;8(12):2357–9.

Part II

Immunogenetics of the Host Response to Infection

Immunodeficiency and Autoimmunity

4

T. Prescott Atkinson

Abbreviations

AD	Autosomal dominant
AIRE	Autoimmune regulator
APDS	Activated PI3K-delta syndrome
APECED	Autoimmune polyendocrinopathy-candidiasis-ectodermal dysplasia
AR	Autosomal recessive
CHARGE syndrome	Coloboma, heart defects, atresia choanae (also known as choanal atresia), growth retardation, genital abnormalities, and ear abnormalities
CHD7	Chromodomain-helicase-DNA-binding protein 7
CMV	Cytomegalovirus
CTLA4	Cytotoxic T-lymphocyte-associated protein 4
DCLRE1c	DNA cross-link repair 1C (also known as Artemis)
GOF	Gain-of-function
IPEX	Immune dysregulation polyendocrinopathy enteropathy X-linked
ITCH	Itchy E3 ubiquitin protein ligase
ITP	Idiopathic thrombocytopenic purpura
JIA	Juvenile idiopathic arthritis
LIG4	DNA ligase 4
LOF	Loss-of-function
LRBA	Lipopolysaccharide (LPS)-responsive vesicle trafficking, beach- and anchor-containing
MDA	Melanoma differentiation-associated protein
NFAT	Nuclear factor of activated T cells
NHEJ1	Nonhomologous end-joining factor 1
PIDD	Primary immune deficiency disorders
PRKDC	Protein kinase, DNA-activated, catalytic polypeptide
pTreg	Peripheral regulatory T cells
RAG	Recombinase activating gene
SCID	Severe combined immunodeficiency
SEMA3E	Semaphorin 3E
STAT	Signal transducer and activator of transcription
TBX1	T-box transcription factor 1
TCR	T cell receptor
TLR	Toll-like receptor
Treg	Regulatory T cell
tTreg	Thymic-derived regulatory T cells
XLA	X-linked agammaglobulinemia

T. Prescott Atkinson
Division of Pediatric Allergy, Asthma and Immunology, University of Alabama at Birmingham, Birmingham, AL, USA
e-mail: patkinson@peds.uab.edu

G. Ragab et al. (eds.), *The Microbiome in Rheumatic Diseases and Infection*,
https://doi.org/10.1007/978-3-319-79026-8_4

Introduction

The primary immunodeficiencies are a group of genetic disorders characterized by defects in immune function and increased susceptibility to infection [1–3]. A subset of these inherited diseases also includes immune dysregulation as a part of the phenotype with resulting systemic inflammation and autoimmunity. The loss of self-tolerance may be due to abnormalities in the development of either central or peripheral tolerance and usually involves either quantitative or qualitative (functional) defects in mature T cells. The largest subset of these disorders is characterized by defects in the development of regulatory T cells (Tregs), but several other less common mechanisms have also been identified. For example, defects in B cell production and function have also been associated with autoimmunity. The genes of the early portion of the classical pathway of complement comprise a third, smaller subset. In this latter group, there is no inherent defect in Treg function; instead it is likely that a defect in the clearance of apoptotic cells and immune complexes produced by deficiencies in the early classical pathway permits the accumulation of self-antigens that overwhelm immune tolerance permitting the development of autoimmunity [4, 5]. Gene defects that selectively affect phagocyte number and function, such as ELANE (chronic or cyclic neutropenia) and CYBB (X-linked chronic granulomatous disease), do not generally lead to autoimmunity per se although associated inflammatory conditions such as the granulomatous enteritis seen in chronic granulomatous disease are well described [6].

Tregs generated in the thymus have been called tTregs (previously "natural" or nTregs) [7, 8]. They comprise 5–10% of recent thymic emigrants and express the cell markers CD4, CD25, and the transcription factor FoxP3 [9, 10]. While the process leading to their generation in the thymus is still poorly understood, it is known that they are positively selected by self-antigens expressed in the thymus under the influence of transcriptional elements such as the product of the autoimmune regulator (*AIRE*) gene and that expression of FoxP3 is essential for their differentiation and maintenance. A smaller subset of FoxP3+ Tregs, designated pTregs (formerly "induced" or iTregs), can be generated peripherally through the differentiation of CD4+ T cells under the influence of IL-2, transforming growth factor (TGF)-beta, and other factors. While tTregs primarily mediate tolerance to self-antigens, pTregs are involved in tolerance to environmental antigens such as those in food or associated with commensal organisms and are therefore primarily generated in the gut [11].

Genes that adversely affect T cell maturation in the thymus can result in a constricted T cell receptor (TCR) repertoire and may lead to decreased Tregs with resulting autoimmunity. The recombinase-activating genes RAG1 and RAG2 are among the best examples of this. On the other hand, genetic defects in genes that are associated with Treg development or T cell function may lead to aberrant cellular responses and/or defective Treg function. Forkhead box P3 (FoxP3), a transcription factor required for Treg development, is the best example of such a gene. The occurrence of autoimmune phenomena in patients with dysfunctional immune responses may be triggered by environmental stimuli as the malfunctioning adaptive immune system produces autoantibodies to cytokines during the immune response to infection [12]. Walter et al. studied a series of patients with RAG mutations (vide infra) and phenotypes with a range of severity from combined immunodeficiency with granulomas and autoimmunity to severe combined immunodeficiency and found that many patients made neutralizing antibodies against α and ω interferons and IL-12. Further, using a mouse model of leaky severe combined immunodeficiency (SCID) with hypomorphic RAG1 mutations (Rag1$^{S723C/S723C}$ (mut/mut) mice), they showed that many of the animals made antibodies to these cytokines after being repeatedly injected with agonists for Toll-like receptor (TLR)3/melanoma differentiation-associated protein (MDA)5, TLR7/8, or TLR9. Thus, exposure to microbial products in these immunocompromised animals triggers the development of autoantibodies that further impair the host immune response to infection. It is also likely that molecular mimicry by microorganisms may be more able to overcome tolerance to similar self-epitopes in patients with dysfunctional immune responses.

Though less well understood, similar quantitative and qualitative defects in B cell number and function may lead to autoimmunity. In this review, we will concentrate on those primary immunodeficiency disorders which are associated with autoimmunity primarily by quantitative or qualitative effects on T cell numbers and function. A summary of the T cell defects associated with autoimmunity is included in Table 4.1.

Table 4.1 Primary immune deficiency disorders with autoimmunity

Autoimmunity due to quantitative T cell defects
Thymic hypoplasia/aplasia
DiGeorge syndrome
Chromosome 22q11.2 deletion syndrome, CHD7 haploinsufficiency, TBX1 deficiency
FOXN1 deficiency
Omenn's syndrome
Near complete LOF mutations in RAG1, RAG2, Artemis (DCLRE1C), IL7RA, RMRP, ADA, DNA ligase IV (LIG4), IL2RG, AK2, or associated with "atypical" DiGeorge syndrome (near complete thymic aplasia)
Immunodeficiency due to hypomorphic mutations (RAG1, RAG2, others)
Autoimmunity due to defective development of central tolerance/thymic education
AIRE deficiency (APECED/APS1)
Autoimmunity due to primary defects in Treg differentiation
FoxP3 deficiency
CD25 deficiency
STAT5B deficiency
ITCH deficiency
Haploinsufficiency of immunoregulatory genes
CTLA-4
NFAT-5
Gain-of-function defects
STAT1 GOF
STAT3 GOF
APDS/mutations in PIK3CD
Other combined immune deficiencies with autoimmunity
LRBA deficiency (CTLA4 expression defect)
IL-10 signaling defects (IL10, IL10RA, IL10RB deficiency)
TCR Signaling defects
LCK deficiency
TRAC (TCRα) deficiency
CD3G deficiency
ORAI-I deficiency
STIM-1 deficiency
Tripeptidyl-peptidase II deficiency
SPENCD/mutations in ACP5
KMT2D, KDM6A deficiency (Kabuki syndrome)
WAS deficiency (Wiskott-Aldrich syndrome)/ Wiskott-Aldrich-like disorder (WIPF1 deficiency)

Autoimmunity due to Quantitative T Cell Defects

DiGeorge syndrome, conotruncal congenital heart malformation with parathyroid and thymic hypoplasia/aplasia due to defective organogenesis during fetal development, leads to variably low thymic T cell production that may range from near normal to extremely decreased, resulting in virtual absence of T cells or severe oligoclonality (Omenn's syndrome) [13]. Mature T cells exiting the thymus do not have an intrinsic functional defect, and the majority of these patients do not suffer from unusual, frequent, or severe infections despite their reduced T cell numbers. DiGeorge patients comprise the largest subset of patients detected in newborn screening for SCID, although the majority of DiGeorge patients have high enough T cell production to pass the screen [14].

The most common cause is 22q11.2 deletion syndrome, which has an estimated incidence of 1:1000 live births [15]. However, monogenic causes are known, including T-box transcription factor 1 (TBX1) (which resides within the chromosome 22q11.2 region), FOXN1, or two genes which in the haploinsufficient state lead to a severe congenital malformation syndrome called CHARGE syndrome (coloboma, heart defects, atresia choanae (also known as choanal atresia), growth retardation, genital abnormalities, and ear abnormalities): CHD7 (chromodomain-helicase-DNA-binding protein 7) and SEMA3E (semaphorin 3E) [15–17]. In a retrospective study of 130 patients with 22q11.2 deletion syndrome without severe immunodeficiency, Tison et al. found an overall prevalence of autoimmunity of 8.5% (primarily cytopenias, hypothyroidism, and juvenile arthritis) [18]. All of the patients who developed autoimmunity were from that fraction with lower numbers of naive T cells. In another study by Jawad et al., a similar rate was found; 20 patients out of 195 (10.5%) (excluding two with ataxia of unknown etiology) with chromosome 22q11.2 deletion syndrome had autoimmunity of some type (principally idiopathic thrombocytopenic purpura (ITP) and juvenile idiopathic arthritis (JIA)) [19]. It is likely that the increased rate of autoimmunity seen in those DiGeorge patients with lower naive T cell numbers is due at least in part to decreased numbers of Tregs, although defective selection in the thymus may also play a role [20].

A second category of primary immune deficiency disorders (PIDD) with decreased T cell production includes those disorders that are due to defects in the initiation and repair of double-stranded DNA breaks that impair TCR rearrangement in precursor T cells within the thymus and B cell receptor (BCR) rearrangement in B cell precursors in the bone marrow [21]. These genes include the recombinase genes RAG1 and RAG2, DCLRE1C (DNA cross-link repair 1C, also known as Artemis), LIG4 (ligase 4), PRKDC (protein kinase, DNA-activated, catalytic polypeptide), and NHEJ1 (nonhomologous end-joining factor 1, also known as Cernunnos). When completely deficient in humans, each of these genes produces SCID, but heterozygous defects that include hypomorphic mutations may permit a leaky phenotype [22–24]. In the best documented examples, which are due to RAG1/RAG2 mutations, increased susceptibility to infection is accompanied by autoimmunity [24–26]. The most common autoimmune manifestations have included alopecia, vitiligo, granulomas, myasthenia gravis, vasculitis, and psoriasis. Granulomatous inflammatory processes have been described that can mimic the granulomatous vasculitides [27, 28]. Analysis of the T and B cell populations in such patients reveals decreased proportions of naive cells and skewed receptor repertoires. As with the patients with DiGeorge syndrome who have more severely decreased T cell numbers, the tendency toward autoimmunity is likely due in part to the decreased thymic output and decreased Treg numbers and diversity, but the mechanisms leading to loss of tolerance are more complex. Specifically, there is also dysregulation in the B cell compartment in these patients which compounds the problem. Another mechanism includes a defect in thymic education from defective thymic architecture and expression of AIRE, the genetic deficiency of which will be discussed next [28–30].

Deficiency in Development of Central Tolerance due to Defects in Thymic Education

Genetic deficiency of AIRE has become the prototypical disorder marking defective thymic education as a cause of a failure in central tolerance [31]. First identified as the cause of autoimmune polyendocrinopathy, candidiasis, and ectodermal dysplasia (APECED) (also called autoimmune polyendocrinopathy syndrome type 1, APS-1), AIRE has been shown to form part of a transcription factor complex that is required for the expression of ectopic proteins within the thymus forming an essential component of the negative thymic selection process for nascent T cells [32, 33]. Deficient individuals developed a characteristic pattern of autoimmunity targeting endocrine glands, typically parathyroid and adrenals, as well as autoantibodies against Th17 cytokines.

The latter turns out to explain their marked propensity for chronic mucocutaneous candidiasis, Th17 immunity being particularly important in the defense against superficial cutaneous and mucous membrane fungal infections [34].

Autoimmunity due to Defects in Treg Development

Defects in the expression of FoxP3, the transcription factor essential for the development of Tregs, or in the expression of CD25, the receptor for IL-2, produce defects in Treg number or function and an increase in autoimmune phenomena. IPEX syndrome (immune dysregulation, polyendocrinopathy, enteropathy, X-linked), first described in 2001, is due to loss-of-function (LOF) mutations in the X-linked FoxP3 gene [35]. Affected patients may develop symptoms of autoimmunity antenatally with severe enteropathy, inflammatory autoimmune skin disease, and other autoimmune disorders, particularly diabetes mellitus, and may be stillborn or become critically ill soon after delivery [36–39]. Although IPEX is not a primary immune deficiency (affected patients' T cells are fully functional though dysregulated), without treatment most patients die from infection related to their inflammatory skin and gastrointestinal tract disease before the age of 2 years. A second disorder has been described with defective FoxP3 expression due to autosomal recessive (AR) loss-of-function (LOF) mutations in the ubiquitin E3 ligase ITCH [40]. ITCH deficiency in a rodent model severely decreased TGF-β-induced FoxP3 expression in developing pTregs and compromised TGF-β -mediated inhibition of T cell proliferation [41, 42]. Affected human patients in the original description, who were homozygous for a truncating mutation in the gene, were members of a large Amish kindred and exhibited a variable combination of clinical features including dysmorphic facies, short stature, relative macrocephaly, chronic lung disease, hepatosplenomegaly, hypotonia, chronic diarrhea, and failure to thrive. Autoimmune features found among affected patients included hypothyroidism, autoimmune hepatitis, diabetes mellitus, and autoimmune enteropathy.

Two PIDD that are characterized by recurrent infections due to defective adaptive immunity as well as deficient Treg development are discussed here. Autosomal recessive deficiency of CD25 (the high affinity IL-2 receptor alpha subunit, CD25RA) is associated with both autoimmunity and immunodeficiency. Sharfe et al. described a 3-year-old boy with a history of consanguinity who suffered from recurrent respiratory infections, including cytomegalovirus (CMV) pneumonitis and candida stomatitis/esophagitis [43]. His lymphocyte mitogen panels demonstrated moderately deficient responses, and he failed to reject a skin graft. There were dense lymphocytic infiltrates in the lungs, liver, and gut. A homozygous four base pair insertion was found in the CD25RA gene that disrupted protein transcription. He was successfully treated with a bone marrow transplant. Caudy et al. described a patient with similar features to IPEX patients with endocrinopathies, eczema, hemolytic anemia, lymphadenopathy, hepatosplenomegaly, and enteropathy who was also confirmed to have CD25 deficiency [44]. They found that while CD4+ FoxP3+ T cell numbers were similar to control subjects, the production of IL-10 from stimulated CD4+ T cells was severely decreased suggesting that CD25 deficiency, in addition to causing a significant combined immunodeficiency, creates an IPEX-like phenotype by suppressing Treg function.

Patients with homozygous or compound heterozygous mutations in STAT5b (signal transduction and activator of transcription 5b) also present with an IPEX-like phenotype and immune deficiency as well as growth hormone-resistant short stature [45, 46]. They exhibit moderate lymphopenia and suffer from severe infections and display features of autoimmunity, including juvenile idiopathic arthritis, autoimmune thyroiditis, and ITP. Because the IL-2 receptor is partly dependent on STAT5b for signaling and IL-2 signaling is important for FoxP3 upregulation, CD4+ CD25+ FoxP3+ Tregs are significantly decreased. Most patients have eczematous skin disease and have developed chronic pulmonary inflammation with lymphoid interstitial pneumonitis and worsening pulmonary fibrosis, which can be fatal.

Autoimmunity by Haploinsufficiency of Immunoregulatory Genes

Haploinsufficiency in a number of different genes has been shown to cause a diverse array of phenotypes with immune dysregulation [47]. Of these, heterozygous LOF alleles in cytotoxic T lymphocyte-associated 4 (CTLA4) have been best described as causing autoimmunity [48, 49]. CTLA4 expressed by Tregs acts as a high-affinity competitor for CD28 in the activation of effector T cells by depleting its ligands CD80 and CD86 from antigen-presenting cells and thus resulting in downregulation of effector T cell activation. Haploinsufficiency of CTLA4 results in immunodeficiency (decreased B cells and hypogammaglobulinemia) and autoimmunity, including autoimmune cytopenias, autoimmune enteropathy, and granulomatous infiltrative lung disease [47–50]. LRBA (Lipopolysaccharide (LPS)-responsive vesicle trafficking, beach- and anchor-containing), expression of which is induced by bacterial lipopolysaccharide in B cells and macrophages, upregulates Treg CTLA4 expression. Homozygous or compound heterozygous deficiency of LRBA includes autoimmunity as part of the phenotype primarily because of impaired Treg CTLA4 expression [51]. As genomic data on patients with undefined immune deficiencies with autoimmunity continue to accumulate, it is likely that other genes will be discovered for which haploinsufficiency is the cause. For example, it has been reported that a heterozygous deletion on chromosome 16 that included the transcription factor nuclear factor of activated T cells 5 (NFAT5) was responsible for such a phenotype in a 19-year-old man [52].

Autoimmunity from Dominant Gain-of-Function (GOF) Mutations

Mutations that produce constitutive activation of immunologic signaling pathways can result in autoimmunity. Some of the best examples include the syndromes created by gain of function (GOF) mutations in STAT proteins, STAT1 and STAT3, and activating mutations in the enzyme phosphatidylinositol-3-kinase delta (PI3 Kinase δ), which produces the activated phosphatidylinositol-3-kinase (PI3K) delta syndrome, (APDS). Because they are key signaling intermediates in cytokine receptor signaling, abnormalities in function in the various STAT family proteins can exert profound effects on immune function [45]. STAT1 among all the known family members exhibits the broadest heterogeneity in phenotypes [45, 53]. Three different functional effects of STAT1 mutations are known—AR homozygous or compound heterozygous LOF mutations, autosomal dominant (AD) LOF mutations, and AD GOF mutations. The LOF mutations cause primary immunodeficiency with particular susceptibility to intracellular pathogens such as mycobacteria and herpesviruses while the GOF mutations add autoimmunity to the immunodeficiency [54–57]. The GOF mutations were first described as the cause of AD chronic mucocutaneous candidiasis that is often associated with hypothyroidism but also occasionally with type I diabetes, cytopenias, vitiligo, and systemic lupus erythematosus [45, 58–60]. Therapy of such patients with the Janus kinase (JAK) inhibitor ruxolitinib has been reported to provide significant immunologic improvement and offers hope for eventual effective avenues of specific therapy for these patients [61]. STAT3 dominant negative and dominant activating mutations present a similar spectrum of phenotypes with the dominant negative mutations responsible for AD Hyper-IgE (Job's) syndrome and AD GOF mutations producing immunodeficiency, short stature, eczema, and autoimmunity [62–64]. Autoimmune features have been reported to include hypothyroidism and type I diabetes, cytopenias, arthritis, and serum autoantibodies.

Phosphatidylinositol-3-kinases are a family of enzymes that are activated following receptor-ligand binding and phosphorylate a membrane phospholipid, phosphatidylinositol-4,5-bisphosphate (PIP_2), to form phosphatidylinositol-3,4,5-trisphosphate (PIP_3), which creates a binding site on the inner leaflet of the plasma membrane for the PH domain on cytoplasmic signaling molecules including the Akt kinase (protein kinase B). Akt is a key activating serine kinase in multiple cellular processes including cell division mediated through the mTOR (mammalian target of rapamycin) pathway [65, 66]. Activating mutations in the catalytic domain of the isoform predominantly found in leukocytes, p110δ, were found to produce a dominant immunodeficiency with features of autoimmunity and a predisposition for persistent Epstein-Barr virus (EBV) viremia and lymphoid malignancies [67, 68]. Affected patients tend to exhibit decreased IgG and increased IgM levels, poor antibody responses, and lymphopenia that worsens with age associated with increased activation-induced lymphocyte apoptosis. Autoimmune features are frequent in APDS patients and have included cytopenias, seronegative arthritis, thyroid disease, pericarditis, sclerosing cholangitis, and glomerulonephritis [69]. Importantly, therapy of APDS patients with mTOR inhibitors such as sirolimus results in improved lymphocyte counts, increased immune function, and decreased peripheral lymphadenopathy and splenomegaly [69].

Autoimmunity with Selective B Cell Deficiencies

Autoimmunity can also be seen in B cell deficiencies, and perhaps the best data supporting this association comes from patients with Bruton's tyrosine kinase (BTK) deficiency (XLA, X-linked agammaglobulinemia) [70, 71]. These patients have a severe but leaky deficiency of B cells in which there is a block in the development of B cells at the pre-B cell stage. However, typically a very small percentage of B cells manage to pass this developmental choke point and develop into mature, functional B cells with an overall highly constricted repertoire exhibiting abnormal V_H and V_L gene utilization and deficient regulation with a high percentage of polyreactive autoantibodies as determined by single cell analysis [72]. Although T cells are thought to be functioning normally in XLA patients, their myeloid cells, which also express BTK protein, have deficient signaling through Toll-like receptors [71]. A recent review of patients in the US Immunodeficiency Network (USIDnet) registry of 179 patients revealed that 5% of patients had hypothyroidism, 3.4% had Crohn's disease/enteritis (considerably higher than the reported incidence of 0.4%), 16% had arthritis (excluding septic arthritis), 4% had anemia, and 2% had ITP/thrombocytopenia [71]. Thus, although it is unclear whether some of these autoimmune features are due to the defect in B cell maturation, the occurrence of relatively high proportions of autoimmune diseases in XLA patients suggests that defects in B cell differentiation and function can contribute to the autoimmunity seen in some types of combined immune deficiency.

Summary

Primary immune deficiencies are increasingly being recognized as underlying disorders in patients presenting with autoimmunity. Almost all of the known examples have been uncovered over the past two decades. A variety of mechanisms have been established, and there is little doubt that more genes and more mechanisms remain to be discovered. The role of microorganisms, both pathogens and elements of the normal microbiome in the various anatomic sites in the human host, is just beginning to be elucidated, but it is likely that microbial triggers play an important part in the development of autoimmunity in many of these disorders of immune function.

References

1. Raje N, Dinakar C. Overview of immunodeficiency disorders. Immunol Allergy Clin North Am. 2015;35(4):599–623. https://doi.org/10.1016/j.iac.2015.07.001.
2. Picard C, et al. Primary immunodeficiency diseases: an update on the classification from the International Union of Immunological Societies Expert Committee for primary immunodeficiency 2015. J Clin Immunol. 2015;19:19.
3. Bousfiha A, et al. The 2015 IUIS phenotypic classification for primary immunodeficiencies. J Clin Immunol. 2015;7:7.
4. Martin M, Blom AM. Complement in removal of the dead – balancing inflammation. Immunol

Rev. 2016;274(1):218–32. https://doi.org/10.1111/imr.12462.
5. Son M, Diamond B, Santiago-Schwarz F. Fundamental role of C1q in autoimmunity and inflammation. Immunol Res. 2015;63(1–3):101–6. https://doi.org/10.1007/s12026-015-8705-6.
6. Uzzan M, et al. Gastrointestinal disorders associated with common variable immune deficiency (CVID) and chronic granulomatous disease (CGD). Curr Gastroenterol Rep. 2016;18(4):17. https://doi.org/10.1007/s11894-016-0491-3.
7. Lu L, Barbi J, Pan F. The regulation of immune tolerance by FOXP3. Nat Rev Immunol. 2017;31(10):75.
8. Palomares O, et al. Mechanisms of immune regulation in allergic diseases: the role of regulatory T and B cells. Immunol Rev. 2017;278(1):219–36. https://doi.org/10.1111/imr.12555.
9. Wang YM, et al. Development and function of Foxp3(+) regulatory T cells. Nephrology (Carlton). 2016;21(2):81–5. https://doi.org/10.1111/nep.12652.
10. Caramalho I, et al. Regulatory T-cell development in the human thymus. Front Immunol. 2015;6:395. https://doi.org/10.3389/fimmu.2015.00395. eCollection 2015.
11. Josefowicz SZ, Lu LF, Rudensky AY. Regulatory T cells: mechanisms of differentiation and function. Annu Rev Immunol. 2012;30:531–64. https://doi.org/10.1146/annurev.immunol.25.022106.141623.
12. Walter JE, et al. Broad-spectrum antibodies against self-antigens and cytokines in RAG deficiency. J Clin Invest. 2015;125(11):4135–48. https://doi.org/10.1172/JCI80477.
13. Davies EG. Immunodeficiency in DiGeorge syndrome and options for treating cases with complete athymia. Front Immunol. 2013;4:322. https://doi.org/10.3389/fimmu.2013.00322.
14. Kwan A, Puck JM. History and current status of newborn screening for severe combined immunodeficiency. Semin Perinatol. 2015;39(3):194–205. https://doi.org/10.1053/j.semperi.2015.03.004.
15. McDonald-McGinn DM, et al. 22q11.2 deletion syndrome. Nat Rev Dis Primers. 2015;1:15071. https://doi.org/10.1038/nrdp.2015.71.
16. Wong MT, et al. CHARGE syndrome: a review of the immunological aspects. Eur J Hum Genet. 2015;23(11):1451–9. https://doi.org/10.1038/ejhg.2015.7.
17. Rota IA, Dhalla F. FOXN1 deficient nude severe combined immunodeficiency. Orphanet J Rare Dis. 2017;12(1):6. https://doi.org/10.1186/s13023-016-0557-1.
18. Tison BE, et al. Autoimmunity in a cohort of 130 pediatric patients with partial DiGeorge syndrome. J Allergy Clin Immunol. 2011;128(5):1115–7e1-3.
19. Jawad AF, et al. Immunologic features of chromosome 22q11.2 deletion syndrome (DiGeorge syndrome/velocardiofacial syndrome). J Pediatr. 2001;139(5):715–23.
20. Ferrando-Martinez S, et al. Low thymic output, peripheral homeostasis deregulation, and hastened regulatory T cells differentiation in children with 22q11.2 deletion syndrome. J Pediatr. 2014;164(4):882–9. https://doi.org/10.1016/j.jpeds.2013.12.013.
21. de Villartay JP. Congenital defects in V(D)J recombination. Br Med Bull. 2015;114(1):157–67. https://doi.org/10.1093/bmb/ldv020.
22. Lee PP, et al. The many faces of Artemis-deficient combined immunodeficiency – two patients with DCLRE1C mutations and a systematic literature review of genotype-phenotype correlation. Clin Immunol. 2013;149(3):464–74. https://doi.org/10.1016/j.clim.2013.08.006.
23. Buck D, et al. Cernunnos, a novel nonhomologous end-joining factor, is mutated in human immunodeficiency with microcephaly. Cell. 2006;124(2):287–99.
24. Chen K, et al. Autoimmunity due to RAG deficiency and estimated disease incidence in RAG1/2 mutations. J Allergy Clin Immunol. 2014;133(3):880–2e10.
25. Notarangelo LD, et al. Human RAG mutations: biochemistry and clinical implications. Nat Rev Immunol. 2016;16(4):234–46. https://doi.org/10.1038/nri.2016.28.
26. Lee YN, et al. Characterization of T and B cell repertoire diversity in patients with RAG deficiency. Sci Immunol. 2016;1(6):eaah6109. https://doi.org/10.1126/sciimmunol.aah6109.
27. De Ravin SS, et al. Hypomorphic rag mutations can cause destructive midline granulomatous disease. Blood. 2010;116(8):1263–71.
28. Mathieu AL, et al. PRKDC mutations associated with immunodeficiency, granuloma, and autoimmune regulator-dependent autoimmunity. J Allergy Clin Immunol. 2015;135(6):1578–88.e5. https://doi.org/10.1016/j.jaci.2015.01.040.
29. Cavadini P, et al. AIRE deficiency in thymus of 2 patients with Omenn syndrome. J Clin Invest. 2005;115(3):728–32.
30. Poliani PL, et al. Early defects in human T-cell development severely affect distribution and maturation of thymic stromal cells: possible implications for the pathophysiology of Omenn syndrome. Blood. 2009;114(1):105–8.
31. Anderson MS, et al. Projection of an immunological self shadow within the thymus by the aire protein. Science. 2002;298(5597):1395–401.
32. Bansal K, et al. The transcriptional regulator aire binds to and activates super-enhancers. Nat Immunol. 2017;18(3):263–73. https://doi.org/10.1038/ni.3675.
33. Villasenor J, Benoist C, Mathis D. AIRE and APECED: molecular insights into an autoimmune disease. Immunol Rev. 2005;204:156–64.
34. Nagamine K, et al. Positional cloning of the APECED gene. Nat Genet. 1997;17(4):393–8.
35. Bennett CL, et al. The immune dysregulation, polyendocrinopathy, enteropathy, X-linked syndrome (IPEX) is caused by mutations of FOXP3. Nat Genet. 2001;27(1):20–1.
36. Reichert SL, McKay EM, Moldenhauer JS. Identification of a novel nonsense mutation in the FOXP3 gene in a fetus with hydrops – expanding

the phenotype of IPEX syndrome. Am J Med Genet A. 2016;170A(1):226–32. https://doi.org/10.1002/ajmg.a.37401.
37. Xavier-da-Silva MM, et al. Fetal-onset IPEX: report of two families and review of literature. Clin Immunol. 2014;156(2):131–40.
38. Hannibal MC, Torgerson T. IPEX syndrome. In: GeneReviews – NCBI bookshelf. Seattle: University of Washington; 2011.
39. van der Vliet HJ, Nieuwenhuis EE. IPEX as a result of mutations in FOXP3. Clin Dev Immunol. 2007;2007:89017.
40. Lohr NJ, et al. Human ITCH E3 ubiquitin ligase deficiency causes syndromic multisystem autoimmune disease. Am J Hum Genet. 2010;86(3):447–53. https://doi.org/10.1016/j.ajhg.2010.01.028.
41. Venuprasad K. Cbl-b and itch: key regulators of peripheral T-cell tolerance. Cancer Res. 2010;70(8):3009–12. https://doi.org/10.1158/0008-5472.CAN-09-4076.
42. Venuprasad K, et al. The E3 ubiquitin ligase itch regulates expression of transcription factor Foxp3 and airway inflammation by enhancing the function of transcription factor TIEG1. Nat Immunol. 2008;9(3):245–53. https://doi.org/10.1038/ni1564.
43. Sharfe N, et al. Human immune disorder arising from mutation of the alpha chain of the interleukin-2 receptor. Proc Natl Acad Sci U S A. 1997;94(7):3168–71.
44. Caudy AA, et al. CD25 deficiency causes an immune dysregulation, polyendocrinopathy, enteropathy, X-linked-like syndrome, and defective IL-10 expression from CD4 lymphocytes. J Allergy Clin Immunol. 2007;119(2):482–7.
45. Lorenzini T, et al. STAT mutations as program switchers: turning primary immunodeficiencies into autoimmune diseases. J Leukoc Biol. 2017;101(1):29–38. https://doi.org/10.1189/jlb.5RI0516-237RR.
46. Casanova JL, Holland SM, Notarangelo LD. Inborn errors of human JAKs and STATs. Immunity. 2012;36(4):515–28.
47. Rieux-Laucat F, Casanova JL. Immunology. Autoimmunity by haploinsufficiency. Science. 2014;345(6204):1560–1. https://doi.org/10.1126/science.1260791.
48. Schubert D, et al. Autosomal dominant immune dysregulation syndrome in humans with CTLA4 mutations. Nat Med. 2014;20(12):1410–6. https://doi.org/10.1038/nm.3746.
49. Kuehn HS, et al. Immune dysregulation in human subjects with heterozygous germline mutations in CTLA4. Science. 2014;345(6204):1623–7. https://doi.org/10.1126/science.1255904.
50. Jouhadi Z, et al. Autosomal dominant immune dysregulation syndrome in humans with CTLA4 mutations. Pediatrics. 2014;134(5):e1458–63. https://doi.org/10.1542/peds.2013-1383.
51. Lo B, et al. Autoimmune disease. Patients with LRBA deficiency show CTLA4 loss and immune dysregulation responsive to abatacept therapy. Science. 2015;349(6246):436–40. https://doi.org/10.1126/science.aaa1663.
52. Boland BS, et al. Immunodeficiency and autoimmune enterocolopathy linked to NFAT5 haploinsufficiency. J Immunol. 2015;194(6):2551–60. https://doi.org/10.4049/jimmunol.1401463.
53. Toubiana J, et al. Heterozygous STAT1 gain-of-function mutations underlie an unexpectedly broad clinical phenotype. Blood. 2016;127(25):3154–64. https://doi.org/10.1182/blood-2015-11-679902.
54. Depner M, et al. The extended clinical phenotype of 26 patients with chronic mucocutaneous candidiasis due to gain-of-function mutations in STAT1. J Clin Immunol. 2015;25:25.
55. Uzel G, et al. Dominant gain-of-function STAT1 mutations in FOXP3 wild-type immune dysregulation-polyendocrinopathy-enteropathy-X-linked-like syndrome. J Allergy Clin Immunol. 2013;131(6):1611–23.
56. Tsumura M, et al. Dominant-negative STAT1 SH2 domain mutations in unrelated patients with Mendelian susceptibility to mycobacterial disease. Hum Mutat. 2012;33(9):1377–87.
57. Boisson-Dupuis S, et al. Inborn errors of human STAT1: allelic heterogeneity governs the diversity of immunological and infectious phenotypes. Curr Opin Immunol. 2012;24(4):364–78.
58. Smeekens SP, et al. STAT1 hyperphosphorylation and defective IL12R/IL23R signaling underlie defective immunity in autosomal dominant chronic mucocutaneous candidiasis. PLoS One. 2011;6(12):e29248.
59. van de Veerdonk FL, et al. STAT1 mutations in autosomal dominant chronic mucocutaneous candidiasis. N Engl J Med. 2011;365(1):54–61.
60. Liu L, et al. Gain-of-function human STAT1 mutations impair IL-17 immunity and underlie chronic mucocutaneous candidiasis. J Exp Med. 2011;208(8):1635–48.
61. Mossner R, et al. Ruxolitinib induces interleukin 17 and ameliorates chronic mucocutaneous candidiasis caused by STAT1 gain-of-function mutation. Clin Infect Dis. 2016;62(7):951–3. https://doi.org/10.1093/cid/ciw020.
62. Vogel TP, Milner JD, Cooper MA. The Ying and Yang of STAT3 in human disease. J Clin Immunol. 2015;35(7):615–23. https://doi.org/10.1007/s10875-015-0187-8.
63. Milner JD, et al. Early-onset lymphoproliferation and autoimmunity caused by germline STAT3 gain-of-function mutations. Blood. 2015;125(4):591–9. https://doi.org/10.1182/blood-2014-09-602763.
64. Milner JD, et al. Autoimmunity, hypogammaglobulinemia, lymphoproliferation, and mycobacterial disease in patients with activating mutations in STAT3. Blood. 2015;125(4):591–9. https://doi.org/10.1182/blood-2014-09-602763.
65. Lucas CL, et al. PI3Kdelta and primary immunodeficiencies. Nat Rev Immunol. 2016;16(11):702–14. https://doi.org/10.1038/nri.2016.93.

66. Heurtier L, Deau MC, Kracker S. Hyper-activated PI3K-delta in immunodeficiency. Oncotarget. 2015;6(21):18242–3.
67. Angulo I, et al. Phosphoinositide 3-kinase delta gene mutation predisposes to respiratory infection and airway damage. Science. 2013;342(6160):866–71. https://doi.org/10.1126/science.1243292.
68. Lucas CL, et al. Dominant-activating germline mutations in the gene encoding the PI(3)K catalytic subunit p110delta result in T cell senescence and human immunodeficiency. Nat Immunol. 2014;15(1):88–97. https://doi.org/10.1038/ni.2771.
69. Coulter TI, et al. Clinical spectrum and features of activated phosphoinositide 3-kinase delta syndrome: a large patient cohort study. J Allergy Clin Immunol. 2017;139(2):597–606.e4. https://doi.org/10.1016/j.jaci.2016.06.021.
70. Corneth OB, Klein Wolterink RG, Hendriks RW. BTK signaling in B cell differentiation and autoimmunity. Curr Top Microbiol Immunol. 2016;393:67–105. https://doi.org/10.1007/82_2015_478.
71. Hernandez-Trujillo VP, et al. Autoimmunity and inflammation in X-linked agammaglobulinemia. J Clin Immunol. 2014;34(6):627–32. https://doi.org/10.1007/s10875-014-0056-x.
72. Ng YS, et al. Bruton's tyrosine kinase is essential for human B cell tolerance. J Exp Med. 2004;200(7):927–34.

5 Immunology of the Microbiome: Implications for Rheumatoid Arthritis and Other Autoimmune Diseases

Daniel M. Altmann, Catherine J. Reynolds, and Rosemary J. Boyton

Abbreviations

GF	Germ-free
IBD	Inflammatory bowel disease
MAMP	Microbe-associated molecular pattern
NOD	Nonobese diabetic
PAMP	Pathogen-associated molecular pattern
PRR	Pattern recognition receptors
RA	Rheumatoid arthritis
SCFA	Short-chain fatty acids
SFB	Segmented filamentous bacteria
TCR	T cell receptor

Background

In rheumatoid arthritis (RA) as in several other inflammatory/immune conditions, there is ongoing interest in the notion that pathogenesis may encompass consequences of microbiota dysbiosis [1–5]. Evidence for this view in RA, discussed in more detail below and in Chap. 15, encompasses strands such as the successful utilization of antimicrobial therapeutics, the impact of microbial environmental differences in rodent models, and the evidence of microbial community differences in periodontal disease and gut microbiota correlating with disease. However, whether microbiota differences are cause or effect of the disease process remains unclear. Nevertheless, such studies, as well as those correlating microbiota phyla, species, or pathways with immune subset differentiation and phenotype, underpin a view that a more thorough grasp of these interactions would facilitate new avenues for therapeutic intervention as well as supplying new biomarkers for disease progression and prognosis.

The search for microbiota species correlating with susceptibility to RA or to other autoimmune or inflammatory conditions rests primarily on the notion, drawn from studies in mice, that specific bacterial species are not only recognized by receptors of the innate and adaptive immune response but can play specific roles in driving the development of polarized immune effector subsets [6]. Keynote examples, as discussed below, were demonstrations of the requirement in the gut microbiota of segmented filamentous bacteria (SFB) for the development of Th17 cells, and of specific clostridial species, especially from phylogenetic cluster IV and XIV, for the development of Tregs [7].

The concept of an equilibrium between the microbial species of the indigenous microbiota and the health status of the host goes back to Metchnikoff, while Lederberg is often credited with initiating the modern concept of microbiome

D. M. Altmann (✉) · C. J. Reynolds · R. J. Boyton
Department of Medicine, Hammersmith Hospital, Imperial College London, London, UK
e-mail: d.altmann@ic.ac.uk

G. Ragab et al. (eds.), *The Microbiome in Rheumatic Diseases and Infection*,
https://doi.org/10.1007/978-3-319-79026-8_5

research—"we should think of each host and its parasites as a superorganism with the respective genomes yoked..." [8].

The ever-increasing granularity that has been attained in characterization of the microbiota—not just bacterial but also viral and fungal—has offered many tantalizing disease correlates, offering hints of causality and prospects for therapeutics. More laborious and challenging has been the process of drafting the new biology of the specific ligand-receptor interactions that might operate at the interface of host and microbiota, determining healthy or pathologic outcomes.

Old-school immunology teaches that this is a body system evolved to differentiate between self and nonself, or, at least, between contexts, such as danger and non-danger. Within this frame of reference, understanding interaction of the immune system with the commensals we carry would appear trivial: we may be colonized by 10^{13}–10^{14} bacteria, but our immune system can ignore them, either because of physical barriers at the mucosa and/or because the immune system has developed with them in place and learnt to ignore them in some form of tolerance or ignorance. However, this viewpoint has become increasingly untenable over several years, as it became clearer that changes to the microbiota could shift susceptibility to inflammatory, autoimmune, and infectious diseases, that these were microbial proteomes just as capable of recognition by receptors of the innate and adaptive immune response as any pathogen, and that these recognition events could result in considerable modulation of immune subset development. This has posed conceptual challenges to aspects of the pre-existing models: the gateway for host defense to signal the presence of a microbial pathogen that must be cleared from the body by triggering an inflammatory response is recognition of microbial products via pattern recognition receptors (PRR). How then could this same machinery be used in the very different context of needing to maintain a homeostatic, mutualistic relationship with microbes that should not trigger an inflammatory response for clearance? The emerging answer is that far from the interaction between microbiota ligands and PRR being some form of dampened version of pathogen recognition, this form of bidirectional host-microbe cross talk may be a key evolutionary function of pattern recognition [9, 10].

Innate Recognition of the Microbiota

How then does one resolve the apparent paradox that we carry a large biomass of pathogen-associated molecular patterns (PAMPs)—expressing symbiotic microbial species, and yet inflammation is rarely triggered by such interactions and no sterilizing immune clearance activated? It is this conundrum that led some in the field to rename PAMPs more correctly microbe-associated molecular patterns (MAMPs) [10]. It is now appreciated that signaling to innate receptors by the microbiota is essential for avoidance of dysbiosis and disease.

One solution was identified several years ago in the zebra fish [11]. It was found that recognition of microbiota-derived LPS by the TLR4/MyD88 complex triggers an intestinal alkaline phosphatase that detoxifies the LPS and attenuates inflammation. In the absence of this pathway, an excessive, inflammatory neutrophil response is triggered.

In mouse studies, much evidence has come from analysis of PRR knockout strains. For example, Nod2 knockout mice show a number of downstream consequences of dysregulated interaction with the microbiota, including changes in microbial composition and impaired ability to clear *Helicobacter hepaticus* [12]. Of studies conducted in TLR knockout strains, loss of TLR5 sensing of bacterial flagellin appears particularly decisive in determination of microbiota homeostasis [13]. Investigation of the gut microbiota and its innate recognition in the type I diabetes of nonobese diabetic (NOD) mice has been particularly interesting. Myd88 −/− NOD mice show distal gut microbiota changes, with a lower *Firmicutes/Bacteroidetes* ratio compared to Myd88 +/+ NOD mice. The Myd88 −/− NOD mice do not develop disease when in specific pathogen-free conditions; however, when housed at germ-free (GF) status, Myd88 −/− NOD mice develop severe disease [14]. This was among the earliest studies that served not only to link causally the environment to microbiota composition and disease but also demonstrated the importance of recognition of the microbiota microbial community by innate immune receptors. Conditional deletion of MyD88 only in Tregs causes a loss in intestinal Tregs, expansion of Th17 cells, and dysbiosis with an expansion of SFB [15].

The Nod-like receptor family (NLR) contributing to inflammasome formation is also implicated: loss of NLRP6, for example, leads to dysbiosis characterized by overrepresentation of *Prevotellaceae* [16]. While findings such as these confirm the existence of a dialogue between host PRRs and the microbiota so as to influence microbial communities and disease phenotypes, there are still many unknowns at the level of the specific annotations of the qualitative differences between those downstream functions that cause elimination of pathogens and those that merely modulate commensal communities. That this is an active, dynamic process is shown by the finding that colonization of mouse gut by SFB leads to expansion of IL-17A-secreting Th17 cells and that this IL-17A in turn recruits neutrophils which recognize and curtail the expansion of SFB [17].

Interaction of Adaptive Immunity with the Microbiota

Mice housed under GF conditions display immune dysregulation at several levels, from cytokine polarization to innate lymphoid cell development, with associated disease susceptibilities [18]. Key insights into mechanisms by which specific microbiota species differences could influence immune function and thus, disease phenotypes, have come from studies examining intestinal lymphoid subsets. Thus far, a number of examples demonstrating the dependence of immune subset differentiation on the presence of a specific bacterial species has been delineated in inbred mice. The assumption is that there may be many such examples to be documented in the mammalian adaptive immune response. The Littman lab initially demonstrated that differentiation of intestinal Th17 cells in mice required the presence of SFB [19]. Dependence on SFB for Th17 disease phenotypes, such as experimental arthritis models, was subsequently shown [20]. Several studies indicate that such subset expansions operate through more or less conventional, peptide-MHC-specific T cell receptor (TCR) immune recognition of microbiota antigens. Interestingly, TCR sequencing of intestinal Th17 cells reveals a highly focused population, specifically targeted on SFB antigens [21]. While any role for specific SFB-like species from human gut remains unclear, using a panel of GF mice monocolonized with individual bacterial species derived from human gut microbiota, it was found that a number of other bacterial species, notably *Bifidobacterium adolescentis*, could promote intestinal, noninflammatory, Th17 development [22]. This proceeded through a somewhat distinct transcriptional pathway from SFB-mediated Th17 expansion. Honda et al. demonstrated requirement for clostridial species in the functional differentiation of Tregs [23]. Subsequent studies showed that a number of other individual bacterial species including some from the Clostridia class and the *Bacteroides* genus could similarly support development of intestinal Tregs [24, 25]. The Mathis-Benoist labs looked for transcriptional profiles that were specific to intestinal Treg cells involved in modulating recognition of the gut microbiota, and found that, both in mice and humans, intestinal Tregs often express RORγT [25]. This was surprising as RORγT has been considered the hallmark transcription factor driving the differentiation of Th17 (pro-inflammatory) effector function. Presence of the intestinal RORγT Treg population was dependent on presence of the gut microbiota since treatment of mice with broad spectrum antibiotics largely ablated this subset. Again using the panel of GF mice monocolonized with individual bacterial species derived from human gut microbiota, it was found that several individual species could largely restore this Treg subset. The bacterial species encompassed both *Firmicutes* and

Bacteroidetes phyla, among them, *Clostridium ramosum*, *Staphylococcus saprophyticus*, and *Bacteroides thetaiotaomicron*.

The cases of SFB and Clostridia demonstrate the principle that microbiota components could influence immune regulation and disease, both through effects on effector function and on immune regulation. Currently lacking is the detail of these relationships: how many different species act in this fashion on various immune subsets, and, most importantly, what is the nature of any of these relationships for human immunity? Possession of this knowledge would greatly enhance the ability to design therapeutic strategies to modulate microbiota-driven effects on autoimmune and inflammatory disease phenotypes. The knowledge gap with respect to human gut-derived species is being somewhat resolved by the aforementioned studies with monocolonized GF mice: analysis of 53, individual human gut-derived bacterial species in this system yields a complex picture, whereby a wide array of host transcriptional and immunological consequences are discerned, although not attributable to specific, simple, correlations with given microbial phyla [26].

The gut microbiota is the largest and most experimentally accessible in the body and offers a clear window onto the local interaction with development of host immune subsets as this site. Still to be fully characterized are the ramifications of this for immunity and disease at other sites or systemically. While the rules for interaction of microbiota species in the gut with the immune system are starting to be understood, much of this knowledge is lacking when it comes to microbiota at other mucosal interfaces.

Implications for Etiology of RA

In terms of the interaction between genetics and environment in RA, arguably the environmental factor that has been most strongly implicated is the microbial environment, not least due to the role of bacterial infections in triggering reactive arthritis [27]. In brief, the evidence in support of a role for the host microbiota in RA etiology may be assembled as follows (see also Chap. 15):

- RA therapeutics have a history of successful application of antibiotic/anti-inflammatory treatments, notably the use from the 1940s onward of sulfasalazine [28].
- Since the 1970s, it has been apparent that rodent models of RA-related joint pathology are strongly influenced by the microbiological status of the colony and facility. The 1979 adjuvant arthritis study by Kohashi et al. found that severe disease developed in 100% of GF rats, while less severe disease developed and was seen in 20% of conventionally housed rats, leading to the conclusion that "a bacterial flora may have some suppressive effect on the development of the disease…possibly through modulation of the immune response." [29]. On the other hand, for the articular disease phenotype of HLA-B27 rats reported by the Taurog lab, GF status prevented disease development [30]. Taken together, the diverse rodent disease model studies appeared to argue that there may be both pathogenic and regulatory immune subsets differentially influenced by the presence or absence of microbiota species.
- A long-standing hypothesis of RA etiology was once termed the "oral sepsis hypothesis" (and led historically to RA being treated by dental extractions) and is more currently construed in terms of a role of periodontitis in general and *Porphyromonas gingivalis* infection in particular in pathogenesis. There is a potential link to pathogenic mechanisms since *P. gingivalis* has a peptidylarginine deaminase that can convert arginine to citrulline [31].
- A New York-based study of microbiota and disease in RA patients by Scher et al. found that in new-onset, untreated RA patients, presence of *Prevotella copri* (and a reduction in *Bacteroides*) was strongly correlated with disease [32]. This was to some extent reiterated in a Japanese RA cohort [33]. A major study in a Chinese RA cohort found no evidence for alterations in abundance of *Prevotella* species but did find that patient microbiota displayed a deficit in *Haemophilus* species and an abundance of *Lactobacillus salivarius* [34].

As discussed above, studies in mouse models show that presence of specific gut commensal species can shape development of immune subsets and disease, including arthritis models [6, 22]. These findings support the notion of a "gut-joint axis," dictating disease susceptibility via the differential impact of microbiota species on the early programming of immune subsets.

The issue of whether one can define a core, healthy, human, microbiota has been highly contentious, not least due to differences in terms and definitions such as whether this core is described both qualitatively and quantitatively [35, 36]. An alternative view is that a core microbiome is more usefully defined in terms of core transcriptional functions and pathways present, rather than purely by the species enumerated that mediate these functions [37]. This emphasizes the need for long-term microbiota research programs to be able to progress beyond the statistical attribution and enumeration of 16S rRNA gene sequences to a more multifaceted omics analysis, encompassing pathway analysis, metabolomics, biochemistry, and transcriptomics, combined with an ability to culture and study individual bacterial species, and then attempt to recapitulate the disease and its modulation in experimental animal models.

Many studies have been reported on associations between dysbiosis and inflammatory/autoimmune disease phenotypes, notably in inflammatory bowel diseases (IBD) including Crohn's disease and ulcerative colitis (see Chap. 19) and in type I diabetes. More or less without exception, these are correlative studies, unable to distinguish between cause or consequence of the disease process. IBD appears to be associated with a reduction in diversity of gut microbiota. Several reports have shown that the microbial populations in the intestine of IBD patients are different from those of healthy individuals [38]. The MetaHIT consortium describe IBD patients as carrying on average, 25% fewer 16S rRNA defined genes than individuals not suffering from IBD [39]. The mechanistic case has for the most part been based on modulation of disease phenotypes in animal models, as described above.

With respect to pathways by which microbiota differences may impact inflammatory disease, attention has focused on the relationship between diet, particularly dietary fiber, microbiota composition (especially the ratio of *Firmicutes* to *Bacteroidetes*), and control of inflammation [40]. A mechanistic link is supplied by the fact that gut microbiota metabolize fiber, thereby increasing the concentration of circulating short-chain fatty acids (SCFAs) [40]. In one recent study [40], mice were fed for 6 weeks with a diet that was either normal, high, or low fiber, and hyperimmunized with allergen, and then subjected to a respiratory allergen challenge. The low-fiber diet was associated with a gut (and lung) microbiota of decreased complexity and dominated by *Firmicutes* and correlated with increased severity of the pulmonary inflammatory response. The high-fiber-associated microbiota could metabolize fiber to generate SCFAs, particularly propionate, detectable in serum and urine. Importantly for consideration of translational initiatives in relation to microbiota control of inflammatory phenotypes, simple administration of propionate in drinking water could to a large extent ameliorate the inflammatory phenotype. Studies such as this support the notion that diet can influence the effect of the microbiota on control of inflammation in disease, that analysis of metabolic products in serum or urine may offer prognostic biomarkers, and that disease might be treated with dietary supplements of this type.

Concluding Remarks: The Implicated Immunological Mechanisms

Thus far, this chapter has described two, non-mutually exclusive routes through which change in the mix and abundance of microbiota species might impact risk of RA and other autoimmune and inflammatory diseases: the first notion is that different species have the ability to preferentially promote the development of immune subsets of particular effector function. This field is currently progressing from initial analysis focused on the intestinal Th17 and Treg compartments, to wider analysis of other innate and adaptive subsets at other sites. From studies in various autoimmune mouse models, these compartmental perturbations may be sufficient to shift the balance to or from disease. The second, related, notion is that microbiota differences lead in turn to local or distant differences in bacterial-derived metabolites such as SCFAs, and these in turn have immune-modulatory properties. Also mentioned has been the observation, worthy of further analysis, that microbiota differences can modulate citrullination of self-proteins with associated impacts on autoantigen recognition. More recent studies suggest an additional mechanism that may link microbiota species to RA pathogenesis: the direct immune recognition by B and T cell receptors of bacterial antigens expressed by species such as *Prevotella copri*, leading to recognition of cross-reactive self-epitopes in synovium [41].

Taken together, recent findings have offered rapid progress in the elucidation of correlates of disease risk among microbiota species, with some clues as to associated mechanism. Such findings offer strong hopes for new microbiota-based therapeutic strategies based on modulation of inflammatory pathways.

References

1. Scher JU, Abramson SB. The microbiome and rheumatoid arthritis. Nat Rev Rheumatol. 2011;7: 569–78.
2. McInnes IB, Schett G. The pathogenesis of rheumatoid arthritis. N Engl J Med. 2011;365(23):2205–19.
3. The Human Microbiome Project Consortium. Structure, function and diversity of the healthy human microbiome. Nature. 2013;486:207–14.
4. The Integrative HMO Research Network Consortium. The integrative human microbiome project: dynamic analysis of microbiome-host omics profiles during periods of human health and disease. Cell Host Microbe. 2014;16:276–89.
5. Honda K, Littman DR. The microbiome in infectious disease and inflammation. Annu Rev Immunol. 2012;30:759–95.
6. Surana NK, Kasper DL. Deciphering the tête-à-tête between the microbiota and the immune system. J Clin Invest. 2014;124(10):4197–203.
7. Nutsch KM, Hsieh CS. T cell tolerance and immunity to commensal bacteria. Curr Opin Immunol. 2012;24(4):385–91.
8. Lederberg J. Infectious history. Science. 2000;288:287–93.
9. Brown RL, Clarke TB. The regulation of host defences to infection by themicrobiota. Immunology. 2017 Jan;150(1):1–6.
10. Chu H, Mazmanian SK. Innate immune recognition of the microbiota promotes host-microbial symbiosis. Nat Immunol. 2013;14(7):668–75.
11. Bates JM, Akerlund J, Mittge E, Guillemin K. Intestinal alkaline phosphatase detoxifies lipopolysaccharide and prevents inflammation in zebrafish in response to the gut microbiota. Cell Host Microbe. 2007;2(6):371–82.
12. Petnicki-Ocwieja T, Hrncir T, Liu YJ, Biswas A, Hudcovic T, Tlaskalova-Hogenova H, Kobayashi KS. Nod2 is required for the regulation of commensal microbiota in the intestine. Proc Natl Acad Sci U S A. 2009;106(37):15813–8.
13. Vijay-Kumar M, Aitken JD, Carvalho FA, Cullender TC, Mwangi S, Srinivasan S, Sitaraman SV, Knight R, Ley RE, Gewirtz AT. Metabolic syndrome and altered gut microbiota in mice lacking toll-like receptor 5. Science. 2010;328(5975):228–31.
14. Burrows MP, Volchkov P, Kobayashi KS, Chervonsky AV. Microbiota regulates type 1 diabetes through toll-like receptors. Proc Natl Acad Sci U S A. 2015;112(32):9973–7. https://doi.org/10.1073/pnas.1508740112.
15. Wang S, Charbonnier LM, Noval Rivas M, Georgiev P, Li N, Gerber G, Bry L, Chatila TA. MyD88 adaptor-dependent microbial sensing by regulatory T cells promotes mucosal tolerance and enforces commensalism. Immunity. 2015;43(2):289–303.
16. Elinav E, Strowig T, Kau AL, Henao-Mejia J, Thaiss CA, Booth CJ, Peaper DR, Bertin J, Eisenbarth SC, Gordon JI, Flavell RA. NLRP6 inflammasome regulates colonic microbial ecology and risk for colitis. Cell. 2011;145(5):745–57.
17. Flannigan KL, Ngo VL, Geem D, Harusato A, Hirota SA, Parkos CA, Lukacs NW, Nusrat A, Gaboriau-Routhiau V, Cerf-Bensussan N, Gewirtz AT, Denning TL. IL-17A-mediated neutrophil recruitment limits expansion of segmented filamentous bacteria. Mucosal Immunol. 2017;10(3):673–84.
18. Hepworth MR, Monticelli LA, Fung TC, Ziegler CG, Grunberg S, Sinha R, Mantegazza AR, Ma HL, Crawford A, Angelosanto JM, Wherry EJ, Koni PA, Bushman FD, Elson CO, Eberl G, Artis D, Sonnenberg GF. Innate lymphoid cells regulate CD4+ T-cell responses to intestinal commensal bacteria. Nature. 2013;498(7452):113–7.
19. Ivanov II, Atarashi K, Manel N, Brodie EL, Shima T, Karaoz U, Wei D, Goldfarb KC, Santee CA, Lynch SV, Tanoue T, Imaoka A, Itoh K, Takeda K, Umesaki Y, Honda K, Littman DR. Induction of intestinal Th17 cells by segmented filamentous bacteria. Cell. 2009;139(3):485–98.
20. Wu HJ, Ivanov II, Darce J, Hattori K, Shima T, Umesaki Y, Littman DR, Benoist C, Mathis D. Gut-residing segmented filamentous bacteria drive autoimmune arthritis via T helper 17 cells. Immunity. 2010;32(6):815–27.

21. Yang Y, Torchinsky MB, Gobert M, Xiong H, Xu M, Linehan JL, Alonzo F, Ng C, Chen A, Lin X, Sczesnak A, Liao JJ, Torres VJ, Jenkins MK, Lafaille JJ, Littman DR. Focused specificity of intestinal TH17 cells towards commensal bacterial antigens. Nature. 2014;510(7503):152–6.
22. Tan TG, Sefik E, Geva-Zatorsky N, Kua L, Naskar D, Teng F, Pasman L, Ortiz-Lopez A, Jupp R, Wu HJ, Kasper DL, Benoist C, Mathis D. Identifying species of symbiont bacteria from the human gut that, alone, can induce intestinal Th17 cells in mice. Proc Natl Acad Sci U S A. 2016;113(50):E8141–50.
23. Atarashi K, Tanoue T, Oshima K, Suda W, Nagano Y, Nishikawa H, Fukuda S, Saito T, Narushima S, Hase K, Kim S, Fritz JV, Wilmes P, Ueha S, Matsushima K, Ohno H, Olle B, Sakaguchi S, Taniguchi T, Morita H, Hattori M, Honda K. Treg induction by a rationally selected mixture of Clostridia strains from the human microbiota. Nature. 2013;500(7461):232–6.
24. Faith JJ, Ahern PP, Ridaura VK, Cheng J, Gordon JI. Identifying gut microbe-host phenotype relationships using combinatorial communities in gnotobiotic mice. Sci Transl Med. 2014;6(220):220–11.
25. Sefik E, Geva-Zatorsky N, Oh S, Konnikova L, Zemmour D, McGuire AM, Burzyn D, Ortiz-Lopez A, Lobera M, Yang J, Ghosh S, Earl A, Snapper SB, Jupp R, Kasper D, Mathis D, Benoist C. Mucosal immunology. Individual intestinal symbionts induce a distinct population of RORγ^+ regulatory T cells. Science. 2015;349(6251):993–7.
26. Geva-Zatorsky N, Sefik E, Kua L, Pasman L, Tan TG, Ortiz-Lopez A, Yanortsang TB, Yang L, Jupp R, Mathis D, Benoist C, Kasper DL. Mining the human gut microbiota for immunomodulatory organisms. Cell. 2017;168(5):928–43.
27. Girschick HJ, Guilherme L, Inman RD, Latsch K, Rihl M, Sherer Y, Shoenfeld Y, Zeidler H, Arienti S, Doria A. Bacterial triggers and autoimmune rheumatic diseases. Clin Exp Rheumatol. 2008;26(1 Suppl 48):S12–7.
28. Neumann VC, Grindulis KA, Hubball S, McConkey B, Wright V. Comparison between penicillamine and sulphasalazine in rheumatoid arthritis: Leeds-Birmingham trial. Br Med J (Clin Res Ed). 1983;287(6399):1099–102.
29. Kohashi O, Kuwata J, Umehara K, Uemura F, Takahashi T, Ozawa A. Susceptibility to adjuvant-induced arthritis among germfree, specific-pathogen-free, and conventional rats. Infect Immun. 1979;26(3):791–4.
30. Rath HC, Herfarth HH, Ikeda JS, Grenther WB, Hamm TE Jr, Balish E, Taurog JD, Hammer RE, Wilson KH, Sartor RB. Normal luminal bacteria, especially Bacteroides species, mediate chronic colitis, gastritis, and arthritis in HLA-B27/human beta2 microglobulin transgenic rats. J Clin Invest. 1996;98(4):945–53.
31. Brusca SB, Abramson SB, Scher JU. Microbiome and mucosal inflammation as extra-articular triggers for rheumatoid arthritis and autoimmunity. Curr Opin Rheumatol. 2014;26:101–7.
32. Scher JU, Sczesnak A, Longman RS, Segata N, Ubeda C, Bielski C, Rostron T, Cerundolo V, Pamer EG, Abramson SB, Huttenhower C, Littman DR. Expansion of intestinal Prevotella copri correlates with enhanced susceptibility to arthritis. Elife. 2013;2:e01202.
33. Maeda Y, Kurakawa T, Umemoto E, Motooka D, Ito Y, Gotoh K, Hirota K, Matsushita M, Furuta Y, Narazaki M, Sakaguchi N, Kayama H, Nakamura S, Iida T, Saeki Y, Kumanogoh A, Sakaguchi S, Takeda K. Dysbiosis contributes to arthritis development via activation of autoreactive T cells in the intestine. Arthritis Rheumatol. 2016;68(11):2646–61.
34. Zhang X, Zhang D, Jia H, Feng Q, Wang D, Liang D, Wu X, Li J, Tang L, Li Y, Lan Z, Chen B, Li Y, Zhong H, Xie H, Jie Z, Chen W, Tang S, Xu X, Wang X, Cai X, Liu S, Xia Y, Li J, Qiao X, Al-Aama JY, Chen H, Wang L, Wu QJ, Zhang F, Zheng W, Li Y, Zhang M, Luo G, Xue W, Xiao L, Li J, Chen W, Xu X, Yin Y, Yang H, Wang J, Kristiansen K, Liu L, Li T, Huang Q, Li Y, Wang J. The oral and gut microbiomes are perturbed in rheumatoid arthritis and partly normalized after treatment. Nat Med. 2015;21(8):895–905.
35. Li K, Bihan M, Methé BA. Analyses of the stability and core taxonomic memberships of the human microbiome. PLoS One. 2013;8(5):e63139. https://doi.org/10.1371/journal.pone.0063139.
36. Turnbaugh PJ, Hamady M, Yatsunenko T, Cantarel BL, Duncan A, Ley RE, Sogin ML, Jones WJ, Roe BA, Affourtit JP, Egholm M, Henrissat B, Heath AC, Knight R, Gordon JI. A core gut microbiome in obese and lean twins. Nature. 2009;457(7228):480–4.
37. Arumugam M, Raes J, Pelletier E, Le Paslier D, Yamada T, Mende DR, Fernandes GR, Tap J, Bruls T, Batto JM, Bertalan M, Borruel N, Casellas F, Fernandez L, Gautier L, Hansen T, Hattori M, Hayashi T, Kleerebezem M, Kurokawa K, Leclerc M, Levenez F, Manichanh C, Nielsen HB, Nielsen T, Pons N, Poulain J, Qin J, Sicheritz-Ponten T, Tims S, Torrents D, Ugarte E, Zoetendal EG, Wang J, Guarner F, Pedersen O, de Vos WM, Brunak S, Doré J, MetaHIT Consortium, Antolín M, Artiguenave F, Blottiere HM, Almeida M, Brechot C, Cara C, Chervaux C, Cultrone A, Delorme C, Denariaz G, Dervyn R, Foerstner KU, Friss C, van de Guchte M, Guedon E, Haimet F, Huber W, van Hylckama-Vlieg J, Jamet A, Juste C, Kaci G, Knol J, Lakhdari O, Layec S, Le Roux K, Maguin E, Mérieux A, Melo Minardi R, M'rini C, Muller J, Oozeer R, Parkhill J, Renault P, Rescigno M, Sanchez N, Sunagawa S, Torrejon A, Turner K, Vandemeulebrouck G, Varela E, Winogradsky Y, Zeller G, Weissenbach J, Ehrlich SD, Bork P. Enterotypes of the human gut microbiome. Nature. 2011;473(7346):174–80.
38. Bäckhed F, Fraser CM, Ringel Y, Sanders ME, Sartor RB, Sherman PM, Versalovic J, Young V, Finlay BB. Defining a healthy human gut microbiome: current concepts, future directions, and clinical applications. Cell Host Microbe. 2012;12(5):611–22.

39. Qin J, Li R, Raes J, Arumugam M, Burgdorf KS, Manichanh C, Nielsen T, Pons N, Levenez F, Yamada T, Mende DR, Li J, Xu J, Li S, Li D, Cao J, Wang B, Liang H, Zheng H, Xie Y, Tap J, Lepage P, Bertalan M, Batto JM, Hansen T, Le Paslier D, Linneberg A, Nielsen HB, Pelletier E, Renault P, Sicheritz-Ponten T, Turner K, Zhu H, Yu C, Li S, Jian M, Zhou Y, Li Y, Zhang X, Li S, Qin N, Yang H, Wang J, Brunak S, Doré J, Guarner F, Kristiansen K, Pedersen O, Parkhill J, Weissenbach J, MetaHIT Consortium, Bork P, Ehrlich SD, Wang J. A human gut microbial gene catalogue established by metagenomic sequencing. Nature. 2010;464(7285):59–65.
40. Trompette A, Gollwitzer ES, Yadava K, Sichelstiel AK, Sprenger N, Ngom-Bru C, Blanchard C, Junt T, Nicod LP, Harris NL, Marsland BJ. Gut microbiota metabolism of dietary fiber influences allergic airway disease and hematopoiesis. Nat Med. 2014;20(2):159–66.
41. Pianta A, Arvikar SL, Strle K, Drouin EE, Wang Q, Costello CE, Steere AC. Two rheumatoid arthritis-specific autoantigens correlate microbial immunity with autoimmune responses in joints. J Clin Invest. 2017;127(8):2946–56.

6 Animal Models of Rheumatoid Arthritis

David R. Webb

Abbreviations

AI	Autoimmune
APCA	Anti-parietal cell antibodies
BSA	Bovine serum albumin
CAIA	Collagen antibody-induced arthritis
CFA	Complete Freund's adjuvant
CIA	Collagen-induced arthritis
GF	Germ-free
IBD	Inflammatory bowel disease
Ig RF	RF-like immunoglobulin
IL	Interleukin
LPS	Lipopolysaccharide
mAB	Monoclonal antibody
MS	Multiple sclerosis
NSAID	Nonsteroidal anti-inflammatory drug
PMN	Polymorphonuclear cell
RA	Rheumatoid arthritis
RF	Rheumatoid factor
SCID	Severe combined immunodeficiency

D. R. Webb
The Department of Integrated Structural and Computational Biology, The Scripps Research Institute, La Jolla, CA, USA
e-mail: dwebb@scripps.edu

Introduction

We are now well into a new century that has brought with it a considerable increase in our understanding of the underlying mechanisms that exist in several of the more prominent autoimmune (AI) diseases. This new understanding has led to a revolution in the treatment of RA, multiple sclerosis, and inflammatory bowel diseases including ulcerative colitis and Crohn's disease [1–6]. Many patients have seen enormous benefits from new therapies that are also recently developed, in particular the use of therapeutic monoclonal antibodies (mAb) [1]. The principal reason for these advances has been the extensive use of animal models that mimic the various pathological aspects of these diseases and in particular the use of the mouse as an experimental tool [6–8]. These models have not only led to an increased understanding of the underlying cellular and molecular mechanisms of AI disease but have also served to establish *Mus musculus* as the test organism in translational studies [6]. It must also be said that the heavy reliance on the mouse as a model of human diseases has its drawbacks as well. It is by now well established that the mouse models have flaws [5, 6, 8–11]. It will be the focus of this brief review to discuss the use of animal models in RA giving both a historical perspective as well as presenting newer information as to what is understood about the pathological basis of RA. In particular, the recent new data

G. Ragab et al. (eds.), *The Microbiome in Rheumatic Diseases and Infection*,
https://doi.org/10.1007/978-3-319-79026-8_6

that speak to the role of bacteria in the induction of RA will be discussed [12, 13].

History of Animal Models of RA

Once it was understood that one of the guiding principles of immunity was the ability to distinguish between "self" and "not self," it was not too great a conceptual step to conclude that autoimmunity must arise as a result of a dysfunction in the immune system causing it to recognize "self"-antigens. Two problems immediately arose from this. First, it raised the question as to the nature of the inciting antigen. And second, in the absence of knowing the inciting antigen, how could one model the disease? Related to these concerns is the question of what makes patients susceptible to RA? We will return to this question later. Early on it was noted that in RA as well as in other AI diseases, there existed autoantibodies which were thought to be the primary pathological element in the development and maintenance of the disease (Fig. 6.1a) [14, 15]. This was due in part to our understanding developed in the early part of the twentieth century as to how antibodies could be induced via immunization with antigen, by vaccination, for example. Thus, the working assumption was that there must be a close correspondence between disease initiation via an unknown, infectious antigenic stimulus and the appearance of the symptoms of the disease itself. Complicating this notion are data from a variety of studies showing that normal individuals produce autoantibodies long before the onset of any autoimmune disease symptoms [12, 13]. Subsequently, as has been reviewed recently by Rosen and Casciola-Rosen [15], it has become possible to think of the

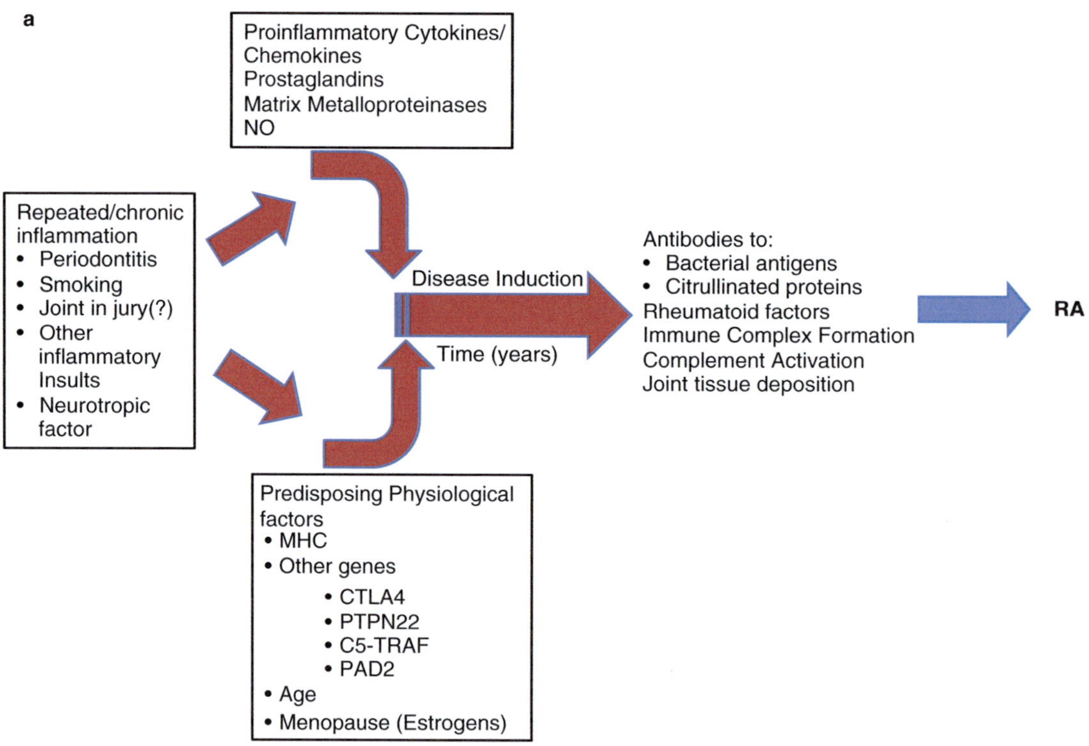

Fig. 6.1 Elements of rheumatoid arthritis (RA) in humans (**a**) and in the primary animal models of rheumatoid arthritis in rodents (**b**). (**a**) RA is a complex disease involving a variety of inflammation driven changes as illustrated here. (**b**) The primary models used to study RA are those in the rat and mouse that have been experimentally designed primarily to mimic the joint destruction, cellular infiltrate, and production of pro-inflammatory mediators that reflect what is seen in humans. Both models have been successfully used to develop drugs that provide symptomatic relief (NSAIDs) as well as disease modification (anti-cytokines, antiproliferative agents)

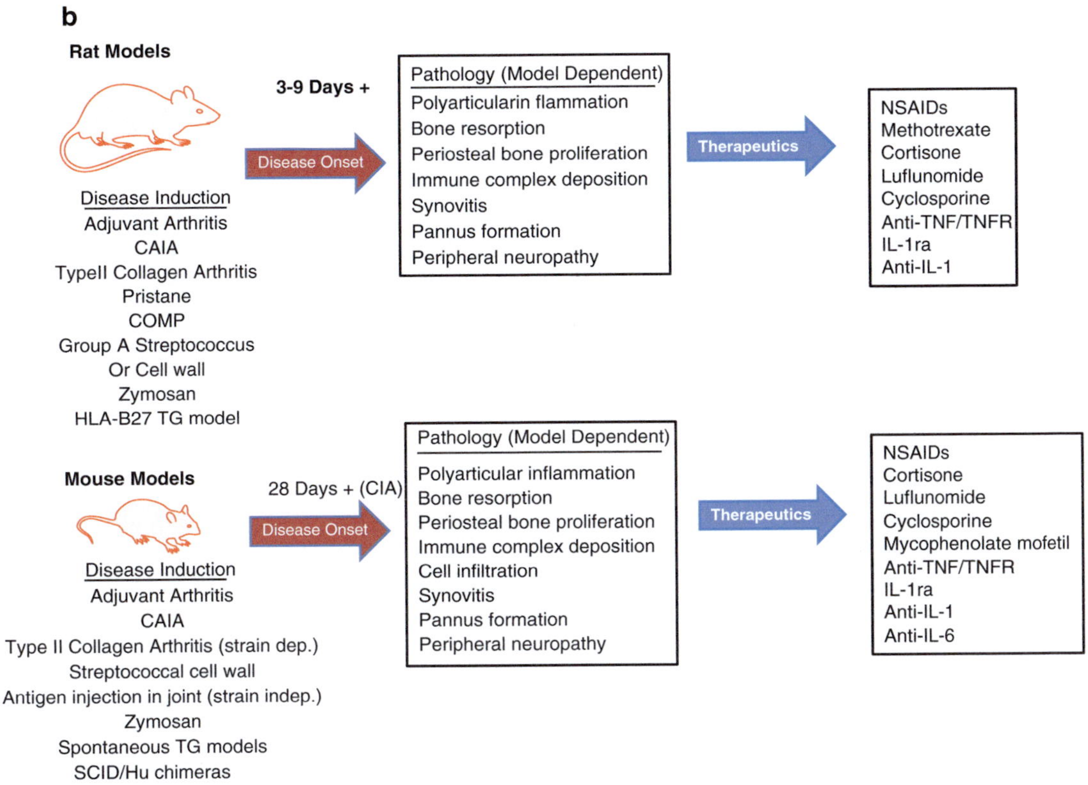

Fig. 6.1 (continued)

development of autoantibodies as part of the "continuum" of initiation and propagation of an immune response with tissue damage feeding into a loop of continuous autoantigen stimulation.

The early discovery of autoantibodies in RA, including the so-called rheumatoid factor (RF), was thought to explain many of the comorbidities that occur in RA patients. It also led researchers to ask how RF might be formed following an appropriate stimulus. As Izui et al. [13] showed many years ago, injection of bacterial lipopolysaccharide (LPS) into mice resulted in the formation of IgM RF in several strains including nude (athymic) mice. It also led to the induction of autoantibodies (anti-DNA, anti-spleen cells, and anti-red blood cells). The thinking in that period was that polyclonal activation of B cells led to the induction of autoreactive B cell clones that generated the RF-like immunoglobulins (Ig RF). While research on the induction of RA using bacterial components has continued up to the present time, during the 1980s there was a shift in focus for researchers interested in developing new therapeutics due to the discovery of the role of soluble factors, first called lymphokines and later cytokines, that were produced in abundance during immune responses of all types [2, 6]. Nevertheless, the recent advent of therapeutic mAbs has allowed investigators to show that depletion of B cells using rituximab in combination with methotrexate or cyclophosphamide will provide significant improvement in a variety of autoimmune human diseases including RA [2, 3, 5, 6].

The discovery and elucidation of the biochemical nature of cytokines changed the focus of many researchers studying RA both in animal models and in patients [1–5]. It became apparent by the early 1990s that the use of monoclonal anti-cytokine antibodies might represent a breakthrough in the understanding and treatment of RA. In particular, the work of Feldmann and his collaborators established first in collagen-induced arthritis (CIA) mouse models of RA, and then in patients, that treatment with anti-TNF mAbs could have profound effects on RA symptoms and disease progression [1, 6, 11]. Later, other researchers, following this lead, have discovered that mAbs to other cytokines such as interleukin 1 (IL-1) and interleukin 6 (IL-6) may also be important therapeutics in treating many patients. In all of these studies, investigators principally used mouse models employing both bacterial components (usually as Freund's adjuvant) as well as tissue proteins such as animal-derived collagen to induce an acute arthritis that developed over a few weeks rather than over years as occurs in human disease [6, 10, 11, 13, 16]. The CIA model has emerged as one of the principal tools for the development of therapeutics based primarily on the work cited above. We will later consider its advantages and disadvantages.

Finally, as alluded to earlier, there is the question of disease susceptibility. Not every patient with RA has periodontal disease, and not every patient with periodontal disease develops RA. Indeed, the prevalence of autoimmune diseases in general is linked to many factors including gender, age, genetics, and type of disease [16, 17]. Beginning in the middle of the 20th century, there was a concerted effort to identify genetic risk factors in RA and other autoimmune diseases. Studies in both mice and humans led to the discovery that the major histocompatibility complex (MHC) is the genetic location of the susceptibility genes associated with the development of autoimmune diseases. The MHC consists of a plethora of genetic loci that have been studied for decades [6, 18]. For our purposes here, it is the class II genes, the HLA-DR genes in humans and genes that are located in the H-2 I region in mice (I-A and I-E), that seem to confer susceptibility [5, 17]. These genes code for cell surface proteins present on antigen-presenting cells that are responsible for displaying antigenic peptides derived from infectious organisms as well as from self-proteins, principally to various T-cell subtypes [18, 19]. This discovery has been a powerful tool to understand the nature of the antigens that induce RA in both animals and humans [11–13, 16].

Animal Models of RA

When discussing animal models of RA, it is important to take cognizance of the different research disciplines that are interested in RA. The immunology community has largely gravitated to mouse models using a variety of approaches outlined in Fig. 6.1b. This was done to explore the fundamental cellular and molecular pathologies that are responsible for the induction and maintenance of RA. It also involved the extensive use of both a variety of strains of mice as well as more recently the use of transgenic mice [5, 13, 14]. In addition, there has been extensive use of genomics comparing both mice and humans not only in terms of genetic susceptibility but also in terms of understanding the role of the microbiome in the induction and exacerbation of the disease. By contrast, pharmacologists that have focused on inflammatory diseases and who are interested in the biochemical pharmacology of diseases have traditionally favored the rat as their research tool [6, 13]. As has been noted by many authors [5, 9, 11, 13], models of RA are invariably acute models of disease with symptoms and pathological changes occurring in a matter of days or weeks in contrast to humans, where the disease may develop over years. In addition, some models are self-limiting so that the disease resolves itself after a period of time.

Thus, while these models have been highly useful in developing a comprehensive view of the disease, not all aspects of human RA may be seen in any one model [5, 8, 9, 12, 13]. Therefore, each animal model must be carefully deployed depending on what the ultimate goal of the given research project might be. There have also developed distinctly different approaches to therapy with initial treatment often focusing on pain management and reduction of inflammation using NSAIDs, corticosteroids, and methotrexate [5, 14]. Only with the more recent advent of the biologics (e.g., anti-TNF) has it become possible to treat the underlying cellular and molecular drivers of disease leading to remarkable reductions in disease manifestations [1, 5, 11, 14, 15, 18, 19].

With that introduction, the remainder of this section will survey the animal models most commonly used, their advantages and disadvantages, and prospects for the future.

Adjuvant-Induced Arthritis in the Rat

This model has proven to be remarkably successful in predicting the likely clinical activity of classic nonsteroidal anti-inflammatory drugs (NSAIDs), in particular those that target the eicosanoid pathways such as the cyclooxygenase I and cyclooxygenase II inhibitors [20]. In this model, disease is induced with complete Freund's adjuvant (CFA) containing inactivated mycobacteria, or with synthetic adjuvants. The primary choice of rat strains is the male Lewis rat as the disease is more variable in females. As with all models, the onset of disease is acute, generally occurring by days 9–10 as evidenced by paw swelling. The model is generally run for a period of 5–7 days following disease onset, and the rats may be treated either prophylactically at the time of injection or therapeutically with the onset of symptoms [14]. The model (Fig. 6.1b) is very consistent in terms of disease onset and progression with reliable pathology and tissue markers. As discussed by Bendele in her excellent review [14], it is characterized by polyarticular inflammation, bone resorption, and periosteal proliferation. Cartilage destruction tends to be milder compared to the inflammation and bone resorption. As is true for most of the animal models discussed herein, the underlying mechanisms of the induced disease are not well understood. As will be discussed later, the most interesting finding may be the interactions with intestinal microbiota [12]. To carry out the detailed analysis of the disease, the animals are typically sacrificed, following which the affected tissues are surgically removed and examined both grossly and by tissue fixation and microscopy. Tissues other than the bones and joints may be affected including the spleen (splenomegaly), liver (hepatomegaly), and the eye (uveitis). These changes also will resolve following treatment with effective drugs or compounds. As suggested earlier, this model is particularly good for studying NSAIDs. Although the newer biologic agents such as anti-TNF will work, they are generally less effective when used alone than, for example, indomethacin [5, 12]. Combinations of both classes of drugs are also effective.

Collagen-Induced Arthritis in the Rat and Mouse

Due to the joint destruction commonly seen in advanced cases of RA (and OA), it is not remarkable that scientists interested in RA at the basic level as well as those interested in more translational research have used antigen induction models of arthritis, principally employing homologous or heterologous type II collagen. This model has been used in both rat and mouse, with the mouse dominating research into the cellular and molecular pathology of the disease (Fig. 6.1b) [1, 5, 20].

In the rat, injection of collagen either with or without an adjuvant results in an arthritis that involves both cellular and humoral aspects of the immune system. It consists of immune complex deposition on articular surfaces, bone resorption, periosteal proliferation of fibroblastoid cells, synovitis, and joint inflammation. In most respects, this model more completely reflects the pathology seen in humans including the formation of a pannus. However, as with the adjuvant model, this is an acute disease occurring on days 10–13 usually after at least two injections of collagen (normally using incomplete FA), this time in female rats. Treatments usually start with disease onset and may last for a week or less. Animals are sacrificed at the termination of the experiments so that the relevant anatomical and histopathological measurements may be made. Here, histopathological changes occur in the knee as well as the paws. The model is sensitive to all forms of therapy including NSAIDs, methotrexate, and the biologics including anti-TNF, anti-TNFR, and IL-1ra (Anakinra) [5, 10, 14].

In the mouse, attention must be paid to the strains used here since not all strains of mice will develop arthritis in response to heterologous (usually bovine) type II collagen exposure. Here the role of the MHC haplotype is critical, and induction of the arthritis also seems to require a humoral as well as a cellular immune response. Mice with an H-2q haplotype, including both the DBA/1J and B10.Q strains, seem to be uniquely susceptible, and the susceptibility maps to the H-2 I region, suggesting a requirement for T cells in disease induction (CD8+ T cells in particular). Interestingly, CFA is nonarthritogenic in mice, thus implicating the type II collagen as the inducing agent. Thus, this model is rather different than the rat CIA model and has become a major research tool in the immunology community interested in RA (Fig. 6.1b) [1, 5, 14, 20]. There are a variety of protocols that have been used for sensitization to collagen, some employing CFA or endotoxin as well as bovine type II collagen. The incidence and severity of disease will vary in up to 100% of animals depending on the protocol, and disease onset generally occurs 4 or more weeks after induction. As noted above, a variety of NSAIDs and biologics are effective as therapeutics in this model including anti-IL-1, -IL-6, -IL-17, IL-1ra, and, of course, anti-TNF or anti-TNFR. These data indicate strong cytokine dependence in the induction and maintenance of this disease model that also seems to reflect the disease seen in humans in terms of both humoral and cellular responses. That is also evident in the systemic, histopathological, and anatomical manifestations of the disease. These include tissue and bone damage (resorption) to feet and knee joints, pannus formation, and fibroblastoid cell proliferation. As opposed to some of the rat models, disease in mice may persist for up to several weeks. It should be noted that cortisone is often not as effective in this model, and due to toxicity to animals, use of methotrexate is not recommended. It has also been the model of choice to study the timing and role of cytokines, T cells, B cells, and monocyte/macrophages in the initiation and maintenance of the disease.

Antigen and/or Antibody-Induced Arthritis Models

As has been pointed out by Benedele [14], most species of laboratory animals subjected to antigen exposure by direct injection into the joint (e.g., cationic proteins such as methylated bovine serum albumin (BSA)) will develop an acute inflammation leading to joint destruction. This appears to involve an Arthus reaction on the articular cartilage with antigen-antibody complexes depositing on the cartilage, resulting in complement activation and cartilage destruction. While this approach has been used with larger laboratory species such as the rabbit so as to obtain larger joint material, the lack of good markers for the various cell types that are involved here limits its utility as a research tool as opposed to using it as a model for therapy. The model can and has been used in the mouse where the response is not strain selective as is the case with collagen models [1].

As was pointed out earlier, the production of autoantibodies to self-type II collagen, citrullinated proteins, and rheumatoid factor (IgG/IgM) are found in both RA and in many of the rat and mouse models. Indeed, serum from a collagen-immunized mouse will induce arthritis in a non-immunized mouse [20, 21]. Also mixtures of type II collagen and anti-collagen antibody will also induce arthritis (collagen antibody-induced arthritis, CAIA) [21]. These models also reveal the role of macrophages and polymorphonuclear leukocytes (PMN); however, there is a lack of T- and B-cell involvement. T cells can be shown to enhance the disease, however. These models are frequently used as research/pharmacological tools to study the role of innate immune responses in RA as opposed to the acquired (lymphocyte dependent) response. As with the antigen-induced models, this approach is not strain specific in the mouse, as virtually 100% of the animals are affected [10, 14].

Genetically Modified Models of Spontaneous Arthritis

There are a variety of models that have employed transgenic technology primarily as tools to help in the exploration of the role of specific genes in RA. The first of these was reported in 1991 and involves the over expression of human TNF [22].

The human TNF-transfected mouse presents with a chronic, inflammatory, erosive polyarthritis.

Anti-TNF therapy completely blocks the disease. In that this is a chronic, non-resolving disease, it more closely resembles the human RA that is also highly responsive to anti-TNF therapy. The model has also been used to study the role of effector cytokines and chemokines in regulating both the inflammation and cartilage and bone destruction. Another transgenic model involves the study of human HLA class II alleles that share a common stretch of amino acids at the HLA-DRB1 locus [22]. In addition to HLA-DR*0401, human CD4, an RA-related autoantigenic protein (HCgp-39), and a HCgp-39 epitope-specific TCR-αβ transgene have all been deployed to study the role of Th1 responses in overcoming self-tolerance that occurs in RA [14, 20]. There are additional spontaneous transgenic models of RA reviewed recently by Asquith et al. [20] all of which explore various cellular and molecular aspects of innate and acquired immunity and the role of self-antigens in disease induction and maintenance.

There are many additional models involving genetic manipulation that are also reported in the literature that have been used not only to explore the role of cytokines, chemokines, and proteolytic enzymes but also to try to tease out possible initiating events that lead to human RA. These include the K/BxN model that implied a role for antibodies to glucose-6-phosphate isomerase in RA [23] and the SKG model that involves a mutation in ZAP-70, a protein kinase involved in T-cell activation, and is induced by environmental stimuli or zymosan [23]. The severe combined immunodeficient (SCID) mouse has been used as a platform to generate so-called SCID-hu chimeric mice that are implanted with human synovial tissue, thus allowing the exploration of the pathology of the human synovium involving cartilage invasion and destruction via the synovial fibroblast. All of the models outlined in this section have been primarily used to explore the cellular and biochemical basis of human RA as understood from studies of human RA pathology and as such are biased to reflect the particular hypothesis being studied. Most of these are not used in a drug discovery setting to explore the use of new therapeutics although they have suggested potentially new therapeutic targets [22].

Animal Models Exploring the Role of Microbe-Induced Inflammation in RA

The rise of genomics as a tool to study the entire microbiome has had a profound effect on the study of the relationship between humans and their environment. This has been particularly profound in the study of the interaction between individuals and their own microbial community. With the advent of modern genomics sequencing tools, it is now possible to accurately assess the microbial species resident in humans and mice in both healthy and disease states. Such studies are having a profound effect on how immunologists view autoimmune diseases of all types [5, 10, 14, 23]. In particular, it has focused attention on the interaction between microbes at mucosal surfaces and the development of autoimmune disease [11, 12, 24]. As outlined in a review by Brusca et al. [12], the usefulness of labels such as commensal, mutualistic, and pathogenic has blurred, and the complexity of the host-microbe interaction is only now coming to be both appreciated and more deeply explored. In this regard, it is now increasingly appreciated that host susceptibility previously noted as being related to the MHC in both mice and humans is likely due to how bacteria on mucosal surfaces interact with the immune system located there.

Long before investigators had the tools to query the microbiota as we can today, there had been interest in the extent to which the microbiota affected animal models of disease. In many cases, this was studied using animals raised in the germ-free (GF) environment. Multiple studies involving spontaneous induction of inflammatory bowel disease (IBD) using a variety of genetic models [25], as well as HLA-B27-transgenic mouse and rat [26] models of spondyloarthritis, a model of multiple sclerosis (MS) due to a T-cell transgene directed against a protein that constitutes the myelin protective sheath [27], and the K/BxN model of RA, all have diminished or absent disease induction in the GF state [28]. Attenuated disease was also observed in the model of SpA induced by injection of SKG (ZAP-70 deficient) mice with the bacterial and fungal sugar curdlan (β-1,3-glucan aggregates)

[29]. Additionally, in most of these studies, the disease can be reintroduced by a limited consortium of bacteria, such as segmented filamentous bacteria in the models of RA [29] and MS [28]. Two studies of the nonobese diabetic model of type I diabetes have demonstrated that GF mice have increased lymphocytic infiltration of the pancreas, although this has not translated into a more aggressive diabetes phenotype [30]. There are some exceptions to these observations. One study of the CIA rat model of RA showed that the disease was not altered one way or the other in the GF state [31], and another showed more severe disease in the same model among rats raised in the GF state [32, 33]. Despite these latter two findings, microbiota from mice that developed arthritis following injection of collagen, compared to that from mice that were resistant to disease induction, was more arthritogenic when transplanted into GF mice [34].

Interestingly, studies of adjuvant- and chemical-induced autoimmunity have often reported the opposite: worsening of the disease in the GF state. This has been reported twice in the adjuvant-induced model of arthritis in F344 rats, which develop disease only in the GF state [35, 36], and has also been observed in the dextran sulfate mouse model of IBD [37]. In contrast, pristane-induced arthritis was less severe in the somewhat cleaner specific pathogen-free facility as compared to the conventional facility [38, 39]. Finally, there were no differences in the severity of arthritis induced by *Mycobacterium* adjuvant or mineral oil in rats raised in the GF environment [31].

It bears emphasis first that not only is the GF state a highly contrived environment that can never be replicated in humans but also that even typical animal housing conditions do not replicate normal human life. Work recently reported by Beura et al. [40] has shown that mice reared in the wild, or under non-barrier conditions, recapitulate the human immune system to a far greater degree than do mice raised in typical specific pathogen-free research facilities. This suggests that as research proceeds in relating the role of the microbiota to the development of RA, these findings must be taken into account. Thus it may be that the best approach in using models of RA in rodents, particularly the mouse, may be to use non-barrier mice and combine it with the type of studies reported by Trombone et al. [24] that uses a model of infection-induced periodontal disease in two selected mouse strains chosen on the basis of one being highly susceptible and the other being resistant to inflammatory periodontal disease. A model of this type may thus offer the best opportunity to understand fundamental aspects of disease induction despite the acute nature of the models.

Conclusions: Translating Animal Work to Human Disease

Although much information has been learned through the study of animal models, it has its limitations. From the standpoint of developing effective therapeutics, the use of the collagen-induced arthritis model in susceptible mouse strains has been notably successful [1, 5, 10]. However, with respect to understanding the pathophysiology of the disease and its microbial alterations, the models fall short. That is, linking the findings using any of the models to a fundamental understanding of the initiation of RA as well as its long-term consequences is far more difficult than testing therapeutic agents. As noted above, all of the animal models are, of necessity, acute, occurring usually within days after various induction protocols and showing a pathology that reflects some, but not necessarily all, of the aspects of the disease under study [41]. In particular, the principal question that the models cannot answer is why does it take a decade or more for the disease to convert from, for example, antibodies to self-proteins (e.g., rheumatoid factor) in the blood to the active pathology that we associate with RA? No animal model is likely to be able to address this question, as the pre-disease state in humans is far longer than the typical animal life span. Nor is it feasible in a laboratory setting to recapitulate the variety of microbial exposures and the genetic and environmental influences on the microbiota that are present in humans. Thus, while the microbiota is clearly essential in animal models of disease, a cautionary note from this author is that a direct connection between intestinal dysbiosis and the development of RA in humans remains to be established. The continued interplay between clinical and experimental studies in humans using the tools of genomics, proteomics, and metabolomics coupled concurrently with animal model studies may offer the best way forward to continue the evolution of both palliative and preventive approaches to RA as well as other autoimmune diseases.

References

1. Feldmann M, Maini RN. Anti-TNFα therapy of rheumatoid arthritis: what have we learned? Annu Rev Immunol. 2001;19:163–96. https://doi.org/10.1146/annurev.immunol.19.1.163.
2. Bouma G, Strober W. The immunological and genetic basis of inflammatory bowel disease. Nat Rev Immunol. 2003;3:521–33. https://doi.org/10.1038/nri1132.
3. Wirtz S, Neufert C, Weigmann B, Neurath MF. Chemically induced mouse models of intestinal inflammation. Nat Protoc. 2007;2:541–6. https://doi.org/10.1038/nprot.2007.41.
4. Honda K, Littman DR. The microbiome in infectious disease and inflammation. Annu Rev Immunol. 2012;30:759–95. https://doi.org/10.1146/annurev-immunol-020711-074937.
5. Webb DR. Animal models of human disease: inflammation. Biochem Pharmacol. 2014;87:121–30. https://doi.org/10.1016/j.bcp.2013.06.014.
6. Sundberg JP, Ward JM, HogenEsch H, Nikitin AY, Treuting PM, Macauley JB, et al. Training pathologists in mouse pathology. Vet Pathol. 2012;49:393–7. https://doi.org/10.1177/0300985810381244.
7. Mestas J, Hughes CCW. Of mice and not men: differences between mouse and human immunology. J Immunol. 2004;172:2731–8. https://doi.org/10.4049/jimmunol.172.5.2731.
8. Rice J. Animal models: not close enough. Nature. 2012;484:S9. https://doi.org/10.1038/nature11102.
9. van der Worp HB, Howells DW, Sena ES, Porritt MJ, Rewell S, O'Collins V, et al. Can animal models of disease reliably inform human studies? PLoS Med. 2010;7:1–8. https://doi.org/10.1371/journal.pmed.1000245.
10. Williams RO. Rodent models of arthritis: relevance for human disease. Clin Exp Immunol. 1998;114:330–2. https://doi.org/10.1046/j.1365-2249.1998.00785.x.
11. Araujo VMA, Melo IM, Lima V. Relationship between periodontitis and rheumatoid arthritis: review of the literature. Mediat Inflamm. 2015;2015:259074. https://doi.org/10.1155/2015/259074.
12. Brusca SB, Abramson SB, Scher JU. Microbiome and mucosal inflammation as extra-articular triggers for rheumatoid arthritis and autoimmunity. Curr Opin Rheumatol. 2014;26:101–7. https://doi.org/10.1097/BOR.0000000000000008.
13. Izui S, Eisenberg RA, Dixon FJ. IgM rheumatoid factors in mice injected with bacterial lipopolysaccharides. J Immunol. 1979;122:2096–102. http://www.ncbi.nlm.nih.gov/pubmed/376732.
14. Bendele A. Animal models of rheumatoid arthritis. J Musculoskelet Neuronal Interact. 2001;1:377–85.
15. Rosen A, Casciola-Rosen L. Autoantigens as partners in initiation and propagation of autoimmune rheumatic diseases. Annu Rev Immunol. 2016;34:395–420. https://doi.org/10.1146/annurev-immunol-032414-112205.
16. Jacobson DL, Gange SJ, Rose NR, Graham NMH. Epidemiology and estimated population burden of selected autoimmune diseases in the United States. Clin Immunol Immunopathol. 1997;84:223–43. https://doi.org/10.1006/clin.1997.4412.
17. Traherne JA. Human MHC architecture and evolution: implications for disease association studies. Int J Immunogenet. 2008;35:179–92. https://doi.org/10.1111/j.1744-313X.2008.00765.x.
18. Firestein G, Panayi G, Wollheim F, editors. Rheumatoid arthritis. 2nd ed. New York: Oxford University Press; 2006.
19. Fries JF, Williams CA, Morfeld D, Singh G, Sibley J. Reduction in long-term disability in patients with rheumatoid arthritis by disease-modifying antirheumatic drug-based treatment strategies. Arthritis Rheum. 1996;39:616–22. https://doi.org/10.1002/art.1780390412.
20. Asquith DL, Miller AM, McInnes IB, Liew FY. Animal models of rheumatoid arthritis. Eur J Immunol. 2009;39:2040–4. https://doi.org/10.1002/eji.200939578.
21. Wooley PH, Luthra HS, Stuart JM, David CS. Type II collagen-induced arthritis in mice. I. Major histocompatibility complex (I region) linkage and antibody correlates. J Exp Med. 1981;154:688–700. https://doi.org/10.1002/art.1780270907.
22. Seki N, Sudo Y, Yoshioka T. Type II collagen-induced murine arthritis. I. Induction and perpetuation of arthritis require synergy between humoral and cell-mediated immunity. J Immunol. 1988;140:1477–84. http://www.jimmunol.org/content/140/5/1477.short.
23. Kollias G, Papadaki P, Apparailly F, Vervoordeldonk MJ, Holmdahl R, Baumans V, et al. Animal models for arthritis: innovative tools for prevention and treatment. Ann Rheum Dis. 2011;70:1357–62. https://doi.org/10.1136/ard.2010.148551.
24. Trombone APF, Ferreira SB, Raimundo FM, De Moura KCR, Avila-Campos MJ, Silva JS, et al. Experimental periodontitis in mice selected for maximal or minimal inflammatory reactions: increased inflammatory immune responsiveness drives increased alveolar bone loss without enhancing the control of periodontal infection. J Periodontal Res. 2009;44:443–51. https://doi.org/10.1111/j.1600-0765.2008.01133.x.
25. Hörmannsperger G, Schaubeck M, Haller D. Intestinal microbiota in animal models of inflammatory diseases. ILAR J. 2015;56:179–91. https://doi.org/10.1093/ilar/ilv019.
26. Rath HC, Herfarth HH, Ikeda JS, Grenther WB, Hamm TE, Balish E, et al. Normal luminal bacteria, especially bacteroides species, mediate chronic colitis, gastritis, and arthritis in HLA-B27/human β2 microglobulin transgenic rats. J Clin Investig. 1996;98:945–53. https://doi.org/10.1172/JCI118878.
27. Berer K, Mues M, Koutrolos M, Rasbi ZA, Boziki M, Johner C, et al. Commensal microbiota and myelin

autoantigen cooperate to trigger autoimmune demyelination - with comments. Nature. 2011;479:538–41. https://doi.org/10.1038/nature10554.

28. Wu HJ, Wu E. The role of gut microbiota in immune homeostasis and autoimmunity. Gut Microbes. 2012;3:4–14. https://doi.org/10.4161/gmic.19320.
29. Rehaume L, Mondot S, De Carcer DA, Velasco J, Benham H, Hasnain S, et al. Host genetic background disrupts the relationship between microbiota and gut mucosal tolerance leading to spondyloarthritis and ileitis after a dectin-1 trigger. Arthritis Rheum. 2013;65:S1152. http://bf4dv7zn3u.search.serialssolutions.com.myaccess.library.utoronto.ca/?url_ver=Z39.88-2004&rft_val_fmt=info:ofi/fmt:kev:mtx:journal&rfr_id=info:sid/Ovid:emed12&rft.genre=article&rft_id=info:doi/10.1002%2Fart.38216&rft_id=info:pmid/&rft.issn=0004-3591.
30. Alam C, Bittoun E, Bhagwat D, Valkonen S, Saari A, Jaakkola U, et al. Effects of a germ-free environment on gut immune regulation and diabetes progression in non-obese diabetic (NOD) mice. Diabetologia. 2011;54:1398–406. https://doi.org/10.1007/s00125-011-2097-5.
31. Bjork J, Kleinau S, Midtvedt T, Klareskog L, Smedegard G. Role of the bowel flora for development of immunity to hsp 65 and arthritis in three experimental models. Scand J Immunol. 1994;40:648–52. https://doi.org/10.1111/j.1365-3083.1994.tb03518.x.
32. Taurog JD, Richardson JA, Croft JT, Simmons WA, Zhou M, Fernández-Sueiro JL, et al. The germfree state prevents development of gut and joint inflammatory disease in HLA-B27 transgenic rats. J Exp Med. 1994;180:2359–64. https://doi.org/10.1084/jem.180.6.2359.
33. Breban M. Immunopathologie actuelle. Rev Rhum Monogr. 2014;81:235–9. https://doi.org/10.1016/j.monrhu.2014.06.002.
34. Liu X, Zeng B, Zhang J, Li W, Mou F, Wang H, et al. Role of the gut microbiome in modulating arthritis progression in mice. Sci Rep. 2016;6:30594. https://doi.org/10.1038/srep30594.
35. Kohashi O, Kohashi Y, Takahashi T, Ozawa A, Shigematsu N. Reverse effect of gram positive bacteria vs. gram negative Bacteria on adjuvant induced arthritis in germfree rats. Microbiol Immunol. 1985;29:487–97. https://doi.org/10.1111/j.1348-0421.1985.tb00851.x.
36. Van Den Broek MF, Van Bruggen MCJ, Koopman JP, Hazenberg MP, Van Den Berg WB. Gut flora induces and maintains resistance against streptococcal cell wall-induced arthritis in F344 rats. Clin Exp Immunol. 1992;88:313–7. https://doi.org/10.1111/j.1365-2249.1992.tb03079.x.
37. Pils MC, Bleich A, Prinz I, Fasnacht N, Bollati-Fogolin M, Schippers A, et al. Commensal gut flora reduces susceptibility to experimentally induced colitis via T-cell-derived interleukin-10. Inflamm Bowel Dis. 2011;17:2038–46. https://doi.org/10.1002/ibd.21587.
38. Thompson SJ, Thompson HS, Harper N, Day MJ, Coad AJ, Elson CJ, et al. Prevention of pristane-induced arthritis by the oral administration of type II collagen. Immunology. 1993;79:152–7. http://www.pubmedcentral.nih.gov/articlerender.fcgi?artid=1422061&tool=pmcentrez&rendertype=abstract.
39. Thompson SJ, Elson CJ. Susceptibility to pristane-induced arthritis is altered with changes in bowel flora. Immunol Lett. 1993;36:227–31. https://doi.org/10.1016/0165-2478(93)90057-9.
40. Beura LK, Hamilton SE, Bi K, Schenkel JM, Odumade OA, Casey KA, et al. Normalizing the environment recapitulates adult human immune traits in laboratory mice. Nature. 2016;532:512–6. https://doi.org/10.1038/nature17655.
41. Roudier J. Association of MHC and rheumatoid arthritis. Association of RA with HLA-DR4: the role of repertoire selection. Arthritis Res. 2000;2:217–20. https://doi.org/10.1186/ar91.

Part III

Infectious Agents

Lyme Disease: Infectious and Noninfectious Features

7

Arthur Weinstein

Abbreviations

CDC US Centers for Disease Control and Prevention
ELISA Enzyme-linked immunosorbent assay
EM Erythema migrans
HLA Human leukocyte antigen
JIA Juvenile idiopathic arthritis
LA Lyme arthritis
LD Lyme disease
LN Lyme neuroborreliosis
PCR Polymerase chain reaction
RA Rheumatoid arthritis

History

In the mid-1970s, there was a peculiar cluster of what appeared to be cases of juvenile idiopathic arthritis (JIA) occurring in the city of Lyme, Connecticut, as well as in two nearby communities. What set off alarm bells was the large number of cases occurring in a limited geographic distribution in a town with a population at the time of 5000, with several cases occurring on the same city block and even the same household [1]. These cases were brought to the attention of a postdoctoral fellow in rheumatology named Allen Steere, who suspected an infectious etiology, although the causative organism was not identified in this original report. Since 25% of the cases also presented with a preceding rash consistent with erythema migrans (EM), already known to be associated with the *Ixodes* tick, an association between these two entities was postulated. Thus, the term Lyme disease (LD) was introduced in 1977 [1]. Four years later, Willy Burgdorfer analyzed the midguts of several *Ixodes dammini* ticks, finding spirochetes in several of them; he also reported that patients with LD had antibodies against them. Thus, the bacteria were given the name *Borrelia burgdorferi*, and it was correctly identified as the causative agent of LD [2]. Since then, substantial progress has been made toward the recognition, diagnosis, and management of this disorder.

A. Weinstein
Clinical Professor Emeritus of Medicine,
Georgetown University, Washington, DC, USA
e-mail: aw89@georgetown.edu

Epidemiology

LD is the most common tick-borne infection in the United States. The numbers reported to the Centers for Disease Control and Prevention (CDC) have remained fairly constant over the past few years at about 25–30,000 per annum (CDC. Reported cases of Lyme disease by year, United States, 2003–2012. 2013. www.cdc.gov/lyme/stats/chartstables/casesbyyear.html, accessed 12/18/2017). However, a CDC analysis

G. Ragab et al. (eds.), *The Microbiome in Rheumatic Diseases and Infection*,
https://doi.org/10.1007/978-3-319-79026-8_7

of medical claim information from a large insurance database suggests that physician diagnosed LD yearly may be up to ten times that reported to the CDC [3]. In the United States, the prevalence remains highest in the Northeast, in the mid-Atlantic region, in the upper Midwest around the Great Lakes, and in the Pacific Northwest, with a small number of states—Connecticut, Massachusetts, Rhode Island, New York, New Jersey, Pennsylvania, Delaware, Maryland, Virginia, Wisconsin, and Minnesota—accounting for about 90% of reported cases. As in the United States, certain areas in Europe such as Sweden [4], Austria, Estonia, Lithuania, the Netherlands, and Slovenia are at higher risk than others [5], although the European literature also postulates under-reporting [6]. There appears to be a bimodal age distribution, with peaks around 5–10 years of age and another from 35–55 years, likely reflecting ages in which humans are most likely to be outdoors [7]. There is a fairly even sex distribution of cases.

Borrelia burgdorferi spp. and Its Transmission

Ixodes ticks transmit *Borrelia* spp. wherever in the world Lyme disease is found. This includes *I. scapularis* in the Northeast, mid-Atlantic, and upper Midwest and *I. pacificus* in the Western United States. Animal reservoir species include small mammals, particularly the white-footed mouse *Peromyscus leucopus* [8].

The *Borrelia* genus are spirochetal bacteria (phylum: *Spirochaetales*) that comprises approximately 20 different species, three of which are most responsible for clinical manifestations of infection: *B. burgdorferi*, *B. afzelii*, and *B. garinii*; the former is mostly responsible for the disease in the United States, while the latter two are largely responsible for the disease in Europe [9]. These bacteria do not directly infect humans but rather can only do so following the bite of the *Ixodes* tick. Despite generally being referred to as a "deer tick," *Ixodes* does not actually feed on deer until its adult life; however, the deer is essential for its life cycle, as this is where mating takes place [10]. As reviewed [10], there are three stages to the *Ixodes* life cycle, with one meal per stage. Adult ticks mate while attached to the deer and then drop to the ground to release their eggs. The eggs themselves are not infected with *Borrelia*, so they hatch into uninfected larvae (first part of life cycle). The larvae feed upon a variety of small animals, including mice, squirrels, and birds. If the host animal happens to be infected with *Borrelia*, the larva will then acquire these bacteria as well. After its meal, regardless of whether it has acquired *Borrelia*, the larva drops to the ground and molts into a nymph (second part of life cycle). The nymph will retain any *Borrelia* acquired as a larva. Like its larva predecessor, the nymph will feed on small animals, the same type of animals infected by the larva. In this manner, the nymph can transmit the bacteria to these animals, thus ensuring reservoirs of infection for the next generation of larva. Nymphs can also feed on humans (and dogs), thus transmitting the infection. The nymph part of the life cycle generally takes place from May through early July, which therefore represents the most likely time for humans to be infected with *Borrelia* [11, 12]. Following their blood meal, nymphs molt into adults (third part of life cycle), which generally feed on large animals such as deer. Adult ticks are generally not considered to be infectious, as deer do not maintain *Borrelia* as efficiently as do the smaller animals. However, as noted above, they are essential for the life cycle, as this is where mating takes place.

Genospecies and Virulence

There are numerous borrelial genospecies, but the most important for the transmission of clinical disease to humans are the under the *B. burgdorferi* sensu lato complex. This includes *B. burgdorferi* sensu stricto, the important genospecies in the United States and Europe, as well as two other species which also cause disease in Europe—*B. afzelii* and *B. garinii*—commonly associated with rashes and neurologic involvement, respectively. In addition, a provisionally named species that causes Lyme borreliosis, *candidatus B. mayonii*, has been recently described from Minnesota in the United States [13]. *Borrelia* spp. are spirochetes with a complex genomic structure consisting of linear chromosomes and linear and circular plasmids [14]. This genetic heterogeneity contributes to antigenic heterogeneity that changes with initial infection and subsequent dissemination. It also likely accounts for virulence factors which lead to differing genospecific invasive potentials and thus differences in disease expression [15, 16].

Mechanism of Transmission

Borrelia spirochetes are resident in the tick midgut. With tick attachment to the host skin and ingestion of a blood meal, the bacteria replicate and migrate through the tick wall and disseminate into the hemocoele and eventually to the salivary glands from which site they are injected into the skin. This process is consequential since it takes 48–72 h for its completion [17, 18]. This is also the time frame for tick engorgement with blood. Therefore, early removal of unengorged ticks is much less likely to result in clinical disease although infection has been occasionally described with shorter duration of attachment.

Potential Role of the Tick Microbiome

Researchers at Yale University have investigated the role of gut microbiota of *I. scapularis* ticks in the efficiency of *B. burgdorferi* to colonize the tick gut epithelium. Perturbation of the larval tick microbiome resulted in decreased *B. burgdorferi* colonization possibly through modulation and decrease of tick transcription factor signal transducer and activator of transcription (STAT) levels and alteration of the gut barrier integrity [19, 20]. The potential clinical or therapeutic implications of these observations are uncertain.

Infectious Features of Early Lyme Disease

Because nymphal ticks are the most common transmission vector, the early features of LD occur most frequently in late spring through the summer and early fall when nymphs are most actively seeking a blood meal. In most cases, borrelial organisms have been detected by culture or borrelial DNA/RNA by polymerase chain reaction (PCR) in blood or affected tissue/fluid, supporting the infectious nature of these manifestations [21–23]. However, clinical diagnosis is generally made without microbiological support as described in section "Lyme Disease Diagnosis".

Erythema Migrans (EM) and Other Rashes

EM is the commonest clinical feature of LD affecting about 70% of reported cases [8, 24]. The true incidence of EM may be significantly higher based on cohort and epidemiological studies. One reason for this is that tick attachment and EM are usually asymptomatic, except for mild pruritus in some cases, and bites may occur at sites not easily visible such as the back or back of the leg. It begins as an erythematous macule or papule within 2 weeks at the site of tick attachment. A cardinal feature of EM is erythematous expansion within days to weeks with or without central clearing. Rarely a vesicular center or ulceration may be seen. The rash generally fades without sequelae. Secondary lesions (disseminated EM) are found in about 20% of patients and are due to hematogenous dissemination of the spirochete. Skin culture positivity and detection of *B. burgdorferi* DNA by PCR at the margin of EM lesions support the infectious nature of this clinical presentation [21]. EM-like lesions not caused by *Borrelia* have been described in the United States. Specifically, in the Southern United States, where LD is rare, the *Amblyomma americanum* tick can spread unknown bacteria that results in a rash clinically indistinguishable from EM called Southern Tick-Associated Rash Illness (STARI), which does not appear to respond well to anti-*borrelial* therapy [25], but which does not necessarily require specific therapy. Other cutaneous lesions including borrelial lymphocytoma (early) and acrodermatitis chronica atrophicans (late) are seen in Europe [26, 27]. The latter is usually caused by *B. afzelii* and is thus more commonly seen in Europe than in the United States; it is characterized by a slowly progressive rash on the extensor surfaces of the extremities frequently occurring at a site of a previous EM rash [9]. At its onset, it typically manifests as bluish-red discoloration with swelling and can enlarge over months to years, eventually resolving with atrophy [6, 8]. In some cases, morphea-like lesions can also occur; this as well appears to be more common in Europe than in the United States [28].

Lyme Neuroborreliosis (LN)

Neurologic features occur with disseminated LD and are seen within weeks to months after a tick bite, especially in patients who were not treated at an earlier stage because EM was not present or not noted or because of misdiagnosis. LN occurs in about 15% of patients with LD and is even commoner in Europe because of the neurotropism of *B. garinii* [8, 24, 29]. The commonest manifestation is cranial neuritis, especially 7th nerve palsy, mimicking Bell's palsy of viral origin. Bilateral facial involvement may occur and is a hallmark of LN. Other neurological features, which may occur simultaneously or separately, include lymphocytic meningitis and painful radiculoneuropathies, motor or sensory. The triad of these three features was described by Bannwarth in the 1940s long before the etiology became known [30].

Other Clinical Features

Lyme carditis is another well-recognized feature of early bacterial dissemination but is now an unusual clinical feature, accounting for only 1% of reported cases. High-grade atrioventricular nodal block (second and third degree) may be seen with accompanying symptoms, even fatality. Acute myopericarditis may rarely occur [8].

Acutely, flu-like constitutional symptoms with predominate headache, myalgias, and arthralgias may occur especially with dissemination. This may be the only early feature of borrelial infection, seen in about 15% of patients, and the presence of these symptoms in a Lyme endemic area in the summertime should raise the suspicion of LD [31].

While LA is considered a late feature of LD when presenting as a monoarthritis, it often begins as an early feature of disseminated infection with intermittent and migratory joint pains, with or without signs of inflammation. During this phase, unusual musculoskeletal features may be seen, including bursitis, tendinitis, temporomandibular joint involvement, and carpal tunnel syndrome. Left untreated, this will eventually evolve to classical LA [32, 33].

Numerous other clinical features have been attributed to LD for which there is incomplete or unconvincing microbiological support. However, ocular complications, including uveitis and keratitis, may rarely occur with borrelial infection.

Infectious Features of Late Lyme Disease

These complications generally occur in borrelial infected individuals who have never received appropriate antibiotic therapy for early LD, often because the early features were unrecognized or misdiagnosed. Appropriate treatment of early LD almost invariably prevents these later features. Microbiological support for many of the later features is often wanting, and even positive PCR results for borrelial DNA in synovial fluid of patients with LA may represent nonviable organisms [34]. Despite this, the diagnosis can be made with a good degree of accuracy by clinical features and laboratory testing for antibodies to borrelial antigens as described below.

Lyme Arthritis

If early borrelial infection is left untreated, about 60% of patients in the United States will develop LA [33]. This late feature usually presents many months after the initial infection and thus may occur in the winter, when early Lyme disease diagnosis is distinctly unusual. Most patients have an inflammatory arthritis affecting one or both knees. The synovial fluid is inflammatory. If the features of early Lyme disease were not present and if a prior history of migrating joint pains was not elicited, then the diagnosis of Lyme arthritis might be missed and other causes of infectious arthritis, idiopathic inflammatory arthritis (including JIA in children), and even crystal arthropathy in the elderly will be considered. Although the pathogenesis is clearly infectious with most patients responding to oral or parenteral antibiotics, it is of interest that viable borrelial organisms are not cultivable from the synovial fluid. Rarely spirochetes may be found in the synovium or enmeshed in a fibrinous synovial exudate. There is evidence that borrelial-triggered inflammations, involving both the innate and adaptive immune systems, are key elements in the pathogenesis of the inflammatory arthritis [33]. Clinically, the onset is often acute, with a marked knee effusion and elevated acute phase reactants. Symptomatic response to antibiotic therapy is seen to occur slowly over weeks to months since the large effusion has resulted in a mechanically disadvantaged knee joint. Physical therapy with quadriceps muscle strengthening can help with rehabilitation.

Late Lyme Neuroborreliosis

True late LN is unusual in the United States, and in fact there is considerable skepticism regarding the diagnosis without adherence to diagnostic guidelines, which include the appropriate clinical picture, often encephalomyelitis with cognitive dysfunction, sleep disturbances, and mood changes, and demonstration of positive intrathecal anti-*Bb* antibody index, often with cerebrospinal fluid (CSF) pleocytosis and/or increased CSF protein [35, 36]. Of course, most patients also have high titers of serum antibodies to *B. burgdorferi*. A chronic distal axonal neuropathy has also been described leading mainly to sensory paresthesias. A much broader variety of more severe neurological complications has been described in Europe, including cranial nerve palsies and paraparesis because of the neurotropism of *B. garinii*. Parenteral antibiotics are recommended for LN, early and late [37].

Noninfectious Features of Lyme Disease

These clinical conditions are associated with prior Lyme disease infection. The causes are not confirmed although it is highly likely that immunological mechanisms play a role in antibiotic-refractory Lyme arthritis.

Recurrent Arthritis: Antibiotic-Refractory Lyme Arthritis

While LA may take many months to resolve after antibiotic therapy, it resolves completely in about 90% of patients. However, in about 10% of patients, joint swelling and pain will recur or persist for months to years. This usually involves the same joint(s) as the original LA, that is, one or both knees [32]. Viable organisms are not found in the synovium or synovial fluid from these joints, and PCR for borrelial DNA is generally negative. Patients with this syndrome have an increased carriage of certain rheumatoid arthritis-associated human leukocyte antigen (HLA) alleles, including HLA-DRB1*0401 and *0101, as well as others, supporting an immunological predisposition [38]. Furthermore, these HLA alleles demonstrated greater capacity to present Borrelia-associated peptides, as compared to HLA alleles not associated with chronic LA, thereby suggesting a mechanism by which infection may progress to chronic arthritis [38]. Autoreactive B and T cell responses can be detected in both antibiotic-responsive and antibiotic-refractory Lyme arthritis, but in antibiotic-refractory Lyme arthritis, there are a number of other immunological features including Th1 inflammatory responses, altered regulatory T cell numbers, and possibly autoimmunity to endothelial cell growth factor [39, 40]. This condition does not respond to repeated or prolonged courses of oral or parenteral antibiotics. Patients can respond to local treatment, including intra-articular corticosteroid injections or synovectomy, or to systemic antirheumatic drugs such as hydroxychloroquine, sulfasalazine, and methotrexate. Eventual resolution is the rule after many months or years [41].

Other Systemic Rheumatic Syndromes Following Lyme Disease

Some patients have been characterized as developing rheumatoid arthritis (RA), psoriatic arthritis, or peripheral spondyloarthropathy months after antibiotic-treated Lyme disease infection [42]. These patients, while clinically resembling autoimmune arthritis, had some serological features that were atypical, including a lack of rheumatoid factor and antibodies to citrullinated proteins in most of the RA patients. Furthermore, four subjects have obtained a drug-free remission. This raises the possibility that at least some of these patients may have an illness in the spectrum of antibiotic-refractory Lyme arthritis.

Posttreatment Lyme Disease Symptoms and Syndrome

A significant minority of patients, from 10% to 15% in clinical trials, have reported residual subjective symptoms following treatment for Lyme disease [43, 44]. In many, these symptoms eventually resolve spontaneously, although some patients have persistent complaints (>6 months). These symptoms are some combination of fatigue, musculoskeletal pain (myalgia and arthralgia), headache, difficulty with concentration and memory, and paresthesias. Although subjective and without physical findings or testing that support structural abnormalities, these complaints can result in significant disability. Since these symptoms are common in the general population, it remains uncertain whether they are truly reflective of prior Lyme disease with some studies supporting that hypothesis [45] and others not [43, 46]. There is no convincing evidence in controlled trials that patients with post-Lyme disease syndrome have ongoing borrelial infection, and they do not respond to aggressive and prolonged antibiotic therapy [47–49]. The cause remains unknown, the symptoms tend to wax and wane chronically, and treatment has been symptomatic.

Controversies Surrounding Chronic Lyme Disease

This widely used term is poorly defined [50, 51]. It should be distinguished from late Lyme disease manifestations. While sometimes referring to posttreatment Lyme disease syndrome as described above, many patients with these clinical symptoms have no clear-cut evidence of prior borrelial infection. The belief that LD is the cause of these symptoms despite evidence to the contrary has been perpetuated by **scientific misconceptions and distortions** including the propensity of LD to cause disability in the absence of objective clinical signs, the insensitivity of currently accepted diagnostic tests for even late features of Lyme disease, the persistence of *B. burgdorferi* within cells or in hidden sites, and the effectiveness of prolonged (months to years) treatments with combinations of antibiotics or alternative and sometimes harmful therapies [52]. Patient advocacy groups, physician proponents, the media (both traditional and social), and even well-intentioned but misled politicians have contributed to these unfortunate pseudoscientific beliefs [53].

Lyme Disease Diagnosis

Principles of Diagnosis

In early LD, positive bacterial cultures can be obtained from the skin, the cerebrospinal spinal fluid, and the blood. However, the yield is low, and cultivation takes many weeks making it an impractical method of diagnosis. The use of PCR to detect the DNA or RNA of viable organisms has proven disappointing because of low yield (blood, spinal fluid) or positivity in the presence of nonviable *Borrelia* (synovial fluid) [21–23, 34].

Therefore, the laboratory methods to support the clinical diagnosis of Lyme disease are indirect and employ serological testing of the immune response to the *Borrelia*. Since antibody responses to an infecting organism may take days to weeks to develop, may not develop at all if early effective treatment is instituted, and may persist for many years after the infection is eradicated, this must be kept in mind when interpreting the "Lyme test" results. Another important feature of the antibody response to *Borrelia*, similar to other infections, is that IgM responses are seen first acutely and IgG antibodies appear weeks to months later with persisting, untreated infection and most commonly with simultaneous diminution of the IgM antibodies.

The standard way to screen for antibodies to *Borrelia* is by a sensitive enzyme-linked immunosorbent assay (ELISA), which detects both IgM and IgG antibodies. Because of the poor specificity of this test, any positive or equivocal result should be followed by the more specific Western blot assay according to the guidelines of the Centers for Disease Control and Prevention [54]. Specifically, false-positive results can result from a variety of causes, including infections with other members of the Spirochaete phyla, the *Borrelia* genus, and even unrelated infections and normal host microbiota [55, 56], as well as from patients with autoimmune diseases such as lupus and rheumatoid arthritis [57]. This two-tiered testing approach has been studied and used for over two decades, for the most part with good success. In these guidelines, an IgM Western blot is positive when any two of the 23 kD, 39 kD, or 41 kD bands are present. An IgG Western blot is positive when any five of the 18 kD, 23 kD, 28 kD, 30 kD, 39 kD, 41 kD, 45 kD, 60 kD, 66 kD, or 93 kD bands are present. Since the criteria for a positive IgG Western blot are much more stringent than for a positive IgM Western blot, it is a much more specific result indicating prior or current exposure to the *borrelial* organism. Patients with late Lyme arthritis almost always exhibit strongly positive IgG Western blots [58].

Single-tiered testing using the C6 peptide antigen of the VlsE borrelial protein has proven to be sensitive and specific for the diagnosis of Lyme disease, reduces the problem of misinterpretation of IgM Western blot results (see below), and is commercially available [59, 60]. It may be particularly advantageous in Europe, as the two-tiered approach appears to be somewhat less sensitive for the detection of the European strains *B. garinii* and *B. afzelii* as compared to *B. burgdorferi* [61].

The CSF is the only body fluid in addition to serum where antibody testing is of proven value. The finding of a high Lyme antibody index, based on the ratio of antibodies in the CSF to serum, can support the diagnosis of neuroborreliosis [35].

Diagnostic Pitfalls

Because antibodies may not be detected in the blood for days to weeks after initial borrelial infection, a negative Lyme ELISA in patients with very early symptoms does not rule out Lyme disease as a cause. Therefore, a patient who presents with classical symptoms beginning with EM in a Lyme disease endemic area in the spring and summer months should be treated for Lyme disease, even without serological testing. On the other hand, since antibodies will eventually appear in untreated patients and even in many patients who have received antibiotics, it may be worthwhile to repeat the test 3–4 weeks later in patients with atypical symptoms such as summer flu or facial palsy without EM to determine if seroconversion has occurred.

A major diagnostic problem is the misuse and misinterpretation of the IgM Western blot result. The criteria were devised for sensitivity for early Lyme disease when the IgG antibodies may not have yet appeared, but not for specificity. Thus, a positive IgM result may indicate early Lyme disease when used in the first 4–6 weeks of symptom onset. In patients with prolonged symptoms, a positive IgM Western blot in the absence of a positive IgG Western blot is more likely to be a false positive and does not indicate Lyme disease infection [62]. Many patients with chronic non-specific symptoms or symptoms of an alternative diagnosis have been labeled as chronic Lyme disease because of a false-positive IgM Western blot result.

Treatment and Prevention of Lyme Disease

Since the first treatment trials of Lyme borreliosis, the organism has not developed resistance to doxycycline or amoxicillin, which remain the mainstays of treatment in adults and young children, respectively. Extensive treatment guidelines have been published by the Infectious Disease Society of North America [63]. In general, one course of oral antibiotics from 2 to 4 weeks is usually sufficient to cure early Lyme disease and prevent later complications [64]. Neuroborreliosis may require intravenous ceftriaxone therapy. Late LA usually responds to one 4-week course of antibiotics, but a second course is sometimes required, e.g., parenteral ceftriaxone. Non-responsiveness to more than two courses of antibiotics suggests alternative diagnoses such as antibiotic-refractory LA or post-Lyme disease syndrome. Rarely, a confounding factor in treatment may be related to coinfection with other organisms such as *Anaplasma phagocytophilum* (which responds to doxycycline), *Babesia microti*, and *Borrelia miyamotoi* or a Powassan virus, all carried by the *Ixodes* tick [63, 65].

Prevention of LD has many approaches, including wearing protective clothing as well as the use of tick repellants. However, most effective is undergoing inspection for ticks and removal when found after being in grassy areas in a Lyme disease endemic region. Removal of ticks prior to their engorgement markedly reduces the likelihood of transmission of *B. burgdorferi* to the skin [66]. Attempted removal of the tick should be done with caution, since the application of torque to the offending tick may result in its decapitation, while nevertheless enabling its mouth to remain embedded in the skin and transmit the disease [67]; crushing the tick may also allow infective agents in its body to enter the bloodstream [67]. Furthermore, one dose of doxycycline 200 mg within 72 h of tick attachment greatly reduces the chance of developing Lyme disease [68]. Although vaccines were developed for Lyme disease and were shown to be relatively effective and safe, none is currently on the market [69, 70].

Conclusions

LD is a tick-borne bacterial infection largely limited to endemic areas in the Northeastern United States and in parts of Europe. The manifestations are protean, and in the absence of the distinctive rash, the diagnosis can be missed. The causative bacteria are highly sensitive to several antibiotics, resulting in generally good outcomes in patients treated during the early localized or early disseminated phase [12]. LD has the potential to develop into an arthritic process, which appears to begin as an infected joint but can evolve into a chronic reactive process. Lessons learned from this illness may help us better understand the pathophysiology of postinfectious and possibly other forms of idiopathic arthritis.

References

1. Steere AC, Malawista SE, Snydman DR, Shope RE, Andiman WA, Ross MR, et al. Lyme arthritis: an epidemic of oligoarticular arthritis in children and adults in three connecticut communities. Arthritis Rheum. 1977;20:7–17.
2. Burgdorfer W. How the discovery of Borrelia burgdorferi came about. Clin Dermatol. 1993;11:335–8.
3. Kuehn BM. CDC estimates 300,000 US cases of Lyme disease annually. JAMA. 2013;310:1110.
4. Orczyk K, Swidrowska-Jaros J, Smolewska E. When a patient suspected with juvenile idiopathic arthritis turns out to be diagnosed with an infectious disease – a review of Lyme arthritis in children. Pediatr Rheumatol Online J. 2017;15:35.
5. Mead PS. Epidemiology of Lyme disease. Infect Dis Clin N Am. 2015;29:187–210.
6. Hofmann H, Fingerle V, Hunfeld KP, Huppertz HI, Krause A, Rauer S, et al. Cutaneous Lyme borreliosis: guideline of the German Dermatology Society. Ger Med Sci. 2017;15:Doc14.
7. Bacon RM, Kugeler KJ, Mead PS, Centers for Disease C, Prevention. Surveillance for Lyme disease – United States, 1992-2006. MMWR Surveill Summ. 2008;57:1–9.

8. Stanek G, Strle F. Lyme borreliosis. Lancet. 2003;362:1639–47.
9. Steere AC, Strle F, Wormser GP, Hu LT, Branda JA, Hovius JW, et al. Lyme borreliosis. Nat Rev Dis Primers. 2016;2:16090.
10. Radolf JD, Caimano MJ, Stevenson B, Hu LT. Of ticks, mice and men: understanding the dual-host lifestyle of Lyme disease spirochaetes. Nat Rev Microbiol. 2012;10:87–99.
11. Anderson JF. Ecology of Lyme disease. Conn Med. 1989;53:343–6.
12. Kowalski TJ, Tata S, Berth W, Mathiason MA, Agger WA. Antibiotic treatment duration and long-term outcomes of patients with early Lyme disease from a Lyme disease-hyperendemic area. Clin Infect Dis. 2010;50:512–20.
13. Pritt BS, Mead PS, Johnson DKH, Neitzel DF, Respicio-Kingry LB, Davis JP, et al. Identification of a novel pathogenic Borrelia species causing Lyme borreliosis with unusually high spirochaetaemia: a descriptive study. Lancet Infect Dis. 2016;16:556–64.
14. Brisson D, Drecktrah D, Eggers CH, Samuels DS. Genetics of Borrelia burgdorferi. Annu Rev Genet. 2012;46:515–36.
15. Wormser GP, Brisson D, Liveris D, Hanincova K, Sandigursky S, Nowakowski J, et al. Borrelia burgdorferi genotype predicts the capacity for hematogenous dissemination during early Lyme disease. J Infect Dis. 2008;198:1358–64.
16. Baranton G, De Martino SJ. Borrelia burgdorferi sensu lato diversity and its influence on pathogenicity in humans. Curr Probl Dermatol. 2009;37:1–17.
17. Piesman J, Gern L. Lyme borreliosis in Europe and North America. Parasitology. 2004;129(Suppl):S191–220.
18. Des Vignes F, Piesman J, Heffernan R, Schulze TL, Stafford KC 3rd, Fish D. Effect of tick removal on transmission of Borrelia burgdorferi and Ehrlichia phagocytophila by Ixodes scapularis nymphs. J Infect Dis. 2001;183:773–8.
19. Narasimhan S, Rajeevan N, Liu L, Zhao YO, Heisig J, Pan J, et al. Gut microbiota of the tick vector Ixodes scapularis modulate colonization of the Lyme disease spirochete. Cell Host Microbe. 2014;15:58–71.
20. Narasimhan S, Fikrig E. Tick microbiome: the force within. Trends Parasitol. 2015;31:315–23.
21. Liveris D, Wang G, Girao G, Byrne DW, Nowakowski J, McKenna D, et al. Quantitative detection of Borrelia burgdorferi in 2-millimeter skin samples of erythema migrans lesions: correlation of results with clinical and laboratory findings. J Clin Microbiol. 2002;40:1249–53.
22. Wormser GP, McKenna D, Carlin J, Nadelman RB, Cavaliere LF, Holmgren D, et al. Brief communication: hematogenous dissemination in early Lyme disease. Ann Intern Med. 2005;142:751–5.
23. Nocton JJ, Dressler F, Rutledge BJ, Rys PN, Persing DH, Steere AC. Detection of Borrelia burgdorferi DNA by polymerase chain reaction in synovial fluid from patients with Lyme arthritis. N Engl J Med. 1994;330:229–34.
24. Borchers AT, Keen CL, Huntley AC, Gershwin ME. Lyme disease: a rigorous review of diagnostic criteria and treatment. J Autoimmun. 2015;57:82–115.
25. Goddard J. Not all erythema migrans lesions are Lyme disease. Am J Med. 2017;130:231–3.
26. Asbrink E, Hovmark A, Olsson I. Clinical manifestations of acrodermatitis chronica atrophicans in 50 Swedish patients. Zentralbl Bakteriol Mikrobiol HygA. 1986;263:253–61.
27. Berglund J, Eitrem R, Ornstein K, Lindberg A, Ringer A, Elmrud H, et al. An epidemiologic study of Lyme disease in southern Sweden. N Engl J Med. 1995;333:1319–27.
28. Moreno C, Kutzner H, Palmedo G, Goerttler E, Carrasco L, Requena L. Interstitial granulomatous dermatitis with histiocytic pseudorosettes: a new histopathologic pattern in cutaneous borreliosis. Detection of Borrelia burgdorferi DNA sequences by a highly sensitive PCR-ELISA. J Am Acad Dermatol. 2003;48:376–84.
29. Hildenbrand P, Craven DE, Jones R, Nemeskal P. Lyme neuroborreliosis: manifestations of a rapidly emerging zoonosis. AJNR Am J Neuroradiol. 2009;30:1079–87.
30. Bannwarth A. Chronische lymphocytare meningitis, entzundliche polyneuritis und "rheumatismus" [Chronic lymphocytic meningitis, inflammatory polyneuritis and 'rheumatism']. Arch Psychiatr Nervenkr. 1941;113:284–376.
31. Aucott J, Morrison C, Munoz B, Rowe PC, Schwarzwalder A, West SK. Diagnostic challenges of early Lyme disease: lessons from a community case series. BMC Infect Dis. 2009;9:79.
32. Steere AC, Schoen RT, Taylor E. The clinical evolution of Lyme arthritis. Ann Intern Med. 1987;107:725–31.
33. Bockenstedt LK, Wormser GP. Review: unraveling Lyme disease. Arthritis Rheumatol. 2014;66:2313–23.
34. Li X, McHugh GA, Damle N, Sikand VK, Glickstein L, Steere AC. Burden and viability of Borrelia burgdorferi in skin and joints of patients with erythema migrans or Lyme arthritis. Arthritis Rheum. 2011;63:2238–47.
35. Steere AC, Berardi VP, Weeks KE, Logigian EL, Ackermann R. Evaluation of the intrathecal antibody response to Borrelia burgdorferi as a diagnostic test for Lyme neuroborreliosis. J Infect Dis. 1990;161:1203–9.
36. Hansen K, Lebech AM. The clinical and epidemiological profile of Lyme neuroborreliosis in Denmark 1985-1990. A prospective study of 187 patients with Borrelia burgdorferi specific intrathecal antibody production. Brain. 1992;115(Pt 2):399–423.
37. Koedel U, Fingerle V, Pfister HW. Lyme neuroborreliosis-epidemiology, diagnosis and management. Nat Rev Neurol. 2015;11:446–56.

38. Steere AC, Klitz W, Drouin EE, Falk BA, Kwok WW, Nepom GT, et al. Antibiotic-refractory Lyme arthritis is associated with HLA-DR molecules that bind a Borrelia burgdorferi peptide. J Exp Med. 2006;203:961–71.
39. Shin JJ, Glickstein LJ, Steere AC. High levels of inflammatory chemokines and cytokines in joint fluid and synovial tissue throughout the course of antibiotic-refractory Lyme arthritis. Arthritis Rheum. 2007;56:1325–35.
40. Vudattu NK, Strle K, Steere AC, Drouin EE. Dysregulation of CD4+CD25(high) T cells in the synovial fluid of patients with antibiotic-refractory Lyme arthritis. Arthritis Rheum. 2013;65:1643–53.
41. Steere AC, Angelis SM. Therapy for Lyme arthritis: strategies for the treatment of antibiotic-refractory arthritis. Arthritis Rheum. 2006;54:3079–86.
42. Arvikar SL, Crowley JT, Sulka KB, Steere AC. Autoimmune arthritides, rheumatoid arthritis, psoriatic arthritis, or peripheral spondyloarthritis following Lyme disease. ArthritisRheumatol. 2017;69:194–202.
43. Cerar D, Cerar T, Ruzic-Sabljic E, Wormser GP, Strle F. Subjective symptoms after treatment of early Lyme disease. Am J Med. 2010;123:79–86.
44. Shadick NA, Phillips CB, Logigian EL, Steere AC, Kaplan RF, Berardi VP, et al. The long-term clinical outcomes of Lyme disease. A population-based retrospective cohort study. Ann Intern Med. 1994;121:560–7.
45. Cairns V, Godwin J. Post-Lyme borreliosis syndrome: a meta-analysis of reported symptoms. Int J Epidemiol. 2005;34:1340–5.
46. Wormser GP, Weitzner E, McKenna D, Nadelman RB, Scavarda C, Farber S, Pakash P, Ash J, Nowakowski J. Long-term assessment of fibromyalgia in patients with cultureconfirmed Lyme disease. Arthritis Rheumatol. 2015;67:837–9.
47. Klempner MS, Hu LT, Evans J, Schmid CH, Johnson GM, Trevino RP, et al. Two controlled trials of antibiotic treatment in patients with persistent symptoms and a history of Lyme disease. N Engl J Med. 2001;345:85–92.
48. Krupp LB, Hyman LG, Grimson R, Coyle PK, Melville P, Ahnn S, et al. Study and treatment of post Lyme disease (STOP-LD): a randomized double masked clinical trial. Neurology. 2003;60: 1923–30.
49. Fallon BA, Keilp JG, Corbera KM, Petkova E, Britton CB, Dwyer E, et al. A randomized, placebo-controlled trial of repeated IV antibiotic therapy for Lyme encephalopathy. Neurology. 2008;70:992–1003.
50. Feder HM Jr, Johnson BJ, O'Connell S, Shapiro ED, Steere AC, Wormser GP, et al. A critical appraisal of "chronic Lyme disease". N Engl J Med. 2007;357:1422–30.
51. Lantos PM. Chronic Lyme disease: the controversies and the science. Expert Rev Anti-Infect Ther. 2011;9:787–97.
52. Marzec NS, Nelson C, Waldron PR, Blackburn BG, Hosain S, Greenhow T, et al. Serious bacterial infections acquired during treatment of patients given a diagnosis of chronic Lyme disease – United States. MMWR Morb Mortal Wkly Rep. 2017;66:607–9.
53. Auwaerter PG, Bakken JS, Dattwyler RJ, Dumler JS, Halperin JJ, McSweegan E, et al. Antiscience and ethical concerns associated with advocacy of Lyme disease. Lancet Infect Dis. 2011;11(9):713.
54. Centers for Disease C, Prevention. Recommendations for test performance and interpretation from the Second National Conference on Serologic Diagnosis of Lyme Disease. MMWR Morb Mortal Wkly Rep. 1995;44:590–1.
55. Magnarelli LA, Anderson JF. Enzyme-linked immunosorbent assays for the detection of class-specific immunoglobulins to Borrelia burgdorferi. Am J Epidemiol. 1988;127:818–25.
56. Magnarelli LA, Miller JN, Anderson JF, Riviere GR. Cross-reactivity of nonspecific treponemal antibody in serologic tests for Lyme disease. J Clin Microbiol. 1990;28:1276–9.
57. Weiss NL, Sadock VA, Sigal LH, Phillips M, Merryman PF, Abramson SB. False positive seroreactivity to Borrelia burgdorferi in systemic lupus erythematosus: the value of immunoblot analysis. Lupus. 1995;4:131–7.
58. Kowal K, Weinstein A. Western blot band intensity analysis. Application to the diagnosis of Lyme arthritis. Arthritis Rheum. 1994;37:1206–11.
59. Branda JA, Aguero-Rosenfeld ME, Ferraro MJ, Johnson BJ, Wormser GP, Steere AC. 2-tiered antibody testing for early and late Lyme disease using only an immunoglobulin G blot with the addition of a VlsE band as the second-tier test. Clin Infect Dis. 2010;50:20–6.
60. Wormser GP, Schriefer M, Aguero-Rosenfeld ME, Levin A, Steere AC, Nadelman RB, et al. Single-tier testing with the C6 peptide ELISA kit compared with two-tier testing for Lyme disease. Diagn Microbiol Infect Dis. 2013;75:9–15.
61. Sanchez E, Vannier E, Wormser GP, Hu LT. Diagnosis, treatment, and prevention of Lyme disease, human granulocytic anaplasmosis, and babesiosis: a review. JAMA. 2016;315:1767–77.
62. Seriburi V, Ndukwe N, Chang Z, Cox ME, Wormser GP. High frequency of false positive IgM immunoblots for Borrelia burgdorferi in clinical practice. Clin Microbiol Infect. 2012;18:1236–40.
63. Wormser GP, Dattwyler RJ, Shapiro ED, Halperin JJ, Steere AC, Klempner MS, et al. The clinical assessment, treatment, and prevention of Lyme disease, human granulocytic anaplasmosis, and babesiosis: clinical practice guidelines by the Infectious Diseases Society of America. Clin Infect Dis. 2006;43:1089–134.
64. Wormser GP, Ramanathan R, Nowakowski J, McKenna D, Holmgren D, Visintainer P, et al. Duration of antibiotic therapy for early Lyme disease.

A randomized, double-blind, placebo-controlled trial. Ann Intern Med. 2003;138:697–704.
65. Hermance ME, Thangamani S. Powassan virus: an emerging arbovirus of public health concern in North America. Vector Borne Zoonotic Dis. 2017;17:453–62.
66. Hayes EB, Piesman J. How can we prevent Lyme disease? N Engl J Med. 2003;348:2424–30.
67. Needham GR. Evaluation of five popular methods for tick removal. Pediatrics. 1985;75:997–1002.
68. Warshafsky S, Lee DH, Francois LK, Nowakowski J, Nadelman RB, Wormser GP. Efficacy of antibiotic prophylaxis for the prevention of Lyme disease: an updated systematic review and meta-analysis. J Antimicrob Chemother. 2010;65:1137–44.
69. Steere AC, Sikand VK, Meurice F, Parenti DL, Fikrig E, Schoen RT, et al. Vaccination against Lyme disease with recombinant Borrelia burgdorferi outer-surface lipoprotein A with adjuvant. Lyme Disease Vaccine Study Group. N Engl J Med. 1998;339: 209–15.
70. Plotkin SA. Need for a new Lyme disease vaccine. N Engl J Med. 2016;375:911–3.

Helicobacter pylori: Immune Responses and Gastric Autoimmunity

8

Maria Kaparakis-Liaskos and Mario M. D'Elios

Abbreviations

AIG	Autoimmune gastritis
AP	Activating protein-1
ATPase	Adenosine triphosphatase
CagA	Cytotoxin-associated protein
cagPAI	cag pathogenicity island
E. coli	*Escherichia coli*
EAIG	Experimental autoimmune gastritis
FasL	Fas ligand
GlcNAc-MurNAc	*N*-Acetyl glucosamine-*N*-acetyl muramic acid
H. pylori	*Helicobacter pylori*
HBD	Human beta-defensin
HLA	Human leukocyte antigen
HP0175	Secreted peptidyl prolyl cis, trans-isomerase of *H. pylori*
HP-NAP	*H. pylori* neutrophil-activating protein
IFN	Interferon
IL	Interleukin
IRF	IFN regulatory factor
IRFs	Interferon regulatory factors
ISGs	Interferon-stimulated genes
LPS	Lipopolysaccharide
MALT	Mucosal-associated lymphoid tissue
MAMP	Microbe-associated molecular pattern
MAPK	Mitogen-activated protein kinase
MCP	Monocyte chemotactic protein
mDAP	*Meso*-diaminopimelate
MMP	Matrix metalloproteinase
NF-κB	Nuclear factor transcription beta
NLR	Nod-like receptor
NOD	Nucleotide-binding oligomerization domain
OMVs	Outer membrane vesicles
PA	Pernicious anaemia
PgdA	Peptidoglycan deacetylase
PRR	Pathogen recognition receptor
RIG	Retinoic acid-inducible gene
TCR	T cell receptor
Th	T helper
TILs	Tumour-infiltrating lymphocytes
TLR	Toll-like receptor
TNF	Tumour necrosis factor
VacA	Vacuolating cytotoxin A

M. Kaparakis-Liaskos
La Trobe University, Melbourne, VIC, Australia
e-mail: m.liaskos@latrobe.edu.au

M. M. D'Elios (✉)
University of Florence, Florence, Italy
e-mail: delios@unifi.it

G. Ragab et al. (eds.), *The Microbiome in Rheumatic Diseases and Infection*,
https://doi.org/10.1007/978-3-319-79026-8_8

Innate Immune Sensing of *H. pylori*

The epithelium is the first line of defence in response to *H. pylori* infection. Host pathogen recognition receptors (PRRs) expressed by epithelial cells are central to initiating and mediating early innate immune responses to *H. pylori* infection. Some of the key host PRRs responsible for the recognition of *H. pylori* microbe-associated molecular patterns (MAMPs) and the subsequent induction of innate immune responses are discussed below.

Detection of *H. pylori* by TLRs

The Toll-like receptors (TLRs) are a family of PRRs that are responsible for the detection of specific MAMPs, such as the recognition of bacterial lipopolysaccharide (LPS) by TLR4, lipoproteins by TLR2 and flagella by TLR5 [1]. Detection of the specific bacterial MAMPs by TLRs results in the induction of a signalling cascade, mediated by the adaptor protein MyD88. This in turn results in the activation of the host transcription factor nuclear factor transcription beta (NF-κB), activating protein-1 (AP-1) and interferon regulatory factors (IRFs). Activation of these inflammatory signalling pathways results in the production of host pro-inflammatory molecules such as interleukin-8 (IL-8) and the release of antimicrobial peptides such as human beta-defensins (HBDs) (reviewed in [1, 2]). The induction of these PRR-mediated signalling cascades ultimately leads to the initiation of an innate immune response via the recruitment of pro-inflammatory cells and immune mediators such as neutrophils, macrophages and dendritic cells to the local tissue. Although human gastric epithelial cells express a limited number of TLRs, namely, TLR2, 4, 5 and 9 [3], TLR expression is upregulated by gastric epithelial cells during *H. pylori* infection, as is the case for TLR4 and its co-receptor MD2 [3, 4].

TLR2 and TLR4

TLR2 detects a wide range of MAMPs including lipoproteins from Gram-negative bacteria and lipoteichoic acid [1, 5], whereas TLR4 specifically detects Gram-negative LPS [6]. Despite the ability of TLRs to detect conserved bacterial MAMPs, *H. pylori* has evolved multiple strategies to avoid immune detection by host TLRs which may contribute to its long-term colonization of the host. Early studies examining the ability of *H. pylori* to mediate innate immune signalling via TLRs in gastric epithelial cells reported that *H. pylori* LPS is atypically recognized by TLR2 and not TLR4 [7–9]. This finding was further supported by studies showing that TLR2-expressing human HEK293 epithelial cells could detect *H. pylori*, whereas TLR4-expressing HEK293 cells were nonresponsive to stimulation with *H. pylori* [10, 11]. It has since been recognized that the *H. pylori* neutrophil-activating protein (HP-NAP) can mediate TLR2-driven responses, as stimulation of TLR2-expressing HEK293 cells with HP-NAP resulted in NF-κB activation in a dose-dependent and TLR2-dependent manner [12].

TLR2 has been implicated in the detection of the *H. pylori* 60 kDa heat-shock protein (HSP-60), a homologue of the *E. coli* GroEL chaperone, which has a role in regulating the attachment of *H. pylori* to the gastric epithelium in addition to its immunostimulatory role [13–16]. Stimulation of human gastric epithelial cells with *H. pylori* HSP-60 resulted in the activation of NF-κB and the production of IL-8 in a TLR-2-dependent manner [13]. However, the ability of HSP-60 to be detected by TLR2 in monocytes is not as clear as there are two conflicting findings regarding the detection of HSP-60 in monocytic cells. Gobert et al. reported that HSP-60 induced the production of IL-6 in RAW 264.7 macrophages via a TLR2-independent mechanism [17], whereas Takenaka et al. demonstrated that TLR2, TLR4 and MyD88 were required to mediate CXCL8 responses to HSP-60 in the gastric epithelial cell line Kato III [13]. Whether the requirement of TLR2 for the recognition of HSP-60 is cell line dependent or not is yet to be determined, and this may be the issue to clarify the conflicting findings.

The ability of TLR2 and TLR4 expressed by immune cells to detect and respond to *H. pylori* has also been investigated. Bone marrow-derived dendritic cells generated from TLR2 and TLR4 knockout animals have impaired IL-6 production in response to *H. pylori*, when compared to DCs from wild-type animals [18]. In contrast, the contribution of TLR2 and TLR4 expressed by macrophages in response to *Helicobacter* infection is less clear. For example, macrophages from TLR2-deficient mice were reported to be nonresponsive to *Helicobacter* stimulation [10, 19]. However, stimulation of wild-type or TLR4-deficient macrophages with *H. pylori* was shown to induce the production of IL-6 and monocyte chemotactic protein-1 (MCP-1) by these cells [10]. A second study reported that TLR4-deficient macrophages had impaired IL-10 and IL-12 production in response to *H. pylori* [19]. Differences in these two reported findings may be attributed to the examination of macrophages isolated from different locations in vivo in addition to differences between LPS-mediated responses in macrophages and epithelial cells [20].

TLR5

Another key bacterial MAMP is its flagella, which is detected by the host PRR TLR5 [21]. Although *H. pylori* expresses four to six unipolar sheathed flagella, it has modified its flagella subunits to avoid immune detection by TLR5. Initial studies examining the immunostimulatory properties of *H. pylori* flagella reported that stimulation of TLR5-expressing HEK293 with purified *H. pylori* flagellin resulted in the activation of NF-κB [9]. However, two subsequent studies reported that *H. pylori* flagellin was not detected by TLR5-expressing epithelial cells, as CXCL8 production and MAPK induction were not detected in response to flagellin stimulation, suggesting that *H. pylori* flagella is able to evade recognition by TLR5 [22, 23]. More recently, it was identified that *H. pylori* flagellin molecules cannot be sensed by TLR5 as they lack the conserved amino acids required for recognition by TLR5 [24].

TLR8 and TLR9

TLR8 and TLR9 specifically detect intracellular foreign nucleic acids, with TLR8 detecting single-stranded RNA [25] and TLR9 detecting unmethylated bacterial CpG DNA [26]. Once *H. pylori* is phagocytosed by human monocytic cells, it activates endosomal TLR8 [27]. In addition, TLR9 has also been implicated in the recognition of *H. pylori* [18]. Specifically, Rad et al. reported that *H. pylori* DNA induced IL-6 and IL-12p40 responses in TLR2/TLR4 knockout dendritic cells, whereas dendritic cells deficient in TLR2, TLR4 and TLR9 displayed abrogated responses to *H. pylori* DNA [18]. The authors concluded that TLR9 was essential for the recognition of *H. pylori* DNA by dendritic cells and significantly contributed to the cytokine production by dendritic cells in response to *H. pylori* [18]. This same study also reported the involvement of the retinoic acid-inducible gene I (RIG-I) in the detection of *H. pylori* RNA, resulting in the induction of type I interferons and interferon-stimulated genes (ISGs) [18].

Nucleotide-Binding Oligomerization Domain

Nucleotide-binding oligomerization domain (NOD)1 is a cytoplasmic host innate immune sensor that specifically detects a muropeptide structure of Gram-negative bacterial peptidoglycan, being *N*-acetyl glucosamine-*N*-acetyl muramic acid (GlcNAc-MurNAc), linked to a tripeptide of which the terminal amino acid is *meso*-diaminopimelate (mDAP) [28, 29]. As NOD1 is expressed by epithelial cells, it was postulated that it has a role in contributing to immune recognition of *H. pylori*. Although *H. pylori* is an extracellular pathogen, it uses its type IV secretion system that is encoded by the cag pathogenicity island (cagPAI) to translocate peptidoglycan into the cytoplasm of the host cell, rendering it accessible to detection by NOD1 [30]. The detection of intracellular *H. pylori* peptidoglycan by NOD1 results in the initiation of a signalling cascade that ultimately leads to the activation of NF-κB [30] and AP-1 [31] and the production of pro-inflammatory molecule IL-8 [30]. Activation of NOD1 by *H. pylori* cagPAI-harbouring strains can also result in the expression of type I interferon (IFN) via IFN regulatory factor 7 (IRF-7) [32] in addition to the production of the antimicrobial peptide human β-defensin 2 (HBD2) [33, 34]. Specifically, the antimicrobial peptide HBD-2 that is upregulated in response to *H. pylori* cagPAI strains is biologically active against *H. pylori* [34] and may therefore contribute to controlling the infection. More recently, it has been shown that activation of the NOD1 pathway in epithelial cells by *H. pylori* enhances pro-inflammatory signalling in response to IFN-γ stimulation by enhancing the production of NOD1- and IFN-γ-regulated chemokines [35]. Using gastric biopsies, the authors identified that there was an increase in NOD1, CXCL8 and IRF1 expression in biopsies from individuals with severe gastritis or gastric tumours compared to gastric tissues from individuals without gastritis [35]. This finding is in contrast to the work by Peek et al. who identified that stimulation of epithelial cells with a *H. pylori* peptidoglycan deacetylase (PgdA) mutant significantly decreases NOD1-dependent NF-κB responses and the induction of autophagy, and infection of Mongolian gerbils with this strain resulted in decreased levels of gastric inflammation and malignancy compared to nonmutant *H. pylori* [36].

NOD1 has also been identified to have a role in inducing the transepithelial migration of neutrophils [37]. In brief, the authors showed that transepithelial migration of neutrophils in response to *H. pylori* infection was less in Caco2 epithelial cells in which NOD1 was knocked down compared to control epithelial cells [37].

In addition to activation of NOD1 via cagPAI-positive *H. pylori* strains, another method exists whereby all *H. pylori* strains irrespective of their cagPAI status can activate NOD1, involving bacterial outer membrane vesicles (OMVs) [38]. OMVs are small nanoparticles ranging between 20 and 250 nm in size and are released by almost all Gram-negative bacteria as part of their normal growth (reviewed in [39]). *H. pylori* releases OMVs both in vitro and in vivo, and these OMVs are capable of entering human epithelial cells in a lipid raft-dependent manner [38]. Upon entry into epithelial cells, peptidoglycan contained within OMVs is accessible to detection via NOD1, which then results in the induction of NF-κB, the production of IL-8 and the upregulation of human beta-defensin (HBD)-2 and HBD-3 [38]. More recently, it was identified that upon entry into human epithelial cells, *H. pylori* OMVs migrate to early endosomes where they are detected via NOD1 and are subsequently degraded via the host cell degradation pathway of autophagy [40]. Blockage of OMV detection via NOD1 or the degradation of OMVs via autophagy inhibits production of IL-8 by these cells [40]. Collectively, these findings reveal that the detection of *H. pylori* OMVs by NOD1 and their subsequent degradation by autophagy are essential to drive and mediate immune responses to *H. pylori* [40].

Inflammasome

Proteins of the Nod-like-receptor (NLR) family regulate the formation of a complex called the inflammasome and the activation of caspase-1, which functions to proteolytically cleave inactive interleukin 1B (IL-1β) and IL-18 to their active forms [41, 42]. In addition to TLRs and NOD1, the inflammasome has more recently been identified as having a role in regulating host immune responses to *H. pylori*. Activation of the inflammasome by *H. pylori* results in caspase-1 cleaving IL-1β and IL-18 precursors to their active forms in vitro [43]. The NLRP3 inflammasome is the most well-characterized inflammasome, and multiple reports have demonstrated that *H. pylori* can activate the NLRP3 inflammasome in immune cells in a cagPAI-dependent manner, resulting in the secretion of IL-1β [44, 45]. More recently, *H. pylori* has been reported to induce activation of the NLRP3 inflammasome in neutrophils [46] and in human monocytic cells (THP-1) [47, 48].

The human cell surface-associated mucin MUC1 that is highly expressed on gastric epithelial cells (reviewed in McGuckin et al. [49]) has been shown to regulate the NF-κB pathway which can subsequently regulate expression of the NLRP3 inflammasome. A study lead by Sutton et al. identified that NLRP3 expression is increased in the gastric tissue of *H. pylori*-infected

MUC1 KO mice. They showed that the activation of the NLRP3 inflammasome by *H. pylori* is tightly regulated by the mucin MUC1, which is essential to limit severe pathology [50].

T Cell Responses in *H. pylori*

Immunity to *Helicobacter* is dependent on T cells [13]. The murine *H. felis* infection model provides a useful model resembling gastric pathological changes in human *H. pylori* infection. *H. felis* infection of B and T cell-deficient mice and T cell-deficient mice does not result in gastric pathology despite high levels of colonization, whereas infection of B cell-deficient mice results in severe gastric alteration, identical to that seen in immunocompetent mice [13]. These results indicate that T cells are required for protection against *Helicobacter* but also that gastric immune-mediated damage is dependent on T cells, and not B cells or antibody secretion.

T-helper (Th) cells can be divided according to their cytokine secretion profile and cytotoxic potential. Th1 cells secrete tumour necrosis factor (TNF)-α and interferon (IFN)-γ, lyse antigen-loaded target cells through mechanisms that are mediated by perforin or FAS (also known as CD95) and elicit macrophage activation. Th2 cells secrete interleukin 4, are involved in down regulation of Th1 cell-mediated inflammatory events and facilitate production of antibodies by B cells. Th17 cells produce IL-17 alone or in combination with IFN-γ. Th17 cells may also secrete IL-6, IL-22 and TNF-α and play a critical role in protection against microbial challenges, particularly extracellular bacteria and fungi [13].

Properties of CD4+ T Cells in *H. pylori*-Related Diseases

In *H. pylori*-infected individuals, Th1 polarization of gastric cell responses occurs and is associated with peptic ulcer disease [13]. T cell clones from the gastric antral mucosa of *H. pylori*-infected patients with or without peptic ulcer display a different preferential antigen specificity. Approximately half of the *H. pylori*-reactive Th cell clones derived from peptic ulcer patients were specific for the cytotoxin-associated protein (CagA), whereas approximately one fourth of *H. pylori*-reactive Th clones from nonulcer gastritis patients were specific for *H. pylori* urease [13]. Upon antigen-specific stimulation, over 80% of the *H. pylori*-reactive Th cells from peptic ulcer disease patients showed a polarized Th1 profile, with high production of IFN-γ and low production of IL-4. Many studies further support the concept that Th1 polarization of the *H. pylori*-specific T cell response is associated with more severe disease [13]. In gastric low-grade mucosal-associated lymphoid tissue (MALT) lymphoma patients, gastric T cells promote neoplastic B cell proliferation via both Th2 cytokines and CD40-CD40 ligand interactions. Moreover gastric T cells from MALT lymphoma patients exhibit defective perforin- and Fas-Fas ligand-mediated killing of B cells [13]. In gastric cancer patients, Th17 responses have been found in the context of gastric mucosa. Most gastric T cell responses are elicited by the secreted peptidyl prolyl cis, trans-isomerase of *H. pylori* (HP0175) in patients with distal gastric adenocarcinoma [13]. Tumour-infiltrating lymphocytes (TILs) are specific for HP0175 not only IL-17 but also IL-21. HP0175-specific TILs expressing helper activity for monocyte matrix metalloproteinase (MMP)-2, MMP-9 and vascular endothelial growth factor production showed poor cytolytic activity. Thus, HP0175, by promoting pro-inflammatory low-cytotoxic TIL response, matrix degradation and pro-angiogenic pathways, may provide a link between *H. pylori* and gastric cancer.

Molecular Mimicry in Gastric Autoimmunity and *H. pylori*

H. pylori infection is frequently associated with gastric autoimmunity. Many studies indicate that most patients with autoimmune gastritis (AIG) have *H. pylori* infection [13]. AIG is characterized by autoimmune- mediated destruction of the secretory glands in the corpus of the stomach, leading to loss of gastric acid producing parietal cells and zymogenic cells, referred to as corpus atrophy. The endpoint of AIG is pernicious anaemia (PA) [13]. There are striking similarities between classical AIG- and *H. pylori*-induced corpus atrophic gastritis [13]. It is of note that early stages of AIG can be successfully treated by *H. pylori* eradication [13]. *H. pylori* induces autoantibodies reactive with gastric mucosal antigens in approximately half of the infected individuals [13]. Gastric H+K+-ATPase, the proton pump located in the secretory canaliculi of the parietal cells, is the autoantigen that drives immunopathology in AIG [13]. H+K+-ATPase has also been identified as the single major autoantigen in chronic *H. pylori* gastritis with corpus atrophy [13]. In mice, *H. pylori* infection induces gastric autoantibodies through mimicry between LPS Lewis blood-group antigens and Lewis antigens on the glycosylated subunit of H+K+-ATPase [13]. However, in humans, *H. pylori*-associated anti-autoantibodies are directed against protein epitopes, and their formation does not involve Lewis mimicry. In humans, *H. pylori* infection leads to the activation of cross-reactive gastric T cells, able to recognize both *H. pylori* peptide antigens and the gastric ATPase autoantigen [13]. Circulating antigastric autoantibodies are not pathogenic themselves but mark ongoing T cell-mediated gastric autoimmunity.

Gastric Th Responses in Gastric Autoimmunity Associated with *H. pylori* Infection

Many T cells are present in the gastric mucosa of AIG patients without previous *H. pylori* [13]. One fourth of the corpus T cells recognized gastric H+K+-ATPase, whereas very few antral T cells (3%) proliferated in response to this autoantigen. Almost all human ATPase-specific T cell clones were CD4+ as in experimental autoimmune gastritis (EAIG), in which administration of depleting anti-CD4 antibodies but not anti-CD8 antibodies reduces the incidence of gastritis [13].

Both gastric T cells reactive to ATPase and T cells reactive to *H. pylori* can be cloned from AIG patients with a concurrent *H. pylori* infection. Very interestingly in these patients, cross-reactive T cells able to recognize both ATPase and *H. pylori* antigens exist [13]. The identification of these cross-reactive *H. pylori*/ATPase-specific T cells has provided a functional mechanism (molecular mimicry) that can explain the association between *H. pylori* infection and corpus atrophic gastritis (Fig. 8.1).

Identification of the Epitopes Recognized by the T Cell Receptor (TCR) of T Cells Specific for *H. pylori*/ ATPase

An elegant approach was used to characterize the TCR specificity of cross-reactive T cells. Firstly, a library of overlapping 15-mer synthetic peptide of human gastric ATPase was used to identify the epitopes recognized by ATPase-specific and *H. pylori*-/ATPase-specific cells from *H. pylori*-infected AIG patients [13]. Secondly, candidate *H. pylori* epitopes were predicted by alignment of identified H+K+-ATPase epitopes with the genomes of the *H. pylori* J99 and 26,695 strains, taking into account the MHC class II peptide-binding motifs of each individual T cell donor. All *H. pylori*/ATPase cross-reactive T cells find their autoantigenic epitope in the α subunit of ATPase, which is much longer (1034 aa) than the β subunit (270 aa) [13]. None of the *H. pylori* peptides recognized by the *H. pylori*/ATPase cross-reactive T cells belong to the known immunodominant *H. pylori* proteins (e.g. vacuolating cytotoxin A (VacA), CagA and Urease), which have been identified as targets of gastric T cells in *H. pylori*-infected patients without gastric autoimmunity [13]. Products of *H. pylori* household genes are the *H. pylori* peptide epitopes recognized by cross-reactive T cells. Antigen-specific stimulation of *H. pylori*/ ATPase-cross-reactive T cells is HLA-DR restricted [13].

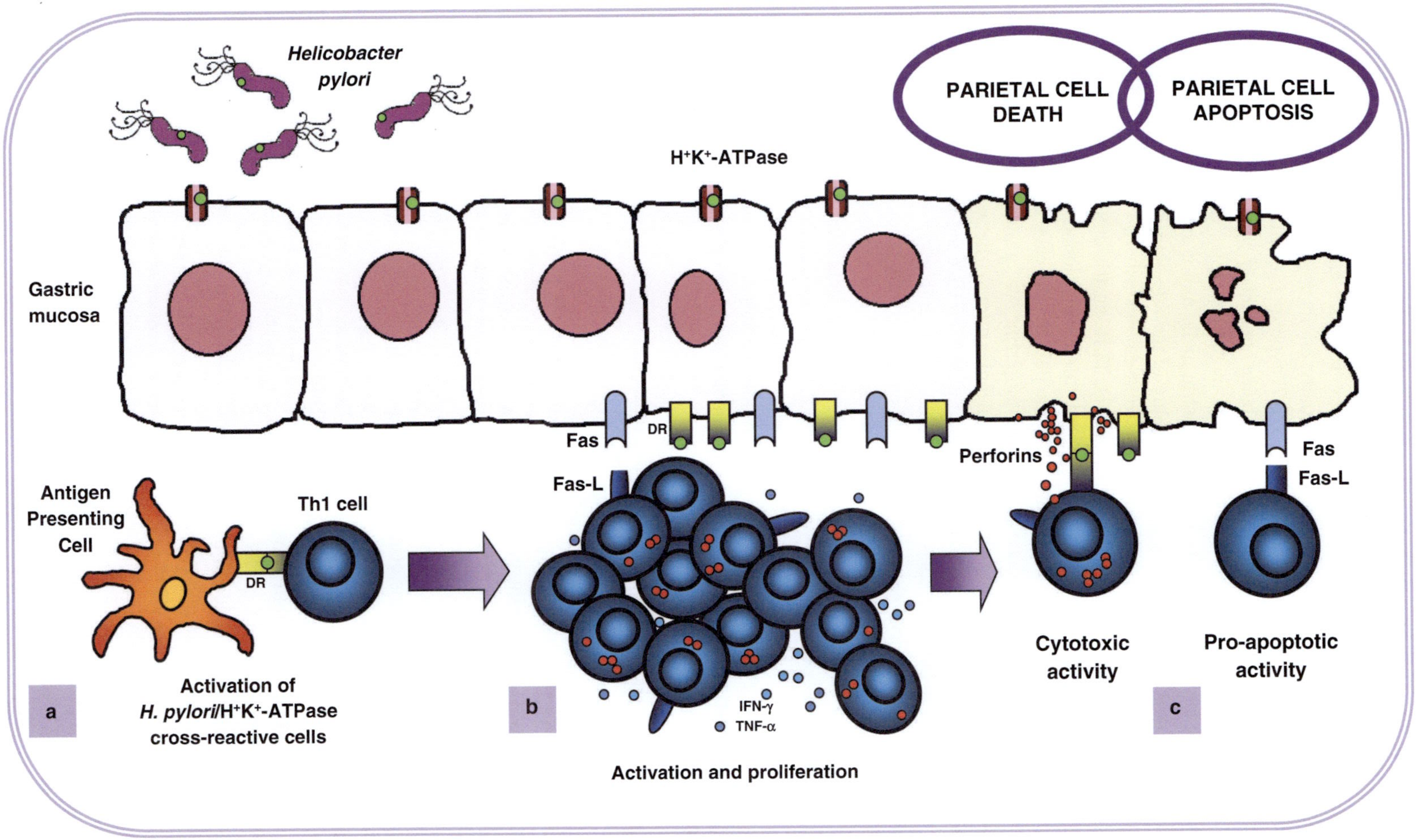

Fig. 8.1 Gastric autoimmunity in *H. pylori* infection. (**a** and **b**) *H. pylori* induces the activation and expansion of *H. pylori*-specific T cells that cross-react with gastric autoantigen (the H+, K+-ATPase) in susceptible individuals by molecular mimicry. (**c**) *H. pylori*-H+, K+-ATPase cross-reactive T cells mediate destruction of gastric mucosa, via cytokine secretion, perforin-mediated cytotoxicity and Fas ligand (FasL)-induced apoptosis

Features of Gastric T Cells in Gastric Autoimmunity Associated or Not with *H. pylori* Infection

All ATPase-reactive gastric T cell or ATPase/*H. pylori* cross-reactive T cell clones from AIG patients have a Th1 phenotype upon activation with the appropriate antigenic peptide. The expression of Fas on gastric epithelial cells is increased by the Th1 cytokines [13], and Fas/FasL interactions contribute to the death of gastric epithelial cells and thereafter leads to gastric atrophy [13]. All the autoreactive and cross-reactive activated ATPase-specific Th clones were able to induce cell death via both Fas-Fas ligand (FasL)-mediated apoptosis and perforin-mediated cytotoxicity against target cells [13]. *H. pylori*-associated anti-gastric autoantibodies have been hypothesized to play a role also for the pathogenesis of Sjogren's syndrome, although further studies are needed to confirm this preliminary observation [51].

Role of *H. pylori* in Damping Autoimmunity

Some *H. pylori* proteins might have inhibitory effects on the immune system. VacA toxin is able to inhibit antigen processing in antigen-presenting cells [52]. VacA indeed is able also to interfere with T cell activation by two different mechanisms. Formation of anion-specific channels by VacA prevents calcium influx from the extracellular milieu. The transcription factor nuclear factor of activated T cells thus fails to translocate to the nucleus and activate key cytokine genes. A second, channel-independent mechanism involves activation of intracellular signalling through the mitogen-activated protein kinases MKK3/6 and p38 and the Rac-specific nucleotide exchange factor, Vav. As a consequence of aberrant Rac activation, disordered actin polymerization is stimulated. The resulting defects in T cell activation may help *H. pylori* to prevent an effective immune response leading to chronic colonization of its gastric niche [53]. Similar damping effects of *H. pylori* have been describing in the context of autoimmunity [54–56].

Conclusions

Helicobacter pylori colonizes mucosa, activates Toll-like and Nod-like receptors and usually elicits a gastric T-helper 1/17 (Th1/Th17) type of immune response. A complex balance between *H. pylori* and immune inhibitory factors, such as VacA, takes part in the gastric niche and is responsible for the chronicity of the infection. Insights into the innate responses against *H. pylori*, dealing with NOD, TLR, gastric epithelial cells, cytokines and immune evasion, have been elucidated. In some infected patients, *H. pylori* promotes the development of gastric autoimmunity via molecular mimicry between *H. pylori* proteins and gastric ATPase autoantigen. On the other hand, in a minority of *H. pylori*-infected patients, *H. pylori* promotes the onset and the promotion of low-grade B cell lymphoma, via an abnormal help for B cell proliferation, mediated by peculiar T cells unable to kill B cells. Thus, the type of the host immune response against *H. pylori* is crucial for the outcome of the infection.

References

1. Akira S, Uematsu S, Takeuchi O. Pathogen recognition and innate immunity. Cell. 2006;124:783–801.
2. O'Neill LA. The interleukin-1 receptor/toll-like receptor superfamily: 10 years of progress. Immunol Rev. 2008;226:10–8.
3. Schmausser B, Andrulis M, Endrich S, Lee SK, Josenhans C, Muller-Hermelink HK, et al. Expression and subcellular distribution of toll-like receptors TLR4, TLR5 and TLR9 on the gastric epithelium in Helicobacter pylori infection. Clin Exp Immunol. 2004;136:521–6.
4. Ishihara S, Rumi MA, Kadowaki Y, Ortega-Cava CF, Yuki T, Yoshino N, et al. Essential role of MD-2 in TLR4-dependent signaling during helicobacter pylori-associated gastritis. J Immunol. 2004;173:1406–16.
5. Takeuchi O, Hoshino K, Kawai T, Sanjo H, Takada H, Ogawa T, et al. Differential roles of TLR2 and TLR4 in recognition of gram-negative and gram-positive bacterial cell wall components. Immunity. 1999;11:443–51.
6. Poltorak A, He X, Smirnova I, Liu MY, Van Huffel C, Du X, et al. Defective LPS signaling in C3H/HeJ and C57BL/10ScCr mice: mutations in Tlr4 gene. Science. 1998;282:2085–8.

7. Chaouche-Drider N, Kaparakis M, Karrar A, Fernandez MI, Carneiro LA, Viala J, et al. A commensal helicobacter sp. of the rodent intestinal flora activates TLR2 and NOD1 responses in epithelial cells. PLoS One. 2009;4:e5396.
8. Lepper PM, Triantafilou M, Schumann C, Schneider EM, Triantafilou K. Lipopolysaccharides from Helicobacter pylori can act as antagonists for toll-like receptor 4. Cell Microbiol. 2005;7:519–28.
9. Smith MF Jr, Mitchell A, Li G, Ding S, Fitzmaurice AM, Ryan K, et al. Toll-like receptor (TLR) 2 and TLR5, but not TLR4, are required for Helicobacter pylori-induced NF-kappa B activation and chemokine expression by epithelial cells. J Biol Chem. 2003;278:32552–60.
10. Mandell L, Moran AP, Cocchiarella A, Houghton J, Taylor N, Fox JG, et al. Intact gram-negative Helicobacter pylori, Helicobacter felis, and Helicobacter hepaticus bacteria activate innate immunity via toll-like receptor 2 but not toll-like receptor 4. Infect Immun. 2004;72:6446–54.
11. Torok AM, Bouton AH, Goldberg JB. Helicobacter pylori induces interleukin-8 secretion by toll-like receptor 2- and toll-like receptor 5-dependent and -independent pathways. Infect Immun. 2005;73:1523–31.
12. Amedei A, Cappon A, Codolo G, Cabrelle A, Polenghi A, Benagiano M, et al. The neutrophil-activating protein of Helicobacter pylori promotes Th1 immune responses. J Clin Invest. 2006;116:1092–101.
13. Takenaka R, Yokota K, Ayada K, Mizuno M, Zhao Y, Fujinami Y, et al. Helicobacter pylori heat-shock protein 60 induces inflammatory responses through the toll-like receptor-triggered pathway in cultured human gastric epithelial cells. Microbiology. 2004;150:3913–22.
14. Ferrero RL, Thiberge JM, Kansau I, Wuscher N, Huerre M, Labigne A. The GroES homolog of Helicobacter pylori confers protective immunity against mucosal infection in mice. Proc Natl Acad Sci U S A. 1995;92:6499–503.
15. Macchia G, Massone A, Burroni D, Covacci A, Censini S, Rappuoli R. The Hsp60 protein of Helicobacter pylori: structure and immune response in patients with gastroduodenal diseases. Mol Microbiol. 1993;9:645–52.
16. Suerbaum S, Thiberge JM, Kansau I, Ferrero RL, Labigne A. Helicobacter pylori hspA-hspB heat-shock gene cluster: nucleotide sequence, expression, putative function and immunogenicity. Mol Microbiol. 1994;14:959–74.
17. Gobert AP, Bambou JC, Werts C, Balloy V, Chignard M, Moran AP, et al. Helicobacter pylori heat shock protein 60 mediates interleukin-6 production by macrophages via a toll-like receptor (TLR)-2-, TLR-4-, and myeloid differentiation factor 88-independent mechanism. J Biol Chem. 2004;279:245–50.
18. Rad R, Ballhorn W, Voland P, Eisenacher K, Mages J, Rad L, et al. Extra- and intracellular pattern recognition receptors cooperate in the recognition of Helicobacter pylori. Gastroenterology. 2009;136(7):2247–57.
19. Obonyo M, Sabet M, Cole SP, Ebmeyer J, Uematsu S, Akira S, et al. Deficiencies of myeloid differentiation factor 88, toll-like receptor 2 (TLR2), or TLR4 produce specific defects in macrophage cytokine secretion induced by Helicobacter pylori. Infect Immun. 2007;75:2408–14.
20. Maeda S, Akanuma M, Mitsuno Y, Hirata Y, Ogura K, Yoshida H, et al. Distinct mechanism of Helicobacter pylori-mediated NF-kappa B activation between gastric cancer cells and monocytic cells. J Biol Chem. 2001;276:44856–64.
21. Hayashi F, Smith KD, Ozinsky A, Hawn TR, Yi EC, Goodlett DR, et al. The innate immune response to bacterial flagellin is mediated by toll-like receptor 5. Nature. 2001;410:1099–103.
22. Gewirtz AT, Yu Y, Krishna US, Israel DA, Lyons SL, Peek RM Jr. Helicobacter pylori flagellin evades toll-like receptor 5-mediated innate immunity. J Infect Dis. 2004;189:1914–20.
23. Lee SK, Stack A, Katzowitsch E, Aizawa SI, Suerbaum S, Josenhans C. Helicobacter pylori flagellins have very low intrinsic activity to stimulate human gastric epithelial cells via TLR5. Microbes Infect. 2003;5:1345–56.
24. Andersen-Nissen E, Smith KD, Strobe KL, Barrett SL, Cookson BT, Logan SM, et al. Evasion of toll-like receptor 5 by flagellated bacteria. Proc Natl Acad Sci U S A. 2005;102:9247–52.
25. Heil F, Hemmi H, Hochrein H, Ampenberger F, Kirschning C, Akira S, et al. Species-specific recognition of single-stranded RNA via toll-like receptor 7 and 8. Science. 2004;303:1526–9.
26. Rutz M, Metzger J, Gellert T, Luppa P, Lipford GB, Wagner H, et al. Toll-like receptor 9 binds single-stranded CpG-DNA in a sequence- and pH-dependent manner. Eur J Immunol. 2004;34:2541–50.
27. Gantier MP, Irving AT, Kaparakis-Liaskos M, Xu D, Evans VA, Cameron PU, et al. Genetic modulation of TLR8 response following bacterial phagocytosis. Hum Mutat. 2010;31:1069–79.
28. Chamaillard M, Hashimoto M, Horie Y, Masumoto J, Qiu S, Saab L, et al. An essential role for NOD1 in host recognition of bacterial peptidoglycan containing diaminopimelic acid. Nat Immunol. 2003;4(7):702.
29. Girardin SE, Boneca IG, Carneiro LA, Antignac A, Jehanno M, Viala J, et al. Nod1 detects a unique muropeptide from gram-negative bacterial peptidoglycan. Science. 2003;300:1584–7.
30. Viala J, Chaput C, Boneca IG, Cardona A, Girardin SE, Moran AP, et al. Nod1 responds to peptidoglycan delivered by the Helicobacter pylori cag pathogenicity island. Nat Immunol. 2004;5:1166–74.
31. Allison CC, Kufer TA, Kremmer E, Kaparakis M, Ferrero RL. Helicobacter pylori induces MAPK phosphorylation and AP-1 activation via a NOD1-dependent mechanism. J Immunol. 2009;183:8099–109.
32. Watanabe T, Asano N, Fichtner-Feigl S, Gorelick PL, Tsuji Y, Matsumoto Y, et al. NOD1 contributes to mouse host defense against Helicobacter pylori via

induction of type I IFN and activation of the ISGF3 signaling pathway. J Clin Invest. 2010;120:1645–62.
33. Boughan PK, Argent RH, Body-Malapel M, Park JH, Ewings KE, Bowie AG, et al. Nucleotide-binding oligomerization domain-1 and epidermal growth factor receptor: critical regulators of beta-defensins during Helicobacter pylori infection. J Biol Chem. 2006;281:11637–48.
34. Grubman A, Kaparakis M, Viala J, Allison C, Badea L, Karrar A, et al. The innate immune molecule, NOD1, regulates direct killing of Helicobacter pylori by antimicrobial peptides. Cell Microbiol. 2010;12:626–39.
35. Allison CC, Ferrand J, McLeod L, Hassan M, Kaparakis-Liaskos M, Grubman A, et al. Nucleotide oligomerization domain 1 enhances IFN-gamma signaling in gastric epithelial cells during Helicobacter pylori infection and exacerbates disease severity. J Immunol. 2013;190:3706–15.
36. Suarez G, Romero-Gallo J, Piazuelo MB, Wang G, Maier RJ, Forsberg LS, et al. Modification of Helicobacter pylori peptidoglycan enhances NOD1 activation and promotes cancer of the stomach. Cancer Res. 2015;75:1749–59.
37. Kim BJ, Kim JY, Hwang ES, Kim JG. Nucleotide binding oligomerization domain 1 is an essential signal transducer in human epithelial cells infected with Helicobacter pylori that induces the transepithelial migration of neutrophils. Gut Liver. 2015;9:358–69.
38. Kaparakis M, Turnbull L, Carneiro L, Firth S, Coleman HA, Parkington HC, et al. Bacterial membrane vesicles deliver peptidoglycan to NOD1 in epithelial cells. Cell Microbiol. 2010;12:372–85.
39. Kaparakis-Liaskos M, Ferrero RL. Immune modulation by bacterial outer membrane vesicles. Nat Rev Immunol. 2015;15:375–87.
40. Irving AT, Mimuro H, Kufer TA, Lo C, Wheeler R, Turner LJ, et al. The immune receptor NOD1 and kinase RIP2 interact with bacterial peptidoglycan on early endosomes to promote autophagy and inflammatory signaling. Cell Host Microbe. 2014;15:623–35.
41. Martinon F, Tschopp J. Inflammatory caspases: linking an intracellular innate immune system to autoinflammatory diseases. Cell. 2004;117:561–74.
42. Strowig T, Henao-Mejia J, Elinav E, Flavell R. Inflammasomes in health and disease. Nature. 2012;481:278–86.
43. Hitzler I, Sayi A, Kohler E, Engler DB, Koch KN, Hardt WD, et al. Caspase-1 has both proinflammatory and regulatory properties in Helicobacter infections, which are differentially mediated by its substrates IL-1beta and IL-18. J Immunol. 2012;188:3594–602.
44. Semper RP, Mejias-Luque R, Gross C, Anderl F, Muller A, Vieth M, et al. Helicobacter pylori-induced IL-1beta secretion in innate immune cells is regulated by the NLRP3 inflammasome and requires the cag pathogenicity island. J Immunol. 2014;193:3566–76.
45. Kim DJ, Park JH, Franchi L, Backert S, Nunez G. The cag pathogenicity island and interaction between TLR2/NOD2 and NLRP3 regulate IL-1beta production in Helicobacter pylori infected dendritic cells. Eur J Immunol. 2013;43:2650–8.
46. Perez-Figueroa E, Torres J, Sanchez-Zauco N, Contreras-Ramos A, Alvarez-Arellano L, Maldonado-Bernal C. Activation of NLRP3 inflammasome in human neutrophils by Helicobacter pylori infection. Innate Immun. 2016;22:103–12.
47. Li X, Liu S, Luo J, Liu A, Tang S, Liu S, et al. Helicobacter pylori induces IL-1beta and IL-18 production in human monocytic cell line through activation of NLRP3 inflammasome via ROS signaling pathway. Pathog Dis. 2015;73:ftu024.
48. Kameoka S, Kameyama T, Hayashi T, Sato S, Ohnishi N, Hayashi T, et al. Helicobacter pylori induces IL-1beta protein through the inflammasome activation in differentiated macrophagic cells. Biomed Res. 2016;37:21–7.
49. McGuckin MA, Linden SK, Sutton P, Florin TH. Mucin dynamics and enteric pathogens. Nat Rev Microbiol. 2011;9:265–78.
50. Ng GZ, Menheniott TR, Every AL, Stent A, Judd LM, Chionh YT, et al. The MUC1 mucin protects against Helicobacter pylori pathogenesis in mice by regulation of the NLRP3 inflammasome. Gut. 2016;65:1087–99.
51. Sorrentino D, Faller G, DeVita S, Avellini C, Labombarda A, Ferraccioli G, et al. Helicobacter pylori associated antigastric autoantibodies: role in Sjogren's syndrome gastritis. Helicobacter. 2004;9:46–53.
52. Molinari M, Salio M, Galli C, Norais N, Rappuoli R, Lanzavecchia A, et al. Selective inhibition of Ii-dependent antigen presentation by Helicobacter pylori toxin VacA. J Exp Med. 1998;187:135–40.
53. Boncristiano M, Paccani SR, Barone S, Ulivieri C, Patrussi L, Ilver D, et al. The Helicobacter pylori vacuolating toxin inhibits T cell activation by two independent mechanisms. J Exp Med. 2003;198:1887–97.
54. Sawalha AH, Schmid WR, Binder SR, Bacino DK, Harley JB. Association between systemic lupus erythematosus and Helicobacter pylori seronegativity. J Rheumatol. 2004;31:1546–50.
55. Rigante D, Esposito S. Infections and systemic lupus erythematosus: binding or sparring partners? Int J Mol Sci. 2015;16:17331–43.
56. Doaty S, Agrawal H, Bauer E, Furst DE. Infection and lupus: which causes which? Curr Rheumatol Rep. 2016;18:13.

9 Rheumatic Complications of *Streptococcus pyogenes*

Guliz Erdem and Edward L. Kaplan

Abbreviations

ARF	Acute rheumatic fever
GAS	Group A streptococcus
MHC	Major histocompatibility complex
PSGN	Post-streptococcal glomerulonephritis
PSRA	Post-streptococcal reactive arthritis
RHD	Rheumatic heart disease

Streptococcus pyogenes or group A streptococcus (GAS) is a Gram-positive coccus that is estimated to cause up to 700 million human infections annually [1, 2]. GAS can cause a variety of infections ranging from pharyngitis and simple skin and soft tissue infections to bacteremia, necrotizing fasciitis, and streptococcal toxic shock syndrome. In addition to acute infections, GAS can cause immune-mediated post-infectious complications. These include acute rheumatic fever, post-streptococcal glomerulonephritis, and reactive arthritis. Precise mechanisms for these non-suppurative sequelae have yet to be elucidated.

G. Erdem (✉)
Nationwide Children's Hospital Medical Center, The Ohio State University, Infectious Diseases Section, Columbus, OH, USA
e-mail: Guliz.erdem@nationwidechildrens.org

E. L. Kaplan
University of Minnesota Medical School, Department of Pediatrics, Minneapolis, MN, USA
e-mail: kapla001@umn.edu

Acute Rheumatic Fever

Acute rheumatic fever (ARF) triggered by GAS is generally considered to be a transient autoimmune disease but has chronic sequelae. In developing areas of the world, ARF and its sequel rheumatic heart disease are estimated to affect nearly 20 million people and remain leading causes of cardiovascular death during the first five decades of life in the twenty-first century [3, 4]. Most of the ARF cases occur in developing countries where the mean incidence of ARF is 19 per 100,000 population [5]. ARF has also been reported both in outbreaks and endemically among US populations [6–8]. ARF occurs most frequently in children 5–15 years of age [1, 9, 10]. The disease usually presents with one or more acute episodes. In 30–50% of cases, ARF may lead to chronic rheumatic heart disease (RHD) with progressive and permanent damage of the cardiac valves, especially the mitral and aortic valves [11].

ARF occurs at a median of 2 weeks after a pharyngeal infection although some have proposed that skin infections may also trigger this immune response, but conclusive data are lacking to support this [3, 12]. The diagnostic criteria for ARF were first developed by T. Duckett Jones in 1944 and have been revised most recently in 2015 [13, 14]. American Heart Association guidelines (Jones criteria) for the diagnosis of rheumatic fever are largely based on clinical manifestations such as arthritis,

G. Ragab et al. (eds.), *The Microbiome in Rheumatic Diseases and Infection*,
https://doi.org/10.1007/978-3-319-79026-8_9

carditis, Sydenham's chorea, subcutaneous nodules, and erythema marginatum [13]. Carditis and Sydenham's chorea could lead to sequelae in affected populations. Carditis occurs in about 60% of ARF patients usually following an initial severe attack [1, 3, 15]. Sydenham's chorea often appears later than the other clinical manifestations. It is characterized by involuntary, rapid, and purposeless movements of the face and limbs and can be associated with emotional lability.

Several hypotheses on the mechanisms by which GAS infection leads to ARF and triggers autoimmunity exist although a definitive explanation remains elusive. ARF and RHD seem to engage both humoral and cellular autoimmunity, most likely due to molecular mimicry and epitope spreading [2]. The theory of molecular mimicry was the result of successful demonstration of cross-reactive antibodies to the M-protein of the streptococcal cell wall and to cardiac myosin [16, 17]. Some antibodies directed against other GAS antigens have been reported to cross-react with host antigens [16, 18, 19]. The autoantibodies which target the valves in rheumatic heart disease and the neuronal cells in Sydenham's chorea are thought to share a common streptococcal epitope, GlcNAc, and target intracellular biomarkers of disease including cardiac myosin in the myocardium and tubulin, a protein in the brain (Fig. 9.1) [18, 20, 21].

The recognition of these antigens while targeting extracellular membrane proteins such as laminin on the valve surface endothelium or lysoganglioside and dopamine receptors in the brain has been postulated to be the basis for molecular mimicry that leads to valve damage in rheumatic heart disease and neuropsychiatric behaviors and involuntary movements in Sydenham's chorea (Fig. 9.2) [18, 21]. In Sydenham's chorea, neurons in the basal ganglia are attacked by antibodies against the group A carbohydrate of *Streptococci* that react with the surface of the neuron. This reaction activates signaling through calcium-/calmodulin-dependent protein kinase type II, which involves an increase in tyrosine hydroxylase in dopaminergic neurons. Receptors, such as the D1 and D2 dopamine receptors, and lysoganglioside might be autoantibody targets on the neuronal cell. This targeting could lead to altered cell signaling and increased levels of

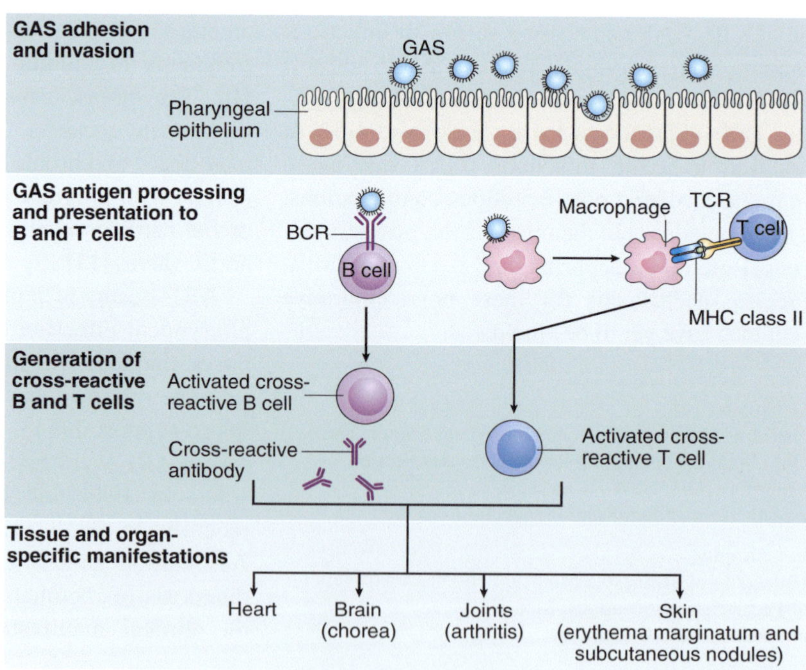

Fig. 9.1 Generation of cross-reactive immune response in ARF. Used with permission from Springer Nature [21]

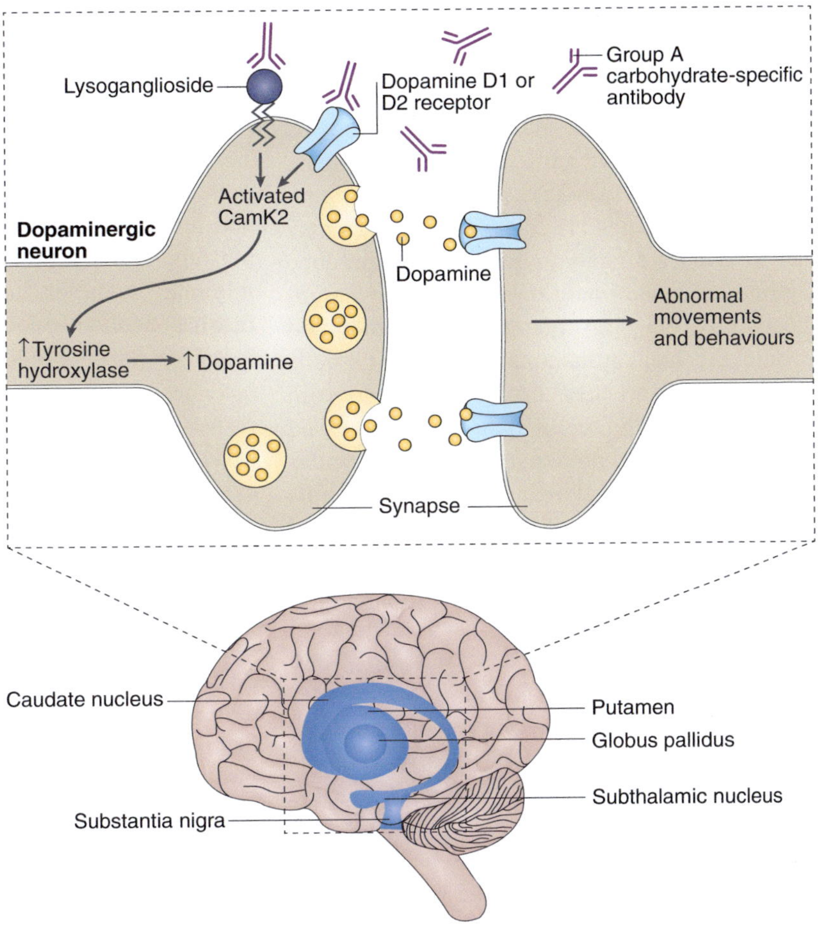

Fig. 9.2 Molecular and cellular basis of Sydenham's chorea. Used with permission from Springer Nature [21]

dopamine, in turn leading to abnormal movements and behaviors (Fig. 9.2) [20]. Antigenic similarity of cardiac myosin and other extracellular matrix proteins or self-cardiac proteins (tropomyosin, keratin, laminin, and vimentin), displaying a coiled-coil structure, with different ARF-associated GAS strains has been reported in several populations including Australian Aborigine, Caucasian, and Thai patients [18–27].

Cell-mediated immunity is also thought to mediate molecular mimicry found in ARF. Peripheral T lymphocytes interacting with adhesion molecules such as vascular cell adhesion molecule-1 infiltrate nonvascular tissues like cardiac valves [8, 15, 25, 26]. Such T cells adhering to valve endothelium and extravasating into the valve are thought to be important in rheumatic heart disease development [18, 27].

Several studies have reported genetic associations with ARF, with some appearing to be major histocompatibility complex (MHC)-related, while others are non-MHC-related, and there are some studies with no association [19, 21, 28–33]. Of these, HLA class II genes represented the strongest association [2]. Genetic polymorphisms in tumor necrosis factor, mannose-binding lectin, and toll-like receptor genes have been also associated with susceptibility to ARF and/or RHD [10]. Another reported linkage is the presence of antiphospholipid antibodies in some patients with rheumatic fever [34]. Anti-endothelial cell antibodies were demonstrated in some RHD patients [35]. These reported findings and associated theories suggest a multifactorial process triggering the autoimmune response. Circulating T cells, activated by GAS exposure, would upregulate adhesion molecules, enabling adhesion to valvular endothelium and subsequent trafficking into valve tissue. This endothelial damage may expose intra-valvular molecular components and perhaps modify cardiac collagen, myosin, laminin, keratin, tropomyosin, and other alpha-coiled coil proteins [18]. These molecules may act as danger signals to local innate immune system cells and could develop greater immunogenicity if posttranslationally modified within the local inflammatory milieu. T cells are normally activated through encounter with antigen-presenting cells that have processed antigens for presentation on MHC molecules within secondary lymphoid organs. If this occurs at ectopic sites, such as within inflamed mucosal or epithelial tissues, or in Aschoff nodules of the heart, T-cell regulation may be perturbed. This dysregulated T-cell activation might favor the emergence of anti-self T-cell clones and sustained production of cytokines such as IFNγ and IL-17, recruiting other inflammatory cells and driving RHD. Chronic valvular inflammation would eventually initiate tissue remodeling, including neovascularization of the normally avascular heart valves. Neovascularization would drive tissue fibrosis and promote easy access for inflammatory cells in future ARF episodes, leading eventually to valve fibrosis and calcification [2].

Adequate antibiotic treatment of documented GAS pharyngitis markedly reduces the incidence of subsequent rheumatic fever, and secondary antimicrobial prophylaxis (either daily oral medication or 3–4 weekly intramuscular benzathine penicillin G) is effective in preventing the recurrence of disease in patients who have had a previous attack of ARF [15, 36–39].

Post-streptococcal Glomerulonephritis

Post-streptococcal glomerulonephritis (PSGN) typically appears 1–3 weeks following pharyngitis and 3–6 weeks following impetigo [2, 10]. PSGN is the most frequent cause of nephritis in children globally with estimated 470,000 cases annually [2]. It mostly affects children between 3 and 12 years of age. PSGN usually has good prognosis in children, but it has been thought to cause chronic renal disease in adults [40].

PSGN is caused by glomerular deposition of immune complexes, complement activation, and temporary amplification of the actions of plasmin. PSGN appears to be a "one hit" immune complex disorder that typically resolves without eliciting an ongoing autoimmune response [41–43]. Two GAS antigens have been implicated as initiators of the immune response: NAPlr, a streptococcal glyceraldehyde 3-phosphate dehydrogenase, and SpeB, a cysteine protease [42, 43].

Post-streptococcal Reactive Arthritis

Post-streptococcal reactive arthritis (PSRA) is diagnosed in patients with polyarthritis who have a recent evidence of streptococcal infection and no other major Jones criteria. The arthritis in PSRA develops within 10 days of streptococcal infection, nonmigratory, usually affects the small joints of hands and/or feet, is not responsive to aspirin/nonsteroidal anti-inflammatory drugs, and usually lasts longer than ARF arthritis [44–46]. M-protein-specific antibodies cross-reacting with the joint cartilage and synovium have been described, and binding of these antibodies to cartilage could lead to complement activation [47]. PSRA shows a bimodal peak between 8–14 years and 21–37 years. Unlike ARF, PSRA is rarely associated with carditis [48].

Notes

GAS cause post-infectious sequelae as ARF and/or RHD, PSGN, and PSRA in susceptible hosts.

The mechanism(s) of disease is unknown, but genetic factors and molecular mimicry between GAS M protein and cardiac myosin may play a role in ARF.

PSGN is caused by immune complexes and complement activation in response to streptococcal antigens. Antibodies generated by GAS infection can mediate cell signaling in neurons, possibly resulting in chorea.

References

1. Carapetis JR, Steer AC, Mulholland EK, Weber M. The global burden of group A streptococcal diseases. Lancet Infect Dis. 2005;5:685–94.
2. Martin WJ, Steer AC, Smeesters PR, Keeble J, Inouye M, Carapetis J, Wicks IP. Post-infectious group A streptococcal autoimmune syndromes and the heart. Autoimmun Rev. 2015;14:710–25.
3. Carapetis JR, McDonald M, Wilson NJ. Acute rheumatic fever. Lancet. 2005;366:155–68.
4. Wyber R, Zuhlke L, Carapetis J. The case for global investment in rheumatic heart-disease control. Bull World Health Organ. 2014;92:768–70.
5. Shulman ST, Stollerman G, Beall B, Dale JB, Tanz RR. Temporal changes in streptococcal M protein types and the near-disappearance of acute rheumatic fever in the United States. Clin Infect Dis. 2006;42:441–7.
6. Veasy LG, Wiedmeier SE, Orsmond GS, Ruttenberg HD, Boucek MM, Roth SJ, et al. Resurgence of acute rheumatic fever in the intermountain area of the United States. NEJM. 1987;316:421–7.
7. Veasy LG, Llyod YT, Daly JA, Korgenski K, Miner L, Bale J, et al. Temporal association of appearance of mucoid strains of *Streptococcus pyogenes* with a continuing high incidence of acute rheumatic fever in Utah. Pediatrics. 2004;113:e168–72.
8. Erdem G, Mizumoto C, Esaki D, Reddy V, Kurahara D, Yamaga K, et al. Group A streptococcal isolates temporally associated with acute rheumatic fever in Hawaii: differences from the continental United States. Clin Infect Dis. 2007;45:e20–4.
9. Tibazarwa KB, Volmink JA, Mayosi BM. Incidence of acute rheumatic fever in the world: a systematic review of population-based studies. Heart. 2008;94:1534–40.
10. Tani LY, Veasy LG, Minich LL, Shaddy RE. Rheumatic fever in children younger than 5 years: is the presentation different? Pediatrics. 2003;112:1065–8.
11. Perricone C, Rinkevich-Shop S, Blank M, Landa-Rouben N, Alessandri C, et al. The autoimmune side of rheumatic fever. IMAJ. 2014;16:654–5.
12. Marijon E, Ou P, Celermajer DS, Ferreira B, Mocumbi AO, Jani D, et al. Prevalence of rheumatic heart disease detected by echocardiographic screening. NEJM. 2007;357:470–6.
13. Gewitz MH, Baltimore RS, Tani LY, Sable CA, Shulman ST, Carapetis J, et al. Revision of the Jones criteria for the diagnosis of acute rheumatic fever in the era of doppler echocardiography: a scientific statement from the American Heart Association. Circulation. 2015;131:1806–18.
14. Remenyi B, Wilson N, Steer A, Ferreira B, Kado J, Kumar K, et al. World Heart Federation criteria for echocardiographic diagnosis of rheumatic heart disease – an evidence-based guideline. Nat Rev Cardiol. 2012;9:297–309.
15. Kaplan EL, Bisno AL. Antecedent streptococcal infection in acute rheumatic fever. Clin Infect Dis. 2006;43:690–2.
16. Paget SA. The microbiome, autoimmunity, and arthritis: cause and effect. Trans Am Clin Climatol Assoc. 2012;123:257–67.
17. van de Rijn I, Zabriskie JB, McCarty M. Group A streptococcal antigens cross-reactive with myocardium. Purification of heart-reactive antibody and isolation and characterization of the streptococcal antigen. J Exp Med. 1977;146:579–99.
18. Cunningham MW. Streptococcus and rheumatic fever. Curr Opin Rheumatol. 2012;24:408–16.
19. Husby G, van de Rijn I, Zabriskie JB, Abdin ZH, Williams RC. Antibodies reacting with cytoplasm of subthalamic and caudate nuclei neurons in chorea and acute rheumatic fever. J Exp Med. 1976;144:1094–110.
20. Chakravarty SD, Zabriskie JB, Gibofsky A. Acute rheumatic fever and streptococci: the quintessential pathogenic trigger of autoimmunity. Clin Rheumatol. 2014;33:893–901.
21. Carapetis JR, Beaton A, Cunningham MW, Guilherme L, Karthikeyan G, Mayosi BM, et al. Acute rheumatic fever and rheumatic heart disease. Nat Rev Dis Primers. 2016;2:1–24.
22. Pruksakorn S, Currie B, Brandt E, Phornphutkul C, Hunsakunachai S, Manmontri A, et al. Identification of T cell auto-epitopes that cross-react with the C-terminal segment of the M protein of group A streptococci. Int Immunol. 1994;6:1235–44.
23. Dale JB, Beachey EH. Epitopes of streptococcal M proteins shared with cardiac myosin. J Exp Med. 1985;162:583–91.
24. Kaplan MH, Suchy ML. Immunologic relation of streptococcal and tissue antigens II. Cross-reaction of antisera to mammalian heart tissue with a cell wall constituent of certain strains of group A streptococci. J Exp Med. 1964;119:643–50.
25. Galvin JE, Hemric ME, Ward K, Cunningham MW. Cytotoxic mAb from rheumatic carditis recognizes heart valves and laminin. J Clin Investig. 2000;106:217–24.
26. Esposito S, Bianchini S, Fastiggi M, Fumagalli M, Andreozzi L, Rigante D. Geoepidemiological hints about *Streptococcus pyogenes* strains in relationship with acute rheumatic fever. Autoimmun Rev. 2015;14:616–21.
27. Musser JM, Shelburne SA III. A decade of molecular pathogenomic analysis of group A streptococcus. J Clin Investig. 2009;119:2455–63.
28. Cunningham MW. Rheumatic fever, autoimmunity, and molecular mimicry: the streptococcal connection. Int Rev Immunol. 2014;33:314–29.
29. Khanna AK, Buskirk DR, Williams RC, Gibofsky A, Crow MK, Menon A, et al. Presence of a non-HLA B cell antigen in rheumatic fever patients and their families as defined by a monoclonal antibody. J Clin Investig. 1989;83:1710–6.
30. Ayoub EM, Barrett DJ, Maclaren NK, Krischer JP. Association of class II human histocompatibility leukocyte antigens with rheumatic fever. J Clin Investig. 1986;77:2019–26.
31. Guilherme L, Weidebach W, Kiss MH, Snitcowsky R, Kalil J. Association of human leukocyte class II

antigens with rheumatic fever or rheumatic heart disease in a Brazilian population. Circulation. 1991;83:1995–8.

32. Maharaj B, Hammond MG, Appadoo B, Leary WP, Pudifin DJ. HLA-A, B, DR, and DQ antigens in black patients with severe chronic rheumatic heart disease. Circulation. 1987;76:259–61.
33. Erdem G, Seifried S. No evidence of human leukocyte antigen gene association with rheumatic fever among children in Samoa. J Pediatr Infect Dis Soc. 2015;4:71–3.
34. da Silva F, de Carvalho J. Rheumatic fever associated with antiphospholipid syndrome: systematic review. J Immunol Res. 2014;2014:614591. https://doi.org/10.1155/2014/614591.
35. Scalzi V, Abu Hadi H, Alessandri C, Croia C, Conti V, Agati L, et al. Anti-endothelial cell antibodies in rheumatic heart disease. Clin Exp Immunol. 2010;161:570–5.
36. Denny FW, Wannamaker LW, Brink WR, Rammelkamp CH, Custer EA. Prevention of rheumatic fever; treatment of the preceding streptococcic infection. JAMA. 1950;143:151–3.
37. Wannamaker LW, Rammelkamp CH, Denny FW, Brink WR, Houser HB, Hahn EO, et al. Prophylaxis of acute rheumatic fever: by treatment of the preceding streptococcal infection with various amounts of depot penicillin. Am J Med. 1951;10:673–95.
38. Markowitz M, Gerber MA. Rheumatic fever: recent outbreaks of an old disease. Conn Med. 1987;51:229–33.
39. Shulman ST, Gerber MA, Tanz RR, Markowitz M. Streptococcal pharyngitis: the case for penicillin therapy. Pediatr Infect Dis J. 1994;13:1–7.
40. Hoyer JR, Michael AF, Fish AJ, Good RA. Acute poststreptococcal glomerulonephritis presenting as hypertensive encephalopathy with minimal urinary abnormalities. Pediatrics. 1967;39:412–7.
41. Lee JL, Naguwa SM, Cheema GS, Gershwin EM. Acute rheumatic fever and its consequences: a persistent threat to developing nations in the twenty-first century. Autoimmun Rev. 2009;9:117–23.
42. Fish AJ, Herdman RC, Michael AF, Pickering RJ, Good RA. Epidemic acute nephritis associated with type 49 streptococcal pyoderma. II. Correlative study of light, immunofluorescent and electron microscopic findings. Am J Med. 1970;48:28–39.
43. Rodriguez-Iturbe B, Batsford S. Pathogenesis of poststreptococcal glomerulonephritis a century after Clemens von Pirquet. Kidney Int. 2007;71:1094–104.
44. Ayoub EM, Ahmed S. Update on complications of group A streptococcal infections. Curr Probl Pediatr. 1997;27:90–101.
45. Pathak H, Marshall T. Post-streptococcal reactive arthritis: where are we now. BMJ Case Rep. 2016;2016:bcr2016215552. https://doi.org/10.1136/bcr-2016-215552.
46. van der Helm-van Mil AHM. Acute rheumatic fever and poststreptococcal reactive arthritis reconsidered. Curr Opin Rheumatol. 2010;22:437–42.
47. Baird RW, Bronze MS, Kraus W, Hill HR, Veasy LG, Dale JB. Epitopes of group A streptococcal M protein shared with antigens of articular cartilage and synovium. J Immunol. 1991;146:3132–7.
48. Walker MJ, Barnett TC, McArthur JD, Cole JN, Gillen CM, Henningham A, et al. Disease manifestations and pathogenic mechanisms of group A streptococcus. Clin Microbiol Rev. 2014;27:264–301.

Mollicutes: Mycoplasma pneumoniae

10

T. Prescott Atkinson

Abbreviations

ADEM	Acute demyelinating encephalomyelitis
CA	Cold agglutinins
GBS	Guillain-Barré syndrome
JIA	Juvenile idiopathic arthritis
Mpn	*Mycoplasma pneumoniae*
SJS	Stevens-Johnson syndrome

Introduction

Mycoplasma pneumoniae (*Mpn*) is a member of the class *Mollicutes* (*mollis*, soft; *cutis*, skin), and like all members of the group, it lacks a cell wall or outer membrane, possessing only a simple lipid bilayer containing, in most members, cholesterol. First isolated in the 1940s by Monroe Eaton and colleagues as the cause of atypical pneumonia, the organism was at first thought to be a virus because it was filterable due to its tiny size (200–700 nm) [1]. Mycoplasmas and related groups within the *Mollicutes* are obligate parasitic bacteria with highly evolved genomes that have lost many genes related to most biosynthetic pathways through reductive evolution from a Gram-positive bacterial ancestor [2, 3]. Interestingly, they use a slightly different genetic code from other bacteria and eukaryotes in which the opal stop codon, UGA, codes for tryptophan. *Mycoplasma genitalium*, a species that is closely related to and probably derived from *Mpn*, possesses the smallest functioning genome known for a cell for a self-replicating organism [4]. *Mpn* has a genome size of 817,276 bp with 757 predicted coding sequences, 36 tRNAs, and 1 tmRNA [5]. Like other members of the *Mollicutes*, *Mpn* is unable to synthesize amino acids, purines, pyrimidines, or cholesterol, and it lacks a functioning tricarboxylic acid cycle for energy production. The restricted metabolome of *Mpn* and other *Mollicutes* underscores their absolute dependence upon their host for most of the biomolecules essential for life.

As discussed in the following sections, infection with *Mpn* has often been associated with different autoimmune phenomena. Common associations have been made with autoimmunity involving the hematologic, dermatologic, musculoskeletal, and neurologic systems among others, and these four systems will be considered in separate following sections. The possible significance of these associations is complicated by the difficulties in accurate diagnosis of *Mpn* infection, which in the past has relied largely on serology. Since antibody to *Mpn*, even of the IgM isotype, is common in the general population,

T. P. Atkinson
Division of Pediatric Allergy, Asthma & Immunology, University of Alabama at Birmingham, Birmingham, AL, USA
e-mail: patkinson@peds.uab.edu

G. Ragab et al. (eds.), *The Microbiome in Rheumatic Diseases and Infection*,
https://doi.org/10.1007/978-3-319-79026-8_10

serologic methods for diagnosis of acute *Mpn* infection can be misleading, akin to trying to diagnose acute Group A streptococcal infection using an antistreptolysin O titer. Furthermore, even after antibiotic treatment of acute infection, the organism can often be cultured from respiratory secretions for many months. However, with the advent of molecular diagnostics, increasingly convincing data are continuing to accumulate linking this and closely related bacteria to autoimmunity.

As an obligate parasite, *Mpn* is under more extreme pressure than many other pathogens to evade the host immune response in order to establish prolonged or even chronic infections. One well-established mechanism is antigenic variation, i.e., changes in the peptide sequence of antigenic proteins, which occurs by intragenomic recombination of repetitive regions, as exemplified by the P1 adhesin, one of the most immunogenic surface molecules [6]. Another is by glycosylation of surface lipids, proteins, and lipoproteins. As with other essential biomolecules, mycoplasmas scavenge host glycans for energy production, limited biosynthesis, and, as has been recently demonstrated for *Mpn*, decoration of their surface lipids [7]. Interestingly, human diacylglycerol and ceramide were also substrates for the most active, and most promiscuous, *Mpn* glycosyltransferase bringing up the possibility that the organism might alter host membrane lipids rendering them more antigenic. N- and O-linked glycosylation of surface lipoproteins have also been shown to occur in *M. pulmonis* and *M. arthritidis*, and this process is likely to be a general one among the *Mollicutes* [8]. Host oligosaccharides with either alpha- or beta-1,4 linkages, not monosaccharides, are needed to support glycosylation, and it appears that rather than UDP-sugars, the mycoplasma glycosyltransferase(s) utilize the energy in the glycan linkage itself to fuel the glycosyltransferase reaction. As with the lipid glycosylation seen with *M. pneumoniae*, this process is quite promiscuous and does not require any obvious peptide motif other than perhaps a nearby lysine residue. Further, the mycoplasmas can utilize glutamine as well as asparagine as an acceptor amino acid in N-linked glycosylation. Thus, the bacteria can cloak their surface lipids and lipoproteins using host-derived carbohydrate, potentially altering immunogenic epitopes and helping to shelter the organism from the host immune system. More importantly for the following discussion, the alteration of host surface lipids and proteins by promiscuous mycoplasmal glycosyltransferases has the potential to create neoantigens that could lead to autoimmunity. Finally, native mycoplasmal glycoproteins and glycolipids may protect the bacterium and at the same time induce autoimmunity by mimicking epitopes of host cell surface molecules. This process of antigenic mimicry is a well-established mechanism for infection-induced autoimmunity for other organisms, and there is some evidence that it is relevant to *Mpn*-induced autoimmune neuropathies as will be discussed below.

Hematologic Manifestations

One of the best documented autoimmune phenomena associated with any microbial organism is *Mpn*-associated development of cold agglutinins (CA), autoantibodies usually of the IgM isotype that bind to the red cell membrane at low temperatures (typically 28–31°F) triggering hemolysis. Although CA can develop in association with other infections, the development of these antibodies has been used for decades as a bedside clinical test for atypical pneumonia due to *Mpn* infection, only more recently having been supplanted by other serologic and most recently by PCR-based tests. The development of CA, usually 2–3 weeks into the illness, is generally proportional to the severity of the illness, and CA can persist at detectable levels in affected individuals for greater than 1 year [9]. In severe cases, fatal hemolytic anemia and renal failure have been reported [10]. The specificity of *Mpn*-associated CA was demonstrated during the 1980s to be directed against the red cell I antigen (branched poly-N-acetyl-lactosamine chains) [11]. These chains may be attached either to glucose ceramide, forming a glycolipid, or to the red cell band 3 glycoprotein, the most abundant red cell surface protein. Later it was demonstrated that the sialylated form of the I antigen is a receptor for *Mpn* (as are other sialoglycoproteins), suggesting that *Mpn* binding to the I antigen creates a neoantigen that triggers CA production, still a likely explanation [12]. The possibility remains, however, that the bound *Mpn* organism may modify the lipid or protein linked to the I antigen, perhaps by glycosylation as discussed in the preceding section, rendering that molecule yet more immunogenic.

Stevens-Johnson Syndrome

A variety of different nonspecific exanthems can be seen with acute *Mpn* infections [13]. However, a bullous mucocutaneous rash meeting criteria for Stevens-Johnson Syndrome (SJS) has been known for over 70 years to be associated with atypical pneumonias and is an occasionally serious complication of acute *Mpn* infection (Fig. 10.1) [14–16]. As with CA, *Mpn*-associated SJS tends to be seen with more severe infections such as community-acquired pneumonia with higher fevers and elevated erythrocyte sedimentation rates, developing relatively late in the course of the disease [17]. However, it can also occur in the context of relatively mild respiratory symptoms, which presents even greater difficulties in diagnosis [18]. *Mpn* has been isolated repeatedly from the skin lesions although many such efforts have failed [18–20], and, interestingly, herpes simplex virus has been occasionally cultured from them [21] as well as from the oral cavity [17]. SJS can occur in localized outbreaks along with epidemics of atypical pneumonia [17, 22]. Genetic analysis of isolates from such localized occurrences has so far failed to suggest that this manifestation of *Mpn* infection is associated with specific strain(s) of *Mpn* [22]. There are also well-documented instances of recurrent disease [23–27].

As a clinical aside, the usual confounding factors are present when SJS develops during a respiratory infection that is being treated with multiple drugs, including antibiotics, as this complication can certainly be due to either the infection or a medication. Thus, it is particularly important for clinicians to be rigorous about the criteria used in the diagnosis of *Mpn* infection in such a patient if mycoplasma infection is a consideration. A single positive IgM or IgG titer may be misleading. Chest films can have significant

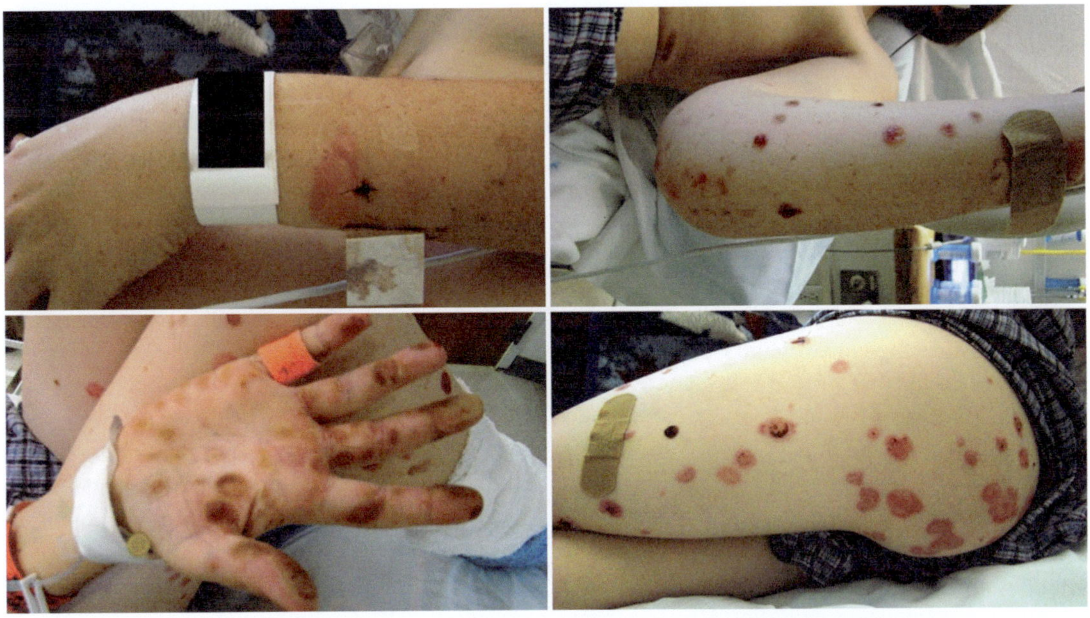

Fig. 10.1 Skin lesions associated with *Mpn*-induced Stevens-Johnson syndrome in a child

findings consistent with *Mpn* infection even with a paucity of symptoms. Respiratory secretions, ideally sputum, should be tested by culture and PCR for the presence of the organism, and an effort should be made to collect acute and convalescent sera for *Mpn* antibodies, even in the absence of severe respiratory symptoms.

Arthritis

The possible role of pathogens and the microbiota in various forms of arthritis will be addressed in depth in Chaps. 15, 16, 17, 18, 19, and 20, but here we will examine some of the data specifically related to *Mpn* infection as a possible cause of adult rheumatoid arthritis (RA) and the various arthritic syndromes collectively termed juvenile idiopathic arthritis (JIA). Mycoplasmas have long been known as a cause of infectious arthritis in humans, particularly in patients with hypogammaglobulinemia [28–31]. They are also well-known causes of chronic arthritis in birds (*M. gallisepticum* and *M. synoviae*), swine (*M. hyorhinis* and *M. hyosynoviae*), goats and sheep (*M. capricolum*), and rodents (*M. arthritidis*) to name but a few examples. Because joint infection with this group of organisms is often low grade and lacks the usual inflammatory signs of septic arthritis, it can even mimic rheumatologic disease [32]. Unsurprisingly, *Mpn* has been repeatedly reported to cause reactive arthritis in association with community-acquired pneumonia [33, 34]. The real question of interest here is whether *Mpn* (or other human mycoplasmas/ureaplasmas) plays a role in any of the various types of chronic adult or juvenile arthritis. It remains an open question [35].

One way in which investigators have attempted to determine whether *Mpn* might play a role in the development of RA has been to examine the prevalence and degree of positivity of circulating antibodies in RA patients compared to non-RA control subjects. In 1975 Cole and colleagues compared antibody titers (as measured by growth inhibition or bactericidal activity) to six species of human mycoplasmas including *Mpn* in a group of 29 RA patients compared to non-RA controls and found no significant differences [36]. However, in a relatively large recent case-control study using modern serologic methods, Ramirez and colleagues found a significant association of antibodies against *Mpn* in 78 RA patients compared to 156 controls [37]. In a review of the incidence of cases of JIA in Manitoba, Canada, between 1975 and 1992, Oen et al. noted a significant correlation between JIA incidence and the periodic increases in *Mpn* infection (diagnosed by serology), which tend to occur every 4–7 years [38]. There was no such correlation noted in the rates of diagnosis of five different respiratory viruses.

The advent of molecular methods of detection of bacteria and viruses appears to offer increased sensitivity and specificity for identification of organisms associated with chronic arthritis. However, these methods suffer from the criticism that they can be overly sensitive and are also susceptible to contamination during sample preparation. Furthermore, the presence of DNA from an organism in, for example, blood or synovial fluid does not necessarily reflect the presence of viable organisms and of course does not necessarily confirm a relationship to disease. Furthermore, many patients with RA are on immunosuppressive medications, which could potentially affect the chances of detection. However, there have been reports of detection of a variety of mycoplasmas including *Mpn* in peripheral blood [39] and synovial fluid [40] of patients with RA. It should also be pointed out that there are also persistent reports of relatively high rates of detection of other species of human mycoplasmas, especially *M. fermentans*, by PCR, culture, and serology in patients with RA compared to controls [39, 41–47].

Since they lack a cell wall, mycoplasmas are unaffected by penicillins and cephalosporins. Varying by species, effective antibiotics generally include tetracyclines, macrolides and ketolides, and quinolones. *Mpn* is sensitive to antibiotics in all three classes, although macrolide resistance is currently on the rise in many countries. Interestingly, there are several placebo-controlled trials of minocycline for rheumatoid arthritis, essentially all of which showed efficacy [48]. In contrast, an early trial with tetracycline and later trials with doxycycline were negative [49–53], albeit one study showed positive results [54]. It is noteworthy that, although the antibiotic spectra of minocycline and doxycycline are similar, minocycline exhibits twice the tissue penetration of doxycycline, and both are several-fold higher in this regard than tetracycline [48], potentially indicating greater capacity of minocycline to treat mycoplasmas present in hard to reach locations such as the synovium. Although this might suggest that there is a microbial etiology for RA, the conclusions that can be drawn from these study results are complicated by the fact that tetracyclines (as well as macrolides) have anti-inflammatory effects that are unrelated to their antimicrobial activities [55].

Neurologic Complications

A large body of literature exists on a variety of neurologic complications, both peripheral and central, which are associated with *Mpn* infection including Guillain-Barré syndrome (GBS), Fisher syndrome, optic neuritis, encephalitis, and acute demyelinating encephalomyelitis (ADEM). One common pathogenic mechanism for those that are thought to have an autoimmune basis is the development of anti-glycolipid antibodies following *Mpn* infection [56]. One common defect that is likely related to the rarity of these conditions and the difficulty in performing prospective studies is that the diagnosis of *Mpn* infection in both case reports and case series is often made with a single antibody determination without positive culture, PCR, or convalescent titers. With that one caveat, there is a convincing amount of data pointing to an association of *Mpn* infection with several different autoimmune neurologic diseases. As noted in the introduction, *Mpn* has been found to have glycosyltransferase(s) that can modify its own and the host's surface glycoprotein and glycolipid glycosylation in a nonspecific manner resulting in immunologic cloaking for the bacterium and, as a bystander effect, in autoimmunity for the host. More direct evidence exists for the role of antigenic mimicry in *Mpn*-induced autoimmune neurologic disorders.

GBS is an acute inflammatory demyelinating polyradiculoneuropathy that is often associated with a preceding infection. The gastrointestinal pathogen *Campylobacter jejuni* is the most common antecedent infection associated with GBS, and much is known about the mechanism by which it induces GBS. The rate of GBS in patients with a *C. jejuni* infection within the preceding 2 weeks is 100 times that of the general population, and 30–40% of GBS cases have had a recent *C. jejuni* infection [57]. Antigenic mimicry of *C. jejuni* antigens with GM1 ganglioside leading to pathogenic autoantibodies is supported by a number of laboratory studies [58]. A similar process of antigenic mimicry is believed to be operative in GBS induced by other microorganisms including *Mpn*. *Mpn* is a relatively uncommon cause of GBS, generally estimated to cause 3–4% of cases [59]. Autoantibodies to galactocerebroside (Gal-C), a major glycolipid constituent of myelin in both the peripheral and central nervous systems, have been hypothesized to play a significant role in *Mpn*-induced autoimmune neuropathies. Rabbits immunized with Gal-C develop an autoimmune neuropathy proving that such antibodies can be pathogenic [60, 61]. Gal-C autoantibodies are present in the majority of GBS associated with *Mpn* infection [62]. Clinical, serologic, and electrophysiologic studies on a large series of GBS patients with and without Gal-C autoantibodies demonstrated that Gal-C autoantibody-positive GBS is more frequently associated with recent *Mpn* infection and with the demyelinating neuropathy variant of GBS with sensory and autonomic neuropathy than with the axonal neuropathy variant [63]. Finally, rabbit anti-Gal-C antibody reacted with several *Mpn* glycolipids by immunostaining indicating that a similar or identical epitope is present on the bacterium [62].

Mpn may be the most common infectious cause of childhood encephalitis. Christie and colleagues published an analysis of 1,988 patients referred to the California Encephalitis Project in which they found evidence of *Mpn* infection in 111 (5.6%) patients, of which 84 (76%) were children [64]. About 84% of these were positive by serology alone, but CSF was positive by PCR in 2%. They concluded that *Mpn* infection is more frequently a cause of encephalitis in children, and in that age group, it was the most common nonviral infectious agent identified. The detection of intrathecal anti-Gal-C antibodies has been detected both in serum and in CSF of patients with *Mpn*-associated encephalitis patients [65]. It has been proposed that detection of intrathecal antibodies to *Mpn*, including cross-reactive antibodies against Gal-C and gangliosides, may constitute significant new methods for diagnosis of *Mpn*-associated encephalitis.

One question of great interest to affected patients and clinicians caring for them is whether antibiotic therapy of a patient with a confirmed *Mpn* infection and an associated extrapulmonary complication such as SJS might result in improvement in the course of this complication. Such data are hard to acquire given the rarity of most of these complications, but it seems reasonable that whether the complication is due to live organisms and/or autoimmunity due to antigenic stimulation from the infection, effective antimicrobial therapy should shorten the course of the disease. In a study of 19 patients with SJS and MPN infections ranging from confirmed to possible, McCormack and colleagues found that a history of antibiotic therapy was significantly associated with confirmed *Mpn* infection, suggesting that such therapy might actually increase the chances of this complication [66]. However, they did not assess the severity of the respiratory symptoms in the infected patients, which might have affected the clinician's decision to treat, and furthermore the antibiotics chosen were all penicillins and cephalosporins, which would not have affected the organism at all. In the patient with SJS associated with a macrolide-resistant *Mpn* infection described by Atkinson and colleagues, there was prolonged illness which included 3 weeks of prodrome; a 3-day hospitalization at an outside hospital which included treatment with IV azithromycin, followed by 7 days of worsening skin disease at the tertiary care hospital; and apparent improvement coincident with initiation of fluoroquinolone therapy [67]. In this case it seemed that the prolonged course might have been due to ineffective therapy of a macrolide-resistant organism with azithromycin. It is noteworthy that there are reports documenting the development of macrolide resistance during therapy of *Mpn* infection in individual patients [68]. Experimental infection of humans with *Mpn* showed that infection-associated cold agglutinins were only seen in the more severely affected patients, who were those without preexisting antibody [69, 70], and more recent studies have suggested that antibiotic therapy improves the course of *Mpn* infection, so it could again be predicted that the development of this common, benign autoimmune manifestation of *Mpn* infection would be blunted by early, effective antibiotic therapy. Some studies have indicated that patients with macrolide-resistant *Mpn* infections treated with macrolides have longer and more severe courses of illness than those infected with macrolide susceptible isolates [71]. However, possibly due to the variability in diagnostic criteria and the impossibility of conducting a clinical trial, systematic review of such reports has not definitely shown benefit of antibiotic therapy [72].

Summary

Mpn, a subtle and sophisticated pathogen that is highly adapted for prolonged infections in humans, has evolved a variety of different mechanisms to evade and distort the host immune response. Numerous basic and clinical studies have convincingly demonstrated that *Mpn* causes a wide array of different autoimmune phenomena. As further studies continue to shed light on the pathogenic mechanisms involved, better understanding of fundamental principles of autoimmune pathogenesis may be forthcoming as well as more efficient strategies of combatting this ubiquitous pathogen.

References

1. Eaton MD, et al. An infectious agent from cases of atypical pneumonia apparently transmissible to cotton rats. Science. 1942;96(2501):518–9.
2. Fadiel A, et al. Mycoplasma genomics: tailoring the genome for minimal life requirements through reductive evolution. Front Biosci. 2007;12:2020–8.

3. Pieper U, et al. Structural evidence for the evolutionary divergence of Mycoplasma from gram-positive bacteria: the histidine-containing phosphocarrier protein. Structure. 1995;3(8):781–90.
4. Su CJ, Baseman JB. Genome size of Mycoplasma genitalium. J Bacteriol. 1990;172(8):4705–7.
5. Desai HP, et al. Complete genome sequence of mycoplasma pneumoniae type 2 reference strain FH using single-molecule real-time sequencing technology. Genome Announc. 2017;5(8):e01629–16. https://doi.org/10.1128/genomeA.01629-16.
6. Dorigo-Zetsma JW, et al. Mycoplasma pneumoniae P1 type 1- and type 2-specific sequences within the P1 cytadhesin gene of individual strains. Infec Immun. 2001;69(9):5612–8.
7. Klement ML, et al. A processive lipid glycosyltransferase in the small human pathogen Mycoplasma pneumoniae: involvement in host immune response. Mol Microbiol. 2007;65(6):1444–57.
8. Daubenspeck JM, et al. General N-and O-linked glycosylation of lipoproteins in Mycoplasmas and role of exogenous oligosaccharide. PLoS One. 2015;10(11):e0143362. https://doi.org/10.1371/journal.pone.0143362. eCollection 2015.
9. Liu C, Eaton MD, Heyl JT. Studies on primary atypical pneumonia. II. Observations concerning the development and immunological characteristics of antibody in patients. J Exp Med. 1959;109(6):545–56.
10. Harwock HJ, Kalmanson GM, Guze LB. Human diseases associated with Mycoplasmas. With an appendix on simple culture techniques. Calif Med. 1972;116(5):1–7.
11. Feizi T, Taylor-Robinson D. Cold agglutinin anti-I and Mycoplasma pneumoniae. Immunology. 1967;13(4):405–9.
12. Hengge UR, et al. Characterization of I/F1 glycoprotein as a receptor for Mycoplasma pneumoniae. Infect Immun. 1992;60(1):79–83.
13. Cherry JD, Hurwitz ES, Welliver RC. Mycoplasma pneumoniae infections and exanthems. J Pediatr. 1975;87(3):369–73. [Review] [34 refs].
14. Prindaville B, et al. Mycoplasma pneumonia—associated mucocutaneous disease in children: dilemmas in classification. Pediatr Dermatol. 2014;31(6):670–5. https://doi.org/10.1111/pde.12482.
15. Ludlam GB, Bridges JB. Association of Stevens-Johnson syndrome with antibody for Mycoplasma pneumoniae. Lancet. 1964;1(7340):958–9.
16. Stanyon JH, Warner WP. Mucosal respiratory syndrome. Can Med Assoc J. 1945;53(5):427–34.
17. Olson D, et al. Outbreak of Mycoplasma pneumoniae-associated Stevens-Johnson syndrome. Pediatrics. 2015;136(2):e386–94. https://doi.org/10.1542/peds.2015-0278.
18. Stutman HR. Stevens-Johnson syndrome and Mycoplasma pneumoniae: evidence for cutaneous infection. J Pediatr. 1987;111(6 Pt 1):845–7.
19. Meseguer MA, de Rafael L, Vidal ML. Stevens-Johnson syndrome with isolation of Mycoplasma pneumoniae from skin lesions. Eur J Clin Microbiol. 1986;5(2):167–8.
20. Lyell A, et al. Mycoplasmas and erythema multiforme. Lancet. 1967;2(7526):1116–8.
21. Fleming PC, et al. Febrile mucocutaneous syndrome with respiratory involvement, associated with isolation of Mycoplasma pneumoniae. Can Med Assoc J. 1967;97(24):1458–9.
22. Watkins LKF, et al. Epidemiology and molecular characteristics of Mycoplasma pneumoniae during an outbreak of M. pneumoniae-associated Stevens-Johnson syndrome. Pediatr Infect Dis J. 2017;36(6):564–71. https://doi.org/10.1097/INF.0000000000001476.
23. Olson D, et al. Characterization of children with recurrent episodes of Stevens-Johnson syndrome. J Pediatr Infect Dis Soc. 2017;6(3):e140–3. https://doi.org/10.1093/jpids/piw085.
24. Wanat KA, et al. Recurrent Stevens-Johnson syndrome secondary to Mycoplasma pneumoniae infection. Cutis. 2014;93(4):E7–8.
25. Campagna C, et al. Mycoplasma pneumoniae-induced recurrent Stevens-Johnson syndrome in children: a case report. Pediatr Dermatol. 2013;30(5):624–6. https://doi.org/10.1111/pde.12177.
26. Daubeney PE, Scopes JW. Recurrent Stevens-Johnson syndrome. J R Soc Med. 1991;84(3):168.
27. Welch KJ, Burke WA, Irons TG. Recurrent erythema multiforme due to Mycoplasma pneumoniae. J Am Acad Dermatol. 1987;17(5 Pt 1):839–40.
28. Sordet C, et al. Bone and joint disease associated with primary immune deficiencies. Joint Bone Spine. 2005;72(6):503–14. [Review] [94 refs].
29. Schaeverbeke T, et al. Mycoplasmas and arthritides. Rev Rhum Engl Ed. 1997;64(2):120–8. [see comments] [Review] [92 refs].
30. Lee AH, Levinson AI, Schumacher HR Jr. Hypogammaglobulinemia and rheumatic disease. Semin Arthritis Rheum. 1993;22(4):252–64.
31. Roifman CM, et al. Increased susceptibility to Mycoplasma infection in patients with hypogammaglobulinemia. Am J Med. 1986;80(4):590–4.
32. Sato H, et al. Hypogammaglobulinemic patient with polyarthritis mimicking rheumatoid arthritis finally diagnosed as septic arthritis caused by Mycoplasma hominis. Intern Med. 2012;51(4):425–9.
33. Lambert HP. Syndrome with joint manifestations in association with Mycoplasma pneumoniae infection. Br Med J. 1968;3(611):156–7.
34. Jones MC. Arthritis and arthralgia in infection with Mycoplasma pneumoniae. Thorax. 1970;25(6):748–50.
35. Taylor-Robinson D, Schaeverbeke T. Mycoplasmas in rheumatoid arthritis and other human arthritides [editorial]. J Clin Pathol. 1996;49(10):781–2.
36. Cole BC, Taylor MB, Ward JR. Studies on the infectious etiology of human rheumatoid arthritis. II. Search for humoral and cell-bound antibodies against mycoplasmal antigens. Arthritis Rheum. 1975;18(5):435–41.

37. Ramirez AS, et al. Relationship between rheumatoid arthritis and Mycoplasma pneumoniae: a case-control study. Rheumatology. 2005;44(7):912–4.
38. Oen K, Fast M, Postl B. Epidemiology of juvenile rheumatoid arthritis in Manitoba, Canada, 1975-92: cycles in incidence. J Rheumatol. 1995;22(4):745–50.
39. Haier J, et al. Detection of mycoplasmal infections in blood of patients with rheumatoid arthritis. Rheumatology (Oxford). 1999;38(6):504–9.
40. Johnson SM, Bruckner F, Collins D. Distribution of Mycoplasma pneumoniae and Mycoplasma salivarium in the synovial fluid of arthritis patients. J Clin Microbiol. 2007;45(3):953–7.
41. Gil C, et al. Presence of Mycoplasma fermentans in the bloodstream of Mexican patients with rheumatoid arthritis and IgM and IgG antibodies against whole microorganism. BMC Musculoskelet Disord. 2009;10:97.
42. Gilroy CB, Keat A, Taylor-Robinson D. The prevalence of Mycoplasma fermentans in patients with inflammatory arthritides. Rheumatology. 2001;40(12):1355–8.
43. Horowitz S, et al. Mycoplasma fermentans in rheumatoid arthritis and other inflammatory arthritides. J Rheumatol. 2000;27(12):2747–53.
44. Schaeverbeke T, et al. Genotypic characterization of seven strains of Mycoplasma fermentans isolated from synovial fluids of patients with arthritis. J Clin Microbiol. 1998;36(5):1226–31.
45. Ataee RA, et al. Simultaneous detection of Mycoplasma pneumoniae, Mycoplasma hominis and Mycoplasma arthritidis in synovial fluid of patients with rheumatoid arthritis by multiplex PCR. Arch Iran Med. 2015;18(6):345–50. doi: 015186/AIM.004.
46. Schaeverbeke T, et al. Systematic detection of mycoplasmas by culture and polymerase chain reaction (PCR) procedures in 209 synovial fluid samples. Br J Rheumatol. 1997;36(3):310–4.
47. Schaeverbeke T, et al. Mycoplasma fermentans, but not M penetrans, detected by PCR assays in synovium from patients with rheumatoid arthritis and other rheumatic disorders. J Clin Pathol. 1996;49(10): 824–8.
48. Cunha BA. New uses for older antibiotics. The 'rediscovery' of four beneficial and cost-effective antimicrobials. Postgrad Med. 1997;101(4):68–70.
49. Skinner M, et al. Tetracycline in the treatment of rheumatoid arthritis. A double blind controlled study. Arthritis Rheum. 1971;14(6):727–32.
50. Pillemer S, et al. Pilot clinical trial of intravenous doxycycline versus placebo for rheumatoid arthritis. J Rheumatol. 2003;30(1):41–3.
51. van der Laan W, et al. Lack of effect of doxycycline on disease activity and joint damage in patients with rheumatoid arthritis. A double blind, placebo controlled trial. J Rheumatol. 2001;28(9):1967–74.
52. St Clair EW, et al. The effects of intravenous doxycycline therapy for rheumatoid arthritis: a randomized, double-blind, placebo-controlled trial. Arthritis Rheum. 2001;44(5):1043–7.
53. Sreekanth VR, et al. Doxycycline in the treatment of rheumatoid arthritis—a pilot study. J Assoc Physicians India. 2000;48(8):804–7.
54. O'Dell JR, Elliott JR, Mallek JA, Mikuls TR, Weaver CA, Glickstein S, Blakely KM, Hausch R, Leff RD. Treatment of early seropositive rheumatoid arthritis: doxycycline plus methotrexate versus methotrexate alone. Arthritis Rheum. 2006;54(2):621–7.
55. Sadarangani SP, Estes LL, Steckelberg JM. Non-anti-infective effects of antimicrobials and their clinical applications: a review. Mayo Clin Proc. 2015;90(1):109–27. https://doi.org/10.1016/j.mayocp.2014.09.006. Epub 2014 Nov 18.
56. Narita M. Pathogenesis of neurologic manifestations of Mycoplasma pneumoniae infection. Pediatr Neurol. 2009;41(3):159–66. https://doi.org/10.1016/j.pediatrneurol.2009.04.012.
57. McCarthy N, Giesecke J. Incidence of Guillain-Barre syndrome following infection with Campylobacter jejuni. Am J Epidemiol. 2001;153(6):610–4.
58. Wijdicks EF, Klein CJ. Guillain-Barre syndrome. Mayo Clin Proc. 2017;92(3):467–79. https://doi.org/10.1016/j.mayocp.2016.12.002.
59. Narita M. Classification of extrapulmonary manifestations due to Mycoplasma pneumoniae infection on the basis of possible pathogenesis. Front Microbiol. 2016;7:23. https://doi.org/10.3389/fmicb.2016.00023. eCollection 2016.
60. Saida T, et al. Experimental allergic neuritis induced by galactocerebroside. Ann Neurol. 1981;9(Suppl):87–101.
61. Saida T, et al. Experimental allergic neuritis induced by sensitization with galactocerebroside. Science. 1979;204(4397):1103–6.
62. Kusunoki S, Shiina M, Kanazawa I. Anti-Gal-C antibodies in GBS subsequent to mycoplasma infection: evidence of molecular mimicry. Neurology. 2001;57(4):736–8.
63. Samukawa M, et al. Clinical features in Guillain-Barre syndrome with anti-Gal-C antibody. J Neurol Sci. 2014;337(1–2):55–60. https://doi.org/10.1016/j.jns.2013.11.016. Epub 2013 Nov 19.
64. Christie LJ, et al. Pediatric encephalitis: what is the role of Mycoplasma pneumoniae? Pediatrics. 2007;120(2):305–13.
65. Meyer Sauteur PM, et al. Antibody responses to Mycoplasma pneumoniae: role in pathogenesis and diagnosis of encephalitis? PLoS Pathog. 2014;10(6):e1003983.
66. McCormack JG. Mycoplasma pneumoniae and the erythema multiforme—Stevens-Johnson syndrome. J Infect. 1981;3(1):32–6.
67. Atkinson TP, et al. Stevens-Johnson syndrome in a boy with macrolide-resistant Mycoplasma pneumoniae pneumonia. Pediatrics. 2011;127(6):e1605–9. https://doi.org/10.1542/peds.2010-2624. Epub 2011 May 2.
68. Suzuki Y, et al. Development of macrolide resistance-associated mutations after macrolide treatment in

children infected with Mycoplasma pneumoniae. J Med Microbiol. 2017;6(10):000582.

69. Smith CB, et al. Mycoplasma pneumoniae infections in volunteers. Ann N Y Acad Sci. 1967;143(1):471–83.
70. Chanock RM, et al. Respiratory disease in volunteers infected with Eaton agent. Proc Natl Acad Sci U S A. 1961;47:887–90.
71. Waites KB, et al. Mycoplasma pneumoniae from the Respiratory Tract and Beyond. Clin Microbiol Rev. 2017;30(3):747–809. https://doi.org/10.1128/CMR.00114-16.
72. Biondi E, et al. Treatment of Mycoplasma pneumonia: a systematic review. Pediatrics. 2014;133(6):1081–90.

11 DNA Viruses in Autoimmune Rheumatic Diseases

Lazaros I. Sakkas and Dimitrios P. Bogdanos

Abbreviations

AAV	ANCA-associated vasculitis
ACPA	Anti-citrullinated protein antibody
AIRD	Autoimmune rheumatic diseases
ANCA	Anti-neutrophil cytoplasmic antibody
ARD	Autoimmune rheumatic disease
CENP-B	Centromere protein B
CMV	Cytomegalovirus
DAS	Disease activity score
DRESS	Drug reaction with eosinophilia and systemic syndrome
dsDNA	Double-stranded DNA
EBV	Epstein-Barr virus
GC	Germinal center
GPA	Granulomatosis with polyangiitis
HBsAg	Hepatitis B surface antigen
HBV	Hepatitis B virus
HHV	Human herpesvirus
HPV	Human papilloma virus
HSV	Herpes simplex virus
IFN	Interferon
LN	Lupus nephritis
MPO	Myeloperoxidase
PBMC	Peripheral blood mononuclear cells
PR3	Proteinase-3
RA	Rheumatoid arthritis
SLE	Systemic lupus erythematosus
SS	Sjogren's syndrome
SSc	Systemic sclerosis
TGF	Transforming growth factor
TNF	Tumor necrosis factor

L. I. Sakkas · D. P. Bogdanos (✉)
Department of Rheumatology and Clinical Immunology, Faculty of Medicine, School of Health Sciences, University of Thessaly, Larissa, Greece
e-mail: bogdanos@med.uth.gr; http://www.autorheumatology.com

Introduction

DNA Viruses and Rheumatic Diseases

Autoimmune rheumatic diseases (AIRDs), such as rheumatoid arthritis (RA), Sjogren's syndrome (SS), systemic lupus erythematosus (SLE), systemic sclerosis (SSc), and anti-neutrophil cytoplasmic antibody (ANCA)-associated vasculitis (AAV), are systemic autoimmune diseases with incompletely understood pathogeneses. Both genetic and environmental factors are implicated, and current thinking is that various environmental factors trigger autoimmunity in an individual with a proper genetic background. Among environmental factors, included are DNA viruses, particularly Epstein-Barr virus (EBV) and human cytomegalovirus (CMV). Apart from these AIRDs, DNA viruses are implicated in other conditions. For instance, EBV and CMV are also triggers of hemophagocytic syndrome in patients receiving biological therapies (Chap. 14) [1].

G. Ragab et al. (eds.), *The Microbiome in Rheumatic Diseases and Infection*,
https://doi.org/10.1007/978-3-319-79026-8_11

They may also be implicated in drug reaction with eosinophilia and systemic syndrome (DRESS), a systemic drug reaction characterized by extensive mucocutaneous rash, fever, lymphadenopathy, organ dysfunction (most often liver dysfunction), and peripheral blood eosinophilia. The pathophysiology of DRESS is incompletely understood but involves reactivation of human herpesvirus (HHV)6, HHV7, CMV, and EBV and a very strong immune response [2].

Herpes Simplex Viruses

Herpes simplex viruses (HSVs) are highly prevalent worldwide and can establish long-term latent infection, a state in which the viral genome persists in cells but does not produce infectious virions, and lytic infection, a state of viral replication and infectious virion shedding [3]. There are no convincing reports on HSV1/2 participation in the pathogenesis of AIRDs, but some data do exist. For instance, HSV1 genome has been detected in salivary glands from three out of 55 SS patients [4]. In addition, there are reports of amino acid sequence homologies between HSV1 proteins and human autoantigens suggesting a possible role for a mechanism of molecular mimicry responsible for HSV-mediated induction of autoimmunity. The immediate-early protein of HSV1 contains multiple homologies to centromere protein B (CENP-B) and the SLE-associated 70 kDa antigen, a component of U1RNP particles (reacting with anti-Sm autoantibodies) [5]. However, HSV1/2 can reactivate and cause infection in immunosuppressed patients with AIRDs [6–8]. Thus, the causality between AIRD and HSV is unclear.

Epstein-Barr Virus

EBV (HHV4) is a γ-herpesvirus, an enveloped virus with double-stranded DNA that infects the vast majority of the adult population worldwide. It enters cells via binding of viral envelope protein gp350 to the CD21 B cell marker. It initially infects epithelial cells and B cells and then stays in latent form (a state in which virus is not replicating and infectious virus is not made) in memory B cells throughout life. During latent infection in B cells, there may be expression of viral nuclear antigens (EBNA1, EBNA2, EBNA3A, EBNA3B, EBNA3C, EBNALP); latent membrane protein (LMP)-1, LMP-2A, and LMP-2B; small nonpolyadenylated RNAs (EBER1, EBER2); microRNAs; and other transcripts (BARTs) (latency III). Latently infected cells may express EBNA1, LMP-1, LMP-2 (latency II), only EBNA1 (latency I), or no viral protein at all (latency 0). EBV may reactivate switching from latent to lytic form, producing infectious virus. The switch from latency to lytic replication is initiated by the expression of the viral immediate-early BZLF1 gene (also known as Z, Zta, Zebra, EB1). Another early lytic antigen essential for viral replication is called "early antigen diffuse."

The main targets of EBV are naïve B cells and B cells undergoing affinity maturation in germinal centers (GCs). Inhibition of B cell apoptosis is the main strategy of EBV. In certain B cells, EBV induces transformational expansion and immortalization as lymphoblastoid cell lines. Antibodies produced by B cells utilize variable (V)-diversity (D)-joining (J) region recombination, which is regulated by recombination-activating genes (RAGs), and EBV induces RAG expression in B cells [9, 10]. EBV antagonizes TGFβ-induced B cell apoptosis by suppressing the pro-apoptotic BIK (Bcl2 interacting killer) [11]. TGFβ induces EBV lytic reactivation by activating BZLF1 gene expression [12, 13].

The ubiquitous presence of EBV along with a significant number of peptides shared between EBV and the human proteome [14] make EBV an attractive environmental causative candidate for various AIRDs.

Rheumatoid Arthritis

RA is characterized by polyarthritis, the presence of rheumatoid factor and anti-citrullinated protein antibodies (ACPAs), and HLA-DRB1* alleles that share a common amino acid sequence (aa 70–74) of the beta chain (shared epitope, HLA-DRB1*SE). ACPAs are directed against various citrullinated proteins, including filaggrin, fibrinogen, α-enolase, fibrin, collagen, vimentin, and others. They appear years before clinical manifestations [15], predict the development of RA in patients with undifferentiated arthritis [16, 17], are specific for RA [reviewed in [18]], and are associated with the disease severity [18, 19].

EBV has long been implicated in the pathogenesis of RA since an increased EBV DNA load was found in peripheral blood from RA patients compared to healthy controls [20], and increased CD8+ T cells recognizing EBV lytic antigen were detected in RA synovial fluid [21], although a systematic review did not find an association of EBV seroprevalence with RA [22]. Subsequent studies linked EBV to ACPAs. Specifically, antibodies to citrullinated peptides derived from EBV proteins were found to be present in sera of RA patients suggesting that EBV infection may trigger the induction of ACPAs. Antiviral citrullinated peptides (VCPs) derived from EBNA1 [23] and EBNA2 [24] were detected in RA. More importantly, antibodies against EBNA1-derived viral citrullinated peptides from RA sera immunoprecipitated an 80 kDa band from EBV-infected cell line [23]. One of these EBNA1-derived viral citrullinated peptides ($EBNA^{35-58cit}$) was a target of ACPAs in RA [25], and by competition assays, anti-$EBNA1_{35-58cit}$ antibodies were highly cross-reactive with citrullinated β_{60-74} fibrin peptide, an immunodominant epitope in ACPA+ RA [26]. Indeed, a large proportion of ACPA-producing plasma cells surrounding GC-like structures in the synovial membrane of RA patients were infected with EBV, as suggested by their co-expression of BFRF1, a protein of early EBV lytic phase [27]. In peripheral blood of severe combined immunodeficiency (SCID) mice transplanted with GC-like structure-containing RA synovial membrane, antibodies against citrullinated EBV peptides were detected and correlated with ACPA [27]. These findings suggest that posttranslationally modified EBV antigens in GC-like structures in RA synovial membrane may trigger ACPA production via cross-reactivity. Citrullinated antigens are likely to be arthritogenic antigens in RA and can promote inflammation through immune complexes with citrullinated proteins, activation of macrophages, and neutrophil extracellular trap formation [28].

EBV can be implicated in RA pathogenesis through other mechanisms. For instance, the EBV gp110, expressed on the budding virion during EBV replication, contains the QKRAA amino acid sequence, which is also present on HLA-DRB1*SE [29], suggesting that the HLA-DRB1*SE may be the target of the immune response. Furthermore, HLA-DRB1*0404, an HLA-DRB1*SE allele, is associated with low T cell responses to EBV gp110, whereas HLA-DRB1*07, an RA protective allele, is associated with high T cell responses to EBV gp110. More importantly, RA disease severity was found to be associated with low T cell responses to gp110 [30].

Another intriguing finding was that the presence of EBV DNA in bone marrow of RA patients was a predictor of a good response to rituximab treatment. EBV DNA was detected by PCR in the bone marrow from RA patients in 15 out of 35 patients treated with rituximab. Of those with EBV, 12/15 (80%) responded, compared to 6/20 (30%) of those without EBV ($p = 0.04$) [31].

Sjogren's Syndrome

SS is characterized by lymphocytic infiltration of exocrine glands, most frequently salivary and lacrimal glands, and the presence of autoantibodies, most frequently SSA. A small percentage of SS patients will go on to develop B cell malignancy.

EBV has a tropism for salivary and lacrimal glands [32]. EBV early antigen antibodies, indicative of viral replication in lytic phase, and EBNA antibodies were found to be correlated with SSA 52 (Ro52) antibodies in SS [33]. GC-like structure-containing SS salivary glands express latent and lytic proteins in B cells and plasma cells, respectively [34]. In particular, perifollicular plasma cells expressing EBV lytic protein display Ro52 immunoreactivity. Furthermore, GC-like structure-containing SS salivary glands transplanted into SCID mice supported the production of both anti-Ro52 abs and anti-EBV antibodies, thus suggesting that EBV may contribute to local autoimmunity in SS [34]. Besides autoimmunity, EBV also affects salivary gland function. The microRNA ebv-miR-BART13, encoded by EBV, is expressed in salivary glands of SS patients and targets STIM1, a sensor of calcium concentration in endoplasmic reticulum, and aquaporin 5, an apical plasma membrane water channel, thus decreasing their function and thus providing a mechanistic link between EBV and salivary gland function in SS [35]. Functional ebv-miR-BART13 can be transferred via exosomes to salivary epithelial cells from B cells [35].

Systemic Lupus Erythematosus

SLE is characterized by multiorgan involvement, including renal involvement with glomerulonephritis, and the presence of many autoantibodies against various antigens. The plethora of autoantibodies against nuclear and other antigens, such as antinuclear antibodies (ANAs), anti-double-stranded DNA (dsDNA) antibodies, anti-Sm antibodies, and anti-phospholipid antibodies (anti-cardiolipin, anti-β2 GPI, lupus anticoagulant) suggests that reduced regulatory function by T and/or B cells and/or hyperactivation of B cells takes place in SLE pathogenesis.

Higher titers of anti-EBV antibodies and 10- to 100-fold higher EBV DNA load were detected in sera of SLE patients compared to controls [36–38]. Higher titers of IgM, IgG, and IgA levels against EBV lytic early antigen diffuse were detected in SLE patients [39, 40] and were inversely correlated with lymphocyte counts [40]. More importantly, EBV latent membrane protein-1 (LMP-1), a CD40 mimic, was detected in renal biopsies from lupus nephritis (LN) patients [41, 42]. EBV-encoded RNA-1 (EBER1), a small RNA that is the most abundant RNA in EBV latent phase, was also detected in LN biopsies [41]. Furthermore, EBV LMP-1 positivity in LN was associated with anti-Sm antibodies [41] and LN classification [42]. EBV-encoded latent membrane protein-2A (LMP-2A) mimics the B cell antigen receptor (BCR) in murine GC. Furthermore, GC B cell-specific LMP-2A expression led to an SLE-like autoimmune phenotype [43], and EBV-encoded LMP-2A induced an anti-Sm response through TLR9 hypersensitivity [44]. However, an EBV-related γ-herpesvirus γHV68 infection strongly inhibited lupus-like disease in mice that spontaneously develop the disease [45].

There are a great number of peptides shared between EBV and the human proteome [14], and molecular mimicry has been documented between SLE autoantigens and EBV antigens. Multiple peptide homologies were detected between EBV and the SLE-associated 70 kDa antigen [5]. A cross-reactivity was found between the Sm B/B′ sequence PPPGMRPP and the EBNA1 sequence PPPGRRP. This EBNA1 peptide is recognized by sera from SLE patients but not from EBV-positive normal individuals. Cross-reactivity was also found between the Sm D1 95–119 peptide and the EBNA1 35–58 peptide [36, 46]. Furthermore, immunization of rabbits with EBNA1 PPPGRRP peptide induced lupus autoimmunity [36]. Also, immunization with EBNA1 peptides or expression of EBNA1 in mice caused IgG antibodies against Sm and dsDNA [47, 48] and leukopenia [47]. Of note, two monoclonal antibodies to EBNA1 cross-reacting with dsDNA bind to the same amino acid viral epitope of EBNA1 [49].

There is an impaired leukocyte response to EBV latent and lytic antigens in SLE [50] which is associated with high anti-EBV antibodies and inversely correlates with SLE disease activity. This may suggest that the high antibody response to EBV may be an attempt to compensate for the impaired T cell response.

Systemic Sclerosis

SSc is a complex disease characterized by extensive fibrosis, vascular fibrointimal proliferation, and autoantibodies. Two main autoantibodies, anti-topoisomerase I (ATA), and anti-centromere autoantibodies (ACA) are associated with diffuse cutaneous (dcSSc) and the limited cutaneous (lcSSc) form of the disease, respectively, and are used in early diagnosis of SSc [51, 52]. The pathogenesis of the disease is incompletely understood, but adaptive immunity responses [51, 53] as well as innate immunity receptors participate in the pathological process [54]. Oligoclonal T cells are found in skin lesions and can promote fibrosis through profibrotic cytokines and cell contact with fibroblasts [55], whereas B cells are hyperactivated, producing autoantibodies with profibrotic actions [53]. Innate immunity, exemplified by type I interferon (IFN) signatures involved in antiviral responses, was detected in the skin and peripheral blood in SSc [56–58]. TLR9, an innate immunity receptor and a sensor of microbial nucleic acids, was upregulated in SSc skin and induced profibrotic responses via TGFβ in fibroblasts [54].

The early EBV lytic transactivator BZLF1 that drives EBV replication, latent genes, and early lytic protein are detected in peripheral blood mononuclear cells (PBMCs), skin fibroblasts, and endothelial cells in SSc suggesting an ongoing EBV infection [59]. In this regard, EBV can impact on both immunity and fibrosis. For instance, EBV can induce anti-Topo I antibodies in B cells from healthy donors [60]. Also, EBV can infect fibroblasts and induce TLR8 and IFN-regulated genes and a profibrotic phenotype, in which EBV replication could be detected in skin fibroblasts, myofibroblasts (activated fibroblasts), and endothelial cells [59]. TGFβ1 expression was upregulated in fibroblasts expressing high levels of BZFL1 [59]. Of note, the BZLF1 increased TGFβ1 production in epithelial cells [61]. TGFβ1 inhibits CpG DNA-induced type I IFN production via ubiquitination of TNF receptor-associated factor 6 (TRAF6) [62]. Thus, on one hand, TGFβ1 dampens the response to EBV, activates BZLF1 gene expression, and induces EBV lytic reactivation, and on the other hand EBV lytic infection upregulates TGFβ1 [12, 13]. Similarly, transfection with BZFL1 induces IL-13 expression, and IL-13 is required at an early stage of EBV-induced proliferation of B cells [63]. Of importance, TGFβ1 and IL-13 are potent profibrotic mediators in SSc [51]. Peripheral blood monocytes from SSc patients and skin macrophages also express BZLF1 and BFRF1, an EBV early lytic protein [64], whereas microarray analysis has revealed that EBV-infected monocytes exhibit upregulation of IFN-regulated genes and TLR8 [64].

There are multiple peptide homologies between EBV immunodominant antigens and SSc autoantigens, and some data suggest the presence of cross-reactive immune responses involving viral/host mimics [65]. The pathogenic significance of these findings and the direct link with the induction of the disease remains obscure.

ANCA Vasculitis

Granulomatosis with polyangiitis (GPA, formerly Wegener's granulomatosis) is the prototype of AAV. GPA is characterized by extravascular granulomas and small vessel vasculitis affecting many organs/systems, most often the respiratory system and kidneys. ANCA in AAV, depending on immunostaining of neutrophils, are classified as cytoplasmic (cANCA) or perinuclear (pANCA) and are directed against proteinase-3 (PR3) or myeloperoxidase (MPO), respectively. Primed with inflammatory mediators, neutrophils express PR3 and MPO on their cell surface and, when stimulated with ANCA, induce endothelial cell death. In experimental models, MPO-ANCA are pathogenic inducing pauci-immune glomerulonephritis and pulmonary capillaritis. However, GPA, apart from small vessel vasculitis and PR3-ANCA, is characterized by granulomas, which suggests T cell involvement as well [66]. GPA granulomatous lesions have GC-like structures capable of antibody production against PR3 [67]. Importantly, EBV-transformed B cells can produce cANCA [68]. In addition, PR3-ANCA and MPO-ANCA may appear transiently in patients with infectious mononucleosis (an acute EBV infection) [69].

Cytomegalovirus

CMV, a β-herpesvirus, is a double-stranded DNA virus which produces latent and lytic infection and infects many cell types, including fibroblasts. An early lytic gene encoding a protein essential for viral replication is called pp52. Once infected, CMV stays for life and can be reactivated when T cell immunity is compromised, most often after organ transplantation. The practicing physician should be vigilant to the fact that CMV in immunocompromised hosts may cause severe and life-threatening disorders, including severe hepatitis, duodenitis, ileocolitis, acute encephalitis, infectious mononucleosis, adult-onset Still's disease, retinitis, pneumonitis, and hemophagocytic syndrome. This acute CMV infection may complicate concomitant treatment of serious manifestations of underlying AIRD [70].

Rheumatoid Arthritis

CMV appears to be implicated in RA pathogenesis. CMV DNA was detected in the synovial membrane from 11 out of 83 patients with RA compared to 2 out of 64 patients with other joint disorders [71]. Latent CMV infection, as detected by CMV seropositivity, was associated with more severe joint damage in RA [72]. Cytotoxic $CD4^{+}CD28^{-}$ T cells are closely associated with CMV seropositivity as well as with cardiovascular disease and are expanded in RA [73, 74]. These findings imply that the increased cardiovascular risk in patients with RA may be due to CMV. Of note, ex vivo T cell responses to CMV lysates were associated with more severe joint damage [75] and with the clinical response to initial disease-modifying antirheumatic drugs in early RA [76]. A higher baseline anti-CMV response predicted inadequate Disease Activity Score (DAS)28 response [76].

Sjogren's Syndrome

There are no convincing data linking CMV to the pathogenesis of SS. The prevalence of IgG anti-CMV antibodies was found to be lower in SS than in controls [33]. Intraperitoneal injections of murine CMV can induce a SS-like disease in autoimmune-prone mice, but the relevance of the murine model results to the human disease is not clear [77].

Systemic Lupus Erythematosus

CMV may be implicated in the pathogenesis of SLE. IgA and IgG antibodies to CMV pp52 early lytic antigen were significantly higher in SLE compared to healthy controls and were positively associated with lymphocyte counts [40]. However, the practicing physician should bear in mind a differential diagnosis of CMV infection in an immunocompromised patient with SLE from CMV causing autoimmunity [78].

Systemic Sclerosis

There are similarities between CMV vasculopathy and SSc vascular disease [79], and vascular factors, such as endothelin, and growth factors, such as TGFβ and platelet-derived growth factor, may provide a mechanistic link between vascular disease and tissue fibrosis. A murine vasculopathy model, resembling SSc vasculopathy, provided evidence that CMV infection alone cannot cause neointima formation but requires the addition of immune dysregulation. For instance, murine CMV-infected mice lacking the IFNγ receptor (IFNγR−/−) subjected to whole-body irradiation developed extensive adventitial and medial inflammatory infiltrates and significant neointima formation in arteries, with proliferation of myofibroblasts and upregulation of TGFβ and platelet-derived growth factor-A and growth factor-B [80].

The frequency of antibodies against specific CMV-encoded antigens, such as UL83, UL57, and UL94, was higher in patients with SSc compared to pathological controls (such as patients with multiple sclerosis) or healthy individuals, but whether these findings are epiphenomena or relevant to the pathogenesis of the disease is not known [81, 82]. There are multiple peptide homologies between CMV and CENP-B which could support a molecular mimicry between CMV and humans [5]. Also, topoisomerase I shares a pentapeptide homology with the CMV UL70 protein [83]. The immune response to CMV can cause vascular injury and fibrosis. For instance, antibodies to CMV-encoded UL94 protein cross-react with the cell membrane tetraspanin transmembrane 4 superfamily member 7 (TM4SF7 or NAG-2) molecule and induce apoptosis of endothelial cells and activation of fibroblasts [84, 85]. Others, however, have been unable to demonstrate immunological cross-reactivity between CMV antigens and SSc-specific autoantigens [82].

ANCA Vasculitis

Studies on the possible role of CMV in AAV are limited. Yet, preliminary results show that CMV may be implicated in GPA. Cytotoxic $CD4^{+}CD28^{-}$ and $CD8^{+}CD28^{-}$ T cell expansions associated with CMV seropositivity were detected in GPA [86, 87] and were linked with increased mortality [87]. Also, concomitant cellular CMV and/or EBV positivity was associated with $CD4^{+}CD28^{-}$ and $CD8^{+}CD28^{-}$ T cells in GPA [88]. Preliminary results showed that $CD4^{+}CD28^{-}$ T cells in CMV-seropositive AAV patients are pro-inflammatory and are expanded and associated with arterial stiffness (carotid to femoral pulse wave velocity). Furthermore, their expansion was attenuated after valacyclovir therapy [89]. Further studies are required in this exciting field.

Human Herpesviruses 6, 7, and 8

The role of these three herpesviruses in AIRD is yet unproven. HHV6 is a double-stranded DNA virus causing latent and lytic infections. An early lytic gene encoding a protein essential for viral replication is called p41. In immunocompromised individuals, HHV6 can cause limbic encephalitis. In one study, cell-free HHV6 DNA was detected in a higher proportion of patients with AIRD (SSc, RA, or SLE) [90]. HHV7 can cause fever and seizures in children. HHV7 prevalence and load in PBMCs did not differ between patients with RA, SLE, or SSc and healthy controls [90]. HHV8 is causally related to Kaposi's sarcoma and to multicentric Castleman's disease, a B cell-proliferative disorder. In immunocompromised individuals, HHV8 can cause fever, splenomegaly and cytopenias, or Kaposi's sarcoma. In one study analyzing cell-free serum, however, HHV8 DNA was not detected in any patient with AIRD (RA, SLE, or SSc) [90].

HHV6, HHV7, and HHV8 do not appear to be involved in the pathogenesis of AIRDs. However, practicing physicians should be aware that HHV6 is associated with severe DRESS [91, 92].

Parvovirus B19

Human parvovirus B19 (parvoB19) is a non-enveloped, single-stranded DNA virus. Its genome encodes two capsid proteins, VP1 and VP2, and a nonstructural protein NS1, which is cytotoxic to host cells. ParvoB19 can infect erythroid progenitor cells and also other cells including endothelial cells [93]. It causes a variety of disorders including erythema infectiosum in children and aplastic anemia and cytopenias in immunocompromised patients.

Acute parvoB19 infection can present with RA-like and SLE-like clinical and serological disease [94–98] and can induce a broad range of autoantibodies, such as rheumatoid factor, ANA, anti-dsDNA, ANCA, and anti-cardiolipin antibodies [98, 99]. ParvoB19-encoded NS1 induces apoptosis of non-permissive cells and cleaves DNA [100, 101]. Furthermore, apoptotic bodies contain targets of common autoantibodies, such as Smith, DNA, histone H4, and phosphatidylserine, which are engulfed and taken up for antigen presentation by differentiated macrophages [101]. Peptide homologies detected between parvoB19 PV1 protein and human cytokeratin and GATA-1, a transcription factor involved in erythropoiesis, could be of pathogenic significance [98].

In RA, parvoB19 seems to modulate cytokine expression, since parvoB19 PV1 protein-stimulated PBMC from RA patients produce less IFNγ than those from healthy controls. Furthermore, plasma IL-10 levels were lower in parvoB19+ RA compared to pavoB19− RA patients but did not differ between parvoB19+ and parvoB19− healthy controls [102].

ParvoB19 does not seem to be involved in SS pathogenesis since no parvoB19 DNA has been detected in peripheral blood from patients with SS [103] or salivary glands [104].

ParvoB19 infection can mimic SLE, particularly patients with cytopenias, pleuritis/pericarditis, or glomerulonephritis [95, 105–109]. ParvoB19 has also been associated with dilated cardiomyopathy and high levels of cytokines IL-17 and IL-6 in SLE patients [110]. ParvoB19 DNA was detected in 17 of 72 SLE patients [103]. However, a recent study found no association of parvoB19 infection (IgM, IgG antibodies, and viral DNA) with the presence or activity of the disease. Yet, an association was found in SLE patients with the presence of anti-phospholipid antibodies [111].

The role of parvoB19 in SSc needs further investigation. ParvoB19 DNA was detected in SSc skin but also in the skin from healthy donors [112]. The virus can infect endothelial cells and fibroblasts [113] and has been found in latency in the bone marrow of SSc patients [114].

Also there is no evidence that parvoB19 is implicated in AAV pathogenesis, although PR3-ANCA and MPO-ANCA may appear transiently (<6 months) during acute parvoB19 infection and lead to misdiagnosis of GPA [69, 99].

Human Papilloma Virus

Human papilloma virus (HPV) is a non-enveloped virus that infects epithelia and has a genome with double-stranded DNA consisting of an early region (E), a late region (L), and an upstream noncoding regulatory region (URR). E1 and E2 proteins modulate viral DNA replication, and L1 and L2 genes encode capsid proteins. There are at least 100 HPV types, with HPV1 and HPV2 causing warts and HPV16 causing cervical dysplasia and cervical cancer [115].

HPV might participate in the pathogenesis of AIRDs since there are peptide homologies between HPV and human proteins which may give rise to autoimmune responses through molecular mimicry [116, 117].

Rheumatoid Arthritis

In RA HPV may trigger the production of ACPAs. The HPV-47 E2 peptide 345–362 is homologous to profilaggrin 306–324, and both citrullinated peptides are targets of ACPA in RA. Furthermore, RA patients with anti-citrullinated HPV-47 E2 345–362 antibodies had higher DAS28 and radiographic progression compared to RA patients without these antibodies [116].

Systemic Lupus Erythematosus

There are peptide homologies between HPV and the SLE autoantigen Ku, complement proteins C4A and C4B, and the B cell signal-transducing surface protein CD19, but their pathogenic relevance is unclear at present [117]. UK women with recent diagnosis of SLE had a high frequency of HPV infection, particularly with HPV-16 variants, and were found to have a higher viral load and frequency of abnormal cervical cytology and squamous intraepithelial lesions [118].

Hepatitis B Virus

Hepatitis B virus (HBV) is a hepatotropic DNA virus causing acute and chronic hepatitis. Only limited data are available on the prevalence of hepatitis B in patients with AIRDs.

HBV Reactivation in Patients with Rheumatic Diseases

HBV may reactivate in patients with hepatitis B surface antigen-negative (HBsAg−) and hepatitis B core antibody-positive (HBcAb+) patients on immunosuppression, particularly with high-dose corticosteroids and cytokine inhibitor biological agents. However, long-term use of methotrexate does not result in HBV reactivation [119]. Better knowledge and more awareness of the risk for HBV reactivation with the different antirheumatic agents and the more recent development of the new-generation oral antivirals have greatly improved the design of screening and therapeutic algorithms in clinical practice [120]. Thus, the US Centers for Disease Control and Prevention recommends screening patients for HBsAg, HBcAb, and hepatitis B surface antibody (HBsAb) before starting immunosuppressive therapy. In a similar vein, the American Association for the Study of Liver Diseases recommends HBV screening before initiation of immunosuppressive therapy. Especially for AIRDs, guidelines for the treatment of RA by the American College of Rheumatology or the European League against Rheumatism also suggest HBV screening and provide recommendations on the management of HBV.

HBV-Associated Polyarteritis Nodosa

The strongest link between HBV and AIRDs is that with polyarteritis nodosa (PAN), a systemic necrotizing vasculitis that predominantly affects medium-sized arteries (Chap. 25). In fact, PAN is the consequence of viral infections, mainly HBV. The incidence of HBV-associated PAN has declined over the past decades following the parallel decline of HBV infection due to prophylactic vaccination. Peripheral neuropathy, recent-onset hypertension resulting from renal vasculopathy, skin nodules, orchitis, and gastrointestinal manifestations, especially those requiring surgery, are more frequent in patients with HBV-associated PAN than in PAN patients without HBV [121]. Overall, HBV infected PAN patients have more severe disease [121]. The pathogenic mechanisms linking HBV with PAN are not entirely resolved. HBsAg/anti-HBs antibody complexes are found in the vascular lesions (especially the recent ones), while such complexes do not appear in healed lesions, suggesting a crucial role played by the immune complexes in the initiation of these vascular lesions [122].

HBV and Other Rheumatic Diseases

HBV patients may rarely (~3%) develop cryoglobulinemic vasculitis with type II or type III cryoglobulinemia [123]. In these patients, cryoglobulinemia is caused by clonal expansion of innate B cells producing a VH1-69-encoded antibody [124].

The presence of chronic HBV infection is endemic in some countries, such as China and Taiwan. A considerable proportion of these patients develop symptoms of polyarthralgia, and serological testing reveals RF positivity, raising the issue of concomitant RA [125]. ACPAs are more specific for RA than RF and should be measured to help in the discrimination of HBV-associated arthropathy from concomitant RA in patients with chronic HBV infection [125]. The presence of SLE in such endemic areas has been reported lower than that in demographically matched non-SLE patients, but the reason for this underrepresentation remains unknown [126].

An increased risk for SS in patients with chronic hepatitis C virus infection but not with HBV has been reported, though more recent data suggest that the risk for SS may be increased in men with HBV rather than in those without chronic viral hepatitis [127]. No association was found between SSc and chronic HBV, although the titers of anti-HBc antibodies were higher in SSc patients compared to controls [128].

Figure 11.1 illustrates individual DNA viruses and their relation with specific autoimmune rheumatic diseases.

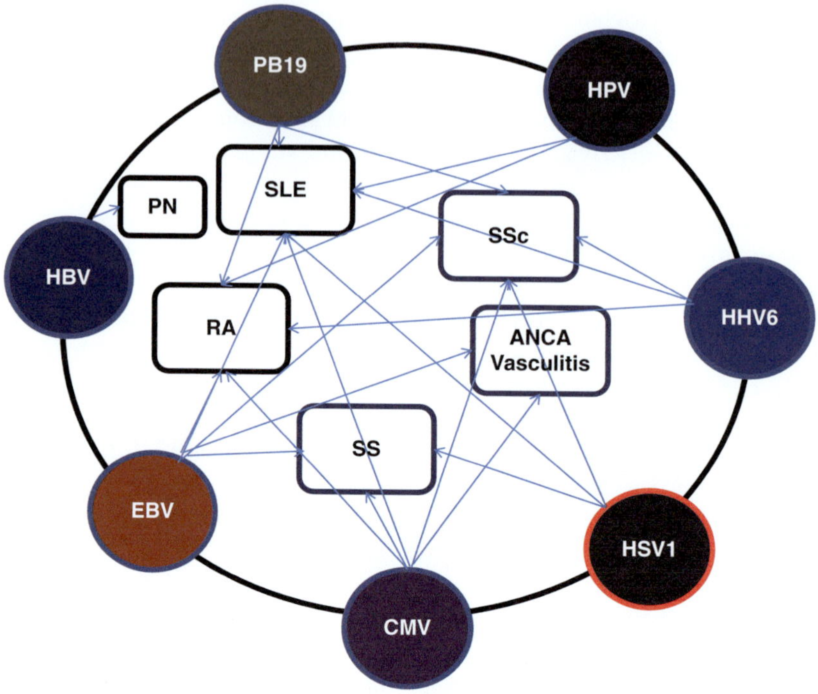

Fig. 11.1 Pathogenic links between DNA viruses and autoimmune rheumatic diseases. *HSV1* herpes simplex virus-1, *EBV* Epstein-Barr virus, *CMV* cytomegalovirus, *HBV* hepatitis B virus, *PB19* parvovirus B19, *HPV* human papillomavirus, *HHV6* human herpesvirus 6, *ANCA* anti-neutrophil cytoplasmic antibody, *RA* rheumatoid arthritis, *SLE* systemic lupus erythematosus, *SS* Sjogren's syndrome, *SSc* systemic sclerosis, *PN* polyarteritis nodosa

Conclusion

Multiple DNA viruses have been linked to a variety of autoimmune diseases. Although not all cases necessarily represent evidence of a causal infection, there is nevertheless strong evidence that EBV is associated with RA and lupus, CMV and *Parvovirus* may be linked to RA, and HBV is clearly implicated in PAN. Furthermore, even in the absence of a causal association, the treating rheumatologist should be aware that in the context of autoimmune diseases and associated treatment, patients are at substantially increased risk of complications associated with infections with DNA viruses.

References

1. Brito-Zeron P, Bosch X, Perez-de-Lis M, Perez-Alvarez R, Fraile G, Gheitasi H, et al. Infection is the major trigger of hemophagocytic syndrome in adult patients treated with biological therapies. Semin Arthritis Rheum. 2016;45(4):391–9.
2. Descamps V, Ranger-Rogez S. DRESS syndrome. Joint Bone Spine. 2014;81(1):15–21.
3. Thellman NM, Triezenberg SJ. Herpes simplex virus establishment, maintenance, and reactivation: in vitro modeling of latency. Pathogens. 2017;6(3):E28.
4. Perrot S, Calvez V, Escande JP, Dupin N, Marcelin AG. Prevalences of herpesviruses DNA sequences in salivary gland biopsies from primary and secondary Sjogren's syndrome using degenerated consensus PCR primers. J Clin Virol. 2003;28(2):165–8.
5. Douvas A, Sobelman S. Multiple overlapping homologies between two rheumatoid antigens and immunosuppressive viruses. Proc Natl Acad Sci U S A. 1991;88(14):6328–32.
6. Witt MN, Braun GS, Ihrler S, Schmid H. Occurrence of HSV-1-induced pneumonitis in patients under standard immunosuppressive therapy for rheumatic, vasculitic, and connective tissue disease. BMC Pulm Med. 2009;9:22.
7. Zhang L, Liu JJ, Li MT. Herpes simplex virus type 1 encephalitis and unusual retinitis in a patient with systemic lupus erythematosus. Lupus. 2013;22(13):1403–8.
8. Curtis JR, Xie F, Yun H, Bernatsky S, Winthrop KL. Real-world comparative risks of herpes virus

infections in tofacitinib and biologic-treated patients with rheumatoid arthritis. Ann Rheum Dis. 2016;75(10):1843–7.

9. Kuhn-Hallek I, Sage DR, Stein L, Groelle H, Fingeroth JD. Expression of recombination activating genes (RAG-1 and RAG-2) in Epstein–Barr virus-bearing B cells. Blood. 1995;85(5):1289–99.
10. Wagner HJ, Scott RS, Buchwald D, Sixbey JW. Peripheral blood lymphocytes express recombination-activating genes 1 and 2 during Epstein–Barr virus-induced infectious mononucleosis. J Infect Dis. 2004;190(5):979–84.
11. Campion EM, Hakimjavadi R, Loughran ST, Phelan S, Smith SM, D'Souza BN, et al. Repression of the proapoptotic cellular BIK/NBK gene by Epstein–Barr virus antagonizes transforming growth factor beta1-induced B-cell apoptosis. J Virol. 2014;88(9):5001–13.
12. Liang CL, Chen JL, Hsu YP, Ou JT, Chang YS. Epstein–Barr virus BZLF1 gene is activated by transforming growth factor-beta through cooperativity of Smads and c-Jun/c-Fos proteins. J Biol Chem. 2002;277(26):23345–57.
13. Iempridee T, Das S, Xu I, Mertz JE. Transforming growth factor beta-induced reactivation of Epstein–Barr virus involves multiple smad-binding elements cooperatively activating expression of the latent-lytic switch BZLF1 gene. J Virol. 2011;85(15):7836–48.
14. Capone G, Calabro M, Lucchese G, Fasano C, Girardi B, Polimeno L, et al. Peptide matching between Epstein–Barr virus and human proteins. Pathog Dis. 2013;69(3):205–12.
15. Nielen MM, van Schaardenburg D, Reesink HW, van de Stadt RJ, van der Horst-Bruinsma IE, de Koning MH, et al. Specific autoantibodies precede the symptoms of rheumatoid arthritis: a study of serial measurements in blood donors. Arthritis Rheum. 2004;50(2):380–6.
16. Barouta G, Katsiari CG, Alexiou I, Liaskos C, Varna A, Bogdanos DP, et al. Anti-MCV antibodies predict radiographic progression in Greek patients with very early (<3 months duration) rheumatoid arthritis. Clin Rheumatol. 2017;36(4):885–94.
17. Sokolove J, Bromberg R, Deane KD, Lahey LJ, Derber LA, Chandra PE, et al. Autoantibody epitope spreading in the pre-clinical phase predicts progression to rheumatoid arthritis. PLoS One. 2012;7(5):e35296.
18. Conigliaro P, Chimenti MS, Triggianese P, Sunzini F, Novelli L, Perricone C, et al. Autoantibodies in inflammatory arthritis. Autoimmun Rev. 2016;15(7):673–83.
19. Alexiou I, Germenis A, Koutroumpas A, Kontogianni A, Theodoridou K, Sakkas LI. Anti-cyclic citrullinated peptide-2 (CCP2) autoantibodies and extra-articular manifestations in Greek patients with rheumatoid arthritis. Clin Rheumatol. 2008;27(4):511–3.
20. Balandraud N, Meynard JB, Auger I, Sovran H, Mugnier B, Reviron D, et al. Epstein–Barr virus load in the peripheral blood of patients with rheumatoid arthritis: accurate quantification using real-time polymerase chain reaction. Arthritis Rheum. 2003;48(5):1223–8.
21. Scotet E, David-Ameline J, Peyrat MA, Moreau-Aubry A, Pinczon D, Lim A, et al. T cell response to Epstein–Barr virus transactivators in chronic rheumatoid arthritis. J Exp Med. 1996;184(5):1791–800.
22. Ball RJ, Avenell A, Aucott L, Hanlon P, Vickers MA. Systematic review and meta-analysis of the sero-epidemiological association between Epstein–Barr virus and rheumatoid arthritis. Arthritis Res Ther. 2015;17:274.
23. Pratesi F, Tommasi C, Anzilotti C, Chimenti D, Migliorini P. Deiminated Epstein–Barr virus nuclear antigen 1 is a target of anti-citrullinated protein antibodies in rheumatoid arthritis. Arthritis Rheum. 2006;54(3):733–41.
24. Pratesi F, Tommasi C, Anzilotti C, Puxeddu I, Sardano E, Di Colo G, et al. Antibodies to a new viral citrullinated peptide, VCP2: fine specificity and correlation with anti-cyclic citrullinated peptide (CCP) and anti-VCP1 antibodies. Clin Exp Immunol. 2011;164(3):337–45.
25. Cornillet M, Sebbag M, Verrouil E, Magyar A, Babos F, Ruyssen-Witrand A, et al. The fibrin-derived citrullinated peptide beta60-74Cit(6)(0),(7)(2),(7)(4) bears the major ACPA epitope recognised by the rheumatoid arthritis-specific anticitrullinated fibrinogen autoantibodies and anti-CCP2 antibodies. Ann Rheum Dis. 2014;73(6):1246–52.
26. Cornillet M, Verrouil E, Cantagrel A, Serre G, Nogueira L. In ACPA-positive RA patients, antibodies to EBNA35-58Cit, a citrullinated peptide from the Epstein–Barr nuclear antigen-1, strongly cross-react with the peptide beta60-74Cit which bears the immunodominant epitope of citrullinated fibrin. Immunol Res. 2015;61(1–2):117–25.
27. Croia C, Serafini B, Bombardieri M, Kelly S, Humby F, Severa M, et al. Epstein–Barr virus persistence and infection of autoreactive plasma cells in synovial lymphoid structures in rheumatoid arthritis. Ann Rheum Dis. 2013;72(9):1559–68.
28. Sakkas LI, Bogdanos DP, Katsiari C, Platsoucas CD. Anti-citrullinated peptides as autoantigens in rheumatoid arthritis-relevance to treatment. Autoimmun Rev. 2014;13(11):1114–20.
29. Roudier J, Petersen J, Rhodes GH, Luka J, Carson DA. Susceptibility to rheumatoid arthritis maps to a T-cell epitope shared by the HLA-Dw4 DR beta-1 chain and the Epstein–Barr virus glycoprotein gp110. Proc Natl Acad Sci U S A. 1989;86(13):5104–8.
30. Balandraud N, Roudier J, Roudier C. Epstein–Barr virus and rheumatoid arthritis. Autoimmun Rev. 2004;3(5):362–7.
31. Magnusson M, Brisslert M, Zendjanchi K, Lindh M, Bokarewa MI. Epstein–Barr virus in bone marrow of rheumatoid arthritis patients predicts response to rituximab treatment. Rheumatology (Oxford). 2010;49(10):1911–9.
32. Fox RI, Pearson G, Vaughan JH. Detection of Epstein–Barr virus-associated antigens and DNA in

salivary gland biopsies from patients with Sjogren's syndrome. J Immunol. 1986;137(10):3162–8.

33. Kivity S, Arango MT, Ehrenfeld M, Tehori O, Shoenfeld Y, Anaya JM, et al. Infection and autoimmunity in Sjogren's syndrome: a clinical study and comprehensive review. J Autoimmun. 2014;51:17–22.
34. Croia C, Astorri E, Murray-Brown W, Willis A, Brokstad KA, Sutcliffe N, et al. Implication of Epstein–Barr virus infection in disease-specific autoreactive B cell activation in ectopic lymphoid structures of Sjogren's syndrome. Arthritis Rheumatol. 2014;66(9):2545–57.
35. Gallo A, Jang SI, Ong HL, Perez P, Tandon M, Ambudkar I, et al. Targeting the Ca(2+) sensor STIM1 by exosomal transfer of Ebv-miR-BART13-3p is associated with Sjogren's syndrome. EBioMedicine. 2016;10:216–26.
36. Toussirot E, Roudier J. Epstein–Barr virus in autoimmune diseases. Best Pract Res Clin Rheumatol. 2008;22(5):883–96.
37. Draborg A, Izarzugaza JM, Houen G. How compelling are the data for Epstein–Barr virus being a trigger for systemic lupus and other autoimmune diseases? Curr Opin Rheumatol. 2016;28(4):398–404.
38. Barzilai O, Sherer Y, Ram M, Izhaky D, Anaya JM, Shoenfeld Y. Epstein–Barr virus and cytomegalovirus in autoimmune diseases: are they truly notorious? A preliminary report. Ann N Y Acad Sci. 2007;1108:567–77.
39. Fattal I, Shental N, Molad Y, Gabrielli A, Pokroy-Shapira E, Oren S, et al. Epstein–Barr virus antibodies mark systemic lupus erythematosus and scleroderma patients negative for anti-DNA. Immunology. 2014;141(2):276–85.
40. Rasmussen NS, Draborg AH, Nielsen CT, Jacobsen S, Houen G. Antibodies to early EBV, CMV, and HHV6 antigens in systemic lupus erythematosus patients. Scand J Rheumatol. 2015;44(2):143–9.
41. Yu XX, Yao CW, Tao JL, Yang C, Luo MN, Li SM, et al. The expression of renal Epstein–Barr virus markers in patients with lupus nephritis. Exp Ther Med. 2014;7(5):1135–40.
42. Ding Y, He X, Liao W, Yi Z, Yang H, Xiang W. The expression of EBV-encoded LMP1 in young patients with lupus nephritis. Int J Clin Exp Med. 2015;8(4):6073–8.
43. Minamitani T, Yasui T, Ma Y, Zhou H, Okuzaki D, Tsai CY, et al. Evasion of affinity-based selection in germinal centers by Epstein–Barr virus LMP2A. Proc Natl Acad Sci U S A. 2015;112(37):11612–7.
44. Wang H, Nicholas MW, Conway KL, Sen P, Diz R, Tisch RM, et al. EBV latent membrane protein 2A induces autoreactive B cell activation and TLR hypersensitivity. J Immunol. 2006;177(5):2793–802.
45. Larson JD, Thurman JM, Rubtsov AV, Claypool D, Marrack P, van Dyk LF, et al. Murine gammaherpesvirus 68 infection protects lupus-prone mice from the development of autoimmunity. Proc Natl Acad Sci U S A. 2012;109(18):E1092–100.
46. Riemekasten G, Marell J, Trebeljahr G, Klein R, Hausdorf G, Haupl T, et al. A novel epitope on the C-terminus of SmD1 is recognized by the majority of sera from patients with systemic lupus erythematosus. J Clin Investig. 1998;102(4):754–63.
47. Poole BD, Gross T, Maier S, Harley JB, James JA. Lupus-like autoantibody development in rabbits and mice after immunization with EBNA-1 fragments. J Autoimmun. 2008;31(4):362–71.
48. Sundar K, Jacques S, Gottlieb P, Villars R, Benito ME, Taylor DK, et al. Expression of the Epstein–Barr virus nuclear antigen-1 (EBNA-1) in the mouse can elicit the production of anti-dsDNA and anti-Sm antibodies. J Autoimmun. 2004;23(2):127–40.
49. Yadav P, Carr MT, Yu R, Mumbey-Wafula A, Spatz LA. Mapping an epitope in EBNA-1 that is recognized by monoclonal antibodies to EBNA-1 that cross-react with dsDNA. Immun Inflamm Dis. 2016;4(3):362–75.
50. Draborg AH, Sandhu N, Larsen N, Lisander Larsen J, Jacobsen S, Houen G. Impaired cytokine responses to Epstein–Barr virus antigens in systemic lupus erythematosus patients. J Immunol Res. 2016;2016:6473204.
51. Sakkas LI, Chikanza IC, Platsoucas CD. Mechanisms of disease: the role of immune cells in the pathogenesis of systemic sclerosis. Nat Clin Pract Rheumatol. 2006;2(12):679–85.
52. Liaskos C, Marou E, Simopoulou T, Barmakoudi M, Efthymiou G, Scheper T, et al. Disease-related autoantibody profile in patients with systemic sclerosis. Autoimmunity. 2017;50:1–8.
53. Sakkas LI, Bogdanos DP. Systemic sclerosis: new evidence re-enforces the role of B cells. Autoimmun Rev. 2016;15(2):155–61.
54. Fang F, Shangguan AJ, Kelly K, Wei J, Gruner K, Ye B, et al. Early growth response 3 (Egr-3) is induced by transforming growth factor-beta and regulates fibrogenic responses. Am J Pathol. 2013;183(4):1197–208.
55. Sakkas LI, Xu B, Artlett CM, Lu S, Jimenez SA, Platsoucas CD. Oligoclonal T cell expansion in the skin of patients with systemic sclerosis. J Immunol. 2002;168(7):3649–59.
56. York MR, Nagai T, Mangini AJ, Lemaire R, van Seventer JM, Lafyatis R. A macrophage marker, Siglec-1, is increased on circulating monocytes in patients with systemic sclerosis and induced by type I interferons and toll-like receptor agonists. Arthritis Rheum. 2007;56(3):1010–20.
57. Kim D, Peck A, Santer D, Patole P, Schwartz SM, Molitor JA, et al. Induction of interferon-alpha by scleroderma sera containing autoantibodies to topoisomerase I: association of higher interferon-alpha activity with lung fibrosis. Arthritis Rheum. 2008;58(7):2163–73.
58. Eloranta ML, Franck-Larsson K, Lovgren T, Kalamajski S, Ronnblom A, Rubin K, et al. Type I interferon system activation and association with

disease manifestations in systemic sclerosis. Ann Rheum Dis. 2010;69(7):1396–402.
59. Farina A, Cirone M, York M, Lenna S, Padilla C, McLaughlin S, et al. Epstein–Barr virus infection induces aberrant TLR activation pathway and fibroblast-myofibroblast conversion in scleroderma. J Investig Dermatol. 2014;134(4):954–64.
60. Hu PQ, Fertig N, Medsger TA Jr, Wright TM. Molecular recognition patterns of serum anti-DNA topoisomerase I antibody in systemic sclerosis. J Immunol. 2004;173(4):2834–41.
61. Cayrol C, Flemington EK. Identification of cellular target genes of the Epstein–Barr virus transactivator Zta: activation of transforming growth factor beta igh3 (TGF-beta igh3) and TGF-beta 1. J Virol. 1995;69(7):4206–12.
62. Naiki Y, Komatsu T, Koide N, Dagvadorj J, Yoshida T, Arditi M, et al. TGF-beta1 inhibits the production of IFN in response to CpG DNA via ubiquitination of TNF receptor-associated factor (TRAF) 6. Innate Immun. 2015;21(7):770–7.
63. Tsai SC, Lin SJ, Chen PW, Luo WY, Yeh TH, Wang HW, et al. EBV Zta protein induces the expression of interleukin-13, promoting the proliferation of EBV-infected B cells and lymphoblastoid cell lines. Blood. 2009;114(1):109–18.
64. Farina A, Peruzzi G, Lacconi V, Lenna S, Quarta S, Rosato E, et al. Epstein–Barr virus lytic infection promotes activation of toll-like receptor 8 innate immune response in systemic sclerosis monocytes. Arthritis Res Ther. 2017;19(1):39.
65. Mahler M, Mierau R, Schlumberger W, Bluthner M. A population of autoantibodies against a centromere-associated protein A major epitope motif cross-reacts with related cryptic epitopes on other nuclear autoantigens and on the Epstein–Barr nuclear antigen 1. J Mol Med (Berl). 2001;79(12):722–31.
66. Kallenberg CG. Advances in pathogenesis and treatment of ANCA-associated vasculitis. Discov Med. 2014;18(99):195–201.
67. Voswinkel J, Mueller A, Kraemer JA, Lamprecht P, Herlyn K, Holl-Ulrich K, et al. B lymphocyte maturation in Wegener's granulomatosis: a comparative analysis of VH genes from endonasal lesions. Ann Rheum Dis. 2006;65(7):859–64.
68. Mayet WJ, Hermann E, Kiefer B, Lehmann H, Manns M, Meyer Zum Buschenfelde KH. In vitro production of anti-neutrophilocyte-cytoplasm-antibodies (ANCA) by Epstein–Barr virus-transformed B-cell lines in Wegener's granulomatosis. Autoimmunity. 1991;11(1):13–9.
69. Hermann J, Demel U, Stunzner D, Daghofer E, Tilz G, Graninger W. Clinical interpretation of antineutrophil cytoplasmic antibodies: parvovirus B19 infection as a pitfall. Ann Rheum Dis. 2005;64(4):641–3.
70. Berman N, Belmont HM. Disseminated cytomegalovirus infection complicating active treatment of systemic lupus erythematosus: an emerging problem. Lupus. 2017;26(4):431–4.
71. Einsele H, Steidle M, Muller CA, Fritz P, Zacher J, Schmidt H, et al. Demonstration of cytomegalovirus (CMV) DNA and anti-CMV response in the synovial membrane and serum of patients with rheumatoid arthritis. J Rheumatol. 1992;19(5):677–81.
72. Pierer M, Rothe K, Quandt D, Schulz A, Rossol M, Scholz R, et al. Association of anticytomegalovirus seropositivity with more severe joint destruction and more frequent joint surgery in rheumatoid arthritis. Arthritis Rheum. 2012;64(6):1740–9.
73. Hooper M, Kallas EG, Coffin D, Campbell D, Evans TG, Looney RJ. Cytomegalovirus seropositivity is associated with the expansion of CD4+CD28− and CD8+CD28− T cells in rheumatoid arthritis. J Rheumatol. 1999;26(7):1452–7.
74. Broadley I, Pera A, Morrow G, Davies KA, Kern F. Expansions of cytotoxic CD4+CD28− T cells drive excess cardiovascular mortality in rheumatoid arthritis and other chronic inflammatory conditions and are triggered by CMV infection. Front Immunol. 2017;8:195.
75. Davis JM 3rd, Knutson KL, Skinner JA, Strausbauch MA, Crowson CS, Therneau TM, et al. A profile of immune response to herpesvirus is associated with radiographic joint damage in rheumatoid arthritis. Arthritis Res Ther. 2012;14(1):R24.
76. Davis JM, Knutson KL, Strausbauch MA, Green AB, Crowson CS, Therneau TM, et al. Immune response profiling in early rheumatoid arthritis: discovery of a novel interaction of treatment response with viral immunity. Arthritis Res Ther. 2013;15(6):R199.
77. Ohyama Y, Carroll VA, Deshmukh U, Gaskin F, Brown MG, Fu SM. Severe focal sialadenitis and dacryoadenitis in NZM2328 mice induced by MCMV: a novel model for human Sjogren's syndrome. J Immunol. 2006;177(10):7391–7.
78. Rozenblyum EV, Allen UD, Silverman ED, Levy DM. Cytomegalovirus infection in childhood-onset systemic lupus erythematosus. Int J Clin Rheumtol. 2013;8(1):137–46.
79. Kahaleh MB, LeRoy EC. Autoimmunity and vascular involvement in systemic sclerosis (SSc). Autoimmunity. 1999;31(3):195–214.
80. Hamamdzic D, Harley RA, Hazen-Martin D, LeRoy EC. MCMV induces neointima in IFN-gammaR−/− mice: intimal cell apoptosis and persistent proliferation of myofibroblasts. BMC Musculoskelet Disord. 2001;2:3.
81. Marou E, Liaskos C, Efthymiou G, Dardiotis E, Daponte A, Scheper T, et al. Increased immunoreactivity against human cytomegalovirus UL83 in systemic sclerosis. Clin Exp Rheumatol. 2017;106(4):31–4.
82. Marou E, Liaskos C, Simopoulou T, Efthymiou G, Dardiotis E, Katsiari C, et al. Human cytomegalovirus (HCMV) UL44 and UL57 specific antibody responses in anti-HCMV-positive patients with systemic sclerosis. Clin Rheumatol. 2017;36(4):863–9.
83. Muryoi T, Kasturi KN, Kafina MJ, Cram DS, Harrison LC, Sasaki T, et al. Antitopoisomerase

I monoclonal autoantibodies from scleroderma patients and tight skin mouse interact with similar epitopes. J Exp Med. 1992;175(4):1103–9.
84. Lunardi C, Bason C, Navone R, Millo E, Damonte G, Corrocher R, et al. Systemic sclerosis immunoglobulin G autoantibodies bind the human cytomegalovirus late protein UL94 and induce apoptosis in human endothelial cells. Nat Med. 2000;6(10):1183–6.
85. Traggiai E, Lunardi C, Bason C, Dolcino M, Tinazzi E, Corrocher R, et al. Generation of anti-NAG-2 mAb from patients' memory B cells: implications for a novel therapeutic strategy in systemic sclerosis. Int Immunol. 2010;22(5):367–74.
86. Morgan MD, Pachnio A, Begum J, Roberts D, Rasmussen N, Neil DA, et al. CD4+CD28− T cell expansion in granulomatosis with polyangiitis (Wegener's) is driven by latent cytomegalovirus infection and is associated with an increased risk of infection and mortality. Arthritis Rheum. 2011;63(7):2127–37.
87. Eriksson P, Sandell C, Backteman K, Ernerudh J. Expansions of CD4+CD28− and CD8+CD28− T cells in granulomatosis with polyangiitis and microscopic polyangiitis are associated with cytomegalovirus infection but not with disease activity. J Rheumatol. 2012;39(9):1840–3.
88. Kerstein A, Schuler S, Cabral-Marques O, Fazio J, Hasler R, Muller A, et al. Environmental factor and inflammation-driven alteration of the total peripheral T-cell compartment in granulomatosis with polyangiitis. J Autoimmun. 2017;78:79–91.
89. Chanouzas D, Dyall L, Dale J, Moss P, Morgan M, Harper L. CD4+CD28− T-cell expansions in ANCA-associated vasculitis and association with arterial stiffness: baseline data from a randomised controlled trial. Lancet. 2015;385(Suppl 1):S30.
90. Broccolo F, Drago F, Cassina G, Fava A, Fusetti L, Matteoli B, et al. Selective reactivation of human herpesvirus 6 in patients with autoimmune connective tissue diseases. J Med Virol. 2013;85(11):1925–34.
91. Tohyama M, Hashimoto K, Yasukawa M, Kimura H, Horikawa T, Nakajima K, et al. Association of human herpesvirus 6 reactivation with the flaring and severity of drug-induced hypersensitivity syndrome. Br J Dermatol. 2007;157(5):934–40.
92. Balci DD, Peker E, Duran N, Dogramaci CA. Sulfasalazine-induced hypersensitivity syndrome in a 15-year-old boy associated with human herpesvirus-6 reactivation. Cutan Ocul Toxicol. 2009;28(1):45–7.
93. von Kietzell K, Pozzuto T, Heilbronn R, Grossl T, Fechner H, Weger S. Antibody-mediated enhancement of parvovirus B19 uptake into endothelial cells mediated by a receptor for complement factor C1q. J Virol. 2014;88(14):8102–15.
94. Woolf AD, Campion GV, Chishick A, Wise S, Cohen BJ, Klouda PT, et al. Clinical manifestations of human parvovirus B19 in adults. Arch Intern Med. 1989;149(5):1153–6.
95. Seve P, Ferry T, Koenig M, Cathebras P, Rousset H, Broussolle C. Lupus-like presentation of parvovirus B19 infection. Semin Arthritis Rheum. 2005;34(4):642–8.
96. Watanabe Y, Inoue Y, Takatani T, Arai H, Yasuda T. Self-limited lupus-like presentation of human parvovirus B19 infection in a 1-year-old girl. Pediatr Int. 2009;51(3):411–2.
97. Narvaez Garcia FJ, Domingo-Domenech E, Castro-Bohorquez FJ, Biosca M, Garcia-Quintana A, Perez-Vega C, et al. Lupus-like presentation of parvovirus B19 infection. Am J Med. 2001;111(7):573–5.
98. Lunardi C, Tinazzi E, Bason C, Dolcino M, Corrocher R, Puccetti A. Human parvovirus B19 infection and autoimmunity. Autoimmun Rev. 2008;8(2):116–20.
99. Chou TN, Hsu TC, Chen RM, Lin LI, Tsay GJ. Parvovirus B19 infection associated with the production of anti-neutrophil cytoplasmic antibody (ANCA) and anticardiolipin antibody (aCL). Lupus. 2000;9(7):551–4.
100. Poole BD, Kivovich V, Gilbert L, Naides SJ. Parvovirus B19 nonstructural protein-induced damage of cellular DNA and resultant apoptosis. Int J Med Sci. 2011;8(2):88–96.
101. Thammasri K, Rauhamaki S, Wang L, Filippou A, Kivovich V, Marjomaki V, et al. Human parvovirus B19 induced apoptotic bodies contain altered self-antigens that are phagocytosed by antigen presenting cells. PLoS One. 2013;8(6):e67179.
102. Naciute M, Mieliauskaite D, Rugiene R, Maciunaite G, Mauricas M, Murovska M, et al. Parvovirus B19 infection modulates the levels of cytokines in the plasma of rheumatoid arthritis patients. Cytokine. 2017;96:41–8.
103. Hsu TC, Tsay GJ. Human parvovirus B19 infection in patients with systemic lupus erythematosus. Rheumatology (Oxford). 2001;40(2):152–7.
104. De Stefano R, Frati E, De Quattro D, Menza L, Manganelli S. Low doses of etanercept can be effective to maintain remission in ankylosing spondylitis patients. Clin Rheumatol. 2014;33(5):707–11.
105. Sugimoto T, Tsuda A, Uzu T, Kashiwagi A. Emerging lupus-like manifestations in acute parvovirus B19 infection. Clin Rheumatol. 2008;27(1):119–20.
106. Chen DY, Chen YM, Lan JL, Tzang BS, Lin CC, Hsu TC. Significant association of past parvovirus B19 infection with cytopenia in both adult-onset Still's disease and systemic lupus erythematosus patients. Clin Chim Acta. 2012;413(9–10):855–60.
107. Cugler T, Carvalho LM, Facincani I, Yamamoto AY, Silva GE, Costa RS, et al. Severe glomerulonephritis and encephalopathy associated with parvovirus B19 infection mimicking systemic lupus erythematosus. Scand J Rheumatol. 2012;41(1):79–81.
108. Cooray M, Manolakos JJ, Wright DS, Haider S, Patel A. Parvovirus infection mimicking systemic lupus erythematosus. CMAJ. 2013;185(15):1342–4.
109. Georges E, Rihova Z, Cmejla R, Decleire PY, Langen C. Parvovirus B19 induced lupus-like syndrome with nephritis. Acta Clin Belg. 2016;71(6):423–5.

110. Chen DY, Chen YM, Tzang BS, Lan JL, Hsu TC. Th17-related cytokines in systemic lupus erythematosus patients with dilated cardiomyopathies: a possible linkage to parvovirus B19 infection. PLoS One. 2014;9(12):e113889.
111. Hod T, Zandman-Goddard G, Langevitz P, Rudnic H, Grossman Z, Rotman-Pikielny P, et al. Does parvovirus infection have a role in systemic lupus erythematosus? Immunol Res. 2017;65(2):447–53.
112. Ohtsuka T, Yamazaki S. Altered prevalence of human parvovirus B19 component genes in systemic sclerosis skin tissue. Br J Dermatol. 2005;152(5):1078–80.
113. Magro CM, Nuovo G, Ferri C, Crowson AN, Giuggioli D, Sebastiani M. Parvoviral infection of endothelial cells and stromal fibroblasts: a possible pathogenetic role in scleroderma. J Cutan Pathol. 2004;31(1):43–50.
114. Ferri C, Zakrzewska K, Longombardo G, Giuggioli D, Storino FA, Pasero G, et al. Parvovirus B19 infection of bone marrow in systemic sclerosis patients. Clin Exp Rheumatol. 1999;17(6):718–20.
115. Graham SV. The human papillomavirus replication cycle, and its links to cancer progression: a comprehensive review. Clin Sci (Lond). 2017;131(17):2201–21.
116. Shi J, Sun X, Zhao Y, Zhao J, Li Z. Prevalence and significance of antibodies to citrullinated human papilloma virus-47 E2345-362 in rheumatoid arthritis. J Autoimmun. 2008;31(2):131–5.
117. Segal Y, Dahan S, Calabro M, Kanduc D, Shoenfeld Y. HPV and systemic lupus erythematosus: a mosaic of potential crossreactions. Immunol Res. 2017;65(2):564–71.
118. Nath R, Mant C, Luxton J, Hughes G, Raju KS, Shepherd P, et al. High risk of human papillomavirus type 16 infections and of development of cervical squamous intraepithelial lesions in systemic lupus erythematosus patients. Arthritis Rheum. 2007;57(4):619–25.
119. Laohapand C, Arromdee E, Tanwandee T. Long-term use of methotrexate does not result in hepatitis B reactivation in rheumatologic patients. Hepatol Int. 2015;9(2):202–8.
120. Koutsianas C, Thomas K, Vassilopoulos D. Hepatitis B reactivation in rheumatic diseases: screening and prevention. Rheum Dis Clin N Am. 2017;43(1):133–49.
121. Pagnoux C, Seror R, Henegar C, Mahr A, Cohen P, Le Guern V, et al. Clinical features and outcomes in 348 patients with polyarteritis nodosa: a systematic retrospective study of patients diagnosed between 1963 and 2005 and entered into the French Vasculitis Study Group Database. Arthritis Rheum. 2010;62(2):616–26.
122. Michalak T. Immune complexes of hepatitis B surface antigen in the pathogenesis of periarteritis nodosa. A study of seven necropsy cases. Am J Pathol. 1978;90(3):619–32.
123. Mazzaro C, Dal Maso L, Urraro T, Mauro E, Castelnovo L, Casarin P, et al. Hepatitis B virus related cryoglobulinemic vasculitis: a multicentre open label study from the Gruppo Italiano di Studio delle Crioglobulinemie - GISC. Dig Liver Dis. 2016;48(7):780–4.
124. Visentini M, Pascolini S, Mitrevski M, Marrapodi R, Del Padre M, Todi L, et al. Hepatitis B virus causes mixed cryoglobulinaemia by driving clonal expansion of innate B-cells producing a VH1-69-encoded antibody. Clin Exp Rheumatol. 2016;34(3 Suppl 97):S28–32.
125. Lim MK, Sheen DH, Lee YJ, Mun YR, Park M, Shim SC. Anti-cyclic citrullinated peptide antibodies distinguish hepatitis B virus (HBV)-associated arthropathy from concomitant rheumatoid arthritis in patients with chronic HBV infection. J Rheumatol. 2009;36(4):712–6.
126. Zhao J, Qiu M, Li M, Lu C, Gu J. Low prevalence of hepatitis B virus infection in patients with systemic lupus erythematosus in southern China. Rheumatol Int. 2010;30(12):1565–70.
127. Yeh CC, Wang WC, Wu CS, Sung FC, Su CT, Shieh YH, et al. Association of Sjogrens syndrome in patients with chronic hepatitis virus infection: a population-based analysis. PLoS One. 2016;11(8):e0161958.
128. Arnson Y, Amital H, Guiducci S, Matucci-Cerinic M, Valentini G, Barzilai O, et al. The role of infections in the immunopathogensis of systemic sclerosis—evidence from serological studies. Ann N Y Acad Sci. 2009;1173:627–32.

RNA Viruses and Autoimmunity: A Short Overview

12

Massimo Galli, Giorgio Bozzi, and Andrea Giacomelli

Abbreviations

AHA	Autoimmune hemolytic anemia
AIDS	Acquired immunodeficiency syndrome
ANA	Antinuclear antibody
Anti-LKM	Anti-liver/kidney microsomal antibodies
CA	Coxsackie A viruses
cART	Combined antiretroviral therapy
CB	Coxsackie B viruses
CD4+ T cells	Helper T lymphocytes
CV	Cryoglobulinemic vasculitis
DCM	Dilated cardiomyopathy
DM	Dermatomyositis
GAD65	Glutamic acid decarboxylase autoantigen
MGN	Membranoproliferative glomerulonephritis
HAV	Hepatitis A virus
HCV	Hepatitis C virus
HIV-1	Human immunodeficiency virus type 1
IRIS	Immune restoration inflammatory syndrome
PM	Polymyositis
PsA	Psoriatic arthritis
RA	Rheumatoid arthritis
RNA	Ribonucleic acid
SLE	Systemic lupus erythematosus
T1D	Type 1 diabetes
TCR	T-cell receptor

M. Galli (✉) · G. Bozzi · A. Giacomelli
Infectious Diseases Unit, University of Milan,
L. Sacco Hospital, Milan, Italy
e-mail: massimo.galli@unimi.it

Enterovirus and Autoimmunity

Enteroviruses belong to the *Picornaviridae* family, comprising non-enveloped, small, single-stranded positive-sense RNA genome viruses. On the basis of their pathogenesis, enteroviruses were originally classified into four groups: polioviruses, coxsackie A viruses (CA), coxsackie B viruses (CB), and echoviruses. Due to the significant overlaps in such taxonomy, enteroviruses (EV) isolated more recently are named with a system of consecutive numbers: EV68, EV69, EV70, EV71, etc. [1]. Enteroviruses are named after their transmission route which is mainly fecal-oral (despite other routes of transmission being present for some species).

The main clinical entities caused almost exclusively by enteroviruses are poliomyelitis, herpangina, hand-foot-and-mouth disease, and epidemic pleurodynia. Other enterovirus-related disorders, such as aseptic meningitis and myopericarditis, may also be caused by other etiological agents.

G. Ragab et al. (eds.), *The Microbiome in Rheumatic Diseases and Infection*,
https://doi.org/10.1007/978-3-319-79026-8_12

Several picornavirus infections showed a strong association with autoimmunity. This is especially true in type 1 diabetes (T1D) and myocarditis. The exact mechanisms inducing autoimmunity remain controversial. Antigenic mimicry, i.e., the shared sequence or tertiary structure between foreign and self-antigens, is the most well-established theory for enterovirus- induced autoimmunity. For example, in a subpopulation of patients with T1D, a molecular mimicry has been found between glutamic acid decarboxylase (GAD65) and protein 2C of coxsackie B-like enteroviruses, suggesting a possible cross-reaction involved in the pathogenesis of the disease [2]. Alternatively, cytopathic infectious agents can cause the release of either sequestered or intracellular autoantigens inducing dual TCR expression (i.e., the induction of T cells bearing receptors potentially responding also against self-tissues) [3].

Viruses have been suggested as a potential environmental trigger of T1D; a disease having a well-documented genetic basis, whose etiology remains to be elucidated. The body of evidence supporting a relationship between viral infections and initiation or acceleration of islet autoimmunity remains largely circumstantial. Among the different possible candidates, the most robust association was established with some enterovirus strains inducing or accelerating the disease in animal models [4].

Higher coxsackievirus-neutralizing antibody titers in serum were reported from recent-onset T1D patients as compared to nondiabetic subjects, and a possible relationship with these viruses was later confirmed using polymerase chain reaction testing, particularly with coxsackie B virus (B4 in particular) [5]. Cross-sectional studies have focused predominantly on recent-onset individuals with T1D, although enterovirus was also identified as a risk factor in prediabetic children and pregnant women. There is still a lack of large prospective studies that establish a clear temporal relation between enterovirus infection and the development of islet autoimmunity.

The possibility of a viral infection specifically affecting pancreatic endocrine cells constitutes a straightforward explanation for the selective demise of beta cells, either through lysis induced by cytopathic viruses or immune-mediated destruction of infected beta cells. Coxsackievirus, however, displays pancreas tropism rather than a preference for islet beta cells; furthermore, direct studies on the pancreas in vivo in order to search for viral infection signatures are limited by the organ's relative inaccessibility [4].

Viral infections are presumed to represent the most common causes of myocarditis in North America and Europe [6]. Viral genomes are detected in the myocardium of a variable proportion of patients with myocarditis and dilated cardiomyopathy (DCM) using molecular techniques. Several lines of evidence support the involvement of autoimmunity in myocarditis. These include the production of antibodies against self-antigens, improvement of myocarditis symptoms with immunosuppressive therapy, and a co-occurrence of myocarditis with other autoimmune diseases [7]. In genetically predisposed mouse strains, viral RNA and inflammation can persist in heart cells for several weeks, triggering myocardial autoimmune reactions [8]. However, there is no direct evidence that this can occur in humans.

Is Hepatitis A Virus a Trigger of Chronic Autoimmune Phenomena?

Like enteroviruses, hepatitis A virus (HAV) is a single-stranded RNA virus belonging to the *Picornaviridae* family. It is transmitted through the fecal-oral route and is the most common cause of acute viral hepatitis, particularly common among children and young adults. Different from other major hepatotropic viruses, it does not sustain a chronic viral hepatitis, as it is systematically cleared after the acute phase [9].

Patients with HAV infection occasionally manifest symptoms consistent with circulating immune complex formation. These include cutaneous vasculitis, arthritis, antinuclear antibody (ANA) production, and cryoglobulinemia. Either IgM or IgG anti-HAV is detected in the cryoglobulins [10]. The symptoms resolve spontaneously with resolution of hepatitis A.

A possible role for HAV as an autoimmune hepatitis trigger has been proposed from a study on relatives of patients with autoimmune chronic active hepatitis [11] and described later in some case reports [12, 13]. The finding of molecular mimicry (cross-reactivity between epitopes of viruses and certain liver antigens) may support the hypothesis of a role for HAV as a trigger of autoimmunity, although this should concern a minority of individuals genetically predisposed, and is influenced by unknown cofactors. In particular, the development of chronic autoimmune hepatitis has been described in patients with a defect in suppressor-inducer T lymphocytes specifically controlling immune responses to the asialoglycoprotein receptor. These predisposed patients might develop specific antibodies directed to the asialoglycoprotein receptor after HAV infection [11]. However, these reports have remained anecdotal.

Hepatitis C Virus and Autoimmunity

HCV is a small, enveloped, positive-sense single-stranded RNA virus of the *Flaviviridae* family. As many as 80–90% of HCV-infected patients have chronic infection defined by persistent serum HCV RNA despite humoral and cellular immune responses [14].

Persistent HCV infection leads to the development of chronic liver disease, cirrhosis, hepatocellular carcinoma, and also a broad spectrum of extrahepatic diseases. HCV infection can in fact subvert the immune system in several ways, ranging from the expansion of selective B-cell subsets to tolerance induction and to the reaction of T cells against apoptosis-derived self-antigens. Cryoglobulins; rheumatoid factor; ANA; and anticardiolipin, antithyroid, and anti-liver/kidney microsomal antibodies (anti-LKM), as well as HCV/anti-HCV immune complex formation and deposition, can be found in infected patients [15]. An association with HCV has been established with cryoglobulinemic vasculitis (CV), membranoproliferative glomerulonephritis (MGN), and porphyria cutanea tarda and also suggested with thyroiditis, Sjogren's syndrome, idiopathic pulmonary fibrosis, polyarthralgias in the setting of positive rheumatoid factor, and some cases of polymyositis/dermatomyositis (PM/DM) (Fig. 12.1) [16].

Cryoglobulins are anti-immunoglobulin immunoglobulins that reversibly precipitate at reduced temperatures. Mixed cryoglobulins

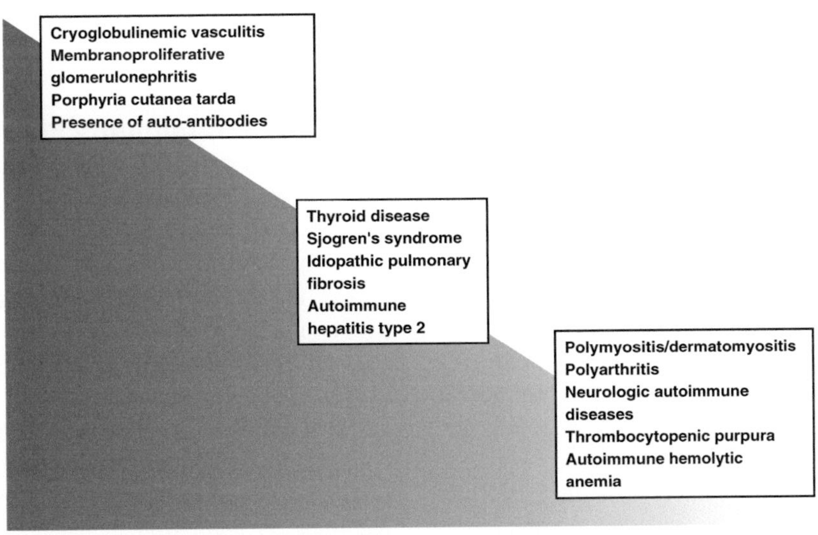

Fig. 12.1 A graphic representation of autoimmune and rheumatic diseases associated with HCV chronic infection, on a gradient based on the association strength, according to literature [15–20]. The left box includes conditions with a definite association with HCV, a high percentage of which occurs in HCV-positive patients. For such diseases, a pathogenic mechanism involving HCV has been described. The middle box encompasses conditions which have some association with HCV chronic infection but have low overall HCV positivity prevalence and/or lack a definite pathogenic link. The right box includes conditions with weak or anecdotal association to HCV

usually contain IgM and IgG immunoglobulins, with the IgM having rheumatoid factor activity directed against IgG molecules. This leads to immune complex formation and cryoprecipitation. The presence of a monoclonal IgM component (type 2 cryoglobulin) may prelude to a progression to frank lymphoma.

HCV infection is the cause of more than 90% of the diagnosed cases of CV, which is a small vessel vasculitis involving mainly the skin, the joints, the peripheral nervous system, and the kidneys. The drivers of B-cell dysregulation during the course of chronic HCV infection are still to be fully characterized [17]. The disease expression is variable, ranging from mild symptoms (purpura, arthralgia) to fulminant life-threatening complications (glomerulonephritis, widespread vasculitis). The prevalent type of glomerulonephritis associated with mixed cryoglobulinemia is membranoproliferative glomerulonephritis (see Chap. 26).

HCV may interfere with the functions and mechanisms of self-recognition both on the immune system and thyroid cells, where HCV may directly destroy thyroid tissue or mimic the structure of some components of thyroid gland, igniting the autoimmune disease. In the course of HCV infection, both hypothyroidism and hyperthyroidism may emerge, Hashimoto's thyroiditis being the most common thyroid disorder observed in patients with HCV infection. Interferon, which has been the mainstay of chronic HCV infection treatment until recently, can be an additional risk factor for the development of thyroid complications. It was advisable for clinicians to monitor thyroid function regularly in patients with chronic HCV and, in particular during treatment, with interferon-based regimens [18].

It has been reported that more than 60% of patients from the Mediterranean area presenting with type 2 autoimmune hepatitis carry anti-HCV antibodies along with the typical anti-LKM autoantibody pattern. However, a very limited proportion of HCV-positive patients have positive anti-LKM [15]. It appears that primary Sjogren's syndrome may only be sporadically associated with HCV infection, and definitive evidence that HCV infection may trigger Sjogren's syndrome is still lacking. Conversely, chronic HCV infection is associated frequently with sialoadenitis and occasionally with sicca syndrome. However, the pathogenic overlap of the increased risk of B-cell malignancies in Sjogren's syndrome and the emergence of an association between HCV infection and monoclonal gammopathies and lymphoproliferative disorders are worth mentioning [19].

Arthritis can be observed along the course of HCV infection and in some cases is associated with mixed cryoglobulinemia. These patients typically present an anti-CCP antibody-negative, nonerosive intermittent oligoarticular arthritis [20].

Non-cryoglobulinemic glomerulonephritis has been associated with HCV, especially in children, and immune-mediated skin diseases, especially oral lichen planus, have been linked to HCV. Neurologic autoimmune diseases, including myelitis and encephalomyelitis, as well as several neuromuscular diseases, have also been reported to occur in HCV infection. The virus might be involved in the pathogenesis of other hematologic entity subsets, such as immune thrombocytopenic purpura (ITP) and autoimmune hemolytic anemia (AHA). Conversely, autoimmune mechanisms have been implicated in thrombocytopenia associated with chronic HCV [19].

HIV and Autoimmunity Before and After Combined Antiretroviral Treatment Introduction

HIV, a member of the genus *Lentivirus*, which is part of the family *Retroviridae*, is the causative agent of acquired immunodeficiency syndrome (AIDS). HIV is a double-stranded RNA virus that infects vital cells of the immune system such as helper T lymphocytes (CD4+ T cells), dendritic cells, and macrophages. HIV infection leads to a progressive decline in the CD4+ T cell count producing a dysregulation in the balance between CD4 and CD8 cells. The use of combined antiretroviral therapy (cART) has revolutionized the life expectancy of infected persons, leading to a growing number of controlled chronic infections.

A link between HIV and rheumatological diseases appeared soon after the appearance of AIDS with the description of painful, disabling asymmetrical inflammatory arthropathy in some AIDS patients [21]. Following the first reports, there have been case series and epidemiological studies describing different clinical manifestations affecting the musculoskeletal system [22]. In the early stage of the HIV infection, when the immune system is only partially impaired, rare cases of autoimmune diseases may develop as in the general population. On the contrary, the loss of competence of the immune system, due to the CD4 cell depletion in the late phases of the disease, leads to an increased incidence of predominantly CD8 T-cell-driven autoimmune diseases, such as psoriasis and diffuse infiltrative lymphocytosis (Sjögren-like) syndrome [22]. Moreover, B cells are continuously stimulated since the early phases of infection, causing the frequent production of autoantibodies (which are present in up to 23% of HIV-infected patients, often without any clinical manifestation) (Fig. 12.2a) [23]. The immune restoration inflammatory syndrome (IRIS) in HIV-infected patients initiating cART is characterized by a paradoxical clinical worsening of a previously known opportunistic disease or the appearance of a new condition after initiating cART. The overall incidence of IRIS is dependent on the population studied and its underlying opportunistic infection burden (Fig. 12.2b) [24].

When immune competence is restored by cART, new onset of autoimmune diseases can occur. Several pathophysiologic hypotheses could explain this phenomenon, including the direct role of viral particles, immune complex-mediated diseases, dysregulation of the B/T lymphocyte interaction [25], molecular mimicry [26], and polyclonal B lymphocyte activation [23]. On the other hand, the partially rescued immune activation control might reduce the autoantibody production. Among the rheumatic manifestations, arthralgia has a prevalence estimates varying widely between 1 and 79%, regardless of whether the studies were carried out in the pre-cART (1.6–45%) or post-cART era [25, 27]. In HIV patients in the pre-cART era, myalgia was reported in 1.7–11% HIV patients [28]. Since the advent of cART, prevalence estimates between 0 and 77% have been reported, while rates of prevalence between 1 and 17% have been reported for fibromyalgia [23, 29]. Thus, the epidemiological data of pre- and post-cART do not allow us to draw clear conclusions on the relationship between actively replicating HIV infection and reactive arthritis. In the studies where HLA data were available, those HIV-infected patients with overlapping features of psoriatic arthritis (PsA) and reactive arthritis were often positive for the HLA-B27 allele [30]. Further confounding factors were derived from the emergence of reactive arthritis reported as a manifestation of IRIS after the introduction of cART [24]. The estimated prevalence rates of PsA among HIV-infected patients have ranged between 0.02% and 5.7% but most commonly were found between 0.02 and 2% [31]. Interestingly, the reports of ankylosing spondylitis, the most common form of seronegative spondyloarthropathy in the Western world, were very few in the pre-cART era [30]. Since cART introduction, when reactive and PsA became less frequent, diseases such as rheumatoid arthritis (RA), osteoporosis, or aseptic bone necrosis became more frequent. The earliest mention of RA and HIV came from pre-cART case reports describing patients with established RA who experienced clinical improvement or remission after the development of HIV [32]. This could be explained by the reduction of the immunogenic autoimmune activity due to the HIV-associated depletion of CD4 lymphocytes, which led to the conclusion that HIV and RA were mutually exclusive diagnoses [32]. ANA is present in up to 23% of HIV-infected persons; nonetheless, few cases of systemic lupus erythematosus (SLE) were described. In the advanced stage of HIV, the severely induced immune depression makes SLE incidence less frequent, probably because CD4 T lymphocytes play a crucial role in SLE pathogenesis [33]. On the contrary, the restoration of the normal immune function could lead to SLE flare. Anticardiolipin antibodies are found in 36–67% of HIV-infected patients; their level is associated with HIV viral load and the degree of immune activation, and

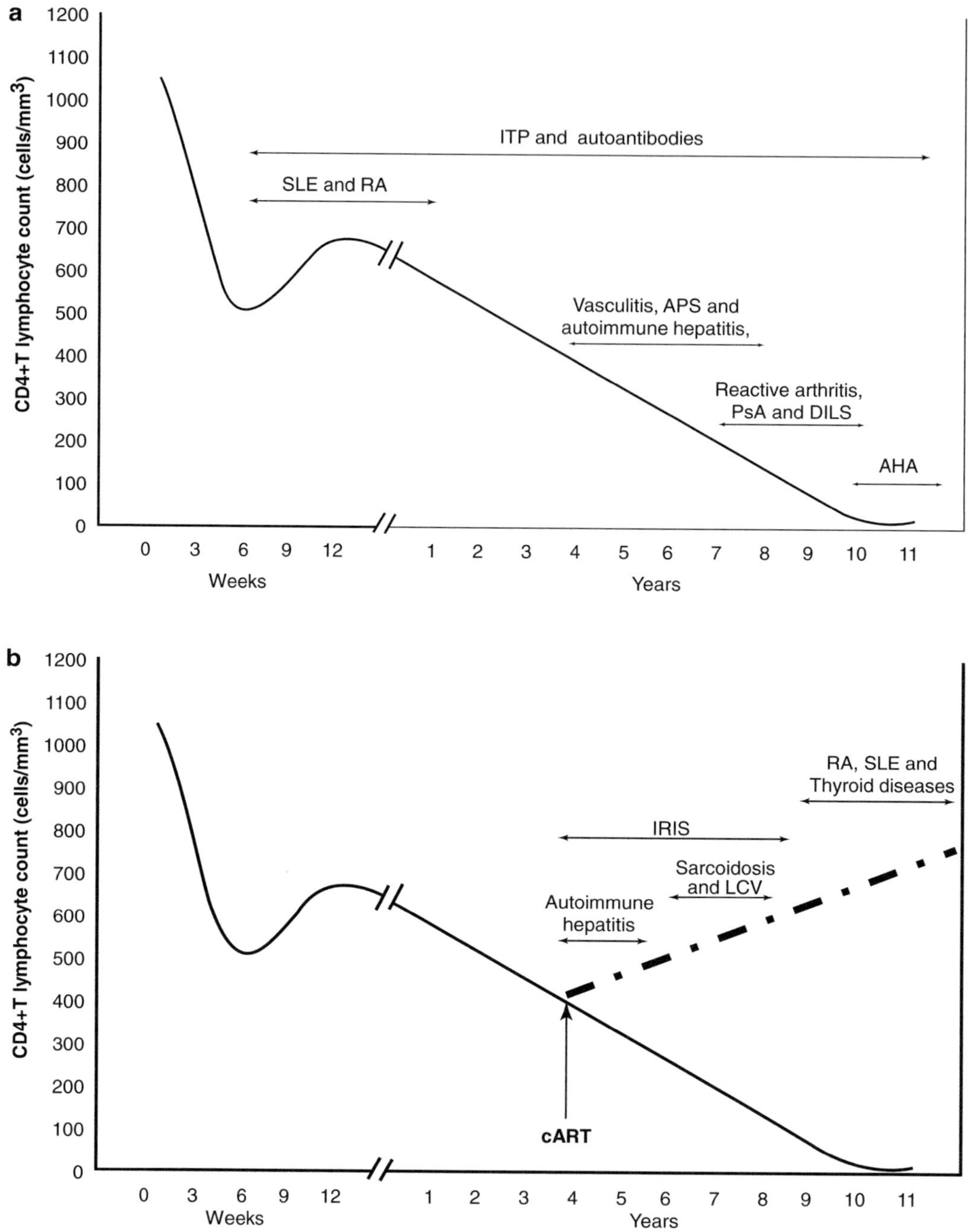

Fig. 12.2 Spectrum of rheumatic diseases in the natural history of HIV infection. (**a**) Rheumatic disease incidence related to CD4 cells declines without treatment intervention. (**b**) Occurrence of rheumatic diseases after cART introduction. ITP could be observed during all the stages of HIV infection, but the introduction of cART has a favorable impact on platelet count. Diseases like SLE and RA seem to improve with uncontrolled HIV infection and could restart when cART leads to immunological recovery. IRIS occurs exclusively after cART introduction manifesting with different phenotypes due to the underlying triggering condition. *SLE* systemic lupus erythematosus, *RA* rheumatoid arthritis, *ITP* immune thrombocytopenic purpura, *APS* antiphospholipid syndrome, *PsA* psoriatic arthritis, *DILS* diffuse infiltrative lymphocytosis syndrome, *AHA* autoimmune hemolytic anemia, *cART* combined antiretroviral therapy, *IRIS* immune restoration inflammatory syndrome, *LCV* leukocytoclastic cutaneous vasculitis

cART reduces the probability of detecting anti-cardiolipin antibodies [34].

The diffuse infiltrative lymphocytosis syndrome is a rheumatic condition mimicking a Sjogren-like multisystem disease, typically causing salivary gland swelling and chronic sicca syndrome. The commonest presentation (88–100% of cases) is bilateral parotid gland enlargement. Its incidence declined following introduction of cART. Antiretroviral treatment improves the symptoms, with adjunctive glucocorticoids required in a minority of cases [35, 36].

Vasculitis is present in up to 1% of HIV-infected people, most usually affecting small- to medium-sized vessels. Etiopathogenetic mechanisms proposed combined immune complex formation and viral tropism for endothelial cells, the latter potentially offering a mechanism by which cART therapy is usually beneficial. Polyarteritis nodosa without concurrent HBV infection may occur at a moderate to advanced level of immunosuppression, and its clinical course seems to be less severe than in non-HIV-infected people, with a favorable evolution on corticosteroids. Henoch-Schonlein purpura, improving with cART introduction, was also described. ANCA-associated vasculitides are extremely rare, notwithstanding ANCA being detected in up to 8% of the patients at an advanced stage of the disease. Leukocytoclastic cutaneous vasculitis, either secondary to the HIV infection itself or caused by direct or immune-mediated damage to the vessel walls, has also been described [37].

Despite a high prevalence of positive direct antiglobulin test (up to 34% of cases), autoimmune hemolytic anemia (AHA) rarely occurs in HIV-infected people; when it does, it usually occurs at an advanced stage of the disease. Here, cART is usually beneficial. On the contrary, ITP was frequently described in HIV-positive patients at all stages of the disease, while decreased platelet production favored by possible viral infection of megakaryocytes is observed in the advanced stage of the disease [38, 39]. Molecular mimicry plays an important role, since cross-reactivity was observed between antibodies directed to GPIIIa platelet surface antigen and an epitope of the Nef viral protein, as well as between antibodies directed to GPIIb/IIIa platelet surface glycoprotein and a particular form of glycosylated viral gp160/120. An increase in platelet count is observed within 3 months of treatment with cART, which is independent of the CD4 cell count but directly correlates with the decrease of the HIV plasma viral load [40].

Since cART introduction, cases of sarcoidosis were described as delayed IRIS manifestation (occurring with a median time of 9 months after cART introduction). In pulmonary forms, alveolitis is usually of CD4 type, with higher CD4/CD8 ratio in the bronchoalveolar lavage compared to blood. The usual evolution is spontaneously favorable or after administration of corticosteroids [41]. Graves' disease and Hashimoto's thyroiditis were also described as a manifestation of delayed IRIS (median time of 17 months from cART introduction) [42]. Autoimmune hepatitis was rarely reported, mainly in IRIS cases requiring temporary cART interruption and immunosuppressive treatment (with corticosteroids and/or azathioprine) [43].

Regarding drugs used to relieve symptoms in rheumatic patients, nonsteroidal anti-inflammatory drugs can be used according to the same guidelines for HIV-negative patients. Methotrexate may be used with careful monitoring of HIV viral loads and CD4 counts. Hydroxychloroquine has been effectively used in HIV-associated arthropathies. The literature on the use of biologic therapies in HIV-infected populations is at the moment limited to case reports and small case series and to the use of rituximab in hematological malignancies [44–46].

Conclusion

RNA viruses are able to elicit autoimmune reactions during acute or chronic infection (Table 12.1). The great majority of these phenomena are transient and strictly related to the acute phase of the disease. In type 1 diabetes, a clear demonstration of a causative role of RNA viruses in triggering autoimmune responses against pancreatic islets of Langerhans has

Table 12.1 Rheumatic diseases associated with RNA viruses and their underlying suggested pathogenic mechanism

RNA viruses	Rheumatic diseases associated	Suggested pathogenic mechanism
Enteroviruses	Myocarditis	Direct infection of myocardium triggering the production of antibodies against self-antigens
	Type 1 diabetes	Molecular mimicry and direct cytopathic effect on beta cells
HAV	Autoimmune hepatitis	Immune complex formation and molecular mimicry
HCV	Vasculitis and membranoproliferative glomerulonephritis	Cryoglobulins
	Thyroiditis and arthritis	Immune complex formation and autoantibodies
	Sialoadenitis and autoimmune hepatitis	Lymphocytic infiltration
HIV	Immune thrombocytopenia	Immune complex, megakaryocyte infection, and molecular mimicry
	Vasculitis	Immune complex formation and viral tropism for endothelial cells
	IRIS	Fast immune system recovery

not been demonstrated. Cryoglobulinemic syndrome during chronic HCV infection is the most extensively studied autoimmune disease and is the only autoimmune manifestation with a clear relation to a viral trigger. In HIV infection, immune system dysregulation is the primary cause of autoimmune disorders. The partial restoration of the immune system after the introduction of antiretroviral therapy could also play a role in the development of autoimmune diseases. In conclusion, a causative role of RNA viruses in the development of major autoimmune conditions has not yet been demonstrated.

Colored Plate "Take-Home Message"

- HIV infection can underlie autoimmune diseases.
- Autoimmune diseases occur in HIV-infected people, most often in a context of good immunological control (except essentially for autoimmune hemolytic anemia) or during IRIS (vasculitis, sarcoidosis, thyroid diseases).
- By improving immune status, cART might favor autoimmune disease onset.
- When necessary, immunosuppressant treatments may be used in this context with good tolerance.
- A close link has been described between *Enterovirus* and autoimmunity, in particular regarding type 1 diabetes.
- Chronic autoimmune liver disease may follow acute hepatitis A infection.

As a consequence of its lymphotropic nature, hepatitis C virus can trigger and sustain a clonal B-cell expansion which causes a wide spectrum of autoimmune/lymphoproliferative disorders, through a multistep process.

References

1. Oberste MS, Maher K, Kilpatrick DR, Pallansch MA. Molecular evolution of the human enteroviruses: correlation of serotype with VP1 sequence and application to picornavirus classification. J Virol. 1999;73(3):1941–8.
2. Vreugdenhil GR, Geluk A, Ottenhoff TH, Melchers WJ, Roep BO, Galama JM. Molecular mimicry in diabetes mellitus: the homologous domain in coxsackie B virus protein 2C and islet autoantigen GAD65 is highly conserved in the coxsackie B-like enteroviruses and binds to the diabetes associated HLA-DR3 molecule. Diabetologia. 1998;41(1):40–6.
3. Massilamany C, Koenig A, Reddy J, Huber S, Buskiewicz I. Autoimmunity in picornavirus infections. Curr Opin Virol. 2016;16:8–14.
4. Coppieters KT, Boettler T, von Herrath M. Virus infections in type 1 diabetes. Cold Spring Harb Perspect Med. 2012;2(1):a007682.
5. Jaïdane H, Hober D. Role of coxsackievirus B4 in the pathogenesis of type 1 diabetes. Diabetes Metab. 2008;34(6 Pt 1):537–48.
6. Huber SA. Viral myocarditis and dilated cardiomyopathy: etiology and pathogenesis. Curr Pharm Des. 2016;22(4):408–26.

7. Cihakova D, Rose NR. Pathogenesis of myocarditis and dilated cardiomyopathy. Adv Immunol. 2008;99:95–114.
8. Rose NR. Myocarditis: infection versus autoimmunity. J Clin Immunol. 2009;29(6):730–7.
9. Trepo C, Zoulim F, Pradat P. Viral hepatitis. Curr Opin Infect Dis. 1999;12:481–90.
10. Shalit M, Wollner S, Levo Y. Cryoglobulinemia in acute type-A hepatitis. Clin Exp Immunol. 1982;47:613–6.
11. Vento S, Garofano T, Di Perri G, et al. Identification of hepatitis A virus as a trigger for autoimmune chronic hepatitis type 1 in susceptible individuals. Lancet. 1991;337:1183–7.
12. Singh G, Palaniappan S, Rotimi O, Hamlin PJ. Autoimmune hepatitis triggered by hepatitis A. Gut. 2007;56:304.
13. Cuthbert JA, Hepatitis A. Old and new. Clin Microbiol Rev. 2001;14(1):38–58. Review. Erratum in: Clin Microbiol Rev 2001;14(3):642.
14. Lingala S, Ghany MG. Natural history of hepatitis C. Gastroenterol Clin N Am. 2015;44(4):717–34. https://doi.org/10.1016/j.gtc.2015.07.003.
15. McMurray RW, Elbourne K. Hepatitis C virus infection and autoimmunity. Semin Arthritis Rheum. 1997;26(4):689–701.
16. Charles ED, Dustin LB. Hepatitis C virus-induced cryoglobulinemia. Kidney Int. 2009;76(8):818–24.
17. Cacoub P, Gragnani L, Comarmond C, Zignego AL. Extrahepatic manifestations of chronic hepatitis C virus infection. Dig Liver Dis. 2014;46(Suppl 5):S165–73.
18. Paroli M, Iannucci G, Accapezzato D. Hepatitis C virus infection and autoimmune diseases. Int J Gen Med. 2012;5:903–7.
19. Jadali Z, Alavian SM. Autoimmune diseases coexisting with hepatitis C virus infection. Iran J Allergy Asthma Immunol. 2010;9(4):191–206.
20. Zuckerman E, Yeshurun D, Rosner I. Management of hepatitis C virus-related arthritis. BioDrugs. 2001;15(9):573–84.
21. Winchester R, Bernstein DH, Fisher HD, et al. The co-occurrence of Reiter's syndrome and acquired immunodeficiency. Ann Intern Med. 1987;106:19–26.
22. Fox C, Walker-Bone K. Evolving spectrum of HIV-associated rheumatic syndromes. Best Pract Res Clin Rheumatol. 2015;29(2):244–58. https://doi.org/10.1016/j.berh.2015.04.019.
23. Marquez J, Restrepo CS, Candia L, et al. Human immunodeficiency virus-associated rheumatic disorders in the HAART era. J Rheumatol. 2004;31:741–6.
24. Murdoch DM, Venter WD, Van Rie A, Feldman C. Immune reconstitution inflammatory syndrome (IRIS): review of common infectious manifestations and treatment options. AIDS Res Ther. 2007;4:9.
25. Parker R, Stein DJ, Jelsma J. Pain in people living with HIV/AIDS: a systematic review. J Int AIDS Soc. 2014;17(1):18719.
26. Oldstone MB, et al. Cell. 1987;50(6):819–20. Erratum in Cell 1987;51(5):878.
27. Medina-Rodriguez F, Guzman C, Jara LJ, et al. Rheumatic manifestations in human immunodeficiency virus positive and negative individuals: a study of 2 populations with similar risk factors. J Rheumatol. 1993;20:1880–4.
28. Berman A, Espinoza LR, Diaz JD, et al. Rheumatic manifestations of human immunodeficiency virus infection. Am J Med. 1988;85:59–64.
29. Kole AK, Roy R, Kole DC. Musculoskeletal and rheumatological disorders in HIV infection: experience in a tertiary referral center. Indian J Sex Transm Dis. 2013;34(2):107–12.
30. Duvic M, Johnson TM, Rapini RP, et al. Acquired immunodeficiency syndrome-associated psoriasis and Reiter's syndrome. Arch Dermatol. 1987;123:1622–32.
31. Achuthan K, Uppal SS. Rheumatological manifestations in 102 cases of HIV infection. J Ind Rheum Ass. 1996;3:43–7.
32. Bijlsma JWJ, Derksen RHWM, Huber-Brunning O, Borleffs JCC. Does AIDS 'cure' rheumatoid arthritis? Ann Rheum Dis. 1988;47:350–1.
33. Rigante D, Mazzoni MB, Esposito S. The cryptic interplay between systemic lupus erythematosus and infections. Autoimmun Rev. 2014;13:96–102.
34. Martinez V, Diemert MC, Braibant M, ALT ANRS CO15 Study Group, et al. Anticardiolipin antibodies in HIV infection are independently associated with antibodies to the membrane proximal external region of gp41 and with cell-associated HIV DNA and immune activation. Clin Infect Dis. 2009;48(1):123–32. https://doi.org/10.1086/595013.
35. Itescu S, Brancato LJ, Winchester R. A sicca syndrome in HIV infection: association with HLA-DR5 and CD8 lymphocytosis. Lancet. 1989;2(8661):466–8.
36. Basu D, Williams F, Ahn C, Reveille J. Changing spectrum of the diffuse infiltrative lymphocytosis syndrome. Arthritis Rheum. 2006;55(3):466–72.
37. Guillevin L. Vasculitides in the context of HIV infection. AIDS. 2008;22(Suppl. 3):S27–33.
38. Galli M, Musicco M, Gervasoni C, et al. No evidence of a higher risk of progression to AIDS in patients with HIV-1-related severe thrombocytopenia. J Acquir Immune Defic Syndr Hum Retrovirol. 1996;12(3):268–75.
39. Franzetti M, Adorni F, Oreni L, et al. Changes in the incidence of severe thrombocytopenia and its predisposing conditions in HIV-infected patients since the introduction of highly active antiretroviral therapy. J Acquir Immune Defic Syndr. 2014;67(5):493–8. https://doi.org/10.1097/QAI.0000000000000347.
40. Ambler KL, Vickars LM, Leger CS, et al. Clinical features, treatment, and outcome of HIV-associated immune thrombocytopenia in the HAART era. Adv Hematol. 2012;2012:910954. https://doi.org/10.1155/2012/910954.

41. Lenner R, Bregman Z, Teirstein AS, DePalo L. Recurrent pulmonary sarcoidosis in HIV-infected patients receiving highly active antiretroviral therapy. Chest. 2001;119(3):978–81.
42. Chen F, Day SL, Metcalfe RA, Sethi G, Kapembwa MS, Brook MG, et al. Characteristics of autoimmune thyroid disease occurring as a late complication of immune reconstitution in patients with advanced human immunodeficiency virus (HIV) disease. Medicine (Baltimore). 2005;84(2):98–106.
43. Murunga E, Andersson M, Rensburg C. Autoimmune hepatitis: manifestation of immune reconstitution inflammatory syndrome in HIV infected patients? Scand J Gastroenterol. 2016;51(7):814–8. https://doi.org/10.3109/00365521.2016.1157888.
44. Maurer TA, Zackheim HS, Tuffanelli L, Berger TG. The use of methotrexate for treatment of psoriasis in patients with HIV infection. J Am Acad Dermatol. 1994;31:372–5.
45. Sperber K, Kalb TH, Stecher VJ, Banerjee R, Mayer L. Inhibition of human immunodeficiency virus type 1 replication by hydroxychloroquine in T cells and monocytes. AIDS Res Hum Retrovir. 1993;9:91–8.
46. Castillo JJ, Echenique IA. Rituximab in combination with chemotherapy versus chemotherapy alone in HIV associated non-Hodgkin lymphoma: a pooled analysis of 15 prospective studies. Am J Hematol. 2012;87:330–3.

13 Autoimmunity and the Paradox of Chagas Disease

Ester Roffe and Philip M. Murphy

Abbreviation

TNF Tumor necrosis factor

Introduction

In the early 1900s, the remarkable Brazilian physician-scientist Carlos Chagas described the epidemiology, causative infectious agent, insect vector, vertebrate reservoir, as well as both the acute and chronic clinical manifestations in humans for the previously unrecognized disease that now bears his name [1]. Chagas' discoveries, which resulted from astute environmental and clinical observations while working under primitive conditions on a malaria control project for a railroad in Minas Gerais in southeast Brazil, represent a landmark in the history of medicine. After noticing that many rural dwellings were infested with hematophagous triatomine bugs from the Reduviid family, also known as kissing bugs for their behavior of taking a blood meal at night from the faces of sleeping humans, Chagas identified a novel trypanosome in bug feces, showed that it could be transmitted to marmoset monkeys by triatomine bug bites, and identified the organism in the blood of a 3-year-old girl. Subsequent studies linked the novel trypanosome to an acute febrile illness as well as to chronic inflammation and dilatation of the heart or gut in about 30% of infected individuals [2]. The mechanism underlying the chronic disease manifestations in part involves inflammation of parasympathetic ganglia resulting in autonomic denervation and impaired visceral muscle contraction [3].

Chronic symptomatic Chagas disease is associated with low to undetectable levels of the pathogen in affected tissues despite high tissue levels of specific humoral and cellular immune responses to both pathogen and host determinants, suggesting the possibility that the underlying pathogenesis may be initiated and maintained by the organism and amplified by autoimmunity [4]. As a chronic inflammatory disease linked precisely to a known infectious agent, the study of autoimmunity in Chagas disease may have general relevance to understanding the immunopathogenic mechanisms and microbiome influences in idiopathic autoimmune diseases.

E. Roffe
Departamento de Bioquímica e Imunologia, Universidade Federal de Minas Gerais, Belo Horizonte, MG, Brazil

P. M. Murphy (✉)
Laboratory of Molecular Immunology, National Institute of Allergy and Infectious Diseases, National Institutes of Health, Bethesda, MD, USA
e-mail: pmm@nih.gov

G. Ragab et al. (eds.), *The Microbiome in Rheumatic Diseases and Infection*, https://doi.org/10.1007/978-3-319-79026-8_13

Trypanosoma cruzi, the Causative Agent of Chagas Disease (Table 13.1)

Table 13.1 Chagas disease at a glance

Cause	Persistent infection with *Trypanosoma cruzi*
Type of infection	Zoonosis
Vector	Triatomine bugs
Mode of transmission	Infected bug feces deposited at pruritic bite site; ingestion of food contaminated with triatomine feces; blood transfusion, organ transplantation, congenital
Reservoir	Wild and domesticated mammals and humans
Epidemiology	Endemic to Latin America, from Mexico to Argentina; North America, Europe, Australia, Russia, and Japan through migration of infected people (mainly by blood transfusion and congenitally)
Prevalence	~10 million (ca. 2015)
Annual mortality	~8000 (ca. 2015)
Pathology	Acute: usually asymptomatic; non-specific febrile illness, Romana's sign. Myocarditis and meningoencephalitis in immunosuppressed people or children under 2 years of age
	Chronic: dilated cardiomyopathy and mega-disease of the GI tract
Pathogenesis	Parasite persistence; Type 1 pathogen-specific cellular immune response; autoreactivity to myosin and other autoantigens; autonomic denervation in the heart and gut
Diagnosis	Detection of organism in blood and tissue; anti-*T. cruzi* antibody detection
Prognosis	~20–30% of infected individuals progress to symptomatic chronic pathology with high mortality
Treatment	Nifurtimox, benznidazole
Prevention	Eradication of vector nests in substandard housing in rural areas; screening of blood supply and organ donations; early diagnosis and treatment of infected pregnant women; pasteurization of food derived from Amazon or other endemic areas

Chagas named the organism he discovered *Trypanosoma cruzi* after his mentor, the Brazilian researcher Oswaldo Cruz. Trypanosomes are a family of over 20 distinct uniflagellate protozoans whose common elongated and tapered shape is conveyed by the genus name (trypano = *Gr.*, drill or bore; soma = *Gr.*, body). *T. cruzi* and *T. brucei* are the only trypanosome species that cause human disease. Although both organisms are transmitted by insect vectors, their biology is otherwise very different. *T. brucei* is an extracellular pathogen endemic to Africa, uses the tsetse fly as vector, and is transmitted bidirectionally between vector and human and other mammalian hosts through the insect proboscis at bite sites [5]. In contrast, *T. cruzi* has both intracellular and extracellular stages, is endemic to Central and South America, uses triatomine bugs as vector, and is transmitted bidirectionally between vector and hosts, to the bug in blood meals taken from the host and to the host in bug feces deposited at the bite site. Although both organisms cause nervous system dysfunction, *T. brucei* mainly affects the central nervous system and is the cause of African sleeping sickness, whereas *T. cruzi* infection affects mainly the peripheral nervous system [6].

During its developmental life cycle (Fig. 13.1), *T. cruzi* assumes a series of morphologically distinct stages defined by the position of the nucleus relative to the flagellum and the kinetoplast (a massive, highly localized collection of mitochondria unique to the Kinetoplastidae, a family of protozoans that includes the trypanosomes). Most prominent are the epimastigote, trypomastigote, and amastigote stages, in which both the kinetoplast and origin of the flagellum are positioned posterior, anterior, and adjacent to the centrally located nucleus, respectively. The terms "mastigote" and "flagellum" are from the Greek and Latin words, respectively, for "whip." Thus, the amastigote lacks a flagellum and is a non-motile intracellular form, whereas trypomastigotes have a long drill-like flagellum and are highly motile, and epimastigotes have a relatively short flagellum. Unlike amastigotes, both epimastigotes and trypomastigotes are extracellular forms; epimastigotes and amastigotes replicate, whereas trypomastigotes do not. Epimastigotes

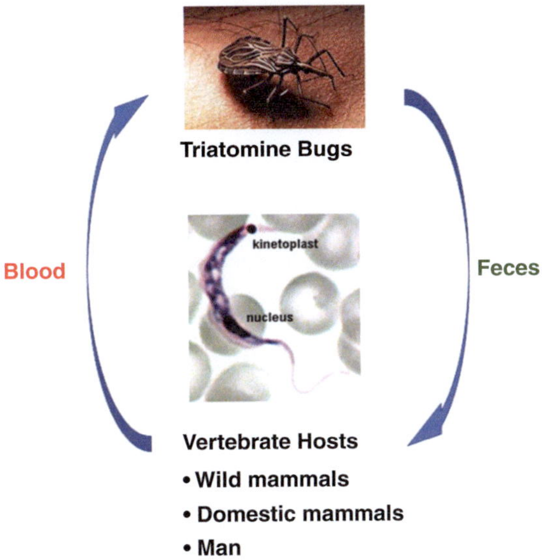

Fig. 13.1 Life cycle of *Trypanosoma cruzi*. *T. cruzi* is able to infect many different cell types of hundreds of wild and domesticated mammals, as well as many different species of Reduviid bugs, accounting for the large reservoir and high prevalence of infection in Latin America, where these bugs are found. Transmission from mammalian host to bug occurs when the bug ingests a blood meal from an infected host. Transmission from bug to human and presumably other mammalian hosts occurs when trypomastigote forms in bug feces are scratched into pruritic bite sites or enter via broken skin or mucosa

are found exclusively in the midgut of the insect vector, whereas trypomastigotes develop in the hindgut and are deposited in bug feces at the pruritic bite site on the human host, where they are scratched into the skin, ultimately entering the bloodstream [7]. Transmission has also been reported from infected food and blood and organ donations, as well as from mother to fetus, and through laboratory accidents [8]. Trypomastigotes can infect virtually all nucleated cells and form cytoplasmic pseudocysts. However, the parasite has a tropism for myocytes [3]. Before being released from the host cell, amastigotes revert to the highly motile trypomastigote form and rupture the cell. Once in the extracellular environment, trypomastigotes are available to a new triatomine bug taking a blood meal from the host, thereby completing the life cycle.

Triatomine bugs are found mainly in rural areas where they come into contact with humans from their nests in infested housing. There is a very large zoonotic reservoir of *T. cruzi* in endemic areas due to the combination of poor housing, the large number of triatomine species that can serve as vectors, and the large number of vertebrates that can serve as hosts. Chagas originally identified the armadillo as a reservoir and it still stands as an important one; however, it is now known that hundreds of mammalian species may contribute, including wild and domesticated species, with humans as an incidental, unnecessary, and unfortunate host [6].

Barriers to Progress in Control of Chagas Disease

The outcome of *T. cruzi* infection is highly variable. In the acute stage, high parasitemia occurs, yet most individuals remain asymptomatic or develop a benign illness usually without coming to medical attention. After a decades-long period of clinical latency called the indeterminate form of the chronic stage, ~20–30% of infected individuals progress to chronic stage pathology, ~two-thirds of which may remain subclinical [2]. Approximately 95% of clinical cases in the chronic stage present with chronic chagasic cardiomyopathy. The remaining ~5% present with gastrointestinal disease affecting mainly the colon and esophagus, which is referred to generically as mega-disease. Megacolon and megaesophagus result from degeneration of the autonomic nervous system and present with constipation and dysphagia, respectively; they are rarely associated with cardiomyopathy. Importantly regarding causation, the characteristic cardiomyopathy of human Chagas disease has been documented in experimentally infected laboratory animals such as rabbits and mice and occurs in naturally infected mammals in the wild [9]. Nevertheless, as with patients, the outcome of *T. cruzi* infection in animal models is variable and depends on many factors, including the species, sex, and genetic background of the host; the strain and cellular tropism of the parasite; as well as the inoculum, the site of inoculation, and the parasite conditions of passage [10].

As with other protozoan infections, there is no vaccine available for *T. cruzi*. Nifurtimox and benznidazole have been used as chemotherapeutic agents in the disease for many years in the USA and Latin America and are recommended for all infected patients, despite the fact that only a minority will develop chronic disease. Benznidazole received accelerated approval by the FDA in 2017 for treatment of infected children 2–12 years of age in the USA. Both agents have significant toxicities which limit compliance, and neither agent has been shown to be effective for the treatment of chagasic cardiomyopathy and mega-disease [8, 11]. Thus, more than a century after its discovery, Chagas disease still represents an unmet medical need and is classified by the World Health Organization as a neglected tropical disease. Nevertheless, there has been progress in reducing transmission through the deployment of vector control programs, screening of the blood supply and organ donors, and improved housing. Still, poverty and habitat encroachment continue to place tens of millions of people at risk for Chagas disease in the Western Hemisphere, where disease prevalence and annual mortality were estimated in 2015 to be ~6.6 million and 8000, respectively [12–14]. Moreover, due to international travel and emigration, Chagas disease is now a global problem. In particular, the prevalence of Chagas disease in the USA, where transmission is virtually nonexistent, is estimated to be ~300,000 from imported cases [15]. Clearly, more basic knowledge is needed regarding host and parasite risk factors for progression to chronic disease, as well as precise mechanisms of immunopathogenesis in Chagas disease to stratify patients for treatment as well as to identify new targets for development of anti-inflammatory and immunomodulatory therapy and vaccines.

Immunopathogenesis of Chagas Disease (Fig. 13.2)

At the vector bite site, *T. cruzi* infects multiple cell types, including macrophages, fibroblasts, endothelial cells, and myocytes, and may cause a localized delayed hypersensitivity reaction called a chagoma. The classic Romana's sign of Chagas disease refers to unilateral periorbital edema caused by a vector bite on the face. Macrophages are able to phagocytose trypomastigotes and are an important innate line of local defense, but the organism may survive by escaping from the phagolysosome [16]. After a burst of local replication lasting several days to weeks, trypomastigotes enter the bloodstream, disseminate, and may establish high levels in the blood in the acute stage. Most acute infections remain subclinical although patients may develop non-specific symptoms, including nausea, vomiting, fever, lymphadenopathy, hepatosplenomegaly, and malaise. Clinical evidence of myocarditis may

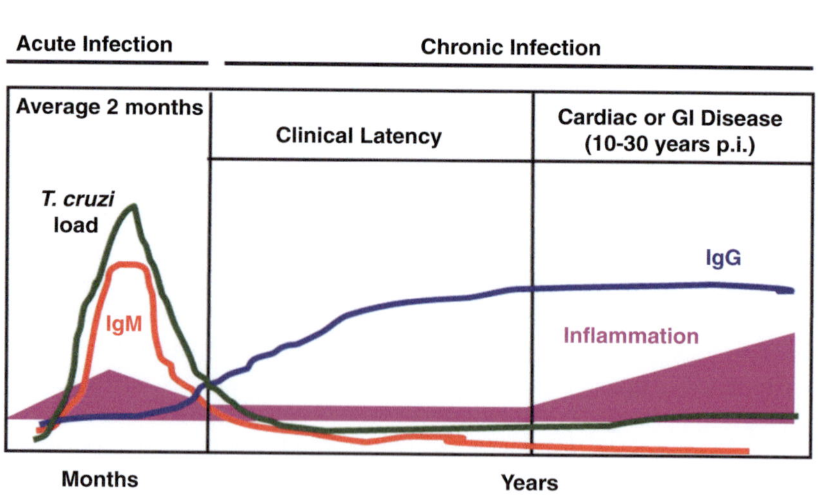

Fig. 13.2 Model time course of key events after *T. cruzi* infection

occur in ~1% of acute infections but with only 1–5% mortality, although, interestingly, clusters of severe disease have been reported in local outbreaks.

The adaptive immune response to *T. cruzi* infection in both patients and experimental animals unfolds slowly but is ultimately highly effective, typically reducing parasitemia to undetectable levels by light microscopy within 3–4 weeks of initial infection and reducing parasite burden in infected tissues to extremely low and often undetectable levels. Critical determinants of parasite control in the acute phase include pathogen-specific IgG, macrophages, Type 1 CD4+ and CD8+ T cells producing interferon-γ, tumor necrosis factor (TNF), and nitric oxide [17], as well as the Th1-associated chemokines CXCL9 and CXCL10 and their shared T cell receptor CXCR3 [18], CCL2 and its macrophage and T cell receptor CCR2 [19], and CCL3 and CCL5 and their shared macrophage and T cell receptor CCR5 [20, 21]. Mice lacking these factors and others are unable to control parasitemia and suffer high mortality in the acute stage of infection [19–21].

Nevertheless, immunocompetent hosts do not achieve sterilizing immunity against *T. cruzi*, and the parasite establishes lifelong persistence in the host at very low levels. The reasons for this are still undefined, but T cell exhaustion, Treg induction, and activation of inhibitory receptors are on the list of possibilities [22–24]. Importantly, the suppressed parasite in the primary host is still capable of causing acute disease with high levels of parasitemia when transferred to a secondary naïve host, indicating that the persisting pathogen has not become avirulent in the primary host [25]. Moreover, parasite burden can increase in chronically infected animals treated with high doses of immunosuppressive agents such as cyclophosphamide [26] and in infected patients under conditions of acquired immunodeficiency such as after human immunodeficiency virus infection or after immunosuppression associated with organ transplantation [27], indicating that in the chronic stage of disease, the parasite is still viable and resistant to or able to elude the immune response, while paradoxically being actively suppressed by it. Nevertheless, reactivation of disease with high parasitemia is rare even in the immunosuppressed patient. Importantly, an infected animal in the chronic stage of infection with a low persistent parasite burden is able to suppress parasitemia after lethal challenge with a second inoculum of the same strain of *T. cruzi* [28], indicating that exhaustion, at least in a systemic sense, cannot be the sole and simple explanation for the failure to achieve sterilizing immunity.

Autoimmunity in Chronic Chagas Disease

Numerous mechanisms collectively contribute to the chronic inflammation and fibrosis that occur in the chronic stage of Chagas disease, with most work focused on cardiomyopathy, the major source of mortality in the disease (Table 13.2). These include direct damage by the parasite, parasite-specific immune responses, non-specific immunity, microvasculopathy, and autoimmunity [29]. The parasite is clearly required for triggering these mechanisms; however, the specific

Table 13.2 Proposed mechanisms of pathogenesis in chronic chagasic cardiomyopathy [2, 6, 16, 29, 30, 35–37]

Pathogen persistence due to evasion of effective immune responses
Escape from phagolysosomes by *T. cruzi*
Death of infected cells ruptured by intracellular development of *T. cruzi* amastigote nests
Oxidative damage to infected cells by intracellular *T. cruzi*
Vasculopathy caused by prostaglandins and bradykinin B2 receptor agonists induced by *T. cruzi*
Death of infected cells targeted directly by Type 1 pathogen-specific cytotoxic T cells
Antibody-dependent cellular cytotoxicity
Death of uninfected bystander cells by toxic mediators released from immune effector cells
Death of infected and uninfected cells by autoimmune effector cells
Fibrosis
Autonomic denervation due to cardiac ganglion inflammation without direct infection of neurons
Immunodominance as a parasite evasion strategy

combination of parasite, host, and environmental factors predictive of progression to chronic disease and the relative contribution of each mechanism to chronic stage pathology have not been clearly delineated.

The importance of parasite persistence for progression to chronic Chagas disease is suggested first and foremost by the presence of parasites specifically in chronic lesions. In human, rare parasites are found in the gut but usually not the heart in patients suffering from chronic gastrointestinal disease if they do not also have chronic chagasic cardiomyopathy and vice versa in patients with chronic chagasic cardiomyopathy who do not also have gastrointestinal disease [30]. In experimental animals, *T. cruzi* infection is clearly the proximal cause of late-onset disease, including chronic cardiomyopathy as well as a form of systemic necrotizing vasculitis that is especially severe in skeletal muscle, resulting in paresis and frank paralysis [31]. T cells predominate in chronic Chagas disease lesions [32]. As in acute infection, both activated CD4 and CD8 subsets are present in chronic infection and are strongly skewed toward production of the Type 1 cytokines interferon-γ and TNF [33]. A high proportion of these cells has been shown to be specific for immunodominant peptides derived from the *T. cruzi* sialidase enzyme [34]. Subdominant epitope determinants have been identified as well in many other parasite proteins [35].

Persistent parasitism may cause damage directly to infected myocytes as they are ruptured by maturing parasite nests. There is no quantitative information on how frequently this occurs, but even low rates could result in massive cumulative damage over the long indeterminate stage of infection. The parasite is also known to release vasoactive substances, including bradykinin B2 receptor agonists and prostaglandins, that may contribute to vasculopathy in Chagas disease resulting in edema formation [36]. Vasculopathy may also involve arteritis and platelet aggregation that together may cause tissue damage from myocardial ischemia [29]. The parasite may also directly injure the myocardium by inducing intracellular oxidative damage and by producing pore-forming hemolysins [29]. Parasite-specific antibodies and cytotoxic T cells, which are found in chagasic tissue, are also likely to contribute to myocyte damage by directly targeting parasite-infected cells [29]. Alternatively, myocyte loss could result indirectly from bystander effects on uninfected myocytes resulting from innate or adaptive mediators generated from specific targeting of parasite-infected cells. A criticism of the parasite persistence theory is that immunopathology is disproportionately high compared to the tissue parasite burden, which by light microscopy may be undetectable in chronic lesions or, if present, not co-localized with inflammatory foci. As a counterargument, more sensitive techniques such as polymerase chain reaction have suggested that pathogen debris may be present in places where intact organisms are not observed microscopically [37]. A second criticism stems from the failure of treatment with benznidazole, including in the recent randomized BENEFIT trial, to reduce cardiac deterioration in chagasic cardiomyopathy despite significantly reducing parasite burden [38].

The neurotoxin theory of Chagas disease postulates that the parasite produces a neurotoxin as an explanation for the parasympathetic neuronal loss that occurs in the gut and heart leading to the characteristic dilatation of mega-disease. However, experimental evidence in support of this theory is lacking [6].

The autoimmunity theory holds that cardiac damage results from a loss of tolerance to cardiac self-antigens. Mechanisms may involve (1) molecular mimicry between structurally similar epitopes of self- and parasite antigens and (2) activation of autoreactive T cells with low affinity for self-antigens by cytokines, interferons, costimulatory pathway activation, and other factors released at sites of parasite- or immunologically induced myocyte damage. Early evidence in favor of an autoimmune basis of Chagas disease included observations that lymphocytes from *T. cruzi*-infected rabbits could kill cardiomyocytes in vitro [39]. This was supported by histopathologic evidence of T cells proximal to necrotic myocytes in the absence of parasite nests. Subsequent studies documented numerous autoantibodies and autoreactive T cells in patients with Chagas disease as well as animal models of *T. cruzi* infection. Prominent among these are autoantibodies to cardiac myosin and arrhythmogenic autoantibodies to β1 and β2 adrenergic receptors and m2 muscarinic acetylcholine receptors [40]. *T. cruzi* proteins with epitope mimics of cardiac myosin include ribosomal P protein and B13 [41, 42]. Autoantibodies may also induce cardiomyocyte damage by antibody-dependent cellular cytotoxicity [43].

However, there is still no conclusive evidence that these autoreactive antibodies and T cells are actually pathogenic in Chagas disease. The prevalence of specific autoimmune responses has not been clearly established prospectively in patients who progress to chronic pathology versus those who do not. Moreover, adoptive transfer experiments of autoreactive T cells purporting to demonstrate development of myocarditis in recipient animals have never recapitulated the severe pathology of chagasic cardiomyopathy or megadisease and have been criticized for not unequivocally excluding the presence of parasites in the transferred cells [6]. An attempt to address this conundrum was made by infecting chicken eggs, which are susceptible to infection with *T. cruzi*, whereas chickens are not [6]. Remarkably, the authors reported that parasite kinetoplast DNA became integrated in the chicken genome and could be transmitted vertically, and that this was associated with fatal cardiomyopathy, suggesting a genetic mechanism of autoimmunity in the absence of replicating parasites. This paper was editorially retracted without concurrence of the authors following extensive investigation of a criticism raised by a reader related to the genetic analysis [6]. Nevertheless, establishing a version of the classic Chagas disease phenotype in chickens in this way is noteworthy. Whether kinetoplast genotoxicity can induce autoimmunity in human Chagas disease is not established. In another line of investigation into the role of autoimmunity, a tolerance protocol using a cardiac myosin-rich fraction purified from outbred mouse heart ventricles was able to attenuate chronic Chagas disease myocarditis after parasite infection of mice [44].

The autoimmune theory makes two clinically important predictions. First, chemotherapy directed against the pathogen may be ineffective as treatment for chronic pathology in Chagas disease. In fact, currently it is; however, there could be many other reasons besides autoimmunity for why a drug might be ineffective even if parasite persistence were the dominant driver of pathogenesis. For example, fibrosis may be sufficiently advanced that it rather than inflammation becomes the dominant pathogenic factor driving cardiomyopathy. There is evidence that benznidazole treatment may ameliorate chronic cardiac pathology in *T. cruzi*-infected mice, and this was associated with reduced parasite burden. However, it was also associated with reduced humoral and cell-mediated autoimmune responses, making it impossible to judge the specific contribution of autoimmunity to the pathology [45]. The second prediction is that *T. cruzi*-based vaccines might induce autoimmunity or exacerbate inflammation [46]. Presently, there is no published evidence in favor of this although myocarditis has been documented in animals actively immunized with subcellular parasite antigens [6]. At present, the risk of inducing autoimmune myocarditis by vaccination is generally regarded as low, and efforts to develop a vaccine for Chagas disease are ongoing.

Conclusion

As with other protozoan pathogens, the complex biology of *T. cruzi* imposes major barriers to progress in understanding disease pathogenesis and in developing effective treatments and prevention measures. These include the genetic diversity of the pathogen, the long period from initial infection to the onset of life-threatening pathology in the chronic stage, the paradox of pathogen persistence despite robust pathogen-specific immune responses, and the difficulty of establishing the relative importance of multiple pathogenic mechanisms to chronic pathology. Ultimately, Chagas disease is a disease of poverty, which identifies an economic and political path toward prevention and ultimately eradication. Intensified efforts to apply modern systems biology approaches to develop algorithms predictive of disease outcome may help to personalize treatment approaches and to identify better vaccine development strategies. The study of autoimmunity in Chagas disease may hold the key to pathogenesis in the chronic stage and may provide new and potentially generalizable insights into how the microbiota may shape the risk of autoimmune disease.

Acknowledgments This work was supported by the Division of Intramural Research of the National Institute of Allergy and Infectious Disease of the National Institutes of Health.

References

1. Chagas C. Nova tripanozomiase humana: estudos sobre a morfolojia e o ciclo evolutivo do Schizotrypanum cruzi n. gen., n. sp., ajente etiolojico de nova entidade morbida do homem. Mem Inst Oswaldo Cruz. 1909;1(2):159–218.
2. Rassi A Jr, Rassi A, Marin-Neto JA. Chagas disease. Lancet. 2010;375(9723):1388–402.
3. Koberle F. Aspectos neurológicos da moléstia de chagas. Arq Neuropsiquiatr. 1967;25(3):159–74.
4. Chagas C. Moléstia de Carlos Chagas ou tireoidite parasitária: nova doença humana transmitida pelo barbeiro. Rev Méd São Paulo. 1911;14:337–56.
5. Franco JR, Simarro PP, Diarra A, Jannin JG. Epidemiology of human African trypanosomiasis. Clin Epidemiol. 2014;6:257–75.
6. Teixeira ARL, Hecht MM, Guimaro MC, Sousa AO, Nitz N. Pathogenesis of Chagas disease: parasite persistence and autoimmunity. Clin Microbiol Rev. 2011;24:592–630.
7. Rey L. Parasitologia - Parasitos e doenças parasitárias do homem nas Américas e na África. [Parasites and parasitic diseases of man in the Americas and Africa]. 2nd ed. Rio de Janeiro: Guanabara Koogan; 1991. p. 731.
8. Bern C. Chagas' disease. N Engl J Med. 2015;373(5):456–66.
9. Chagas C. Nova espécie mórbida do homem, produzida por um trypanosoma (Trypanosoma cruzi). Bras Med. 1909;23:161.
10. Scharfstein J, Gomes JAS, Correa-Oliveira R. Back to the future in Chagas disease: from animal models to patient cohort studies, progress in immunopathogenesis research. Mem Inst Oswaldo Cruz. 2009;104(Suppl. 1):187–98.
11. Bern C, Montgomery SP, Herwaldt BL, Rassi A Jr, Marin-Neto JA, Dantas RO, Maguire JH, Acquatella H, Morillo C, Kirchhoff LV, Gilman RH, Reyes PA, Salvatella R, Moore AC. Evaluation and treatment of Chagas disease in the United States: a systematic review. JAMA. 2007;298:2171–81.
12. GBD 2015 Disease and Injury Incidence and Prevalence Collaborators. Global, regional, and national incidence, prevalence, and years lived with disability for 310 diseases and injuries, 1990–2015: a systematic analysis for the Global Burden of Disease Study 2015. Lancet. 2016;388(10053):1545–602.
13. Chagas disease (American trypanosomiasis) Fact sheet N°340. World Health Organization; 2013. Archived from the original on 27 February 2014. http://www.who.int/mediacentre/factsheets/fs340/en/.
14. GBD 2015 Mortality and Causes of Death Collaborators. Global, regional, and national life expectancy, all-cause mortality, and cause-specific mortality for 249 causes of death, 1980–2015: a systematic analysis for the Global Burden of Disease Study 2015. Lancet. 2016;388(10053):1459–544.
15. Montgomery SP, Starr MC, Cantey PT, Edwards MS, Meymandi SK. Neglected parasitic infections in the United States: Chagas disease. Am J Trop Med Hyg. 2014;90(5):814–8.
16. Cardoso MS, Reis-Cunha JL, Bartholomeu DC. Evasion of the immune response by Trypanosoma cruzi during acute infection. Front Immunol. 2015;6:659.
17. Teixeira MM, Gazzinelli RT, Silva JS. Chemokines, inflammation and Trypanosoma cruzi infection. Trends Parasitol. 2002;18(6):262–5.
18. Hardison JL, Wrightsman RA, Carpenter PM, Lane TE, Manning JE. The chemokines CXCL9 and CXCL10 promote a protective immune response but do not contribute to cardiac inflammation following infection with Trypanosoma cruzi. Infect Immun. 2006;74(1):125–34.
19. Hardison JL, Kuziel WA, Manning JE, Lane TE. Chemokine CC receptor 2 is important for acute control of cardiac parasitism but does not contribute to cardiac inflammation after infection with Trypanosoma cruzi. J Infect Dis. 2006;193(11):1584–8.
20. Machado FS, Koyama NS, Carregaro V, Ferreira BR, Milanezi CM, Teixeira MM, Rossi MA, Silva JS. CCR5 plays a critical role in the development of myocarditis and host protection in mice infected with Trypanosoma cruzi. J Infect Dis. 2005;191(4):627–36.
21. Hardison JL, Wrightsman RA, Carpenter PM, Kuziel WA, Lane TE, Manning JE. The CC chemokine receptor 5 is important in control of parasite replication and acute cardiac inflammation following infection with Trypanosoma cruzi. Infect Immun. 2006;74(1):135–43.
22. Albareda MC, Laucella SA, Alvarez MG, Armenti AH, Bertochi G, Tarleton RL, Postan M. Trypanosoma cruzi modulates the profile of memory CD8+ T cells in chronic Chagas' disease patients. Int Immunol. 2006;18(3):465–71.
23. Bonney KM, Taylor JM, Thorp EB, Epting CL, Engman DM. Depletion of regulatory T cells decreases cardiac parasitosis and inflammation in experimental Chagas disease. Parasitol Res. 2015;114(3):1167–78.
24. Arguello RJ, Albareda MC, Alvarez MG, Bertocchi G, Armenti AH, Vigliano C, Meckert PC, Tarleton

RL, Laucella SA. Inhibitory receptors are expressed by Trypanosoma cruzi-specific effector T cells and in hearts of subjects with chronic Chagas disease. PLoS One. 2012;7(5):e35966.
25. Andrade SG, Campos RF, Sobral KS, Magalhães JB, Guedes RS, Guerreiro ML. Reinfections with strains of Trypanosoma cruzi, of different biodemes as a factor of aggravation of myocarditis and myositis in mice. Rev Soc Bras Med Trop. 2006;39(1):1–8.
26. Pereira ME, Santos LM, Araújo MS, Brener Z. Recrudescence induced by cyclophosphamide of chronic Trypanosoma cruzi infection in mice is influenced by the parasite strain. Mem Inst Oswaldo Cruz. 1996;91(1):71–4.
27. Bern C. Chagas disease in the immunosuppressed host. Curr Opin Infect Dis. 2012;25(4):450–7.
28. Parodi C, Padilla AM, Basombrío MA. Protective immunity against Trypanosoma cruzi. Mem Inst Oswaldo Cruz. 2009;104(Suppl. I):288–94.
29. Bonney K, Engman DM. Autoimmune pathogenesis of Chagas heart disease: looking back, looking ahead. Am J Pathol. 2015;185(6):1537–47.
30. Tarleton RL. Parasite persistence in the aetiology of Chagas disease. Int J Parasitol. 2001;31(5–6):550–4.
31. Roffê E, Marino AP, Weaver J, Wan W, de Araújo FF, Hoffman V, Santiago HC, Murphy PM. Trypanosoma cruzi causes paralyzing systemic necrotizing Vasculitis driven by pathogen-specific type I immunity in mice. Infect Immun. 2016;84(4):1123–36.
32. Higuchi ML, Gutierrez PS, Aiello VD, Palomino S, Bocchi E, Kalil J, Bellotti G, Pileggi F. Immunohistochemical characterization of infiltrating cells in human chronic chagasic myocarditis: comparison with myocardial rejection process. Virchows Arch A Pathol Anat Histopathol. 1993;423(3):157–60.
33. Gomes JA, Bahia-Oliveira LM, Rocha MO, Martins-Filho OA, Gazzinelli G, Correa-Oliveira R. Evidence that development of severe cardiomyopathy in human Chagas' disease is due to a Th1-specific immune response. Infect Immun. 2003;71(3):1185–93.
34. Martin DL, Weatherly DB, Laucella SA, Cabinian MA, Crim MT, Sullivan S, Heiges M, Craven SH, Rosenberg CS, Collins MH, Sette A, Postan M, Tarleton RL. CD8+ T-cell responses to Trypanosoma cruzi are highly focused on strain-variant trans-sialidase epitopes. PLoS Pathog. 2006;2(8):e77.
35. Rodrigues MM, Alencar BC, Claser C, Tzelepis F. Immunodominance: a new hypothesis to explain parasite escape and host/parasite equilibrium leading to the chronic phase of Chagas' disease? Braz J Med Biol Res. 2009;42(3):220–3.
36. Scharfstein J, Andrade D. Infection-associated vasculopathy in experimental chagas disease pathogenic roles of endothelin and kinin pathways. Adv Parasitol. 2011;76:101–27.
37. Tarleton RL, Zhang L. Chagas disease etiology: autoimmunity or parasite persistence? Parasitol Today. 1999;15:94–9.
38. Morillo CA, Marin-Neto JA, Avezum A, Sosa-Estani S, Rassi A Jr, Rosas F, Villena E, Quiroz R, Bonilla R, Britto C, Guhl F, Velazquez E, Bonilla L, Meeks B, Rao-Melacini P, Pogue J, Mattos A, Lazdins J, Rassi A, Connolly SJ, Yusuf S, BENEFIT Investigators. Randomized trial of benznidazole for chronic Chagas' cardiomyopathy. N Engl J Med. 2015;373(14):1295–306.
39. Santos-Buch CA, Teixeira AR. The immunology of experimental Chagas' disease. 3. Rejection of allogeneic heart cells in vitro. J Exp Med. 1974;140(1):38–53.
40. Borda ES, Sterin-Borda L. Antiadrenergic and muscarinic receptor antibodies in Chagas' cardiomyopathy. Int J Cardiol. 1996;54(2):149–56.
41. Motrán CC, Fretes RE, Cerbán FM, Rivarola HW, Vottero de Cima E. Immunization with the C-terminal region of Trypanosoma cruzi ribosomal P1 and P2 proteins induces long-term duration cross-reactive antibodies with heart functional and structural alterations in young and aged mice. Clin Immunol. 2000;97(2):89–94.
42. Cunha-Neto E, Coelho V, Guilherme L, Fiorelli A, Stolf N, Kalil J. Autoimmunity in Chagas' disease. Identification of cardiac myosin-B13 Trypanosoma cruzi protein crossreactive T cell clones in heart lesions of a chronic Chagas' cardiomyopathy patient. J Clin Investig. 1996;98(8):1709–12.
43. Laguens RP, Meckert PC, Chambó JG. Antiheart antibody-dependent cytotoxicity in the sera of mice chronically infected with Trypanosoma cruzi. Infect Immun. 1988;56(4):993–7.
44. Pontes-de-Carvalho L, Santana CC, Soares MB, Oliveira GG, Cunha-Neto E, Ribeiro-dos-Santos R. Experimental chronic Chagas' disease myocarditis is an autoimmune disease preventable by induction of immunological tolerance to myocardial antigens. J Autoimmun. 2002;18:131–8.
45. Garcia S, Ramos CO, Senra JF, Vilas-Boas F, Rodrigues MM, Campos-de-Carvalho AC, Ribeiro-Dos-Santos R, Soares MB. Treatment with benznidazole during the chronic phase of experimental Chagas' disease decreases cardiac alterations. Antimicrob Agents Chemother. 2005;49(4):1521–8.
46. Ruiz AM, Esteva M, Cabeza Meckert P, Laguens RP, Segura EL. Protective immunity and pathology induced by inoculation of mice with different subcellular fractions of Trypanosoma cruzi. Acta Trop. 1985;42(4):299–309.

Part IV

The Role of Infectious Agents in Rheumatic Diseases

14 Macrophage Activation Syndrome

Esraa M. Eloseily and Randy Q. Cron

Abbreviations

AIDS	Acquired immunodeficiency syndrome
APC	Antigen-presenting cell
CsA	Cyclosporine A
CTL	Cytotoxic T lymphocyte
CTLA-4	Cytotoxic T-lymphocyte-associated protein 4
DIC	Disseminated intravascular coagulopathy
EBV	Epstein-Barr virus
fHLH	Familial hemophagocytic lymphohistiocytosis
FSTL-1	Follistatin-like 1
G-CSF	Granulocyte colony-stimulating factor
GM-CSF	Granulocyte-macrophage colony-stimulating factor
HAV	Hepatitis A virus
HBV	Hepatitis B virus
HCV	Hepatitis C virus
HIV	Human immunodeficiency virus
HLH	Hemophagocytic lymphohistiocytosis
HS	HScore
HSCT	Hematopoietic stem cell transplant
ICU	Intensive care unit
IFN-γ	interferon-gamma
IL	Interleukin
IL-18BP	Interleukin-18-binding protein
IL-1Ra	Interleukin-1 receptor antagonist
IVIg	Intravenous immunoglobulin
MAS	Macrophage activation syndrome
NK cell	Natural killer cell
sCD163	Soluble haptoglobin receptor
sCD25	Soluble interleukin-2 receptor alpha chain
sHLH	Secondary hemophagocytic lymphohistiocytosis
sJIA	Systemic juvenile idiopathic arthritis
SLE	Systemic lupus erythematosus
Th1	T-helper 1
TLR	Toll-like receptor
TNF	Tumor necrosis factor
USA	United States of America
XLP	X-linked lymphoproliferative disease

E. M. Eloseily
Assiut University Children's Hospital, Assiut, Egypt

R. Q. Cron (✉)
University of Alabama at Birmingham,
Birmingham, AL, USA
e-mail: rcron@peds.uab.edu

Introduction

HLH/MAS is thought to be a multisystem inflammatory disorder resulting from a pro-inflammatory "cytokine storm" from excessively activated

G. Ragab et al. (eds.), *The Microbiome in Rheumatic Diseases and Infection*,
https://doi.org/10.1007/978-3-319-79026-8_14

lymphocytes and macrophages [1]. Hemophagocytic syndromes are divided into primary and secondary forms. Primary cases are rare (1 in 50,000 live births), commonly present in the first year of life, and are often triggered by infection [2]. They include familial, or primary, forms of hemophagocytic lymphohistiocytosis (fHLH) that have specific genetic homozygous or compound heterozygous loss-of-function mutations in perforin-mediated cytolytic pathway proteins (e.g., *PRF1*, *STX11*, *UNC13D*, *UNC18-2*) employed by CD8 T cells and natural killer (NK) cells [3–6]. Children with certain immunodeficiency syndromes, such as Chédiak-Higashi syndrome, type II Hermansky-Pudlak syndrome, and type II Griscelli syndrome [7], have associated genetic defects in cytolysis and are also at risk for developing fHLH. Specific X-linked immunodeficiencies (signaling-lymphocytic-activation-molecule-associated protein (SAP) and X-linked inhibitor of apoptosis (XIAP) deficiencies) are also associated with Epstein-Barr virus (EBV) triggered HLH [8–10].

Acquired or secondary forms of HLH (sHLH) are usually associated with conditions that cause chronic immune dysregulation, such as rheumatologic diseases [e.g., systemic juvenile idiopathic arthritis (sJIA), systemic lupus erythematosus (SLE)] and certain malignancies (e.g., leukemias, lymphomas). Infectious agents, particularly EBV and other herpesvirus family members, may be the sHLH trigger, although identifiable infections are not always present [7]. In addition, up to 40% of sHLH and macrophage activation syndrome (MAS) patients have been found to possess heterozygous (some dominant negative) mutations in known fHLH genes. Thus, some investigators consider MAS, sHLH, and fHLH to lie on a spectrum of disease [11].

In the clinical setting, the distinction between primary and secondary forms of HLH is less clear and even considered artificial by some. It was initially used to differentiate the primary, more fatal, infantile presentations from the secondary forms, which were considered to present later in life and to have better prognoses. However, it is now known that primary genetic forms can present later in life, even during adulthood [12, 13]. Furthermore, in some studies, only 40% of primary HLH cases are found to have recognized genetic mutations. Moreover, both primary and secondary HLH are known to be precipitated by infections [14, 15]. Finally, as mentioned previously, many patients with sHLH have heterozygous mutations in known fHLH-associated genes, thus blurring the distinction between fHLH and sHLH. Regardless of terminology, the individual patient needs to be treated appropriately. At present, most clinicians would agree that clear-cut infantile cases of fHLH will need bone marrow transplantation, typically preceded by an aggressive chemotherapeutic regimen which includes etoposide and corticosteroids. In addition, identified infectious triggers should also be treated appropriately. For all other children and adults with HLH, the most appropriate treatment remains unclear. Etoposide is quite toxic, often leading to pancytopenia itself and increasing the risk of secondary sepsis as well as increased risk of secondary malignancies [14, 16]. Novel approaches have been anecdotally reported to dampen the overly exuberant immune response and control the cytokine storm and associated multiorgan dysfunction. Most notably, targeting of specific pro-inflammatory cytokines [e.g., interleukin-1 (IL-1) and interferon-gamma (IFN-γ)] seems promising and lacks the toxicity associated with traditional chemotherapeutic approaches [17, 18].

Despite advances in the current treatment protocols, the cure rate for HLH is low. Untreated cases of fHLH have a median survival of less than 2–6 months after diagnosis [19]. In a nationwide registry of pediatric patients with HLH in Korea, the 5-year overall survival rate was 68% (38% in the familial group and 81% in the presumed secondary group) [20]. The prognosis for cases of sHLH varies depending on the underlying etiology, for example, the mortality rate is reported to be lower in cases associated with rheumatic diseases (8–22%) and greater when it is associated with malignancy. The median overall survival is about 36–67% [21–23].

Pathophysiology and Cytokine Storm

MAS/HLH develops as a "cytokine storm" which is often triggered by infectious, rheumatologic, and oncologic diseases [24]. Although not well defined, the pro-inflammatory cytokines associated with MAS/HLH likely include IL-1, IL-6, IL-12, IL-18, IFN-γ, and tumor necrosis factor (TNF) [25, 26] (Table 14.1). Also IL-27, macrophage colony-stimulating factor (M-CSF), and granulocyte-macrophage colony-stimulating factor (GM-CSF) may be increased [27–29]. Furthermore, chemokines, such as IL-8/CXCL8, MIG/CXCL9, IP10/CXCL10, I-TAC/CXCL11, MCP-1/CCL2, MIP-1α/CCL3, and MIP-1β/CCL4, have been reported to be increased [26, 30–32]. Both cytokines and chemokines activate the immune system, perpetuating the ongoing cytokine storm. On the other arm, levels of anti-inflammatory cytokines, such as IL-10 and IL-18-binding protein (IL-18BP), are also increased but might not be sufficient to terminate the ongoing inflammation [33, 34]. Mazodier et al. described a discrepancy between the increase in IL-18 and its antagonist IL-18BP that lead to abnormally high levels of free IL-18 [33]. Similarly, the natural antagonist to IL-1, IL-1 receptor antagonist (IL-1Ra), has been noted to be elevated during MAS/HLH, and a recombinant form of IL-1Ra has been reported by several groups to be an effective therapy for MAS/HLH/cytokine storm syndrome [35–37].

Table 14.1 Cytokines in HLH and their potential roles [38–47]

Cytokine/chemokine	Related features of HLH
TNF	Fever, cachexia, neurological symptoms, depression of hematopoiesis, elevated transaminases, hypoalbuminemia, hypofibrinogenemia, hypertriglyceridemia, disseminated intravascular coagulopathy (DIC), suppression of natural killer (NK) cell activity
IL-1	Fever, depression of hematopoiesis, coagulopathy due to plasminogen activation, hyperferritinemia, acute phase proteins, T-cell activation
IFN-γ	Fever, hemophagocytosis, depression of hematopoiesis, DIC, hypoalbuminemia, liver damage, hypertriglyceridemia, macrophage activation, stimulation of antigen presentation, stimulation of CD4 T-helper 1 (Th1) response
IL-18	Liver pathology, prolonged exposure suppression of NK cell activity
IL-10	Suppression of T-cell activation, inhibition of Th1 cytokine production, regulation of hemophagocytosis, modulation of immune-mediating pathology
IL-6	Fever, anemia, acute phase proteins, renal impairment, T-cell activation and infiltration, suppression of NK cell activity

The etiology of the cytokine storm is not entirely clear. Since fHLH is associated with biallelic defects in gene products involved in the perforin-mediated cytolytic pathway used by NK cells and CD8 T lymphocytes [48, 49], the inability to clear the antigenic stimulus and thus turn off the inflammatory response has been hypothesized to result in hypercytokinemia [50]. Recently, the inability of CD8 T cells and NK cells to lyse antigen-presenting cells (APCs) via the perforin-mediated cytolytic pathway was shown to prolong (by fivefold) the engagement time between the lytic lymphocyte and the APC. This prolonged interaction resulted in increased levels of pro-inflammatory cytokines. For up to 40% of sHLH cases, single-copy mutations in these same perforin pathway genes have been reported. Some of the mutants have been demonstrated to act as complete or partial dominant-negative mutants [51–53], resulting in sHLH in older children and adults [53, 54], the oldest reported case being a 62-year-old patient [55]. One heterozygous mutation in *RAB27A* identified in two unrelated sHLH patients was shown to act in a partial dominant-negative fashion and delayed cytolytic granule polarization to the immunologic synapse between NK cells and their target cells. This was also associated with an increase in IFN-γ production, mimicking the situation described for homozygous defects in perforin or granzyme B. Moreover, increased IL-6 production has been shown to decrease cytolytic activity of NK cells, further exacerbating the lytic defect and resultant production of pro-inflammatory cytokines.

In a healthy individual, exposure of most cells to many intracellular pathogens will normally initiate an inflammatory cascade, frequently leading to release of Th1 cytokines (IFN-γ, TNF) that will activate macrophages, NK cells, and cytolytic T cells. NK and cytolytic T cells release granules that contain perforin and granzymes [49]. Perforin is a key cytolytic protein that causes osmotic lysis of the target cell [56] and is also necessary for the uptake of granzymes by the target cell that will then catalyze cleavage of multiple protein substrates, including caspases which then trigger cell apoptosis. All the genetic defects described in fHLH involve either inadequate levels of perforin itself or improper granule exocytosis leading to impaired apoptosis of the target cell, improper removal of the stimulating antigen, and ultimately ongoing inflammation.

However, other pathways lacking cytolytic pathway gene defects can lead to the final endpoint of HLH or MAS. In a murine model of MAS, it was shown that repeated stimulation of toll-like receptor 9 (TLR9) produced MAS on a normal genetic background, without exogenous antigen. Interestingly, the TLR9-induced MAS model was IFN-γ dependent in some aspects of disease; however, lymphocytes were not required for the pathogenesis [57]. On the other hand, a state of inflammation may also reduce the lytic capacity of NK cells and CD8 T cells [58–60], resulting in cytokine storm due to frustrated phagocytosis. This was illustrated in a study where T-cell-directed immunotherapy for refractory leukemia resulted in cytokine storm and an MAS-like presentation [61]. All the aforementioned pathways have led to the proposal that MAS is due to a combination of genetic predisposition and a hyperinflammatory state reducing cytolytic function, put into action by a trigger (e.g., infection, cancer, immunodeficiency, autoimmunity, and autoinflammation) [19, 53, 62–64]. At some point a threshold level of hypercytokinemia is reached at which the body is incapable of balancing the cytokine storm with anti-inflammatory products, such as IL-10, IL-1Ra, IL-18BP, and others. This is then believed to trigger the multiorgan dysfunction resulting in clinical HLH.

Clinical Picture

Initial symptoms of HLH/MAS are usually nonspecific. The cardinal feature is unremitting high fever. However, therapeutic targeting of pro-inflammatory cytokines (e.g., IL-1, IL-6) to treat underlying rheumatic diseases that often result in MAS (e.g., sJIA) makes fever not an absolute finding in all cases. This is attributed to the powerful antipyretic effect of biologics such as inhibitors of IL-1, IL-6, and TNF. On examination, many patients have hepatomegaly, splenomegaly, or both, and up to 50% of MAS/HLH patients have central nervous system involvement ranging from mild confusion to seizures or frank coma [65]. Different forms of rash can occur, often erythematous or purpuric. Patients can have progressive hepatic dysfunction and ultimately multiorgan failure. DIC-like features are often present and are partly explained by liver dysfunction, fibrinogen consumption, and thrombocytopenia [66]. This highlights the challenges in distinguishing microbial sepsis-induced DIC from HLH in the intensive care unit (ICU). Despite the similarities these two conditions share in clinical presentations, they are frequently treated differently: broad spectrum antibiotics (sepsis) versus immunosuppression (HLH), respectively [67]. As HLH is not a diagnosis of exclusion, and infections are common triggers of HLH, it is important to treat both infection and, if present, the associated cytokine storm of HLH.

Classification Criteria

MAS/HLH can be difficult to diagnose, especially in the early stages where it can be easily misdiagnosed as shock or multiorgan dysfunction due to sepsis. In addition, MAS may be confused with an underlying disease flare, as in the case of sJIA. Because MAS can have a high mortality rate in children with sJIA (~8–22%) [68–70], sensitive diagnostic criteria are needed to assist with early detection, allowing for appropriate and timely therapy. Because of the different diseases associated with MAS/HLH, different diagnostic and classification criteria have been proposed over the years, such as HLH-04, SLE-MAS criteria, the HScore, and the novel 2016 criteria for MAS complicating sJIA (Table 14.2). Some of these criteria are disease specific (e.g., sJIA, SLE) and can be both sensitive and specific, whereas others encompass all potential HLH-associated diagnoses, but tend to have lower sensitivities overall. Clinically, and outside of clinical trials,

Table 14.2 Published criteria for MAS and HLH

HLH-2004 diagnostic	2009 preliminary diagnostic guidelines for MAS complicating cSLE	2005 preliminary diagnostic guidelines for MAS complicating sJIA	2016 classification criteria for MAS complicating sJIA
a. Molecular diagnosis b. Diagnostic criteria • Fever • Splenomegaly • Cytopenia (at least two of three lineages: • Hemoglobin <90 gm/l, • Platelets <100 × 10^9/l, • Neutrophils <1.0 × 10^9/l • Hypertriglyceridemia and/or • Hypofibrinogenemia (triglycerides ≥265 mg/dl, fibrinogen ≤1.5 gm/l) • Hemophagocytosis BM, spleen, or lymph nodes • Low or absent NK cell activity • Ferritin ≥500 ng/ml • Soluble CD25 ≥ 2400 units	a. Clinical criteria • Fever (>38 C) • Hepatomegaly (≥3 cm below the costal arch) • Splenomegaly (≥3 cm below the costal arch) • Hemorrhagic manifestations • Central nervous system dysfunction b. Laboratory criteria • Cytopenia affecting two or more cell lineages (WBC ≤4.0 × 10^9/l, hemoglobin ≤90 gm/l or platelet count ≤150 × 10^9/l) • Increased AST (>40 units/l) • Increased LDH (>567 units/l) • Hypofibrinogenemia • (fibrinogen ≤1.5 gm/l) • Hypertriglyceridemia (triglycerides >178 mg/dl) • Hyperferritinemia (ferritin >500 mg/l)	a. Laboratory criteria • Decreased platelet count (≤262 × 10^9/l) • Elevated levels of AST (>59 U/l) • Decreased WBC count (≤4.0 × 10^9/l) • Hypofibrinogenemia (≤2.5 g/l) b. Clinical criteria • Central nervous system dysfunction • Hemorrhages • Hepatomegaly (≥3 cm below the costal arch)	A febrile patient with known or suspected sJIA is classified as having MAS if the following criteria are met: Ferritin >684 ng/ml and any two of the following: • Platelet count ≤181 × 10^9/l • AST >48 U/l • Triglycerides >156 mg/dl • Fibrinogen ≤360 mg/dl
Implementation			
The diagnosis of HLH can be established in the presence of a molecular diagnosis consistent with HLH or by meeting five of eight clinical and laboratory diagnostic criteria	The diagnosis of MAS requires the simultaneous presence of at least one clinical criterion and at least two laboratory criteria. Bone marrow aspiration for evidence of macrophage hemophagocytosis may be required only in doubtful cases	The diagnosis of MAS requires the presence of at least two laboratory criteria or the presence of at least one laboratory criterion and one clinical criterion. Bone marrow aspiration for evidence of macrophage hemophagocytosis may be required only in doubtful cases	See above *Laboratory abnormalities should not be otherwise explained by the patient's condition, such as concomitant immune-mediated thrombocytopenia, infectious hepatitis, visceral leishmaniasis, or familial hyperlipidemia*

Adapted from Henter et al. [11], Ravelli et al. [71], Parodi et al. [72], Ravelli et al. [73]
AST aspartate aminotransferase, *BM* bone marrow, *HLH* hemophagocytic lymphohistiocytosis, *jSLE* juvenile systemic lupus erythematosus, *LDH* lactate dehydrogenase, *MAS* macrophage activation syndrome, *NK* natural killer, *sJIA* systemic juvenile idiopathic arthritis, *WBC* white blood cells

the various criteria are useful for clinicians to strongly consider MAS/HLH diagnostically so that appropriate therapy can be initiated as soon as possible to result in optimal outcomes.

MAS as a Part of sJIA (sJIA-MAS)

HLH-2004 Diagnostic Guidelines

Due to the fact that MAS resembles fHLH in its clinical presentation, HLH-2004 diagnostic guidelines were initially used to diagnose MAS. Those guidelines were developed to diagnose genetic homozygous/compound heterozygous cases of fHLH [11]. The main deficiencies regarding the HLH-2004 criteria for diagnosing MAS in patients with sJIA are due to the underlying inflammatory nature of sJIA versus fHLH. In active sJIA, one would expect elevated levels of white blood cell counts, platelets, and fibrinogen as part of the inflammatory process. Accordingly, a drop in their levels, which could still be in the normal limits as regards to the HLH-2004 criteria, should raise the suspicion of MAS. Also the underlying inflammatory process leads to elevated levels of ferritin [74]; therefore, the cutoff of ferritin >500 ng/ml in the HLH-2004 guidelines makes it difficult to distinguish MAS complicating sJIA from an sJIA flare. Adding to the shortcomings of HLH-2004 guidelines overall are the lack of availability and timely results of certain criteria, such as NK cell activity or sCD25 levels in many centers [25, 75, 76].

Preliminary Diagnostic Criteria for MAS Complicating sJIA

Eventually, preliminary diagnostic criteria were introduced for sJIA-MAS comparing it to sJIA flare [71], which yielded better results in identifying MAS among sJIA patients when compared to HLH-2004 diagnostic guidelines [77]. However, these new criteria had their own shortcomings. The study that led to the criteria development was lacking in some important laboratory parameters, including some of the important MAS markers such as ferritin, lactate dehydrogenase, and triglycerides [25, 75, 76]. Moreover, they were based on a relatively small sampling of patients, and they were not validated. These shortcomings were an impetus to develop new sJIA-specific MAS criteria.

2016 Classification Criteria for Macrophage Activation Syndrome Complicating Systemic Juvenile Idiopathic Arthritis

The deficiencies in the previous guidelines have pushed for the development of more accurate criteria for sJIA-MAS. Recently, novel classification criteria have been introduced. These were the result of an international collaborative effort combining expert consensus, evidence compiled from the medical literature, and analysis of real patients. The development of the 2016 criteria was conducted under the auspices of the European League Against Rheumatism, the American College of Rheumatology, and the Paediatric Rheumatology International Trials Organization [73]. Based on the common consensus that clinical criteria of MAS are often delayed and/or difficult to distinguish from an underlying disease flare, the 2016 sJIA-MAS criteria are based primarily on laboratory parameters with fever as the only clinical criterion [76]. These criteria are relatively simple yet proved to be both highly sensitive and specific. However, the criteria are not ideal in the setting of children with sJIA who are being actively treated with IL-1 or IL-6 blockade. Ultimately, simple criteria that are not necessarily disease specific but maintain high sensitivity and specificity for establishing an MAS/HLH diagnosis are needed.

MAS as Part of Systemic Lupus Erythematosus (SLE-MAS)

Childhood SLE (cSLE) cases complicated by MAS have been reported with increasing frequency in the recent years. As an SLE disease flare itself often results in pancytopenia, diagnostic criteria for MAS in the setting of SLE are complicated. Accordingly, it has been suggested that cSLE-MAS may be under-recognized [78]. Preliminary guidelines for SLE-MAS were proposed in 2009. A study was conducted based on a multinational survey and data analyzing 38 patients with cSLE-MAS [72]. Patients who had evidence of macrophage hemophagocytosis on bone marrow aspiration were considered to have definite MAS, and those who did not were considered to have probable MAS. The sensitivity, specificity, and the area under the receiver operating characteristic curve of various clinical and laboratory parameters were compared in SLE patients with MAS versus patients with active juvenile SLE without MAS. The best diagnostic performance was obtained using the simultaneous presence of any one or more clinical criteria and any two or more laboratory criteria, which had a sensitivity of 92.1% and a specificity of 90.9% (Table 14.2). The demonstration of macrophage hemophagocytosis in the bone marrow aspirate was considered necessary for confirmation of doubtful cases only. Those results have led to the practical recommendation that in the clinical setting, MAS should be suspected in a patient with cSLE presenting with unexplained fever and cytopenia associated with hyperferritinemia. Both HLH-2004 criteria and preliminary diagnostic guidelines for sJIA-MAS were tested in the study but were found to be inaccurate for detecting cSLE-MAS. Interestingly, about two-thirds of the patients with cSLE-MAS developed it within 1 month of SLE diagnosis. The frequency of ICU admission was 43.7%, and the mortality rate was 11.4%.

Generic MAS Criteria/HScore

In 2014, Fardet et al. developed and partially validated a diagnostic score for the broader category of reactive hemophagocytic syndrome (HS), called the HScore [79], which can be used to estimate an individual's risk of having reactive hemophagocytic syndrome, or HLH. This score was created and tested using a multicenter retrospective cohort of 312 patients scrutinizing 10 explanatory variables that were issued from a previous Delphi survey involving 24 HLH experts from 13 countries [80]. After showing positive associations of each variable with an HLH diagnosis, multivariate logistic regression was used to assess their independent contributions to the outcome. Following calculating each variable's threshold value, the coefficients resulting from multiple logistic regression analysis were used to assign score points to each one. The performance of the score was assessed using developmental and validation data sets. The HScore revealed excellent diagnostic performance and discriminative ability in both developmental and validation data sets. The probability of having HLH ranged from <1% with an HScore of ≤90 to >99% with an HScore of ≥250.

The HScore has some limitations including the heterogeneity of the underlying diseases (a high proportion had cancer-associated HLH), the retrospective manner of the data collection, and the small sample size (only 10% of the entire study population) of the validation data set. As the study included only adults with reactive HLH, the applicability in children, particularly those with sJIA-MAS, is questionable. Adding to its limitations in pediatric cases, some of the criteria in the HScore might not be practically applicable in children. For example, the definition of the item, "Known underlying immunosuppression," lists some medications that are used infrequently in children with sJIA, such as cyclosporine A and azathioprine, and at the same time it does not mention the newer more widely used cytokine antagonists that have been associated with the occurrence of MAS [25, 81, 82]. Moreover, bone marrow aspirates in a search for hemophagocytosis are not frequently performed in children with sJIA-MAS, as it is not considered mandatory in either the HLH-2004 guidelines [11] or the preliminary MAS guidelines [71]. In fact, absence of hemophagocytosis does not rule out MAS, and the procedure should not delay appropriate therapy. Furthermore, the underlying inflammatory nature of sJIA that is associated with marked thrombocytosis makes the threshold level for the platelet count (110,000/mm^3) too low for identifying MAS in the setting of sJIA. It is the relative drop in platelets count, rather than an absolute decrease below a certain threshold, that is more useful to make an early diagnosis [77]. Thus, the HScore is likely more valuable in diagnosing adults with HLH, particularly those with associated leukemias and lymphomas.

New Biomarkers

A new promising laboratory marker of MAS is soluble CD163 (sCD163). Its expression is restricted to the macrophage/monocyte lineage only, unlike ferritin and soluble CD25 (IL-2 receptor α-chain), which are produced by a number of tissues and cell types, including the liver, spleen, heart, kidney, and T cells under a variety of nonspecific inflammatory conditions. sCD163 has been mainly evaluated in MAS, where combination testing of sCD25 and sCD163 identified patients with subclinical MAS [83]. Further studies to evaluate its role in HLH not associated with autoimmune diseases are required. Moreover, like sCD25, the testing is not currently available in a timely fashion in most centers around the world.

Another novel biomarker, follistatin-related protein 1 (FSTL-1) was reported by Gorelik et al. to be elevated in active sJIA with higher levels during MAS. FSTL-1 levels correlated with sCD25 and ferritin levels, and FSTL-1 normalized after treatment. Perhaps more importantly, Gorelik et al. also reported that in their small cohort (28 sJIA patients) a ferritin to ESR ratio > 80 had the highest sensitivity and specificity (100% and 100%, respectively) in distinguishing between MAS and new-onset sJIA disease flare [84]. As ferritin rises due to inflammation in MAS/HLH, and the ESR tends to drop as fibrinogen (an important driver of high ESRs) is consumed during coagulopathy, a simple ratio of ferritin to ESR may prove to be a simple and valuable tool in getting clinicians to consider a diagnosis of MAS/HLH in their febrile hospitalized patients.

Although the serum IL-18 level is also not routinely available clinically, it may also serve as a distinguishing biomarker for sJIA patients who develop MAS. Comparing cytokine patterns between sJIA-MAS patients, EBV-HLH, Kawasaki disease, and healthy age-matched controls, Shimizu et al. reported that IL-18 concentrations during sJIA-MAS were significantly higher compared to the others, and they correlated with measures of disease activity (CRP, ferritin, LDH, and other cytokines). In addition, serum neopterin and sTNF-RII levels were significantly higher during MAS compared to sJIA flares [85]. Other reports also showed that IL-18 levels were significantly elevated in sJIA [86, 87] and the patients with high levels were more likely to develop MAS [88]. Furthermore, sphingomyelinase was found to be elevated in HLH cases [89]. Thus, a variety of new biomarkers may help identify MAS among sJIA patients.

Genetic Associations

Genetic HLH has been commonly classified into two groups: fHLH which are a group of autosomal recessive disorders, and immunodeficiency syndromes related HLH. Of the immunodeficiency syndromes, Chediak-Higashi, Griscelli, and Hermansky-Pudlak are associated with a variable degree of albinism/hypopigmentation of the skin or hair and platelet dysfunction which can assist in identifying potential cases of HLH (Table 14.3) [2, 90–92]. Interestingly, up to 40% of sHLH cases possess heterozygous mutations in these same fHLH-associated gene products. Thus, the overall underlying genetic risk for sHLH may be rather striking.

In addition to underlying inflammatory states (e.g., sJIA, leukemia) and genetic predispositions (e.g., perforin deficiency), infections (some from the commensal human microbiome) are frequently significant contributing factors in lowering the threshold required to develop a cytokine storm syndrome capable of resulting in HLH/MAS (Table 14.4). HLH has been associated with a vast variety of infections, with EBV as the most commonly reported trigger. Both familial (fHLH) and sporadic or secondary (sHLH) cases of HLH are often precipitated by acute infections. It is also important to note that an underlying precipitating infection for HLH can be masked, as the HLH clinical picture can mimic an infectious process or

Table 14.3 Genetic associations with HLH

HLH type	Chromosome	Gene	Protein	Function
Familial HLH				
fHLH1	9q21.3–22	Unknown	Unknown	Unknown
fHLH2	10q22	PRF1	Perforin	Apoptosis and cytotoxicity
fHLH3	17q25.1	UNC13D	Mammalian uncoordinated-13–4 (Munc13–4)	Exocytosis of granules
fHLH4	6q24	STX11	Syntaxin11	Generation of granules with SNAP23
fHLH5	19p13.3–2	STXBP2	Mammalian uncoordinated-18–2 (Munc18–2)	Vesicle fusion
Immunodeficiency				
CD27 deficiency	12p13	CD27	TNF receptor superfamily 7 (TNFRSF7)	Lymphocyte costimulatory molecule
Chediak-Higashi	1q42.1–2	LYST	Lysosomal trafficking regulator	Transport of lysosomes
Griscelli, type 2	15q21	RAB27A	Ras-related protein Rab-27A	Granule exocytosis
Hermansky-Pudlak, type 2	5q14.1	AP3B1	AP-3 complex subunit beta-1	AP3βchain: traffic from Golgi to granules
Hermansky-Pudlak, type 9	15q21.1	BLOC1S6	Biogenesis of lysosome-related organelles complex 1 subunit 6	Intracellular vesicle trafficking
ITK deficiency	5q33.3	ITK	IL-2-inducible T-cell kinase	T-cell development, proliferation, and differentiation
NLRC4 mutation (autoinflammation with recurrent MAS)	2p22.3	NLRC4	NOD-like receptor family, caspase recruitment domain-containing 4	Caspase recruitment and innate immune response
IL-2R-gamma deficiency	10p15–14	IL2RA	IL-2R	T-cell activation and regulation
SCID (common γ chain def)	Xq13	IL-2RG	IL-2R	T-cell activation and regulation
Wiskott-Aldrich	Xp11.23–22	WAS	Wiskott-Aldrich syndrome protein (WASp)	Cytoskeleton
X-linked lymphoproliferative (XLP) type 1	Xq25	SH2D1A	SH2 domain-containing protein 1A(SAP)	Activation of lymphocytes
X-linked lymphoproliferative (XLP) type 2	Xq25	XIAP	Baculoviral IAP repeat-containing protein 4 (BIRC4)	Inhibition of apoptosis
ADA deficiency	20q13.11	ADA	Adenosine deaminase	Metabolism of purine nucleosides
PNP deficiency	14q13.1	PNP	Purine nucleoside phosphorylase	Metabolism of purine nucleosides
DiGeorge syndrome	22q11.2	DCGR	Unknown	Various
XL-O-EDA-ID	Xq28	NEMO	NEMO protein	Inflammation, immunity, cell survival, and signaling pathways
XLA	Xq21.3-q22	BTK	BTK protein	B-cell maturation and proliferation

(continued)

Table 14.3 (continued)

HLH type	Chromosome	Gene	Protein	Function
Hyper-IgD syndrome	12q24	MVK	Mevalonate kinase	Isoprenoid and sterol synthesis
Lysinuric protein intolerance	14q11.2	SLC7A7	Light subunit of a cationic amino acid transporter	Transport of amino acid
Multiple sulfatase def.	3p26	SUMF1	FGE	Transcriptional activation of sulfatase
Methylmalonic aciduria (cobalamin deficiency) cblC type, with homocystinuria	1p34.1	MMACHC	Methylmalonic aciduria and homocystinuria type C protein	Binding and intracellular trafficking of cobalamin
Holt-Oram syndrome	12q24.1	TBX5	T-box 5 protein	Promotes cardiomyocyte differentiation
XMEN syndrome	Xq21.1	MAGT1	Magnesium transporter 1	T-cell activation via T-cell receptor
Others				
IRF5 polymorphisms	7q32.1	IRF5	Interferon regulatory factor 5	Role in the toll-like receptor signaling pathway and activation of pro-inflammatory cytokine genes

Table 14.4 Infectious triggers of MAS/HLH

Infectious triggers	Virus nucleic acid	Examples
Viral	DNA	EBV [93], CMV [94–97], HHV6 [98], HHV-8 [99–101], varicella zoster [102], HSV1 [103], HSV2 [104], adenovirus [105, 106], herpes simplex [107, 108], parvovirus B19 [109, 110], HBV [111]
	RNA	Hepatitis A [112, 113]/C [111, 114–116], HIV-1 [117–119], influenza H1N1 [54, 120–126], parainfluenza [127], mumps [128], measles [129], measles vaccine [130], rubella [131], enterovirus [132], human T-lymphotropic virus [133], rotavirus [134]
Zoonotic viruses	RNA	Flavivirus (dengue fever) [135–138], Crimean-Congo hemorrhagic fever virus [139], hantaviruses [140, 141], bunyavirus [142], hepatitis E virus [143], influenza A virus H5N1 subtype [144], SARS coronavirus [145]
Bacterial	*Mycoplasma pneumoniae* [146, 147], *Salmonella typhi* [148], *Staphylococcus aureus* [149, 150], *Klebsiella pneumoniae* [151], *Aeromonas hydrophila* [151], *Fusobacterium* sp. [152], *Chlamydia pneumoniae* [153], *Legionella pneumophila* [152], *Mycobacterium tuberculosis* [154, 155], *Mycobacterium bovis*—weakened form (bacillus Calmette-Guérin) [156, 157], intravesical BCG [158], *Acinetobacter baumannii* [159], *Escherichia coli* [160], *M. leprae* [161], *Abiotrophia defectiva* in endocarditis patient [162]	
Zoonotic bacteria	*Anaplasma phagocytophilum* [163], *Bartonella henselae* [164], *Borrelia burgdorferi* (Lyme disease) [165], *Brucella* sp. [166–168], *Campylobacter* sp. [169], *Capnocytophaga* sp. [170], *Clostridium* sp. [171, 172],*Coxiella burnetii* [173, 174], *Ehrlichia chaffeensis* and *Ehrlichia ewingii* [175–177], *Leptospira* sp. [178, 179], *Listeria monocytogenes* [180], *Mycobacterium avium complex* [181, 182], *Orientia tsutsugamushi* [183], *Rickettsia* spp. [184], *Salmonella* sp. (excluding *S. typhi*) [185]	
Protozoal/zoonotic protozoa	*Leishmania* sp. [186–188], *Toxoplasma gondii* [189, 190], *Babesia* sp. [191], *Plasmodium falciparum* [192], *Plasmodium vivax* [193, 194], *Strongyloides stercoralis* [152]	
Fungal	*Pneumocystis jiroveci* [62], *Candida* sp. [195], *Aspergillus* sp. [62], *Fusarium verticillioides* [62]	
Zoonotic fungi	*Cryptococcus neoformans* [196], *Histoplasma capsulatum* [197–199], *Penicillium marneffei* [23, 200, 201]	

an overwhelming septicemia. It is important nonetheless to detect and remedy any underlying treatable infection in the setting of HLH.

Virus-Associated Hemophagocytic Syndrome

EBV

Epidemiology As previously mentioned, EBV is the most commonly reported trigger of HLH [93], with the highest incidence in East Asia [202]. This could be explained by the more pathogenic strains of EBV in this part of the world [203] and also by the higher prevalence of EBV and EBV-infected T cells in Asians [204]. EBV-associated HLH (EBV-HLH) cases have also been described in the USA and Europe [205]. Most EBV-HLH cases occur in apparently immunocompetent children and adolescents [206]; however, it can also occur in the setting of primary/genetic forms (fHLH) [207], immunodeficiency disorders (e.g., XLP) [208], and secondary forms, including acute infections (e.g., infectious mononucleosis) [209] and lymphoproliferative disorders (e.g., NK cell and T-cell leukemias and lymphomas) [210].

Pathophysiology The mechanism by which EBV induces HLH has not been fully explained. During primary infection, EBV typically infects and replicates in B cells, whereas a function of EBV-specific cytotoxic T cells is the regulation of the infected B cells and the production of memory cells. On rare occasions, EBV may infect T cells and NK cells via CD21. CD21 is expressed on the surface of these cells and induces persistent EBV infection, with monoclonal or oligoclonal proliferation resulting in chronic active EBV infection, lymphoproliferative disorders, and fulminant EBV-HLH [211–213]. Infection of CD8 T cells with EBV results in a cytokine storm with the release of pro-inflammatory and Th1-type cytokines [214], including TNF and IFN-γ, leading to widespread lymphohistiocytic activation [215]. The resultant cytokine storm tends to be more prominent than those observed in non-EBV-HLH [216]. In addition, impaired function of T cells or NK cells is thought to provide a phenotypic presentation of HLH resulting from EBV via any genetic mutation involved in the T-cell and/or NK cell activation pathways [217, 218].

Diagnosis Serologic testing can help differentiate primary EBV infection from a reactivation process, although they have limitations such as delay in positivity and difficulty in result interpretation. Real-time PCR is used to measure the EBV viral load which can help predict prognosis and response to treatment [219]. EBV PCR levels are usually higher than those seen in uncomplicated cases of EBV infectious mononucleosis [220]. Other techniques are available to determine the involvement of T cells or NK cells in helping to confirm the diagnosis. T-cell receptor (TCR) gene rearrangement is detectable in half of the patients with EBV-HLH using Southern blotting and/or PCR analyses. It is hypothesized that the presence and change of TCR gene clonality probably plays a prognostic role for EBV-HLH [90]. Sandberg et al. [221] recently reported that Southern blot analysis could be replaced by BIOMED-2 multiplex PCR in routine testing of T-cell clonality. The EuroClonality (BIOMED-2) consortium developed a uniform reporting system for the description of the results and conclusions of Ig/TCR clonality assays to help improve the general performance level of clonality assessment and interpretation in cases with suspected lymphoproliferations [222]. It was reported that TCR gene clonality with BIOMED-2 multiplex PCR [223] is highly sensitive for detecting T-cell clonality and is useful in predicting response to treatment in EBV-HLH cases [223]. Interestingly, it was found that male patients with EBV-HLH may have mutations in the *SH2D1A* gene which is classically associated with X-linked lymphoproliferative syndrome (XLPS). XLPS is a syndrome of immunodeficiency to EBV virus. Therefore, it is recommended to test for XLPS in male patients with EBV-HLH [224]. It is also recommended to test for other genetic conditions such as fHLH, especially in male patients under

1 year of age, and in those with HLH in a sibling or with consanguineous parents, or when HLH is recurrent or unresponsive to treatment.

Prognosis Of all the viruses associated with HLH, EBV-HLH carries one of the worst prognoses. In a nationwide survey in Japan to identify prognostic factors in children with EBV-HLH, Kogawa et al. [225] found that most of the clinical and laboratory parameters including EBV load, NK cell activity against EBV-infected cells, and the presence of clonality at the onset of disease were not associated with a poor outcome. Nevertheless, Matsuda et al. showed that change of clonality can be a good marker of disease activity in childhood EBV-HLH [223]. It is also reported that hyperbilirubinemia and hyperferritinemia at the time of diagnosis were significantly associated with a poor outcome. Henter et al. also reported that hyperbilirubinemia and hyperferritinemia at diagnosis, and thrombocytopenia and hyperferritinemia 2 weeks after the initiation of treatment, adversely affect the outcome of HLH [226]. Better outcome is speculated to be associated with going into remission within 8 weeks of treatment initiation [225]. Huang et al. reported that hypoalbuminemia is an independent predictor for HLH in childhood EBV-associated disease [227].

Treatment Antiviral therapy with acyclovir, ganciclovir, or cidofovir is generally ineffective as monotherapy in infectious mononucleosis and EBV-HLH [228]. However, aggressive therapy including immunochemotherapy and allogenic stem cell transplantation has radically improved the prognosis. The optimal treatment strategy [229] for EBV-HLH consists of immunosuppressive medications that inhibit overactive T-cell and NK cell responses [i.e., corticosteroids, cyclosporine A, intravenous immunoglobulin (IVIg), antithymocyte globulins, etoposide, and plasma or blood exchange transfusions] [229, 230]. Hematopoietic stem cell transplantation (HSCT) is the last treatment resort for refractory forms of EBV-HLH, and in the case of EBV infection occurring in genetic forms of HLH [231]. Despite the fact that reports have shown that HSCT is effective in treating patients with refractory EBV-HLH [232], it should be compared to immunochemotherapy in a randomized study to provide evidence for which approach is superior and/or safer [233].

In 2007, Balamuth et al. [230] reported that adding rituximab to the HLH-2004 treatment protocol improves its efficacy. Rituximab is a monoclonal antibody against CD20 on the surface of B cells. Because EBV targets B cells in the initial phase of the disease, rituximab's elimination of B cells is thought to inhibit the extent of the infection. In addition, B cells may be a target in EBV-HLH, and rituximab may reduce morbidity and mortality by reducing the circulating B-cell population and the EBV load [234]. Rituximab seems to be most effective in the setting of XLPS patients infected with EBV but is likely less effective when EBV is capable of infecting the T-cell pool. Nonetheless, the addition of rituximab to the treatment repertoire of EBV-HLH provides an opportunity to tailor therapy specific to the patient (personalized medicine approach).

Other Herpes Viruses

Following EBV, cytomegalovirus (CMV) and human herpes virus (HHV) 8 are the next most common of the herpesviruses to be associated with HLH. CMV infection has been associated with HLH in otherwise healthy patients [96, 235], premature infants [97], patients with inflammatory bowel disease [236, 237], rheumatological diseases [238, 239], cancer [240], and in transplant recipients [241, 242]. In a series of 171 patients undergoing HSCT, HLH was observed in 7 (4%) of them and was triggered by CMV in 3 cases [243]. In a Japanese registry with CMV-HLH diagnosed at less than a year of age (1986–2002), four of the five infants died, suggesting that younger age may be associated with a worse prognosis [244]. The use of specific anti-CMV therapy, such as CMV hyperimmune globulin, foscarnet, or ganciclovir, has been associated with recovery in selected cases [96, 236–238, 242].

Human Herpes Virus 8

HHV-8 has been associated with HLH, mostly in the setting of Kaposi sarcoma [245], multicentric Castleman disease [246], or lymphoproliferative disorder [247], as well as in immunocompromised hosts (HIV) [99], transplant recipients [248], and, rarely, in immunocompetent hosts [100, 101]. In a prospective cohort of 44 patients with Castleman disease and human immunodeficiency virus (HIV), 4 (9%) had HLH [246]. Intriguingly, in this series, the levels of IL-8 and IFN-γ were increased, though the cytokine levels of many known inflammatory markers were not. In this study, all patients recovered after treatment with splenectomy, etoposide, and rituximab [249]. Ganciclovir and foscarnet have also been associated with recovery in some HHV8-HPS cases. Finally, all other herpes viruses [102–104, 250] with the exception of HHV-7 have been associated with HLH.

Neonatal Infection-Associated HLH

Due to the lack of disease awareness among many physicians, HLH presenting within the first 4 weeks of life is rarely recognized. It could either pass undiagnosed or be diagnosed late in the course, or even at autopsy. Neonatal HLH differs from HLH in older children in etiology, manifestations, and laboratory findings. In a nationwide survey in Japan published in 2009, 20 neonates were diagnosed with HLH within 4 weeks after birth; 6 (30%) of them were diagnosed with fHLH, and 6 (30%) were diagnosed with herpes simplex virus-associated HLH (HSV-HLH) [251]. The overall survival rate of these 20 patients was 28.6% for fHLH and severe combined immunodeficiency (SCID)-HLH, and 33.3% for HSV-HLH, despite acyclovir treatment. Although uncommon in HLH of older children, enterovirus (echovirus and coxsackievirus) and HSV have been associated with fatal or fulminant neonatal HLH [252, 253]. This mandates early treatment with high-dose acyclovir in suspected cases without awaiting viral studies results.

HIV

HLH can be associated with HIV [117] infection [the etiology of acquired immunodeficiency syndrome (AIDS)] in different settings. HLH can occur either with HIV alone or with a variety of underlying associated disorders. HLH has been reported in acute or late stages of HIV infection, in the setting of immune reconstitution inflammatory syndromes (IRIS), and in association with HIV-associated malignancies or infections (both opportunistic and non-opportunistic) [254]. HLH has even been reported as the initial presentation of HIV infection [118], which suggests a direct role for HIV in triggering HLH [195].

Due to the fact that both HIV and HLH share many similar clinical and biological findings, it is likely that this association is also underdiagnosed. In one study, hemophagocytosis was observed in 20% of 56 autopsy cases of HIV-positive patients [255]. Around 10% of bone marrow biopsies in HIV patients before highly active antiretroviral therapy (HAART) initiation revealed hemophagocytosis [256]. In adult cases with acute HIV infection, HLH was associated with low CD4 T-cell counts (<200 cells/μL) in almost two-thirds of the cases. In addition, a lower CD4 T-cell count was associated with a worse prognosis [257].

Influenza

The association of HLH with influenza has been described with seasonal [122, 258–262], avian [263, 264], and swine (non-pandemic) influenza [265]. It has also been associated with both immunocompromised [258–261] and otherwise healthy children [122, 266]. In a prospective pediatric study, which included 32 children hospitalized with seasonal influenza, one case had a fatal outcome [262]. Interestingly, patients with severe H5N1 avian influenza have clinical pictures and laboratory findings similar to HLH; these consist mainly of encephalitis [267], organ dysfunction with hemophagocytosis [268], bone marrow suppression [268, 269], and cytokine storm [270, 271]. The most common characteristic pathological picture seen on autopsy and biopsy in such cases is hemophagocytosis [264, 271, 272].

Clinical studies have found that mutations in some viral genes (NS1, PB2, HA, and NA) are significantly related to cytokine release, and it has been shown that recombinant hemagglutinin (H5) from H5N1 virus may suppress perforin expression and reduce the cytotoxicity of CD8 T cells, including their ability to kill H5-bearing cells leading to marked lymphoproliferation and IFN-γ hyperproduction with macrophage overactivation [273]. Considering the high mortality caused by H5N1-HLH, the resistance to many antivirals by H5N1, and the similarity between HLH and severe flu infections have led some to suggest the use of a modified HLH-94 protocol [274] with a shorter course of etoposide and dexamethasone in such cases. However, in a randomized study from Vietnam, all patients with H5N1-HLH died despite receiving corticosteroids [275].

Recently, a study was done on 16 cases of fatal influenza A (H1N1) infection who met 44 and 81% of modified HLH-2004 and MAS criteria, respectively. Five subjects (36%) carried one of three different heterozygous *LYST* mutations, two of whom also possessed the relatively common p.A91V *PRF1* mutation, which was shown to mildly decrease NK cell cytolytic function. Several patients also carried rare variants in other genes previously observed in patients with MAS. The high percentage of HLH gene mutations suggests they are risk factors for mortality among individuals with influenza A (H1N1) infection [276].

Parvovirus

HLH has been reported in approximately 30 cases of parvovirus B19 infection; most of them had hereditary spherocytosis as the underlying disease, and less than 50% were children [106, 109, 110, 277, 278]. Of these patients, 22 survived, of whom 16 did not receive any treatment. This suggests a better prognosis of parvovirus-HLH than that with other viral infections.

Hepatitis Viruses

Fulminant viral hepatitis may mimic and even cause HLH. Hepatitis A virus (HAV) is more frequently associated with HLH than other hepatotropic viruses, including HBV and HCV. Fifteen cases (including children) have been described in the literature, mainly in Asia; three of these patients also had a concurrent rheumatological disease (sJIA or the related adult onset Still disease), and two also had hepatitis C. Four patients survived without specific treatment. The others received corticosteroids with or without IVIg. Overall, 11 of the 15 had a good outcome [112, 113, 279].

Enterovirus

Twelve cases of pediatric enterovirus-related HLH have been described. Four patients had an underlying disease (Hodgkin and non-Hodgkin lymphoma, acute lymphoblastic leukemia, JIA) and had a higher mortality rate (75%). Ten patients received IVIg (six in combination with corticosteroids), but only seven patients survived [132]. Other viruses associated have been associated with HLH (Table 14.4), for most of which varying courses of corticosteroids and IVIg have been used. Interestingly, HLH may contribute to the high mortality rate associated with certain hemorrhagic fever viruses, such as those causing Dengue fever and Ebola.

Bacteria-Associated Hemophagocytic Syndrome

Of the bacterial pathogens, intracellular organisms have most commonly been the precipitating bacterial agents of HLH. The pathophysiology is probably related to the host lymphocytes and monocytes producing high levels of activating cytokines. Defective NK cell and cytotoxic T-cell function is also hypothesized to play a role in the pathophysiology [2].

HLH has been reported with disseminated *Mycobacterium tuberculosis* (TB) infection. It can occur in otherwise healthy patients [280], in end-stage renal disease patients receiving hemodialysis [281], in those who had undergone renal transplantation [164], or who had malignancy [282], HIV/AIDS [283], or sarcoidosis [284]. In a review of 36 cases by Brastianos et al., 83% of cases had evidence of extrapulmonary tuberculosis. The mortality rate was approximately 50% which portrays the poor outcome of TB-HLH, although antituberculous and immunomodulatory therapy (consisting of high-dose corticosteroids, IVIg, antithymocyte globulin, cyclosporine A, epipodophyllotoxin, or plasma exchange) may lead to better outcomes [155]. Early diagnosis and timely administration of antituberculous treatment are crucial in these patients. Moreover, one reported case of HLH occurred after childhood vaccination with the bacillus Calmette-Guérin [157].

HLH has also been described in association with brucellosis, with *Brucella melitensis* being the most frequently isolated species [168]. Leptospirosis has been reported with HLH and has required treatment with corticosteroids, IVIg, or etoposide, in addition to antibiotic treatment [179]. Reports have also related *Rickettsia* and *Ehrlichia* to HLH, and the prognosis seems to be influenced by the specific *Rickettsia* species, patient's immunologic status, and delay in antibiotic therapy or corticosteroid therapy [184]. Also, MAS following urinary tract infection with *Acinetobacter baumannii* was reported for the first time in a previously healthy 3-year-old child; recovery occurred without any cytotoxic treatment or immunotherapy, using only multiple doses of GCSF and red blood cell/platelet transfusions [159]. Just like viruses, a large array of additional bacterial infections has been associated with HLH (Table 14.4), but a propensity for intracellular invasion is a common theme to many of these triggers.

Parasitic and Fungal Infection-Associated Hemophagocytic Syndrome

Leishmania infection has been associated with HLH (particularly *Leishmania donovani* and *Leishmania infantum*), but considering that it presents with organomegaly and pancytopenia, it can also just mimic the syndrome of HLH. This is of importance in non-endemic areas, where visceral leishmaniasis is unlikely considered as a differential diagnosis, and repeated bone marrow smears are often required to identify Leishmania species by means of PCR with species-specific probes [285]. While specific treatment with amphotericin B is usually sufficient to control HLH, fatal outcomes have been seen with undiagnosed Leishmania cases treated as HLH [188]. History of travel to endemic areas is also of utmost importance for suspecting HLH secondary to certain parasitic infections such as malaria, toxoplasma, babesia, and strongyloides.

Yeast infections (Candida sp., Cryptococcus sp., and Pneumocystis sp.) and molds (Histoplasma sp., Aspergillus sp., and Fusarium sp.) have been associated with HLH, most commonly during HIV infection, malignancy, prolonged corticosteroid administration, and transplantation [196, 286, 287]. Disseminated *Penicillium marneffei* infection is common among HIV-infected patients in Southeast Asia. The first case of penicilliosis-HLH was reported in a Thai HIV-infected child in 2001, with complete recovery after antifungal and IVIg therapy [200].

Treatment Options for MAS/HLH

In addition to treating any underlying infection, treatment designed to dampen the cytokine storm associated with MAS/HLH is critical for improving survival (Table 14.5). Some researchers reported the success of high-dose corticosteroids alone [25, 288] in treating sJIA-MAS. While the fundamental role of corticosteroids in the therapy of this disease is not doubted [25, 69, 70], current regimens usually add more aggressive treatment to corticosteroids including cyclophosphamide [289], which has not gained wide use in this condition; cyclosporine A (CsA), which is currently the most commonly added medicine to corticosteroids [290, 291]; and etoposide-based regimens, such as HLH-94 and HLH-2004 [11], which have their not insignificant mortality rates during the pre- and post-bone marrow transplant periods [292]. Of the biologics, IVIg has been used, particularly for infection-associated sHLH, but IVIg must be given early in disease to be effective [293]. Furthermore, IVIg has been shown to be ineffective in some reports [17]. Antithymocyte

Table 14.5 Treatment options for HLH

Antimicrobials	Conventional treatment	Biological therapies	Future targets
Antivirals Antibiotics Antimycotics Amphotericin B	Corticosteroids Cyclosporine-A HSCT Etoposide Cyclophosphamide Methotrexate *Others:* Plasmapheresis	*Intravenous immunoglobulins* *Cytokine-targeting drugs:* • IL-1 blockade Anakinra Rilonacept Canakinumab • IL-6 blockade Tocilizumab • TNF-α blockade Etanercept Infliximab Adalimumab • IFN-γ blockade *Anti-CD20:* • Rituximab *T-cell-targeting drugs:* • Antithymocyte globulins • Alemtuzumab (anti-CD52) • Daclizumab (anti-CD25)	JAK inhibition TLR blockade Administration of IL-10 or IL-18BP PPAR-γ or PD-1 agonists Targeting DCs or Ag presentation Blocking alarmins (HMGB1, IL-33, etc.)

globulin has been used successfully in two patients with probable MAS [294], but it carries a significant risk of serious infections and mortality.

Recently, newer more targeted biologic therapies have provided a more targeted and effective option in treating sJIA-MAS. While there was some initial excitement about TNF blockers with reports on their success in treating many cases of MAS including several children with sJIA [295–303], reports of TNF inhibitors triggering MAS diminished enthusiasm for this therapy [304–310]. Knowing that cause and effect is certainly difficult to prove in these situations, the fact that MAS did develop in the setting of TNF inhibition is concerning [311, 312]. This has led to focusing on therapy directed at two other pro-inflammatory cytokines, IL-1 and IL-6.

The IL-1 receptor antagonist anakinra was shown to be highly effective for sJIA [313, 314]. MAS and sJIA flare share many clinical and laboratory features. Moreover in addition to the 10% risk of developing overt MAS as part of sJIA, another 30–40% of sJIA patients may have occult or subclinical MAS during flare that can eventually lead to overt MAS [68, 83]. This suggested that anakinra would also be a valuable treatment for sJIA-MAS. There are several reports of dramatically successful use of anakinra in cases of sJIA-MAS after failing to respond to corticosteroids and CsA [313, 315–317].

Anakinra is regarded as a generally safe drug because it is a recombinant human protein with a short half-life (approximately 4 h) [318] and a wide therapeutic window (1–48 mg/kg/day) [35, 317]. However, cases of hepatitis attributed to anakinra in children with sJIA have been reported [319]. Moreover, though cause and effect are difficult to establish, there has been a suggestion that anakinra triggered MAS in two children with sJIA [320, 321]. In a large case series of 46 sJIA patients treated with anakinra at disease onset, anakinra was a potential MAS trigger in five children at doses of 1–2 mg/kg/day [313]. However, dose escalation of anakinra often seemed to help control MAS, and none of the children had to permanently stop the anakinra [313]. More research is needed to define the role of anakinra in sJIA-MAS and other forms of sHLH.

IL-6 blockade, via an anti-IL-6 receptor monoclonal antibody (tocilizumab), has also proven successful in treating sJIA [322]. However, a case report of MAS attributed to IL-6 blockade [323] underscores the need for further studies to define its role in the treatment of sJIA-MAS. IL-6 blockade, however, has been successfully used in treating cytokine storm syndrome associated with chimeric antigen receptor

(CAR) T-cell-directed therapy against resistant leukemia [324]. Other biologic therapies are being explored. Co-stimulatory blockade with cytotoxic T-lymphocyte-associated protein 4-immunoglobulin (CTLA-4-Ig) has been anecdotally beneficial in children with severe sJIA [317], but its role in treating MAS is unknown. Nevertheless, there is building evidence that biologic therapies, particularly IL-1 inhibitors, are a welcome addition to corticosteroids and CsA in treating MAS associated with sJIA [17]. Finally, rituximab has recently been reported to lead to remission in a sizable percentage of children with refractory sJIA [325], in addition to its effectiveness in treating EBV-HLH [230, 326].

HSCT

The first report of successful HSCT in HLH was reported in 1986 [327]. HSCT tends to be more frequently used in familial cases of HLH, but it is used in secondary cases as well. While several studies have shown that HSCT is the best option for permanent disease control or cure [328–332], the overall transplant morbidity and mortality is still high (~45%) and it is not uncommon for patients to develop recurrence of HLH before a suitable donor is identified. Moreover, autologous and allogeneic HSCT have been reported to induce HLH in transplanted patients, probably due to the increased risk of infection imposed by the immunosuppressive conditioning regimen with an estimated risk of 4% in a recent cohort [333]. This risk appeared to be reduced in etoposide-containing conditioning regimens [333]. The current era of biologic therapies has reduced the need for HSCT.

In the future, autologous HSCT combined with gene therapy to correct the genetic defects might be applicable. Carmo et al. have shown that transfer of a functional perforin gene (Prf1) into autologous hematopoietic stem cells from perforin-deficient mice restored perforin expression, partially repaired the cytotoxic defect, and attenuated HLH symptoms after viral challenge, provided that at least 30% engraftment was attained [334]. Similarly, Rivat et al. showed that in a mouse model of XLP, gene transfer also restored SAP expression and normalized cytotoxic function [335].

IFN-γ Blockade

IFN-γ has been shown to play a pivotal role in several HLH models. Its neutralization has substantially improved survival in HLH animal models [336, 337] and an MAS model using IL-6 transgenic mice [338]. Levels of both IFN-γ and IFN-γ -induced chemokines such as CXCL10 and CXCL9 are elevated in children with HLH [339]. Moreover, sJIA-MAS is commonly triggered by viral infections which are known to activate IFN-γ-associated pathways. Furthermore, numerous IFN-γ-producing T cells were found in close proximity to activated hemophagocytic histiocytes in a study of inflammatory infiltrates in tissues affected by MAS [340], and children with MAS show increased levels of neopterin, which is known to be released by interferon-stimulated macrophages [26]. A longitudinal study of the cytokine changes in patients with sJIA showed that levels of IFN-γ and IFN-γ-induced chemokines (particularly, CXCL9) markedly increased with the beginning of clinical MAS and returned to normal with its resolution. Furthermore, they were strongly correlated with many laboratory features associated with MAS [338]. These findings highlighted IFN-γ as an appealing targeted and potentially less toxic therapeutic option in HLH, and a clinical trial evaluating NI-0501, which is an anti-IFN-γ monoclonal antibody that binds to and neutralizes human IFN-γ, is underway [341]. Recently, a report on this trial showed promising results [18].

However, some recent studies question the potential of IFN-γ blocking therapy in MAS. First, Tesi et al. reported two cases of HLH in children with novel IFN-γ receptor mutations associated with IFN-γ deficiency, findings which highlight the significance of IFN-γ-independent mechanisms in the immune pathology of HLH and warrant that other novel therapies, beside anti-IFN-γ therapy, be investigated [342]. Additionally, sJIA patients were found to have normal levels of IFN-γ independent of disease activity [343], which suggests that this cytokine does not always play an essential role in disease pathogenesis.

Janus Kinase Inhibition

Because targeting individual cytokines might be insufficient during severe hypercytokinemia, cytokine signaling pathways can be targeted to avoid an imbalance in the cytokine network. Janus kinases control the signaling of many cytokines, notably IFN-γ, IL-2, and IL-6. Thus, inhibition of Janus kinases via ruxolitinib for example may serve this purpose. Das et al. reported that in rodent models of primary and secondary HLH, treatment with the JAK1/2 inhibitor ruxolitinib significantly lessened the clinical and laboratory manifestations, including weight loss, organomegaly, anemia, thrombocytopenia, hypercytokinemia, and tissue inflammation. Importantly, ruxolitinib treatment also significantly improved survival in this model [344]. Similarly, Maschalidi et al. reported that JAK1/2 inhibition in $Prf1^{-/-}$ and $Rab27a^{-/-}$ mice with full-blown HLH syndrome has led to recovery in both models [345].

Other Targets

Peroxisome proliferator-activated receptor-γ agonists have also been presented as potential agents. They interfere with the activation of the NFκB pathway and exert both a broad anti-inflammatory effect and antiviral capacities [346, 347]. Based on research in HLH animal models, other targets for future therapy have been proposed. These include the induction of T-cell exhaustion through the stimulation of inhibitory receptors like programmed cell death 1 (PDCD1/PD-1), restoring cytokine balances by the anti-inflammatory IL-10 or IL-18BP, halting chronic TLR activation by TLR antagonists or blocking TLR signaling pathways, and targeting dendritic cells as the main drivers of ongoing antigen stimulation or suppressing antigen presentation itself [348, 349].

Over the past few years, more has been revealed about the role of IL-18 in the pathogenesis of sJIA and MAS. It has been shown that patients with sJIA have significantly higher levels of IL-18 [85–87] as opposed to other rheumatic diseases such as SLE or rheumatoid arthritis [350, 351]. sJIA patients with high levels of IL-18 are more likely to develop systemic features of the disease and are more prone to develop MAS [85]. Interestingly, the development of MAS in these patients is associated with a further rise in IL-18 levels [85]. IL-18 has also been found to correlate with ferritin in adult onset Still disease [86]. Therefore, IL-18 has been suggested as a promising biomarker for MAS. Another interesting field of growing research is in the role of IL-18-binding protein (IL-18BP) which is a naturally occurring protein that counter-regulates the activity of IL-18. Imbalance between IL-18 and IL-18BP, leading to higher levels of unbound IL-18, has been found in patients with increased disease severity [33, 86, 352]. The administration of synthetic IL-18BP in perforin-deficient mice infected with murine CMV ameliorated liver damage but has not shown an effect on the pro-inflammatory cytokine levels or on the overall survival [353]. Based on these findings, further work is needed to demonstrate the role of IL-18 and IL-18BP in MAS. Along these lines, IL-18BP was shown to be beneficial in treating refractory MAS in a child with an NLRC4 mutation [354].

Recently, neutralizing antibodies and antagonists targeting the alarmin HMGB1 (high mobility group box 1) were proposed as potential therapeutic options, aiming to reduce the immunostimulatory load of necrosis- and pyroptosis-derived danger signals. Models of systemic sterile and infectious inflammation have demonstrated the efficacy of this strategy [355]. Moreover, blocking the alarmin IL-33, via its receptor ST2/IL-1RL1, is also a potential therapy [356] [43]. Overall, the future is looking brighter for a variety of potential therapeutics to treat HLH/MAS in a patient-specific fashion.

References

1. Canna SW, Behrens EM. Making sense of the cytokine storm: a conceptual framework for understanding, diagnosing, and treating hemophagocytic syndromes. Pediatr Clin N Am. 2012;59(2):329–44.
2. Janka GE. Familial and acquired hemophagocytic lymphohistiocytosis. Annu Rev Med. 2012;63:233–46.
3. Feldmann J, Callebaut I, Raposo G, Certain S, Bacq D, Dumont C, et al. Munc13-4 is essential for cytolytic granules fusion and is mutated in a form of familial hemophagocytic lymphohistiocytosis (FHL3). Cell. 2003;115(4):461–73.

4. Zur Stadt U, Rohr J, Seifert W, Koch F, Grieve S, Pagel J, et al. Familial hemophagocytic lymphohistiocytosis type 5 (FHL-5) is caused by mutations in Munc18-2 and impaired binding to syntaxin 11. Am J Hum Genet. 2009;85(4):482–92.
5. zur Stadt U, Schmidt S, Kasper B, Beutel K, Diler AS, Henter J-I, et al. Linkage of familial hemophagocytic lymphohistiocytosis (FHL) type-4 to chromosome 6q24 and identification of mutations in syntaxin 11. Hum Mol Genet. 2005;14(6):827–34.
6. Stepp SE, Dufourcq-Lagelouse R, Le Deist F, Bhawan S, Certain S, Mathew PA, et al. Perforin gene defects in familial hemophagocytic lymphohistiocytosis. Science. 1999;286(5446):1957–9.
7. Emmenegger U, Schaer D, Larroche C, Neftel K. Haemophagocytic syndromes in adults: current concepts and challenges ahead. Swiss Med Wkly. 2005;135(21–22):299–314.
8. Arico M, Imashuku S, Clementi R, Hibi S, Teramura T, Danesino C, et al. Hemophagocytic lymphohistiocytosis due to germline mutations in SH2D1A, the X-linked lymphoproliferative disease gene. Blood. 2001;97(4):1131–3.
9. Marsh RA, Satake N, Biroschak J, Jacobs T, Johnson J, Jordan MB, et al. STX11 mutations and clinical phenotypes of familial hemophagocytic lymphohistiocytosis in North America. Pediatr Blood Cancer. 2010;55(1):134–40.
10. Rigaud S, Fondaneche MC, Lambert N, Pasquier B, Mateo V, Soulas P, et al. XIAP deficiency in humans causes an X-linked lymphoproliferative syndrome. Nature. 2006;444(7115):110–4.
11. Henter JI, Horne A, Arico M, Egeler RM, Filipovich AH, Imashuku S, et al. HLH-2004: diagnostic and therapeutic guidelines for hemophagocytic lymphohistiocytosis. Pediatr Blood Cancer. 2007;48(2):124–31.
12. Allen M, De Fusco C, Legrand F, Clementi R, Conter V, Danesino C, et al. Familial hemophagocytic lymphohistiocytosis: how late can the onset be? Haematologica. 2001;86(5):499–503.
13. Ueda I, Kurokawa Y, Koike K, Ito S, Sakata A, Matsumora T, et al. Late-onset cases of familial hemophagocytic lymphohistiocytosis with missense perforin gene mutations. Am J Hematol. 2007;82(6):427–32.
14. Henter JI, Ehrnst A, Andersson J, Elinder G. Familial hemophagocytic lymphohistiocytosis and viral infections. Acta Paediatr. 1993;82(4):369–72.
15. Henter JI, Elinder G, Lubeck PO, Ost A. Myelodysplastic syndrome following epipodophyllotoxin therapy in familial hemophagocytic lymphohistiocytosis. Pediatr Hematol Oncol. 1993;10(2):163–8.
16. Imashuku S. Etoposide-related secondary acute myeloid leukemia (t-AML) in hemophagocytic lymphohistiocytosis. Pediatr Blood Cancer. 2007;48(2):121–3.
17. Miettunen PM, Narendran A, Jayanthan A, Behrens EM, Cron RQ. Successful treatment of severe paediatric rheumatic disease-associated macrophage activation syndrome with interleukin-1 inhibition following conventional immunosuppressive therapy: case series with 12 patients. Rheumatology. 2011;50(2):417–9.
18. Jordan M, Locatelli F, Allen C, De Benedetti F, Grom AA, Ballabio M, et al. editors. A novel targeted approach to the treatment of hemophagocytic lymphohistiocytosis (HLH) with an anti-interferon gamma (IFN gamma) monoclonal antibody (mAb), NI-0501: first results from a pilot phase 2 study in children with primary HLH. Blood; 2015. AMER SOC HEMATOLOGY 2021 L ST NW, SUITE 900, WASHINGTON, DC 20036 USA.
19. Zhang K, Filipovich AH, Johnson J, Marsh RA, Villanueva J. In: Adam MP, Ardinger HH, Pagon RA, Wallace SE, Bean LJH, Stephens K, et al. editors. Hemophagocytic Lymphohistiocytosis, familial. Seattle: GeneReviews((R)); 1993.
20. Koh KN, Im HJ, Chung NG, Cho B, Kang HJ, Shin HY, et al. Clinical features, genetics, and outcome of pediatric patients with hemophagocytic lymphohistiocytosis in Korea: report of a nationwide survey from Korea histiocytosis working party. Eur J Haematol. 2015;94(1):51–9.
21. Lehmberg K, Sprekels B, Nichols KE, Woessmann W, Muller I, Suttorp M, et al. Malignancy-associated haemophagocytic lymphohistiocytosis in children and adolescents. Br J Haematol. 2015;170(4):539–49.
22. Celkan T, Berrak S, Kazanci E, Özyürek E, Ünal S, Uçar C, et al. Malignancy-associated hemophagocytic lymphohistiocytosis in pediatric cases: a multicenter study from Turkey. Turk J Pediatr. 2009;51(3):207.
23. Veerakul G, Sanpakit K, Tanphaichitr VS, Mahasandana C, Jirarattanasopa N. Secondary hemophagocytic lymphohistiocytosis in children: an analysis of etiology and outcome. J Med Assoc Thailand. 2002;85:S530–41.
24. Grom AA, Mellins ED. Macrophage activation syndrome: advances towards understanding pathogenesis. Curr Opin Rheumatol. 2010;22(5):561.
25. Ravelli A, Grom AA, Behrens EM, Cron RQ. Macrophage activation syndrome as part of systemic juvenile idiopathic arthritis: diagnosis, genetics, pathophysiology and treatment. Genes Immun. 2012;13(4):289–98.
26. Put K, Avau A, Brisse E, Mitera T, Put S, Proost P, et al. Cytokines in systemic juvenile idiopathic arthritis and haemophagocytic lymphohistiocytosis: tipping the balance between interleukin-18 and interferon-γ. Rheumatology. 2015;54(8):1507–17.
27. Akashi K, Hayashi S, Gondo H, Mizuno S, Harada M, Tamura K, et al. Involvement of interferon-γ and macrophage colony-stimulating factor in pathogenesis of haemophagocytic lymphohistiocytosis in adults. Br J Haematol. 1994;87(2):243–50.
28. Kuriyama T, Takenaka K, Kohno K, Yamauchi T, Daitoku S, Yoshimoto G, et al. Engulfment

of hematopoietic stem cells caused by down-regulation of CD47 is critical in the pathogenesis of hemophagocytic lymphohistiocytosis. Blood. 2012;120(19):4058–67.
29. Nold-Petry CA, Lehrnbecher T, Jarisch A, Schwabe D, Pfeilschifter JM, Muhl H, et al. Failure of interferon γ to induce the anti-inflammatory interleukin 18 binding protein in familial hemophagocytosis. PLoS One. 2010;5(1):e8663.
30. Bracaglia C, Marafon DP, Caiello I, de Graaf K, Guilhot F, Ferlin W, et al. High levels of interferon-gamma (IFNγ) in macrophage activation syndrome (MAS) and CXCL9 levels as a biomarker for IFNγ production in MAS. Pediatr Rheumatol. 2015;13(1):1.
31. Tamura K, Kanazawa T, Tsukada S, Kobayashi T, Kawamura M, Morikawa A. Increased serum monocyte chemoattractant protein-1, macrophage inflammatory protein-1β, and interleukin-8 concentrations in hemophagocytic lymphohistiocytosis. Pediatr Blood Cancer. 2008;51(5):662–8.
32. Teruya-Feldstein J, Setsuda J, Yao X, Kingma DW, Straus S, Tosato G, et al. MIP-1alpha expression in tissues from patients with hemophagocytic syndrome. Lab Investig. 1999;79(12):1583–90.
33. Mazodier K, Marin V, Novick D, Farnarier C, Robitail S, Schleinitz N, et al. Severe imbalance of IL-18/IL-18BP in patients with secondary hemophagocytic syndrome. Blood. 2005;106(10):3483–9.
34. Osugi Y, Hara J, Tagawa S, Takai K, Hosoi G, Matsuda Y, et al. Cytokine production regulating Th1 and Th2 cytokines in hemophagocytic lymphohistiocytosis. Blood. 1997;89(11):4100–3.
35. Fisher CJ, Dhainaut J-FA, Opal SM, Pribble JP, Balk RA, Slotman GJ, et al. Recombinant human interleukin 1 receptor antagonist in the treatment of patients with sepsis syndrome: results from a randomized, double-blind, placebo-controlled trial. JAMA. 1994;271(23):1836–43.
36. Shakoory B, Carcillo JA, Chatham WW, Amdur RL, Zhao H, Dinarello CA, et al. Interleukin-1 receptor blockade is associated with reduced mortality in sepsis patients with features of macrophage activation syndrome: reanalysis of a prior phase III trial. Crit Care Med. 2016;44(2):275–81.
37. Opal SM, Fisher CJ Jr, Dhainaut JF, Vincent JL, Brase R, Lowry SF, et al. Confirmatory interleukin-1 receptor antagonist trial in severe sepsis: a phase III, randomized, double-blind, placebo-controlled, multicenter trial. The Interleukin-1 Receptor Antagonist Sepsis Investigator Group. Crit Care Med. 1997;25(7):1115–24.
38. Créput C, Galicier L, Buyse S, Azoulay E. Understanding organ dysfunction in hemophagocytic lymphohistiocytosis. Intensive Care Med. 2008;34(7):1177–87.
39. Henter J, Elinder G, Soder O, Hansson M, Andersson B, Andersson U. Hypercytokinemia in familial hemophagocytic lymphohistiocytosis. Blood. 1991;78(11):2918–22.
40. Lachmann HJ, Quartier P, So A, Hawkins PN. The emerging role of interleukin-1β in autoinflammatory diseases. Arthritis Rheum. 2011;63(2):314–24.
41. Sieni E, Cetica V, Mastrodicasa E, Pende D, Moretta L, Griffiths G, et al. Familial hemophagocytic lymphohistiocytosis: a model for understanding the human machinery of cellular cytotoxicity. Cell Mol Life Sci. 2012;69(1):29–40.
42. Avau A, Put K, Wouters CH, Matthys P. Cytokine balance and cytokine-driven natural killer cell dysfunction in systemic juvenile idiopathic arthritis. Cytokine Growth Factor Rev. 2015;26(1):35–45.
43. Brisse E, Matthys P, Wouters CH. Understanding the spectrum of haemophagocytic lymphohistiocytosis: update on diagnostic challenges and therapeutic options. Br J Haematol. 2016;174(2):175–87.
44. De Kerguenec C, Hillaire S, Molinié V, Gardin C, Degott C, Erlinger S, et al. Hepatic manifestations of hemophagocytic syndrome: a study of 30 cases. Am J Gastroenterol. 2001;96(3):852–7.
45. Dinarello C, Novick D, Kim S, Kaplanski G. Interleukin-18 and IL-18 binding protein. Front Immunol. 2013;4:289.
46. Moore KW, de Waal Malefyt R, Coffman RL, O'Garra A. Interleukin-10 and the interleukin-10 receptor. Annu Rev Immunol. 2001;19(1):683–765.
47. Janka GE. Familial and acquired hemophagocytic lymphohistiocytosis. Eur J Pediatr. 2007;166(2):95–109.
48. Jenkins MR, Rudd-Schmidt JA, Lopez JA, Ramsbottom KM, Mannering SI, Andrews DM, et al. Failed CTL/NK cell killing and cytokine hypersecretion are directly linked through prolonged synapse time. J Exp Med. 2015;212(3):307–17.
49. Janka G. Hemophagocytic lymphohistiocytosis: when the immune system runs amok. Klin Padiatr. 2009;221(05):278–85.
50. Grom AA. Natural killer cell dysfunction: a common pathway in systemic-onset juvenile rheumatoid arthritis, macrophage activation syndrome, and hemophagocytic lymphohistiocytosis? Arthritis Rheum. 2004;50(3):689–98.
51. Saltzman RW, Monaco-Shawver L, Zhang K, Sullivan KE, Filipovich AH, Orange JS. Novel mutation in syntaxin-binding protein 2 (STXBP2) prevents IL-2-induced natural killer cell cytotoxicity. J Allergy Clin Immunol. 2012;129(6):1666.
52. Spessott WA, Sanmillan ML, McCormick ME, Patel N, Villanueva J, Zhang K, et al. Hemophagocytic lymphohistiocytosis caused by dominant-negative mutations in STXBP2 that inhibit SNARE-mediated membrane fusion. Blood. 2015;125(10):1566–77.
53. Zhang M, Behrens EM, Atkinson TP, Shakoory B, Grom AA, Cron RQ. Genetic defects in cytolysis in macrophage activation syndrome. Curr Rheumatol Rep. 2014;16(9):1–8.
54. Zhang X-Y, Ye X-W, Feng D-X, Han J, Li D, Zhang C. Hemophagocytic lymphohistiocytosis induced by severe pandemic influenza A (H1N1)

2009 virus infection: a case report. Case Rep Med. 2011;2011:1–3.
55. Nagafuji K, Nonami A, Kumano T, Kikushige Y, Yoshimoto G, Takenaka K, et al. Perforin gene mutations in adult-onset hemophagocytic lymphohistiocytosis. Haematologica. 2007;92(7):978–81.
56. Lichtenheld MG, Olsen KJ, Lu P, Lowrey DM, Hameed A, Hengartner H, et al. Structure and function of human perforin. Nature. 1988;335(6189):448–51.
57. Behrens EM, Canna SW, Slade K, Rao S, Kreiger PA, Paessler M, et al. Repeated TLR9 stimulation results in macrophage activation syndrome–like disease in mice. J Clin Investig. 2011;121(6):2264–77.
58. Sullivan KE, Delaat CA, Douglas SD, Filipovich AH. Defective natural killer cell function in patients with hemophagocytic lymphohistiocytosis and in first degree relatives. Pediatr Res. 1998;44(4):465–8.
59. Villanueva J, Lee S, Giannini EH, Graham TB, Passo MH, Filipovich A, et al. Natural killer cell dysfunction is a distinguishing feature of systemic onset juvenile rheumatoid arthritis and macrophage activation syndrome. Arthritis Res Ther. 2004;7(1):1.
60. Caiello I, Minnone G, Holzinger D, Vogl T, Prencipe G, Manzo A, et al. IL-6 amplifies TLR mediated cytokine and chemokine production: implications for the pathogenesis of rheumatic inflammatory diseases. PLoS One. 2014;9(10):e107886.
61. Maude SL, Frey N, Shaw PA, Aplenc R, Barrett DM, Bunin NJ, et al. Chimeric antigen receptor T cells for sustained remissions in leukemia. N Engl J Med. 2014;371(16):1507–17.
62. Zhang L, Zhou J, Sokol L. Hereditary and acquired hemophagocytic lymphohistiocytosis. Cancer Control. 2014;21(4):301–12.
63. Schulert GS, Grom AA. Macrophage activation syndrome and cytokine-directed therapies. Best Pract Res Clin Rheumatol. 2014;28(2):277–92.
64. Weaver LK, Behrens EM. Hyperinflammation, rather than hemophagocytosis, is the common link between macrophage activation syndrome and hemophagocytic lymphohistiocytosis. Curr Opin Rheumatol. 2014;26(5):562.
65. Minoia F, Davì S, Horne A, Demirkaya E, Bovis F, Li C, et al. Clinical features, treatment, and outcome of macrophage activation syndrome complicating systemic juvenile idiopathic arthritis: a multinational, multicenter study of 362 patients. Arthritis Rheumatol. 2014;66(11):3160–9.
66. Tsuda H, Shirono K. Serum lipids in adult patients with hemophagocytic syndrome. Am J Hematol. 1996;53(4):285.
67. Prendki V, Stirnemann J, Lemoine M, Lohez M, Aras N, Ganne-Carrié N, et al. Prevalence and clinical significance of Küpffer cell hyperplasia with hemophagocytosis in liver biopsies. Am J Surg Pathol. 2011;35(3):337–45.
68. Behrens EM, Beukelman T, Paessler M, Cron RQ. Occult macrophage activation syndrome in patients with systemic juvenile idiopathic arthritis. J Rheumatol. 2007;34(5):1133–8.
69. Sawhney S, Woo P, Murray K. Macrophage activation syndrome: a potentially fatal complication of rheumatic disorders. Arch Dis Child. 2001;85(5):421–6.
70. Stephan J, Koné-Paut I, Galambrun C, Mouy R, Bader-Meunier B, Prieur AM. Reactive haemophagocytic syndrome in children with inflammatory disorders. A retrospective study of 24 patients. Rheumatology. 2001;40(11):1285–92.
71. Ravelli A, Magni-Manzoni S, Pistorio A, Besana C, Foti T, Ruperto N, et al. Preliminary diagnostic guidelines for macrophage activation syndrome complicating systemic juvenile idiopathic arthritis. J Pediatr. 2005;146(5):598–604.
72. Parodi A, Davì S, Pringe AB, Pistorio A, Ruperto N, Magni-Manzoni S, et al. Macrophage activation syndrome in juvenile systemic lupus erythematosus: a multinational multicenter study of thirty-eight patients. Arthritis Rheum. 2009;60(11):3388–99.
73. Ravelli A, Minoia F, Davi S, Horne A, Bovis F, Pistorio A, et al. 2016 classification criteria for macrophage activation syndrome complicating systemic juvenile idiopathic arthritis: a European league against rheumatism/American College of rheumatology/paediatric rheumatology international trials organisation collaborative initiative. Arthritis Rheumatol. 2016;68(3):566–76.
74. Pelkonen P, Swanljung K, Siimes M. Ferritinemia as an indicator of systemic disease activity in children with systemic juvenile rheumatoid arthritis. Acta Paediatr. 1986;75(1):64–8.
75. Davì S, Lattanzi B, Demirkaya E, Rosina S, Bracciolini G, Novelli A. Toward the development of new diagnostic criteria for macrophage activation syndrome in systemic juvenile idiopathic arthritis. Ann Paediatr Rheumatol. 2012;1:1–7.
76. Kelly A, Ramanan AV. Recognition and management of macrophage activation syndrome in juvenile arthritis. Curr Opin Rheumatol. 2007;19(5):477–81.
77. Davì S, Minoia F, Pistorio A, Horne A, Consolaro A, Rosina S, et al. Performance of current guidelines for diagnosis of macrophage activation syndrome complicating systemic juvenile idiopathic arthritis. Arthritis Rheumatol. 2014;66(10):2871–80.
78. Pringe A, Trail L, Ruperto N, Buoncompagni A, Loy A, Breda L, et al. Review: macrophage activation syndrome in juvenile systemic lupus erythematosus: an under-recognized complication? Lupus. 2007;16(8):587–92.
79. Fardet L, Galicier L, Lambotte O, Marzac C, Aumont C, Chahwan D, et al. Development and validation of the HScore, a score for the diagnosis of reactive hemophagocytic syndrome. Arthritis Rheumatol. 2014;66(9):2613–20.
80. Hejblum G, Lambotte O, Galicier L, Coppo P, Marzac C, Aumont C, et al. A web-based Delphi study for eliciting helpful criteria in the positive diagnosis of hemophagocytic syndrome in adult patients. PLoS One. 2014;9(4):e94024.

81. De Benedetti F, Brunner HI, Ruperto N, Kenwright A, Wright S, Calvo I, et al. Randomized trial of tocilizumab in systemic juvenile idiopathic arthritis. N Engl J Med. 2012;367(25):2385–95.
82. Ruperto N, Brunner HI, Quartier P, Constantin T, Wulffraat N, Horneff G, et al. Two randomized trials of canakinumab in systemic juvenile idiopathic arthritis. N Engl J Med. 2012;367(25):2396–406.
83. Bleesing J, Prada A, Siegel DM, Villanueva J, Olson J, Ilowite NT, et al. The diagnostic significance of soluble CD163 and soluble interleukin-2 receptor α-chain in macrophage activation syndrome and untreated new-onset systemic juvenile idiopathic arthritis. Arthritis Rheum. 2007;56(3):965–71.
84. Gorelik M, Fall N, Altaye M, Barnes MG, Thompson SD, Grom AA, et al. Follistatin-like protein 1 and the ferritin/erythrocyte sedimentation rate ratio are potential biomarkers for dysregulated gene expression and macrophage activation syndrome in systemic juvenile idiopathic arthritis. J Rheumatol. 2013;40(7):1191–9.
85. Shimizu M, Yokoyama T, Yamada K, Kaneda H, Wada H, Wada T, et al. Distinct cytokine profiles of systemic-onset juvenile idiopathic arthritis-associated macrophage activation syndrome with particular emphasis on the role of interleukin-18 in its pathogenesis. Rheumatology. 2010;49(9):1645–53.
86. Kawashima M, Yamamura M, Taniai M, Yamauchi H, Tanimoto T, Kurimoto M, et al. Levels of interleukin-18 and its binding inhibitors in the blood circulation of patients with adult-onset Still's disease. Arthritis Rheum. 2001;44(3):550–60.
87. Maeno N, Takei S, Imanaka H, Yamamoto K, Kuriwaki K, Kawano Y, et al. Increased interleukin-18 expression in bone marrow of a patient with systemic juvenile idiopathic arthritis and unrecognized macrophage-activation syndrome. Arthritis Rheum. 2004;50(6):1935–8.
88. Shimizu M, Nakagishi Y, Inoue N, Mizuta M, Ko G, Saikawa Y, et al. Interleukin-18 for predicting the development of macrophage activation syndrome in systemic juvenile idiopathic arthritis. Clin Immunol. 2015;160(2):277–81.
89. Jenkins RW, Clarke CJ, Lucas JT, Shabbir M, Wu BX, Simbari F, et al. Evaluation of the role of secretory sphingomyelinase and bioactive sphingolipids as biomarkers in hemophagocytic lymphohistiocytosis. Am J Hematol. 2013;88(11):E265–E72.
90. Ishii E. Hemophagocytic lymphohistiocytosis in children: pathogenesis and treatment. Front Pediatr. 2016;4:47.
91. Cron RQ, Davi S, Minoia F, Ravelli A. Clinical features and correct diagnosis of macrophage activation syndrome. Expert Rev Clin Immunol. 2015;11(9):1043–53.
92. Yanagimachi M, Goto H, Miyamae T, Kadota K, Imagawa T, Mori M, et al. Association of IRF5 polymorphisms with susceptibility to hemophagocytic lymphohistiocytosis in children. J Clin Immunol. 2011;31(6):946–51.
93. Chen C, Huang Y, Jaing T, Hung I, Yang C, Chang L, et al. Hemophagocytic syndrome: a review of 18 pediatric cases. J Microbiol Immunol Infect. 2004;37(3):157.
94. Risdall RJ, McKenna RW, Nesbit ME, Krivit W, Balfour HH, Simmons RL, et al. Virus-associated hemophagocytic syndrome A benign histiocytic proliferation distinct from malignant histiocytosis. Cancer. 1979;44(3):993–1002.
95. Burgio GR, Aricó M, Marconi M, Lanfranchi A, Caselli D, Ugazio AG. Spontaneous NBT reduction by monocytes as a marker of disease activity in children with histiocytosis. Br J Haematol. 1990;74(2):146–50.
96. Oloomi Z, Moayeri H. Cytomegalovirus infection-associated hemophagocytic syndrome. Arch Iran Med. 2006;9:284–7.
97. Maruyama K, Koizumi T, Hirato J. Cytomegalovirus associated hemophagocytic lymphohistiocytosis in a premature infant. Pediatr Int. 2006;48(6):648–50.
98. Hoang MP, Dawson DB, Rogers ZR, Scheuermann RH, Rogers BB. Polymerase chain reaction amplification of archival material for Epstein-Barr virus, cytomegalovirus, human herpesvirus 6, and parvovirus B19 in children with bone marrow hemophagocytosis. Hum Pathol. 1998;29(10):1074–7.
99. Fardet L, Blum L, Kerob D, Agbalika F, Galicier L, Dupuy A, et al. Human herpesvirus 8-associated hemophagocytic lymphohistiocytosis in human immunodeficiency virus-infected patients. Clin Infect Dis. 2003;37(2):285–91.
100. Grossman WJ, Radhi M, Schauer D, Gerday E, Grose C, Goldman FD. Development of hemophagocytic lymphohistiocytosis in triplets infected with HHV-8. Blood. 2005;106(4):1203–6.
101. Re A, Facchetti F, Borlenghi E, Cattaneo C, Capucci M, Ungari M, et al. Fatal hemophagocytic syndrome related to active human herpesvirus-8/Kaposi sarcoma-associated herpesvirus infection in human immunodeficiency virus-negative, non-transplant patients without related malignancies. Eur J Haematol. 2007;78(4):361–4.
102. van der Werff ten Bosch J, Kollen WJ, Ball LM, Brinkman D, Vossen AC, Lankester AC, et al. Atypical varicella zoster infection associated with hemophagocytic lymphohistiocytosis. Pediatr Blood Cancer. 2009;53(2):226–8.
103. Yamada K, Yamamoto Y, Uchiyama A, Ito R, Aoki Y, Uchida Y, et al. Successful treatment of neonatal herpes simplex-type 1 infection complicated by hemophagocytic lymphohistiocytosis and acute liver failure. Tohoku J Exp Med. 2008;214(1):1–5.
104. Ramasamy K, Lim Z, Savvas M, Salisbury J, Dokal I, Mufti G, et al. Disseminated herpes virus (HSV-2) infection with rhabdomyolysis and hemophagocytic lymphohistiocytosis in a patient with bone marrow failure syndrome. Ann Hematol. 2006;85(9):629–30.
105. Levy J, Wodell R, August C, Bayever E. Adenovirus-related hemophagocytic syndrome after bone mar-

row transplantation. Bone Marrow Transplant. 1990;6(5):349–52.
106. Ardalan M, Shoja M, Tubbs R, Esmaili H, Keyvani H. Postrenal transplant hemophagocytic lymphohistiocytosis and thrombotic microangiopathy associated with parvovirus b19 infection. Am J Transplant. 2008;8(6):1340–4.
107. Wada Y, Kai M, Tanaka H, Shimizu N, Shimatani M, Oshima T. Computed tomography findings of the liver in a neonate with Herpes simplex virus-associated hemophagocytic lymphohistiocytosis. Pediatr Int. 2011;53(5):773–6.
108. Yamaguchi K, Yamamoto A, Hisano M, Natori M, Murashima A. Herpes Simplex Virus 2–Associated Hemophagocytic Lymphohistiocytosis in a pregnant patient. Obstet Gynecol. 2005;105(5, Part 2):1241–4.
109. Yilmaz S, Oren H, Demircioglu F, Firinci F, Korkmaz A, Irken G. Parvovirus B19: a cause for aplastic crisis and hemophagocytic lymphohistiocytosis. Pediatr Blood Cancer. 2006;47(6):861.
110. Dutta U, Mittal S, Ratho RK, Das A. Acute liver failure and severe hemophagocytosis secondary to parvovirus B19 infection. Indian J Gastroenterol. 2005;24(3):118.
111. Faurschou M, Nielsen OJ, Hansen PB, Juhl BR, Hasselbalch H. Fatal virus-associated hemophagocytic syndrome associated with coexistent chronic active hepatitis B and acute hepatitis C virus infection. Am J Hematol. 1999;61(2):135–8.
112. Tuon FF, Gomes VS, Amato VS, Graf ME, Fonseca GHH, Lazari C, et al. Hemophagocytic syndrome associated with hepatitis A: case report and literature review. Rev Inst Med Trop Sao Paulo. 2008;50(2):123–7.
113. Russo RA, Rosenzweig SD, Katsicas MM. Hepatitis A-associated macrophage activation syndrome in children with systemic juvenile idiopathic arthritis: report of 2 cases. J Rheumatol. 2008;35(1):166–8.
114. Tierney Jr LM, Thabet A, Nishino H. Case 10-2011: a woman with fever, confusion, liver failure, anemia, and thrombocytopenia. N Engl J Med. 2011;364(13):1259–70.
115. Akamatsu N, Sugawara Y, Tamura S, Matsui Y, Hasegawa K, Imamura H, et al., editors. Hemophagocytic syndrome after adult-to-adult living donor liver transplantation. Amsterdam: Elsevier; 2006.
116. Pease DF, Mathew J, Hepatitis C. Virus associated hemophagocytic lymphohistiocytosis: case report and literature review. J Hematol. 2013;2(2):76–8.
117. Doyle T, Bhagani S, Cwynarski K. Haemophagocytic syndrome and HIV. Curr Opin Infect Dis. 2009;22(1):1–6.
118. Sun H-Y, Chen M-Y, Fang C-T, Hsieh S-M, Hung C-C, Chang S-C. Hemophagocytic lymphohistiocytosis: an unusual initial presentation of acute HIV infection. J Acquir Immune Defic Syndr. 2004;37(4):1539–40.
119. Park K-H, Yu H-S, Jung S-I, Shin D-H, Shin J-H. Acute human immunodeficiency virus syndrome presenting with hemophagocytic lymphohistiocytosis. Yonsei Med J. 2008;49(2):325–8.
120. Harms PW, Schmidt LA, Smith LB, Newton DW, Pletneva MA, Walters LL, et al. Autopsy findings in eight patients with fatal H1N1 influenza. Am J Clin Pathol. 2010;134(1):27–35.
121. Lai S, Merritt BY, Chen L, Zhou X, Green LK. Hemophagocytic lymphohistiocytosis associated with influenza A (H1N1) infection in a patient with chronic lymphocytic leukemia: an autopsy case report and review of the literature. Ann Diagn Pathol. 2012;16(6):477–84.
122. Mou SS, Nakagawa TA, Riemer EC, McLean TW, Hines MH, Shetty AK. Hemophagocytic lymphohistiocytosis complicating influenza A infection. Pediatrics. 2006;118(1):e216–9.
123. Özdemir H, Ciftci E, Ince EÜ, Ertem M, Ince E, Dogru Ü. Hemophagocytic lymphohistiocytosis associated with 2009 pandemic influenza A (H1N1) virus infection. J Pediatr Hematol Oncol. 2011;33(2):135–7.
124. Shrestha B, Omran A, Rong P, Wang W. Report of a fatal pediatric case of hemophagocytic lymphohistiocytosis associated with pandemic influenza A (H1N1) infection in 2009. Pediatr Neonatol. 2015;56(3):189–92.
125. Willekens C, Cornelius A, Guerry M-J, Wacrenier A, Fourrier F. Fulminant hemophagocytic lymphohistiocytosis induced by pandemic A (H1N1) influenza: a case report. J Med Case Rep. 2011;5(1):1.
126. Zheng Y, Yang Y, Zhao W, Wang H. Novel swine-origin influenza A (H1N1) virus-associated hemophagocytic syndrome—a first case report. Am J Trop Med Hyg. 2010;82(4):743–5.
127. Beffermann N, Pilcante J, Sarmiento M. Acquired hemophagocytic syndrome related to parainfluenza virus infection: case report. J Med Case Rep. 2015;9(1):1.
128. Xing Q, Xing P. Mumps caused hemophagocytic syndrome: a rare case report. Am J Emerg Med. 2013;31(6):1000.e1–2.
129. Iaria C, Leonardi MS, Buda A, Toro ML, Cascio A. Measles and secondary hemophagocytic lymphohistiocytosis. Emerg Infect Dis. 2012;18(9):1529.
130. Otagiri T, Mitsui T, Kawakami T, Katsuura M, Maeda K, Ikegami T, et al. Haemophagocytic lymphohistiocytosis following measles vaccination. Eur J Pediatr. 2002;161(9):494–6.
131. Koubaa M, Marrakchi C, Maaloul I, Makni S, Berrajah L, Elloumi M, et al. Rubella associated with hemophagocytic syndrome. First report in a male and review of the literature. Mediterranean J Hematol Infect Dis. 2012;4(1):e2012050.
132. Katsibardi K, Moschovi MA, Theodoridou M, Spanakis N, Kalabalikis P, Tsakris A, et al. Enterovirus-associated hemophagocytic syndrome in children with malignancy: report of three cases and review of the literature. Eur J Pediatr. 2008;167(1):97–102.

133. Nagao T, Takahashi N, Saitoh H, Noguchi S, Guo Y, Ito M, et al. Adult T-cell leukemia-lymphoma developed from an HTLV-1 carrier during treatment of B-cell lymphoma-associated hemophagocytic syndrome. [Rinsho ketsueki] Jpn J Clin Hematol. 2012;53(12):2008–12.
134. Takahashi S, Oki J, Miyamoto A, Koyano S, Ito K, Azuma H, et al. Encephalopathy associated with haemophagocytic lymphohistiocytosis following rotavirus infection. Eur J Pediatr. 1999;158(2):133–7.
135. Ray S, Kundu S, Saha M, Chakrabarti P. Hemophagocytic syndrome in classic dengue fever. J Global Infect Dis. 2011;3(4):399.
136. Koshy M, Mishra AK, Agrawal B, Kurup AR, Hansdak SG. Dengue fever complicated by hemophagocytosis. Oxford Med Case Rep. 2016;2016(6):121–4.
137. Ab-Rahman HA, Rahim H, AbuBakar S, Wong P-F. Macrophage activation syndrome-associated markers in severe dengue. Int J Med Sci. 2016;13(3):179.
138. Sam S-S, Omar SFS, Teoh B-T, Abd-Jamil J, AbuBakar S. Review of dengue hemorrhagic fever fatal cases seen among adults: a retrospective study. PLoS Negl Trop Dis. 2013;7(5):e2194.
139. Erduran E, Cakir M. Reactive hemophagocytic lymphohistiocytosis and Crimean-Congo hemorrhagic fever. Int J Infect Dis. 2010;14:e349.
140. Baty V, Schuhmacher H, Bourgoin C, Latger V, Buisine J, May T, et al. Hemophagocytic syndrome and hemorrhagic fever with renal syndrome. Presse Méd. 1998;27(31):1577.
141. Lee JJ, Chung IJ, Shin DH, Cho SH, Cho D, Ryang DW, et al. Hemorrhagic fever with renal syndrome presenting with hemophagocytic lymphohistiocytosis. Emerg Infect Dis. 2002;8(2):209–10.
142. Lin L, Xu Y-Z, Wu X-M, Ge H-F, Feng J-X, Chen M-F, et al. A rare fatal case of a novel bunyavirus-associated hemophagocytic lymphohistiocytosis. J Infect Dev Countries. 2016;10(05):533–6.
143. Kamihira T, Yano K, Tamada Y, Matsumoto T, Miyazato M, Nagaoka S, et al. Case of domestically infected hepatitis E with marked thrombocytopenia. Nihon Shokakibyo Gakkai Zasshi. 2008;105(6):841–6.
144. Lu M, Xie Z, Gao Z, Wang C, Li N, Li M, et al. Histopathologic study of avian influenza H5N1 infection in humans. Zhonghua bing li xue za zhi. 2008;37(3):145–9.
145. Pei F, Zheng J, Gao Z, Zhong Y, Fang W, Gong E, et al. Lung pathology and pathogenesis of severe acute respiratory syndrome: a report of six full autopsies. Zhonghua bing li xue za zhi: Chin J Pathol. 2005;34(10):656–60.
146. Yoshiyama M, Kounami S, Nakayama K, Aoyagi N, Yoshikawa N. Clinical assessment of Mycoplasma pneumoniae-associated hemophagocytic lymphohistiocytosis. Pediatr Int. 2008;50(4):432–5.
147. Ishida Y, Hiroi K, Tauchi H, Oto Y, Tokuda K, Kida K. Hemophagocytic lymphohistiocytosis secondary to Mycoplasma pneumoniae infection. Pediatr Int. 2004;46(2):174–7.
148. Non LR, Patel R, Esmaeeli A, Despotovic V. Typhoid fever complicated by hemophagocytic lymphohistiocytosis and rhabdomyolysis. Am J Trop Med Hyg. 2015;93(5):1068–9.
149. Sniderman JD, Cuvelier GD, Veroukis S, Hansen G. Toxic epidermal necrolysis and hemophagocytic lymphohistiocytosis: a case report and literature review. Clin Case Rep. 2015;3(2):121–5.
150. Dube R, Kar SS, Mahapatro S, Ray R. Infection associated hemophagocytic lymphohistiocytosis: a case report. Indian J Clin Pract. 2013;24(2).
151. Tseng Y-T, Sheng W-H, Lin B-H, Lin C-W, Wang J-T, Chen Y-C, et al. Causes, clinical symptoms, and outcomes of infectious diseases associated with hemophagocytic lymphohistiocytosis in Taiwanese adults. J Microbiol Immunol Infect. 2011;44(3):191–7.
152. Rouphael NG, Talati NJ, Vaughan C, Cunningham K, Moreira R, Gould C. Infections associated with haemophagocytic syndrome. Lancet Infect Dis. 2007;7(12):814–22.
153. Yagi K, Kano G, Shibata M, Sakamoto I, Matsui H, Imashuku S. Chlamydia pneumoniae infection-related hemophagocytic lymphohistiocytosis and acute encephalitis and poliomyelitis-like flaccid paralysis. Pediatr Blood Cancer. 2011;56(5):853–5.
154. Maheshwari P, Chhabra R, Yadav P. Perinatal tuberculosis associated hemophagocytic lymphohistiocytosis. Indian J Pediatr. 2012;79(9):1228–9.
155. Brastianos PK, Swanson JW, Torbenson M, Sperati J, Karakousis PC. Tuberculosis-associated haemophagocytic syndrome. Lancet Infect Dis. 2006;6(7):447–54.
156. Wali Y, Beshlawi I. BCG lymphadenitis in neonates with familial hemophagocytic lymphohistiocytosis. Pediatr Infect Dis J. 2012;31(3):324.
157. Rositto A, Molinaro L, Larralde M, Ranalletta M, Drut R. Disseminated cutaneous eruption after BCG vaccination. Pediatr Dermatol. 1996;13(6):451–4.
158. Schleinitz N, Bernit E, Harle J-R. Severe hemophagocytic syndrome after intravesical BCG instillation. Am J Med. 2002;112(7):593–4.
159. Gosh J, Roy M, Bala A. Infection associated with hemophagocytic lymphohistiocytosis triggered by nosocomial infection. Oman Med J. 2009;24(3):223–5.
160. Chang C-C, Hsiao P-J, Chiu C-C, Chen Y-C, Lin S-H, Wu C-C, et al. Catastrophic hemophagocytic lymphohistiocytosis in a young man with nephrotic syndrome. Clin Chim Acta. 2015;439:168–71.
161. Saidi W, Gammoudi R, Korbi M, Aounallah A, Boussofara L, Ghariani N, et al. Hemophagocytic lymphohistiocytosis: an unusual complication of leprosy. Int J Dermatol. 2015;54(9):1054–9.
162. Kiernan TJ, O'Flaherty N, Gilmore R, Ho E, Hickey M, Tolan M, et al. Abiotrophia defectiva endocarditis and associated hemophagocytic syndrome—a first case report and review of the literature. Int J Infect Dis. 2008;12(5):478–82.

163. Dumler JS. The biological basis of severe outcomes in Anaplasma phagocytophilum infection. FEMS Immunol Med Microbiol. 2012;64(1):13–20.
164. Karras A, Thervet E, Legendre C. Hemophagocytic syndrome in renal transplant recipients: report of 17 cases and review of literature. Transplantation. 2004;77(2):238–43.
165. Cantero-Hinojosa J, D'iez-Ruiz A, Santos-Perez J, Aguilar-Martinez J, Ramos-Jimenez A. Lyme disease associated with hemophagocytic syndrome. J Mol Med. 1993;71(8):620.
166. Akbayram S, Dogan M, Akgun C, Peker E, Parlak M, Caksen H, et al. An analysis of children with brucellosis associated with pancytopenia. Pediatr Hematol Oncol. 2011;28(3):203–8.
167. Erduran E, Makuloglu M, Mutlu M. A rare hematological manifestation of brucellosis: reactive hemophagocytic syndrome. J Microbiol Immunol Infect. 2010;43(2):159–62.
168. Sari I, Altuntas F, Hacioglu S, Kocyigit I, Sevinc A, Sacar S, et al. A multicenter retrospective study defining the clinical and hematological manifestations of brucellosis and pancytopenia in a large series: hematological malignancies, the unusual cause of pancytopenia in patients with brucellosis. Am J Hematol. 2008;83(4):334–9.
169. Anstead GM, Jorgensen JH, Craig FE, Blaser MJ, Patterson TF. Thermophilic multidrug-resistant Campylobacter fetus infection with hypersplenism and histiocytic phagocytosis in a patient with acquired immunodeficiency syndrome. Clin Infect Dis. 2001;32(2):295–6.
170. Tamura A, Matsunobu T, Kurita A, Shiotani A. Hemophagocytic syndrome in the course of sudden sensorineural hearing loss. ORL. 2012;74(4):211–4.
171. Ramon I, Libert M, Guillaume M-P, Corazza F, Karmali R. Recurrent haemophagocytic syndrome in an HIV-infected patient. Acta Clin Belg. 2010;65(4):276–8.
172. Chinen K, Ohkura Y, Matsubara O, Tsuchiya E. Hemophagocytic syndrome associated with clostridial infection in a pancreatic carcinoma patient. Pathol Res Pract. 2004;200(3):241–5.
173. Harris P, Dixit R, Norton R. Coxiella burnetii causing haemophagocytic syndrome: a rare complication of an unusual pathogen. Infection. 2011;39(6):579–82.
174. Hufnagel M, Niemeyer C, Zimmerhackl LB, Tüchelmann T, Sauter S, Brandis M. Hemophagocytosis: a complication of acute Q fever in a child. Clin Infect Dis. 1995;21(4):1029–31.
175. Hanson D, Walter AW, Powell J. Ehrlichia-induced hemophagocytic lymphohistiocytosis in two children. Pediatr Blood Cancer. 2011;56(4):661–3.
176. Burns S, Saylors R, Mian A. Hemophagocytic lymphohistiocytosis secondary to Ehrlichia chaffeensis infection: a case report. J Pediatr Hematol Oncol. 2010;32(4):e142–3.
177. Abbott KC, Vukelja SJ, Smith CE, McAllister CK, Konkol KA, O'rourke TJ, et al. Hemophagocytic syndrome: a cause of pancytopenia in human ehrlichiosis. Am J Hematol. 1991;38(3):230–4.
178. Krishnamurthy S, Mahadevan S, Mandal J, Basu D. Leptospirosis in association with hemophagocytic syndrome: a rare presentation. Indian J Pediatr. 2013;80(6):524–5. https://doi.org/10.1007/s12098-012-0863-0.
179. Niller H. Myelodysplastic syndrome (MDS) as a late stage of subclinical hemophagocytic lymphohistiocytosis (HLH): a putative role for Leptospira infection. A hypothesis. Acta Microbiol Immunol Hung. 2010;57(3):181–9.
180. Lambotte O, Fihman V, Poyart C, Buzyn A, Berche P, Soumelis V. Listeria monocytogenes skin infection with cerebritis and haemophagocytosis syndrome in a bone marrow transplant recipient. J Infect. 2005;50(4):356–8.
181. Pellegrin J, Merlio J, Lacoste D, Barbeau P, Brossard G, Beylot J, et al. Syndrome of macrophagic activation with hemophagocytosis in human immunodeficiency virus infection. Rev Med interne. 1992;13(6):438–40.
182. Yang W, Fu L, Lan J, Shen G, Chou G, Tseng C, et al. Mycobacterium avium complex-associated hemophagocytic syndrome in systemic lupus erythematosus patient: report of one case. Lupus. 2003;12(4):312–6.
183. Valsalan R, Kosaraju K, Sohanlal T, Kumar PP. Hemophagocytosis in scrub typhus. J Postgrad Med. 2010;56(4):301.
184. Cascio A, Giordano S, Dones P, Venezia S, Iaria C, Ziino O. Haemophagocytic syndrome and rickettsial diseases. J Med Microbiol. 2011;60(4):537–42.
185. Gutiérrez-Ravé PV, Luque MR, Ayerza LM, Cañavate IM, Prados MD. Reactive hemophagocytic syndrome: analysis of a series of 7 cases. Med Clin. 1990;94(4):130–4.
186. Guo X, Chen N, Wang T, Zhou C, Li Q, Gao J. Visceral leishmaniasis associated hemophagocytic lymphohistiocytosis: report of four childhood cases. Zhonghua er ke za zhi. 2011;49(7):550–3.
187. Rajagopala S, Dutta U, Chandra KP, Bhatia P, Varma N, Kochhar R. Visceral leishmaniasis associated hemophagocytic lymphohistiocytosis–case report and systematic review. J Infect. 2008;56(5):381–8.
188. Gagnaire M-H, Galambrun C, Stéphan JL. Hemophagocytic syndrome: a misleading complication of visceral leishmaniasis in children—a series of 12 cases. Pediatrics. 2000;106(4):e58.
189. Arslan F, Batirel A, Ramazan M, Ozer S, Mert A. Macrophage activation syndrome triggered by primary disseminated toxoplasmosis. Scand J Infect Dis. 2012;44(12):1001–4.
190. Briand P, Gangneux J, Favaretto G, Ly-Sunnaram B, Godard M, Robert-Gangneux F, et al. Hemophagocytic syndrome and toxoplasmic primo-infection. Ann Biol Clin. 2008;66(2):199–205. https://doi.org/10.1684/abc.2008.0209.
191. Gupta P, Hurley RW, Helseth PH, Goodman JL, Hammerschmidt DE. Pancytopenia due

to hemophagocytic syndrome as the presenting manifestation of babesiosis. Am J Hematol. 1995;50(1):60–2.
192. Bhagat M, Kanhere S, Kadakia P, Phadke V, George R, Chaudhari K. Haemophagocytic lymphohistiocytosis: a cause of unresponsive malaria in a 5-year-old girl. Paediatr Int Child Health. 2015;35(4):333–6. https://doi.org/10.1080/20469047.2015.1109227.
193. Saribeyoglu ET, Anak S, Agaoglu L, Boral O, Unuvar A, Devecioglu O. Secondary hemophagocytic lymphohistiocytosis induced by malaria infection in a child with Langerhans cell histiocytosis. Pediatr Hematol Oncol. 2004;21(3):267–72.
194. Ullah W, Abdullah HMA, Qadir S, Shahzad MA. Haemophagocytic lymphohistiocytosis (HLH): a rare but potentially fatal association with Plasmodium vivax malaria. BMJ Case Rep. 2016;2016:bcr2016215366.
195. Bhatia S, Bauer F, Bilgrami SA. Candidiasis-associated hemophagocytic lymphohistiocytosis in a patient infected with human immunodeficiency virus. Clin Infect Dis. 2003;37(11):):e161–6.
196. Numata K, Tsutsumi H, Wakai S, Tachi N, Chiba S. A child case of haemophagocytic syndrome associated with cryptococcal meningoencephalitis. J Infect. 1998;36(1):118–9.
197. Majluf-Cruz A, Hurtado MR, Souto-Meirino C, del Río CC, Simon J. Hemophagocytic syndrome associated with histoplasmosis in the acquired immunodeficiency syndrome: description of 3 cases and review of the literature. Sangre. 1993;38(1):51–5.
198. Quijano G, Siminovich M, Drut R. Histopathologic findings in the lymphoid and reticuloendothelial system in pediatric HIV infection: a postmortem study. Pediatr Pathol Lab Med. 1997;17(6):845–56.
199. Keller FG, Kurtzberg J. Disseminated histoplasmosis: a cause of infection-associated hemophagocytic syndrome. J Pediatr Hematol Oncol. 1994;16(4):368–71.
200. Chokephaibulkit K, Veerakul G, Vanprapar N, Chaiprasert A, Tanphaichitr V, Chearskul S. Penicilliosis-associated hemophagocytic syndrome in a human immunodeficiency virus-infected child: the first case report in children. J Med Assoc Thai. 2001;84(3):426–9.
201. Chim C, Fong C, Ma S, Wong S, Yuen K. Reactive hemophagocytic syndrome associated with Penicillium marneffei infection. Am J Med. 1998;104(2):196–7.
202. Elazary AS, Wolf DG, Amir G, Avni B, Rund D, Yehuda DB, et al. Severe Epstein–Barr virus-associated hemophagocytic syndrome in six adult patients. J Clin Virol. 2007;40(2):156–9.
203. Tabata Y, Hibi S, Teramura T, Kuriyama K, Yagi T, Todo S, et al. Molecular analysis of latent membrane protein 1 in patients with Epstein-Barr virus-associated hemophagocytic lymphohistiocytosis in Japan. Leuk Lymphoma. 2000;38(3–4):373–80.
204. Kawaguchi H, Miyashita T, Herbst H, Niedobitek G, Asada M, Tsuchida M, et al. Epstein-Barr virus-infected T lymphocytes in Epstein-Barr virus-associated hemophagocytic syndrome. J Clin Investig. 1993;92(3):1444.
205. Beutel K, Gross-Wieltsch U, Wiesel T, Stadt UZ, Janka G, Wagner HJ. Infection of T lymphocytes in Epstein-Barr virus-associated hemophagocytic lymphohistiocytosis in children of non-Asian origin. Pediatr Blood Cancer. 2009;53(2):184–90.
206. Imashuku S. Clinical features and treatment strategies of Epstein–Barr virus-associated hemophagocytic lymphohistiocytosis. Crit Rev Oncol Hematol. 2002;44(3):259–72.
207. Cho HS, Park YN, Lyu CJ, Park SM, Oh SH, Yang CH, et al. EBV-elicited familial hemophagocytic lymphohistiocytosis. Yonsei Med J. 1997;38:245–8.
208. Purtilo D, Yang JS, Cassel C, Harper R, Stephenson S, Landing B, et al. X-linked recessive progressive combined variable immunodeficiency (Duncan's disease). Lancet. 1975;305(7913):935–41.
209. Christensson B, Braconier JH, Winqvist I, Relander T, Dictor M. Fulminant course of infectious mononucleosis with virus-associated hemophagocytic syndrome. Scand J Infect Dis. 1987;19(3):373–9.
210. Akashi K, Mizuno S-I. Epstein-Barr virus-infected natural killer cell leukemia. Leuk Lymphoma. 2000;40(1–2):57–66.
211. Ohshima K, Suzumiya J, Sugihara M, Nagafuchi S, Ohga S, Kikuchi M. Clinicopathological study of severe chronic active Epstein-Barr virus infection that developed in association with lymphoproliferative disorder and/or hemophagocytic syndrome. Pathol Int. 1998;48(12):934–43.
212. Su I-J, Wang C-H, Cheng A-L, Chen R-L. Hemophagocytic syndrome in Epstein-Barr virus-associated T-lymphoproliferative disorders: disease spectrum, pathogenesis, and management. Leuk Lymphoma. 1995;19(5–6):401–6.
213. Lindemann TL, Greene JS. Persistent cervical lymphadenopathy in an adolescent with Epstein–Barr induced hemophagocytic syndrome: manifestations of a rare but often fatal disease. Int J Pediatr Otorhinolaryngol. 2005;69(7):1011–4.
214. Chuang H-C, Lay J-D, Hsieh W-C, Wang H-C, Chang Y, Chuang S-E, et al. Epstein-Barr virus LMP1 inhibits the expression of SAP gene and upregulates Th1 cytokines in the pathogenesis of hemophagocytic syndrome. Blood. 2005;106(9):3090–6.
215. Kasahara Y, Yachie A. Cell type specific infection of Epstein–Barr virus (EBV) in EBV-associated hemophagocytic lymphohistiocytosis and chronic active EBV infection. Crit Rev Oncol Hematol. 2002;44(3):283–94.
216. Imashuku S, Hibi S, Tabata Y, Sako M, Sekine Y, Hirayama K, et al. Biomarker and morphological characteristics of Epstein-Barr virus-related hemophagocytic lymphohistiocytosis. Med Pediatr Oncol. 1998;31(3):131–7.
217. Nazaruk RA, Rochford R, Hobbs MV, Cannon MJ. Functional diversity of the CD8+ T-cell response to Epstein-Barr virus (EBV): implications for the

pathogenesis of EBV-associated lymphoproliferative disorders. Blood. 1998;91(10):3875–83.
218. Hatta K, Morimoto A, Ishii E, Kimura H, Ueda I, Hibi S, et al. Association of transforming growth factor-β1 gene polymorphism in the development of Epstein-Barr virus-related hematologic diseases. Haematologica. 2007;92(11):1470–4.
219. Teramura T, Tabata Y, Yagi T, Morimoto A, Hibi S, Imashuku S. Quantitative analysis of cell-free Epstein-Barr virus genome copy number in patients with EBV-associated hemophagocytic lymphohistiocytosis. Leuk Lymphoma. 2002;43(1):173–9.
220. Kimura H, Hoshino Y, Hara S, Nishikawa K, Sako M, Hirayama M, et al. Viral load in Epstein-Barr virus-associated hemophagocytic syndrome. Microbiol Immunol. 2002;46(8):579–82.
221. Sandberg Y, van Gastel-Mol EJ, Verhaaf B, Lam KH, van Dongen JJ, Langerak AW. BIOMED-2 multiplex immunoglobulin/T-cell receptor polymerase chain reaction protocols can reliably replace Southern blot analysis in routine clonality diagnostics. J Mol Diagn. 2005;7(4):495–503.
222. Langerak AW, Groenen PJ, Bruggemann M, Beldjord K, Bellan C, Bonello L, et al. EuroClonality/BIOMED-2 guidelines for interpretation and reporting of Ig/TCR clonality testing in suspected lymphoproliferations. Leukemia. 2012;26(10):2159–71.
223. Matsuda K, Nakazawa Y, Yanagisawa R, Honda T, Ishii E, Koike K. Detection of T-cell receptor gene rearrangement in children with Epstein–Barr virus-associated hemophagocytic lymphohistiocytosis using the BIOMED-2 multiplex polymerase chain reaction combined with GeneScan analysis. Clin Chim Acta. 2011;412(17):1554–8.
224. Kelesidis T, Humphries R, Terashita D, Eshaghian S, Territo MC, Said J, et al. Epstein–Barr virus-associated hemophagocytic lymphohistiocytosis in Los Angeles county. J Med Virol. 2012;84(5):777–85.
225. Kogawa K, Sato H, Asano T, Ohga S, Kudo K, Morimoto A, et al. Prognostic factors of Epstein–Barr virus-associated hemophagocytic lymphohistiocytosis in children: report of the Japan Histiocytosis Study Group. Pediatr Blood Cancer. 2014;61(7):1257–62.
226. Trottestam H, Berglöf E, Horne A, Onelöv E, Beutel K, Lehmberg K, et al. Risk factors for early death in children with haemophagocytic lymphohistiocytosis. Acta Paediatr. 2012;101(3):313–8.
227. Huang SC, Chen JS, Cheng CN, Yang YJ. Hypoalbuminaemia is an independent predictor for hemophagocytic lymphohistiocytosis in childhood Epstein–Barr virus-associated infectious mononucleosis. Eur J Haematol. 2012;89(5):417–22.
228. Bakhshi S, Pautu JL. EBV-associated hemophagocytic lymphohistiocytosis with spontaneous regression. Indian Pediatr. 2005;42(12):1253.
229. Imashuku S, Tabata Y, Teramura T, Hibi S. Treatment strategies for Epstein-Barr virus-associated hemophagocytic lymphohistiocytosis (EBV-HLH). Leuk Lymphoma. 2000;39(1–2):37–49.
230. Balamuth NJ, Nichols KE, Paessler M, Teachey DT. Use of rituximab in conjunction with immunosuppressive chemotherapy as a novel therapy for Epstein Barr virus-associated hemophagocytic lymphohistiocytosis. J Pediatr Hematol Oncol. 2007;29(8):569–73.
231. Imashuku S, Hibi S, Todo S, Sako M, Inoue M, Kawa K, et al. Allogeneic hematopoietic stem cell transplantation for patients with hemophagocytic syndrome (HPS) in Japan. Bone Marrow Transplant. 1999;23(6):569–72.
232. Ohga S, Kudo K, Ishii E, Honjo S, Morimoto A, Osugi Y, et al. Hematopoietic stem cell transplantation for familial hemophagocytic lymphohistiocytosis and Epstein–Barr virus-associated hemophagocytic lymphohistiocytosis in Japan. Pediatr Blood Cancer. 2010;54(2):299–306.
233. Qin Q, Xie Z, Shen Y, Yang S, Liu C, Huang Z, et al. Assessment of immunochemotherapy and stem cell transplantation on EBV-associated hemophagocytic lymphohistiocytosis in children: a systematic review and meta analysis. Eur Rev Med Pharmacol Sci. 2012;16(5):672–8.
234. Milone MC, Tsai DE, Hodinka RL, Silverman LB, Malbran A, Wasik MA, et al. Treatment of primary Epstein-Barr virus infection in patients with X-linked lymphoproliferative disease using B-cell–directed therapy. Blood. 2005;105(3):994–6.
235. Danish EH, Dahms BB, Kumar ML. Cytomegalovirus-associated hemophagocytic syndrome. Pediatrics. 1985;75(2):280–3.
236. Kohara MM, Blum RN. Cytomegalovirus Ileitis and Hemophagocytic syndrome associated with use of anti—tumor necrosis factor—α antibody. Clin Infect Dis. 2006;42(5):733–4.
237. Koketsu S-I, Watanabe T, Hori N, Umetani N, Takazawa Y, Nagawa H. Hemophagocytic syndrome caused by fulminant ulcerative colitis and cytomegalovirus infection: report of a case. Dis Colon Rectum. 2004;47(7):1250–5.
238. Amenomori M, Migita K, Miyashita T, Yoshida S, Ito M, Eguchi K, et al. Cytomegalovirus-associated hemophagocytic syndrome in a patient with adult onset Still's disease. Clin Exp Rheumatol. 2005;23(1):100–2.
239. Sakamoto O, Ando M, Yoshimatsu S, Kohrogi H, Suga M, Ando M. Systemic lupus erythematosus complicated by cytomegalovirus-induced hemophagocytic syndrome and colitis. Intern Med. 2002;41(2):151–5.
240. Devecioglu O, Anak S, Atay D, Aktan P, Devecioglu E, Ozalp B, et al. Pediatric acute lymphoblastic leukemia complicated by secondary hemophagocytic lymphohistiocytosis. Pediatr Blood Cancer. 2009;53(3):491–2.
241. Sato M, Matsushima T, Takada S, Hatsumi N, Kim K, Sakuraya M, et al. Fulminant, CMV-associated, haemophagocytic syndrome following unrelated bone marrow transplantation. Bone Marrow Transplant. 1998;22(12):1219.

242. Hardikar W, Pang K, Al-Hebbi H, Curtis N, Couper R. Successful treatment of cytomegalovirus-associated haemophagocytic syndrome following paediatric orthotopic liver transplantation. J Paediatr Child Health. 2006;42(6):389–91.
243. Abdelkefi A, Jamil WB, Torjman L, Ladeb S, Ksouri H, Lakhal A, et al. Hemophagocytic syndrome after hematopoietic stem cell transplantation: a prospective observational study. Int J Hematol. 2009;89(3):368–73.
244. Imashuku S, Ueda I, Teramura T, Mori K, Morimoto A, Sako M, et al. Occurrence of haemophagocytic lymphohistiocytosis at less than 1 year of age: analysis of 96 patients. Eur J Pediatr. 2005;164(5):315–9.
245. Uneda S, Murata S, Sonoki T, Matsuoka H, Nakakuma H. Successful treatment with liposomal doxorubicin for widespread Kaposi's sarcoma and human herpesvirus-8 related severe hemophagocytic syndrome in a patient with acquired immunodeficiency syndrome. Int J Hematol. 2009;89(2):195–200.
246. Stebbing J, Ngan S, Ibrahim H, Charles P, Nelson M, Kelleher P, et al. The successful treatment of haemophagocytic syndrome in patients with human immunodeficiency virus-associated multicentric Castleman's disease. Clin Exp Immunol. 2008;154(3):399–405.
247. Pastore RD, Chadburn A, Kripas C, Schattner EJ. Novel association of haemophagocytic syndrome with Kaposi's sarcoma-associated herpesvirus-related primary effusion lymphoma. Br J Haematol. 2000;111(4):1112–5.
248. Bossini N, Sandrini S, Setti G, Luppi M, Maiorca P, Maffei C, et al. Successful treatment with liposomal doxorubicin and foscarnet in a patient with widespread Kaposi's sarcoma and human herpes virus 8-related, serious hemophagocytic syndrome, after renal transplantation. G ital Nefrol. 2004;22(3):281–6.
249. Corbellino M, Bestetti G, Scalamogna C, Calattini S, Galazzi M, Meroni L, et al. Long-term remission of Kaposi sarcoma–associated herpesvirus-related multicentric Castleman disease with anti-CD20 monoclonal antibody therapy. Blood. 2001;98(12):3473–5.
250. Tanaka H, Nishimura T, Hakui M, Sugimoto H, Tanaka-Taya K, Yamanishi K. Human herpesvirus 6-associated hemophagocytic syndrome in a healthy adult. Emerg Infect Dis. 2002;8(1):87.
251. Suzuki N, Morimoto A, Ohga S, Kudo K, Ishida Y, Ishii E, et al. Characteristics of hemophagocytic lymphohistiocytosis in neonates: a nationwide survey in Japan. J Pediatr. 2009;155(2):235–8.e1.
252. Whitley R. Neonatal herpes simplex virus infection. Curr Opin Infect Dis. 2004;17(3):243–6.
253. Rittichier KR, Bryan PA, Bassett KE, Taggart EW, Enriquez FR, Hillyard DR, et al. Diagnosis and outcomes of enterovirus infections in young infants. Pediatr Infect Dis J. 2005;24(6):546–50.
254. Albrecht H, Schafer H, Stellbrink H-J, Greten H. Epstein-Barr virus-associated hemophagocytic syndrome. Arch Pathol Lab Med. 1997;121(8):853.
255. Niedt G, Schinella R. Acquired immunodeficiency syndrome. Clinicopathologic study of 56 autopsies. Arch Pathol Lab Med. 1985;109(8):727–34.
256. Sailler L, Duchayne E, Marchou B, Brousset P, Pris J, Massip P, et al. Etiological aspects of reactive hemophagocytoses: retrospective study in 99 patients. Rev Med Interne. 1996;18(11):855–64.
257. Maakaroun NR, Moanna A, Jacob JT, Albrecht H. Viral infections associated with haemophagocytic syndrome. Rev Med Virol. 2010;20(2):93–105.
258. Potter M, Foot A, Oakhill A. Influenza A and the virus associated haemophagocytic syndrome: cluster of three cases in children with acute leukaemia. J Clin Pathol. 1991;44(4):297–9.
259. Imashuku S. Differential diagnosis of hemophagocytic syndrome: underlying disorders and selection of the most effective treatment. Int J Hematol. 1997;66(2):135–51.
260. Cunney RJ, Bialachowski A, Thornley D, Smaill FM, Pennie RA. An outbreak of influenza A in a neonatal intensive care unit. Infect Control Hosp Epidemiol. 2000;21(7):449–54.
261. Ando M, Miyazaki E, Hiroshige S, Ashihara Y, Okubo T, Ueo M, et al. Virus associated hemophagocytic syndrome accompanied by acute respiratory failure caused by influenza A (H3N2). Intern Med. 2006;45(20):1183–6.
262. Deerojanawong J, Prapphal N, Poovorawan Y. Prevalence, clinical presentations and complications among hospitalized children with influenza pneumonia. Jpn J Infect Dis. 2008;61:446–9.
263. To K-F, Chan PK, Chan K-F, Lee W-K, Lam W-Y, Wong K-F, et al. Pathology of fatal human infection associated with avian influenza A H5N1 virus. J Med Virol. 2001;63(3):242–6.
264. Zhang Z, Zhang J, Huang K, Li K-S, Yuen K-Y, Guan Y, et al. Systemic infection of avian influenza A virus H5N1 subtype in humans. Hum Pathol. 2009;40(5):735–9.
265. Kimura K, Adlakha A, Simon PM. Fatal case of swine influenza virus in an immunocompetent host. Mayo Clin Proc. 1998;73(3):243–5.
266. Watanabe T, Okazaki E, Shibuya H. Influenza A virus-associated encephalopathy with haemophagocytic syndrome. Eur J Pediatr. 2003;162(11):799–800.
267. de Jong MD, Cam BV, Qui PT, Hien VM, Thanh TT, Hue NB, et al. Fatal avian influenza A (H5N1) in a child presenting with diarrhea followed by coma. N Engl J Med. 2005;352(7):686–91.
268. Chokephaibulkit K, Uiprasertkul M, Puthavathana P, Chearskul P, Auewarakul P, Dowell SF, et al. A child with avian influenza A (H5N1) infection. Pediatr Infect Dis J. 2005;24(2):162–6.
269. Peiris J, Yu W, Leung C, Cheung C, Ng W, Nicholls JA, et al. Re-emergence of fatal human influenza A subtype H5N1 disease. Lancet. 2004;363(9409):617–9.

270. Cheung CY, Poon LL, Lau AS, Luk W, Lau YL, Shortridge KF, et al. Induction of proinflammatory cytokines in human macrophages by influenza A (H5N1) viruses: a mechanism for the unusual severity of human disease? Lancet. 2002;360(9348):1831–7.
271. Chan PK. Outbreak of avian influenza A (H5N1) virus infection in Hong Kong in 1997. Clin Infect Dis. 2002;34(Suppl 2):S58–64.
272. Ng WF, To KF, Lam WW, Ng TK, Lee KC. The comparative pathology of severe acute respiratory syndrome and avian influenza A subtype H5N1—a review. Hum Pathol. 2006;37(4):381–90.
273. Hsieh SM, Chang SC. Insufficient perforin expression in CD8+ T cells in response to hemagglutinin from avian influenza (H5N1) virus. J Immunol. 2006;176(8):4530–3.
274. Henter JI, Chow CB, Leung CW, Lau YL. Cytotoxic therapy for severe avian influenza A (H5N1) infection. Lancet. 2006;367(9513):870–3.
275. Beigel JH, Farrar J, Han AM, Hayden FG, Hyer R, de Jong MD, et al. Avian influenza A (H5N1) infection in humans. N Engl J Med. 2005;353(13):1374–85.
276. Schulert GS, Zhang M, Fall N, Husami A, Kissell D, Hanosh A, et al. Whole-exome sequencing reveals mutations in genes linked to hemophagocytic lymphohistiocytosis and macrophage activation syndrome in fatal cases of H1N1 influenza. J Infect Dis. 2016;213(7):1180–8.
277. Kaya Z, Ozturk G, Gursel T, Bozdayi G. Spontaneous resolution of hemophagocytic syndrome and disseminated intravascular coagulation associated with parvovirus b19 infection in a previously healthy child. Jpn J Infect Dis. 2005;58(3):149–51.
278. Larroche C, Scieux C, Honderlick P, Piette AM, Morinet F, Bletry O. Spontaneous resolution of hemophagocytic syndrome associated with acute parvovirus B19 infection and concomitant Epstein-Barr virus reactivation in an otherwise healthy adult. Eur J Clin Microbiol Infect Dis. 2002;21(10):739–42.
279. Watanabe M, Shibuya A, Okuno J, Maeda T, Tamama S, Saigenji K. Hepatitis A virus infection associated with hemophagocytic syndrome: report of two cases. Intern Med. 2002;41(12):1188–92.
280. Verma T, Aggarwal S. Childhood tuberculosis presenting with haemophagocytic syndrome. Indian J Hematol Blood Transfus. 2012;28(3):178–80.
281. Yang C, Lee J, Kim Y, Kim P, Lee S, Kim B, et al. Tuberculosis-associated hemophagocytic syndrome in a hemodialysis patient: case report and review of the literature. Nephron. 1996;72(4):690–2.
282. Ruiz-argüelles GJ, Arizpe-Bravo D, Garces-Eisele J, Sanchez-Sosa S, Ruiz-argüelles A, Ponce-de-Leon S. Tuberculosis-associated fatal hemophagocytic syndrome in a patient with lymphoma treated with fludarabine. Leuk Lymphoma. 1998;28(5–6):599–602.
283. Baraldes MA, Domingo P, Gonzalez MJ, Aventin A, Coll P. Tuberculosis-associated hemophagocytic syndrome in patients with acquired immunodeficiency syndrome. Arch Intern Med. 1998;158(2):194–5.
284. Lam K, Ng W, Chan A. Miliary tuberculosis with splenic rupture: a fatal case with hemophagocytic syndrome and possible association with long standing sarcoidosis. Pathology. 1994;26(4):493–6.
285. Cascio A, Pernice L, Barberi G, Delfino D, Biondo C, Beninati C, et al. Secondary hemophagocytic lymphohistiocytosis in zoonoses. A systematic review. Eur Rev Med Pharmacol Sci. 2012;16(10):1324–37.
286. Koduri PR, Chundi V, DeMarais P, Mizock BA, Patel AR, Weinstein RA. Reactive hemophagocytic syndrome: a new presentation of disseminated histoplasmosis in patients with AIDS. Clin Infect Dis. 1995;21(6):1463–5.
287. De Lavaissière M, Manceron V, Bourée P, Garçon L, Bisaro F, Delfraissy J-F, et al. Reconstitution inflammatory syndrome related to histoplasmosis, with a hemophagocytic syndrome in HIV infection. J Infect. 2009;58(3):245–7.
288. Hadchouel M, Prieur A-M, Griscelli C. Acute hemorrhagic, hepatic, and neurologic manifestations in juvenile rheumatoid arthritis: possible relationship to drugs or infection. J Pediatr. 1985;106(4):561–6.
289. Wallace CA, Sherry DD. Trial of intravenous pulse cyclophosphamide and methylprednisolone in the treatment of severe systemic-onset juvenile rheumatoid arthritis. Arthritis Rheum. 1997;40(10):1852–5.
290. Mouy R, Stephan J-L, Pillet P, Haddad E, Hubert P, Prieur A-M. Efficacy of cyclosporine A in the treatment of macrophage activation syndrome in juvenile arthritis: report of five cases. J Pediatr. 1996;129(5):750–4.
291. Ravelli A, De Benedetti F, Viola S, Martini A. Macrophage activation syndrome in systemic juvenile rheumatoid arthritis successfully treated with cyclosporine. J Pediatr. 1996;128(2):275–8.
292. Henter J-I, Samuelsson-Horne A, Arico M, Egeler RM, Elinder G, Filipovich AH, et al. Treatment of hemophagocytic lymphohistiocytosis with HLH-94 immunochemotherapy and bone marrow transplantation. Blood. 2002;100(7):2367–73.
293. Emmenegger U, Spaeth PJ, Neftel KA. Intravenous immunoglobulin for hemophagocytic lymphohistiocytosis? J Clin Oncol. 2002;20(2):599–601.
294. Coca A, Bundy KW, Marston B, Huggins J, Looney RJ. Macrophage activation syndrome: serological markers and treatment with anti-thymocyte globulin. Clin Immunol. 2009;132(1):10–8.
295. Aeberli D, Oertle S, Mauron H, Reichenbach S, Jordi B, Villiger PM. Inhibition of the TNF pathway: use of infliximab and etanercept as remission-inducing agents in cases of therapy-resistant chronic inflammatory disorders. Swiss Med Wkly. 2002;132(29–30):414–22.
296. Emmenegger U, Reimers A, Frey U, Fux C, Bihl F, Semela D, et al. Reactive macrophage activation syndrome: a simple screening strategy and its potential in early treatment initiation. Swiss Med Wkly. 2002;132(17/18):230–6.
297. Henzan T, Nagafuji K, Tsukamoto H, Miyamoto T, Gondo H, Imashuku S, et al. Success with infliximab

in treating refractory hemophagocytic lymphohistiocytosis. Am J Hematol. 2006;81(1):59–61.
298. Maeshima K, Ishii K, Iwakura M, Akamine M, Hamasaki H, Abe I, et al. Adult-onset Still's disease with macrophage activation syndrome successfully treated with a combination of methotrexate and etanercept. Mod Rheumatol. 2012;22(1):137–41.
299. Makay B, Yılmaz Ş, Türkyılmaz Z, Ünal N, Ören H, Ünsal E. Etanercept for therapy-resistant macrophage activation syndrome. Pediatr Blood Cancer. 2008;50(2):419–21.
300. Prahalad S, Bove KE, Dickens D, Lovell DJ, Grom AA. Etanercept in the treatment of macrophage activation syndrome. J Rheumatol. 2001;28(9):2120–4.
301. Sellmer A, Stausbøl-Grøn B, Krag-Olsen B, Herlin T. Successful use of infliximab in macrophage activation syndrome with severe CNS involvement. Scand J Rheumatol. 2011;40(2):156–7.
302. Takahashi N, Naniwa T, Banno S. Successful use of etanercept in the treatment of acute lupus hemophagocytic syndrome. Mod Rheumatol. 2008;18(1):72–5.
303. Verbsky JW, Grossman WJ. Hemophagocytic lymphohistiocytosis: diagnosis, pathophysiology, treatment, and future perspectives. Ann Med. 2006;38(1):20–31.
304. Chauveau E, Terrier F, Casassus-Buihle D, Moncoucy X, Oddes B. Macrophage activation syndrome after treatment with infliximab for fistulated Crohn's disease. Presse Med. 2005;34(8):583–4.
305. Kaneko K, Kaburaki M, Muraoka S, Tanaka N, Yamamoto T, Kusunoki Y, et al. Exacerbation of adult-onset Still's disease, possibly related to elevation of serum tumor necrosis factor-alpha after etanercept administration. Int J Rheum Dis. 2010;13(4):e67–e9.
306. Kimura Y, Pinho P, Walco G, Higgins G, Hummell D, Szer I, et al. Etanercept treatment in patients with refractory systemic onset juvenile rheumatoid arthritis. J Rheumatol. 2005;32(5):935–42.
307. Ramanan AV, Schneider R. Macrophage activation syndrome following initiation of etanercept in a child with systemic onset juvenile rheumatoid arthritis. J Rheumatol. 2003;30(2):401–3.
308. Sandhu C, Chesney A, Piliotis E, Buckstein R, Koren S. Macrophage activation syndrome after etanercept treatment. J Rheumatol. 2007;34(1):241.
309. Sterba G, Sterba Y, Stempel C, Blank J, Azor E, Gomez L. Macrophage activation syndrome induced by etanercept in a patient with systemic sclerosis. Isr Med Assoc J. 2010;12(7):443.
310. Stern A, Riley R, Buckley L. Worsening of macrophage activation syndrome in a patient with adult onset Still's disease after initiation of etanercept therapy. J Clin Rheumatol. 2001;7(4):252–6.
311. Agarwal S, Moodley J, Goel GA, Theil KS, Mahmood SS, Lang RS. A rare trigger for macrophage activation syndrome. Rheumatol Int. 2011;31(3):405–7.
312. Moltó A, Mateo L, Lloveras N, Olivé A, Minguez S. Visceral leishmaniasis and macrophagic activation syndrome in a patient with rheumatoid arthritis under treatment with adalimumab. Joint Bone Spine. 2010;77(3):271–3.
313. Nigrovic PA, Mannion M, Prince FH, Zeft A, Rabinovich CE, Van Rossum MA, et al. Anakinra as first-line disease-modifying therapy in systemic juvenile idiopathic arthritis: report of forty-six patients from an international multicenter series. Arthritis Rheum. 2011;63(2):545–55.
314. Pascual V, Allantaz F, Arce E, Punaro M, Banchereau J. Role of interleukin-1 (IL-1) in the pathogenesis of systemic onset juvenile idiopathic arthritis and clinical response to IL-1 blockade. J Exp Med. 2005;201(9):1479–86.
315. Bruck N, Suttorp M, Kabus M, Heubner G, Gahr M, Pessler F. Rapid and sustained remission of systemic juvenile idiopathic arthritis-associated macrophage activation syndrome through treatment with anakinra and corticosteroids. J Clin Rheumatol. 2011;17(1):23–7.
316. Kelly A, Ramanan AV. A case of macrophage activation syndrome successfully treated with anakinra. Nat Clin Pract Rheumatol. 2008;4(11):615–20.
317. Record JL, Beukelman T, Cron RQ. Combination therapy of abatacept and anakinra in children with refractory systemic juvenile idiopathic arthritis: a retrospective case series. J Rheumatol. 2011;38(1):180–1.
318. Clark SR, McMahon CJ, Gueorguieva I, Rowland M, Scarth S, Georgiou R, et al. Interleukin-1 receptor antagonist penetrates human brain at experimentally therapeutic concentrations. J Cereb Blood Flow Metab. 2008;28(2):387–94.
319. Canna S, Frankovich J, Higgins G, Narkewicz MR, Nash SR, Hollister JR, et al. Acute hepatitis in three patients with systemic juvenile idiopathic arthritis taking interleukin-1 receptor antagonist. Pediatr Rheumatol. 2009;7(1):1.
320. Lurati A, Teruzzi B, Salmaso A, Demarco G, Pontikati I, Gattinara M, et al. Macrophage activation syndrome (MAS) during anti-IL1 receptor therapy (anakinra) in a patient affected by systemic onset idiopathic juvenile arthritis (soJIA): a report and review of the literature. Pediatr Rheumatol Online J. 2005;3(2):79–85.
321. Zeft A, Hollister R, LaFleur B, Sampath P, Soep J, McNally B, et al. Anakinra for systemic juvenile arthritis: the Rocky Mountain experience. J Clin Rheumatol. 2009;15(4):161–4.
322. Yokota S, Imagawa T, Mori M, Miyamae T, Aihara Y, Takei S, et al. Efficacy and safety of tocilizumab in patients with systemic-onset juvenile idiopathic arthritis: a randomised, double-blind, placebo-controlled, withdrawal phase III trial. Lancet. 2008;371(9617):998–1006.
323. Mizutani S, Kuroda J, Shimura Y, Kobayashi T, Tsutsumi Y, Yamashita M, et al. Cyclosporine A for chemotherapy-resistant subcutaneous panniculitis-

like T cell lymphoma with hemophagocytic syndrome. Acta Haematol. 2011;126(1):8–12.

324. Brudno JN, Kochenderfer JN. Toxicities of chimeric antigen receptor T cells: recognition and management. Blood. 2016;127(26):3321–30.
325. Alexeeva EI, Valieva SI, Bzarova TM, Semikina EL, Isaeva KB, Lisitsyn AO, et al. Efficacy and safety of repeat courses of rituximab treatment in patients with severe refractory juvenile idiopathic arthritis. Clin Rheumatol. 2011;30(9):1163–72.
326. Bosman G, Langemeijer SC, Hebeda K, Raemaekers J, Pickkers P, van der Velden W. The role of rituximab in a case of EBV-related lymphoproliferative disease presenting with haemophagocytosis. Neth J Med. 2009;67(8):364–5.
327. Fischer A, Cerf-Bensussan N, Blanche S, Le Deist F, Bremard-Oury C, Leverger G, et al. Allogeneic bone marrow transplantation for erythrophagocytic lymphohistiocytosis. J Pediatr. 1986;108(2):267–70.
328. Baker K, Filipovich A, Gross T, Grossman W, Hale G, Hayashi R, et al. Unrelated donor hematopoietic cell transplantation for hemophagocytic lymphohistiocytosis. Bone Marrow Transplant. 2008;42(3):175–80.
329. Baker KS, DeLaat CA, Steinbuch M, Gross TG, Shapiro RS, Loechelt B, et al. Successful correction of hemophagocytic lymphohistiocytosis with related or unrelated bone marrow transplantation. Blood. 1997;89(10):3857–63.
330. Blanche S, Caniglia M, Girault D, Landman J, Griscelli C, Fischer A. Treatment of hemophagocytic lymphohistiocytosis with chemotherapy and bone marrow transplantation: a single-center study of 22 cases. Blood. 1991;78(1):51–4.
331. Dürken M, Horstmann M, Bieling P, Erttmann R, Kabisch H, Löliger C, et al. Improved outcome in haemophagocytic lymphohistiocytosis after bone marrow transplantation from related and unrelated donors: a single-centre experience of 12 patients. Br J Haematol. 1999;106(4):1052–8.
332. Dürken M, Finckenstein FG, Janka GE. Bone marrow transplantation in hemophagocytic lymphohistiocytosis. Leuk Lymphoma. 2001;41(1–2):89–95.
333. Kobayashi R, Tanaka J, Hashino S, Ota S, Torimoto Y, Kakinoki Y, et al. Etoposide-containing conditioning regimen reduces the occurrence of hemophagocytic lymphohistiocytosis after SCT. Bone Marrow Transplant. 2014;49(2):254–7.
334. Carmo M, Risma KA, Arumugam P, Tiwari S, Hontz AE, Montiel-Equihua CA, et al. Perforin gene transfer into hematopoietic stem cells improves immune dysregulation in murine models of perforin deficiency. Mol Ther. 2015;23(4):737–45.
335. Rivat C, Booth C, Alonso-Ferrero M, Blundell M, Sebire NJ, Thrasher AJ, et al. SAP gene transfer restores cellular and humoral immune function in a murine model of X-linked lymphoproliferative disease. Blood. 2013;121(7):1073–6.
336. Jordan MB, Hildeman D, Kappler J, Marrack P. An animal model of hemophagocytic lymphohistiocytosis (HLH): CD8+ T cells and interferon gamma are essential for the disorder. Blood. 2004;104(3):735–43.
337. Schmid JP, Ho CH, Chrétien F, Lefebvre JM, Pivert G, Kosco-Vilbois M, et al. Neutralization of IFNγ defeats haemophagocytosis in LCMV-infected perforin-and Rab27a-deficient mice. EMBO Mol Med. 2009;1(2):112–24.
338. Bracaglia C, Caiello I, De Graaf K, D'Ario G, Guilhot F, Ferlin W, et al. Interferon-gamma (IFNy) in macrophage activation syndrome (MAS) associated with systemic juvenile idiopathic arthritis (sJIA). High levels in patients and a role in a murine mas model. Pediatr Rheumatol. 2014;12(1):1.
339. Takada H, Takahata Y, Nomura A, Ohga S, Mizuno Y, Hara T. Increased serum levels of interferon-γ-inducible protein 10 and monokine induced by gamma interferon in patients with haemophagocytic lymphohistiocytosis. Clin Exp Immunol. 2003;133(3):448–53.
340. Billiau AD, Roskams T, Van Damme-Lombaerts R, Matthys P, Wouters C. Macrophage activation syndrome: characteristic findings on liver biopsy illustrating the key role of activated, IFN-γ-producing lymphocytes and IL-6-and TNF-α-producing macrophages. Blood. 2005;105(4):1648–51.
341. Science UnLo. 2016. https://clinicaltrials.gov/ct2/show/NCT01818492.
342. Tesi B, Sieni E, Neves C, Romano F, Cetica V, Cordeiro AI, et al. Hemophagocytic lymphohistiocytosis in 2 patients with underlying IFN-[gamma] receptor deficiency. J Allergy Clin Immunol. 2015;135(6):1638.
343. Sikora KA, Fall N, Thornton S, Grom AA. The limited role of interferon-γ in systemic juvenile idiopathic arthritis cannot be explained by cellular hyporesponsiveness. Arthritis Rheum. 2012;64(11):3799–808.
344. Das R, Guan P, Sprague L, Verbist K, Tedrick P, An QA, et al. Janus kinase inhibition lessens inflammation and ameliorates disease in murine models of hemophagocytic lymphohistiocytosis. Blood. 2016;127(13):1666–75.
345. Maschalidi S, Sepulveda FE, Garrigue A, Fischer A, de Saint Basile G. Therapeutic effect of JAK1/2 blockade on the manifestations of hemophagocytic lymphohistiocytosis in mice. Blood. 2016;128(1):60–71. https://doi.org/10.1182/blood-2016-02-700013.
346. Chuang HC, Lay JD, Hsieh WC, Su IJ. Pathogenesis and mechanism of disease progression from hemophagocytic lymphohistiocytosis to Epstein–Barr virus-associated T-cell lymphoma: nuclear factor-κB pathway as a potential therapeutic target. Cancer Sci. 2007;98(9):1281–7.
347. Hsieh W-C, Lan B-S, Chen Y-L, Chang Y, Chuang H-C, Su I-J. Efficacy of peroxisome proliferator activated receptor agonist in the treatment of virus-associated haemophagocytic syndrome in a rabbit model. Antivir Ther. 2010;15(1):71–81.

348. Yang J, Huck SP, McHugh RS, Hermans IF, Ronchese F. Perforin-dependent elimination of dendritic cells regulates the expansion of antigen-specific CD8+ T cells in vivo. Proc Natl Acad Sci U S A. 2006;103(1):147–52.
349. Brisse E, Wouters CH, Matthys P. Hemophagocytic lymphohistiocytosis (HLH): a heterogeneous spectrum of cytokine-driven immune disorders. Cytokine Growth Factor Rev. 2015;26(3):263–80.
350. Favilli F, Anzilotti C, Martinelli L, Quattroni P, De Martino S, Pratesi F, et al. IL-18 activity in systemic lupus erythematosus. Ann N Y Acad Sci. 2009;1173:301–9.
351. Novick D, Elbirt D, Miller G, Dinarello CA, Rubinstein M, Sthoeger ZM. High circulating levels of free interleukin-18 in patients with active SLE in the presence of elevated levels of interleukin-18 binding protein. J Autoimmun. 2010;34(2):121–6.
352. Dinarello CA. Interleukin-18 and the pathogenesis of inflammatory diseases. Semin Nephrol. 2007;27(1):98–114.
353. Chiossone L, Audonnet S, Chetaille B, Chasson L, Farnarier C, Berda-Haddad Y, et al. Protection from inflammatory organ damage in a murine model of hemophagocytic lymphohistiocytosis using treatment with IL-18 binding protein. Front Immunol. 2012;3:239.
354. Canna SW, Girard C, Malle L, de Jesus A, Romberg N, Kelsen J, et al. Life-threatening NLRC4-associated hyperinflammation successfully treated with IL-18 inhibition. J Allergy Clin Immunol. 2017;139(5):1698–701.
355. Palmblad K, Schierbeck H, Sundberg E, Horne AC, Harris HE, Henter JI, et al. High systemic levels of the cytokine-inducing HMGB1 isoform secreted in severe macrophage activation syndrome. Mol Med. 2014;20:538–47.
356. Rood JE, Rao S, Paessler M, Kreiger PA, Chu N, Stelekati E, et al. ST2 contributes to T-cell hyperactivation and fatal hemophagocytic lymphohistiocytosis in mice. Blood. 2016;127(4):426–35.

15 Rheumatoid Arthritis

Matthew L. Stoll, S. Louis Bridges Jr., and Maria I. Danila

Abbreviations

ACPA	Anti-cyclic citrullinated peptide antibody
CRA	Chronic rheumatoid arthritis
DAS	Disease activity score
DC	Dendritic cells
HC	Healthy control
IL	Interleukin
JIA	Juvenile idiopathic arthritis
MMP	Matrix metalloproteinase
NORA	New-onset rheumatoid arthritis
NSAID	Nonsteroidal anti-inflammatory drug
OA	Osteoarthritis
PAD	Peptidylarginine deiminase
PD	Periodontal disease
PPAD	*P. gingivalis* peptidylarginine deiminase
RA	Rheumatoid arthritis
SE	Shared epitope
SRP	Scaling and root planning
TNFi	Tumor necrosis factor inhibitor

M. L. Stoll (✉)
University of Alabama at Birmingham, Department of Pediatrics, Birmingham, AL, USA
e-mail: mstoll@peds.uab.edu

S. L. Bridges Jr.
Division of Clinical Immunology and Rheumatology, Comprehensive Arthritis, Musculoskeletal, Bone, and Autoimmunity Center, UAB, The University of Alabama at Birmingham, Birmingham, AL, USA

M. I. Danila
University of Alabama at Birmingham, Division of Clinical Immunology and Rheumatology, Birmingham, AL, USA

Introduction

The concept that rheumatoid arthritis (RA) could be mediated by infections is more than 100 years old, since Bailey suggested that the disease was likely mediated by bacterial toxins and indicated that the offending bacterium may reside in the gastrointestinal tract [1]. Indeed, the RA infection theory was the rationale for the development of sulfasalazine in the 1940s [2] as well as for several of the early trials evaluating antibiotics as a therapeutic tool (Table 15.1). Over the ensuing decades, the concept that RA was mediated by infections largely fell out of favor, because no single organism was clearly identified using candidate organism approaches. The pendulum has swung back. Beginning with the study by Vaahtovuo et al. [3], multiple investigators have used culture-independent technology to query mucosal populations at several different body surfaces, finding abnormalities that in many cases have been remarkably consistent and which lead to the conclusion that the oral and enteric microbiota predispose to the development of RA and the formation of its hallmark antibody, anti-cyclic citrullinated peptide antibodies (ACPAs).

G. Ragab et al. (eds.), *The Microbiome in Rheumatic Diseases and Infection*,
https://doi.org/10.1007/978-3-319-79026-8_15

Table 15.1 Antibiotic trials in RA. [12–14]

Study	Patient population	Blinding	Dose (n)[a]	Comparator (n)	Duration	Outcome
Antimycobacterials—rifampicin						
Borg et al. [83]	Duration < 12 months, naïve to DMARDs or CS	Unclear	600 mg QD [9]	HCQ 400 mg QD [7]	12 months	Favored HCQ group in multiple markers of disease activity
Fluoroquinolones—levofloxacin						
Ogrendik [84]	On MTX	DB	500 mg daily [38]	PCB [38]	6 months	Favored levofloxacin group in multiple markers of disease activity
Macrolides—clarithromycin						
Ogrendik [85]	Duration < 3 years, failed 1–4 DMARDs	DB	500 mg QD [41]	PCB [40]	6 months	ACR20 24/41 (59%) CM vs 13/40 (33%) PCB, $p < 0.001$
Saviola et al. [86]	Not taking DMARDs	SB	500 mg BID × 14 days, then QD + MTX, prednisone [16]	Placebo + MTX, prednisone [16]	1 month	ACR70 10/16 (62%) CM vs 4/16 (25%) PCB, $p = 0.033$
Macrolides—roxithromycin						
Ogrendik [87]	Duration <1 year, naïve to DMARDs	DB	300 mg QD [16]	PCB [15]	3 months	ACR20 response in 12/16 (75%) roxithromycin vs 3/15 (20%) PCB, $p = 0.002$
Ogrendik and Karagoz [88]	Failed 1–4 DMARDs	DB	300 mg daily [50]	PCB [50]	6 months	ACR20 response in 30/50 (60%) roxithromycin 17/50 (34%) PCB, $p = 0.009$
Tetracyclines—doxycycline						
Sreekanth et al. [89]	Not taking DMARDs	SB	100 mg BID [15]	MTX 7.5 mg weekly [14]	6 months	Non-statistically significant improvement in MTX arm in several markers of active arthritis
St. Clair et al. [90]	Duration 6 months–12 years	DB	200 mg IV daily × 3 weeks, then weekly [10]	PCB [10]	4 weeks	No differences between the groups
Van der Laan et al. [91]	Stable DMARD therapy for ≥10 months	DB, crossover	50 mg BID [48][b]	PCB [18]	36 weeks	No change in a number of markers of active arthritis
Pillemer et al. [92]	Any	DB	300 mg IV daily [10]	PCB IV [13]	12 weeks	ACR50 in 1/10 (10%) doxycycline vs 0/13 with PCB ($p = 0.43$)
O'Dell et al. [75]	Duration <1 year, naïve to DMARDs	DB	100 mg BID [24] or 20 mg BID [18]	Placebo [24]	2 years	ACR50 response in 10/24 (42%) high-dose, 7/18 (39%) low-dose, and 3/24 (12%) PCB, $p = 0.03$
Tetracyclines—minocycline						
Kloppenburg et al. [93]	Failed ≥1 DMARD	DB	100 mg BID [40]	PCB [40]	26 weeks	Favored minocycline in multiple markers of disease activity

Tilley et al. [94]	Failed ≤1 DMARD for inefficacy	DB	50 mg BID [109]	PCB [110]	48 weeks	Improvements in joint swelling (54% vs 39%, $p = 0.023$) and tenderness (56% vs 41%, $p = 0.021$)
O'Dell et al. [95]	Duration <1 year, naïve to DMARDs	DB	100 mg BID [23]	PCB [23]	6 months	Response seen in 15/23 (65%) minocycline vs 3/23 (13%) PCB, $p < 0.001$
O'Dell et al. [96]	Duration <1 year, naïve to DMARDs	DB	100 mg BID [30]	HCQ 200 mg BID [30]	2 years	ACR50 response in 18/30 (60%) minocycline vs 10/30 (33%) HCQ, $p = 0.04$
Tetracyclines—tetracycline						
Skinner et al. [97]	Any	DB	250 mg QD [15]	PCB [15]	54 weeks	No differences between the groups
Tetracyclines plus lincosamides—tetracycline/clindamycin						
Gompels et al. [98]	Duration >6 months, on DMARD	SB	Clindamycin 900 mg IV weekly × 1 month, then q2 weeks + tetracycline 250 mg 3× weekly [11]	No additional therapy [10]	12 months	ACR20 of 5/11 (45%) antibiotics vs 0/10 controls, $p = 0.04$
Smith et al. [99]	Failed ≥1 DMARD	DB	Clindamycin variable dose + tetracycline BID 3× weekly [12]	PCB [8]	25 weeks	ACR20 in 2/12 (17%) antibiotics vs 0/8 PCB, NS
Nitroimidazole—metronidazole						
Harkness et al. [100]	Any	DB	400 mg BID [10]	PCB [10]	6 weeks	No differences in markers of active arthritis
Marshall et al. [101]	Any	DB	400 mg TID [24]	PCB [26]	24 weeks	Improved articular index and pain score in metronidazole completers, but >75% withdrew due to AEs
Nitroimidazole—ornidazole						
Ogrendik et al. [102]	Not specified	Double	1000 mg daily [53] or 500 mg daily [55]	PCB [52]	3 months	Favored both groups of ornidazole in multiple markers of disease activity
Sulfonamides—sulfamethoxazole alone						
Ash et al. [103]	Not taking DMARDs	SB, crossover	2 g daily [23]	PCB [23]	6 months	Favored SFX group in multiple markers of disease activity

(continued)

Table 15.1 (continued)

Study	Patient population	Blinding	Dose (n)[a]	Comparator (n)	Duration	Outcome
Sulfonamides—sulfamethoxazole/trimethoprim						
Wojtulewski et al. [104]	Not taking DMARDs	DB	40 mg/kg BID [24]	Ketoprofen 50 mg TID [23]	8 weeks	No differences between the groups
Sulfonamides—sulfasalazine						
Neumann et al. [105]	No DMARDs in 3 months prior to enrolment	Unclear	2000 mg daily [31]	D-penicillamine 500 mg daily [32]	4 months	SSZ was equivalent to D-penicillamine
Pullar et al. [106]	Naïve to DMARDs	DB	3000 mg daily [30]	PCB [30]	24 weeks	Favored SSZ group in multiple markers of disease activity
Pinals et al. [107]	No DMARDs in 3 months prior to enrolment	DB	1500 mg BID [50]	PCB [36]	15 weeks	Favored SSZ group in multiple markers of disease activity
Williams et al. [108]	Duration >6 months, no DMARDs	DB	500 mg QID [69]	PCB [51]	37 weeks	ITT analysis favored SSZ group over placebo in multiple markers of disease activity
Hannonen et al. [109]	Duration <1 year, naïve to DMARDs	DB	2000 mg daily [38]	PCB [40]	48 weeks	Favored SSZ group in multiple markers of disease activity

[a]All drugs were administered orally unless indicated otherwise

[b]Due to crossover design, not all of the 48 were on the medication for the entire treatment period

BID twice daily, *CM* clarithromycin, *DB* double-blinded, *DMARD* disease-modifying antirheumatic drug, *ITT* intention to treat, *MTX* methotrexate, *NS* not significant, *PCB* placebo, *QD* daily, *QID* four times daily, *SB* single-blinded (assessor only), *SFX* sulfamethoxazole, *SSZ* sulfasalazine, *TID* three times daily

Fecal Microbiota in RA

Multiple studies have evaluated the contents of the fecal microbiota in RA (Table 15.2). There is substantial heterogeneity in the published studies, primarily in the methodology used to identify the bacteria, the geographic location of the subjects, the use of immunomodulatory medications in the RA patients, and the source of the controls. The first three studies to evaluate the microbiota as a whole used fecal culture followed by various analytic techniques to identify anaerobic and aerobic organisms, as well as to identify a limited number of specific organisms through traditional methods [4–6]. These studies were limited in their ability to identify the vast majority of the bacteria present in the intestinal tract, and not surprisingly, few differences emerged. Shinebaum [4] reported increased *C. perfringens* in RA patients, a finding that was subsequently thought to be secondary to the use of nonsteroidal anti-inflammatory drugs (NSAIDs) on the basis of the observation that RA patients and osteoarthritis (OA) patients on NSAIDs had similar burden of this organism and both patient populations had a higher abundance of *C. perfringens* as compared to OA patients not taking NSAIDs [6]. Severijnen reported higher frequency of what was termed "coccoid rods" in RA patients [5]. None of these studies identified any bacteria that were lower in patients.

Although still widely used in clinical medicine, culture is a suboptimal modality to differentiate all of the components of a complex community of bacteria. It is generally cited that only about 20% of intestinal bacteria can be cultured [7]. Although the number may in fact be higher [8], culture and identification is nevertheless a highly labor-intensive approach; it has been estimated that to culture and identify the fecal community of bacteria would take about one person-year of laboratory effort [9]. In contrast, the process of sequencing of 16S ribosomal DNA and its analysis can be completed in a few days.

Thus, as the technology became available, genetic tools were used to compare the fecal microbiota of RA patients and controls. The first such study to do so was published by Vaahtovuo et al. [3]. This study was nevertheless limited by the use of specific genetic probes, rather than pan-bacterial markers that have since become state of the art. In addition, this early study was possibly limited by the use of patients with fibromyalgia as controls, as it has not been established whether their microbiota is representative of healthy adults. They observed four probe sets of bacteria to be reduced in RA ([1] *Bacteroides/Porphyromonas/Prevotella*, [2] *B. fragilis*, [3] *Bifidobacterium*, [4] *Eubacterium rectale–Clostridium coccoides* group) and did not identify any elevated probes. Today, we recognize that inclusion of both *Bacteroides* and *Prevotella* in a single probe set is a limitation, as these two genera constitute two distinct enterotypes, which tend to be inversely correlated with one another [10].

All subsequent studies used either sequencing of the 16S ribosomal DNA, whole-genome sequencing, or a combination of these approaches. As discussed elsewhere (Chap. 3), these approaches constitute far more comprehensive and relatively unbiased approaches to query the microbiota. The first of these metagenomics studies was the groundbreaking work published by Scher and colleagues in 2013 evaluating populations of subjects with new-onset RA (NORA), long-standing or chronic RA (CRA), and healthy controls (HC) [11]. This study also included subjects with psoriatic arthritis, which is the topic of a different chapter (Chap. 18). One of the key findings was a striking increase in the abundance of a single organism, *Prevotella copri*, which had a fecal abundance upwards of 50% in some subjects and greater than 5% in 33/44 (75%) of NORA subjects compared to 6/28 (21%) of HC. Fecal carriage of *P. copri* was higher in RA patients without versus with the shared epitope (SE), a 5 amino acid sequence motif in residues 70–74 of the HLA-DRβ chain (QKRAA, QRRAA, or RRRAA) that is the genetic factor that confers the highest risk for RA susceptibility [12]. This latter finding suggests that the abundance of *P. copri* above a certain threshold may be needed to overcome the lack of genetic predisposition to RA. Interestingly, the abundance of *P. copri* in subjects with CRA was similar to that of healthy controls.

Table 15.2 Fecal microbiota in RA

Study	Methods	Population	Depleted bacteria	Enriched bacteria	Additional findings	Location
Shinebaum et al. [4]	Culture and gram-staining	NORA ($n = 25$), HC ($n = 25$)	None	*Clostridium perfringens*	Associated with disease activity	Edinburgh, UK
Severijnen et al. [5]	Culture and gram-staining	CRA ($n = 10$), HC ($n = 10$)	None	Coccoid rods, aerobic organisms	Differences in aerobes were abrogated when pts on SSZ and d-PCN were removed	Rotterdam, Netherlands
Dearlove et al. [6]	Culture and gram-staining	NORA ($n = 22$), OA ($n = 48$)	None	None	Association with *C. perfringens* likely due to NSAIDs	Harrogate and Leeds, UK
Vaahtovuo et al. [3]	Targeted 16S	NORA ($n = 51$), FM ($n = 40$)	Four probes: [1] *Bacteroides/Porphyromonas/Prevotella*, [2] *B. fragilis*, [3] *Bifidobacterium*, [4] *Eubacterium rectale–Clostridium coccoides* group	None	None	Turku, Finland
Scher et al. [11]	16S and WGS	NORA ($n = 44$), CRA ($n = 26$), HC ($n = 28$)	*Bacteroides*	*Prevotella copri*	NORA patients had lower alpha diversity, depending on measure used	New York City, NY, USA
Zhang et al. [15]	WGS	NORA ($n = 94$), HC ($n = 80$), relatives ($n = 17$)	*K. pneumoniae, Megamonas hypermegale, Sutterella wadsworthensis, Bifidobacterium bifidum*	*Bacteroides, Eggerthella lenta, Clostridium asparagiforme*		Beijing, China
Chen et al. [14]	16S	CRA ($n = 40$), FDR ($n = 15$), HC ($n = 17$)	*Faecalibacterium*	Actinobacteria phylum; *Collinsella* and *Eggerthella*	Lower alpha diversity in CRA patients	Rochester, MN, USA
Maeda et al. [13]	16S	NORA ($n = 17$), HC ($n = 14$)	*None*	*Prevotella copri*		Osaka, Japan

CRA chronic rheumatoid arthritis, *FDR* first-degree relatives, *FM* fibromyalgia, *HC* healthy controls, *NORA* new-onset rheumatoid arthritis, *OA* osteoarthritis, *WGS* whole-genome sequencing

A subsequent study of NORA patients likewise suggested a role for intestinal *P. copri* in the etiopathogenesis of RA. Maeda et al. studied 17 subjects with NORA and 14 HC [13]. Principal component analysis of the sequencing of the 16S rDNA identified four clusters. One dominated by *Prevotella* was comprised only of RA patients. Most of the *Prevotella* sequences aligned closely with *P. copri*, and patients in the *Prevotella* cluster had elevated inflammatory markers when compared to patients in the remaining clusters.

A Chinese study of NORA patients did not identify significant differences in the abundance of fecal *P. copri* between patients and controls, indicating that geographic differences in genetics and diet likely also play important roles in determining microbial contributions to arthritis. In this study, 94 NORA patients and 80 HC underwent metagenomic shotgun sequencing. Taxa abundant in RA patients included *Eggerthella lenta* and *Clostridium asparagiforme*, while those abundant in controls included *Klebsiella pneumoniae*, *Megamonas hypermegale*, *Sutterella wadsworthensis*, and *Bifidobacterium bifidum*. Longitudinal evaluation of treated RA participants showed that baseline levels of some bacteria, particularly those containing certain virulence factors, were predictive of response to therapy. Using repeat specimens from 40 patients following initiation of therapy, the authors showed that changes in the gut microbiota did not correlate very well with response to therapy.

A North American study of CRA patients showed RA patients to be deficient in fecal *Faecalibacterium prausnitzii* and abundant for rare bacteria within the Actinobacteria phylum, primarily *Collinsella* and *Eggerthella* [14]. The latter finding is consistent with the study by Zhang et al. [15]. As discussed elsewhere (Chap. 19) in this textbook, *F. prausnitzii* has been shown to be decreased in adult and pediatric patients with inflammatory bowel disease [16], as well as in children with enthesitis-related arthritis [17, 18]. Its role in arthritis has been attributed to a variety of potential factors, such as its effects of development of regulatory T cells [19] and on the health of the enterocytes [20].

In summary, multiple studies have evaluated the fecal microbiota in RA patients. All of the studies that used sequencing methods to identify bacteria have identified substantial differences between RA patients and controls. Moreover, two of them, despite geographic heterogeneity, demonstrated depletion of *Bacteroides* [3, 11] and two showed increased abundance of *P. copri* [11, 13], findings which have not been observed in patients with CRA [11, 14]. The only exception to these general findings was a study conducted in China, in which *Bacteroides* was enriched in RA patients [15]. Additional commonalities described in this body of work include that two of these studies demonstrated expansion of a rare genus called *Eggerthella* [14, 15]. Finally, both studies that reported on the within-group (alpha) diversity of the samples demonstrated decreased diversity in RA patients, although in one of these studies, this finding was dependent upon the metric used [11, 14].

Several studies provided mechanisms by which the associated bacteria may predispose to arthritis. For example, one of the findings by Chen et al. was that a rare genus within the Actinobacteria phylum, *Collinsella*, was enriched in RA patients [14]. As part of the study, the authors introduced this organism into the collagen-induced arthritis model, finding that addition of *Collinsella* increased the frequency albeit not the severity of arthritis. They also found that mouse dendritic cells (DC) pre-cultured with *Collinsella* demonstrated more robust responses to collagen as compared to DC not cultured with *Collinsella* and that *Collinsella* increased the permeability of the CACO-2 intestinal cell line. Taken together, they proposed that a combination of decreased *Faecalibacterium* and increased *Collinsella* resulted in increased intestinal permeability, potentially permitting microbial components to enter the lamina propria and trigger dysfunctional immunity. Likewise, Scher et al. demonstrated that colonization of antibiotic-depleted mice with *P. copri*, the most abundant organism in their study, resulted in increased colitis induced by dextran sulfate [11]. Maeda et al. used fecal transplant to test the ability of *Prevotella* to induce arthritis in SKG mice injected with zymosan, finding that microbiota containing *Prevotella* were associated with the development of arthritis while microbiota lacking *Prevotella*—whether derived from RA patients or healthy controls—did not [13]. The *Prevotella*-exposed mice also had increased numbers of CD4+ and CD4 + IL-17+ T cells in the large intestine, and T cells derived from regional lymph nodes in these mice showed enhanced Th17 responses compared to T cells derived from mice exposed to control microbiota.

Thus, studies of the fecal microbiota in RA patients indicate expansion of *P. copri* in NORA patients and also show in animal systems that *P. copri* is pro-inflammatory and immunogenic. Pianta et al. demonstrated that *P. copri* is immunogenic in humans as well [21]. They used liquid chromatography mass spectroscopy to identify the peptidome from HLA-DR+ antigen-presenting cells. Among them was a peptide that matched to a portion of a 27-kD protein from *P. copri* (Pc-p27). Production of interferon-gamma following in vitro exposure to this peptide was observed in T cells from 17/40 (42%) of RA patients compared to 0/15 healthy controls and 0/10 patients with Lyme arthritis. Likewise, RA patients demonstrated increased levels of IgA antibodies against both the peptide and whole bacteria, with the levels of these antibodies correlating with those of inflammatory cytokines. Thus, *P. copri* is not only abundant in NORA but also appears to trigger mucosal immune reactions.

While there is compelling evidence that *P. copri* is likely involved in the initiation of RA, there are still multiple unanswered questions. It is not known what drives the expansion of *Prevotella*, nor what factors cause it evidently to return to normal in patients with long-standing disease. Would prevention of this expansion of *P. copri* be able to prevent this disease from starting, and would eradication of *P. copri* be a therapeutic option? The latter seems unlikely, in light of the absence of any studies showing expansion of this organism in patients with long-standing disease. Additionally, if *P. copri* induces mucosal immunity and inflammation, as the study by Scher suggested [11], why is subclinical gut inflammation a rare finding in patients with RA, as compared to patients with spondyloarthritis [22, 23]?

Periodontal Disease and Associated Microbiota in RA

The gut is not the only habitat that has been associated with RA; the oral microbiota may also play an important role in the disease, particularly in the context of periodontal disease (PD). PD is fundamentally an infectious and inflammatory process [24, 25]. An early step in the initiation of PD is the development of a biofilm consisting of oral bacteria. This biofilm permits the expansion of pathogenic organisms, such as *Porphyromonas gingivalis*, that are not ordinarily present on the gingival surface in significant quantities [25]. *P. gingivalis* is a gram-negative anaerobic coccobacillus that can both elude host immune responses and cause local tissue destruction [25]. Deep sequencing of the gingival microbiota revealed that *P. gingivalis* is only present in subjects with PD, even among RA patients [26]. The host responds to the microbial challenge by generating an immunologic response, consisting of various innate and adaptive mediators of inflammation. This results in plaque formation and local gingival inflammation. As this progresses, the connective tissue attachment to the tooth is damaged, followed by the development of bone destruction [24]. Treatment of periodontitis typically consists of a procedure called scaling and root planning (SRP), which consists of physical removal of the plaque, which is the nidus of the inflammatory process [27].

There is abundant epidemiologic evidence of an association between RA and PD [26, 28–31]. For example, a cross-sectional study conducted through the National Health and Nutrition Examination Survey III consisting of 4461 North American participants showed that RA patients were more likely to have PD compared to those without RA (OR 1.82 following adjustment for multiple potential confounders, including smoking status, 95% CI 1.04–3.20) [28]. Likewise, a cross-sectional study of 852 non-smoking adults in India referred for periodontal evaluation showed an incidence of RA of 4.4%, compared to 1% in the general population [29]. Small studies have found such an association as well [26, 30, 31], including those that were limited to patients with newly diagnosed disease [26, 31].

There are many potential explanations for this association. One potential association is that this reflects confounding by cigarette smoking. That is, cigarette smoking is a well-known risk factor for RA [32] and is also a risk factor for PD [33], so the association between RA and PD could potentially reflect confounding by the shared risk factor of cigarette smoking. Arguing against this possibility is that the large studies discussed above took smoking into account, either through statistical adjustment [28] or by excluding smokers [29], yet the association holds. Furthermore, as discussed below, it is plausible that cigarette smoking is not simply a shared risk factor for PD and RA, but drives the increased risk of RA through the intermediary of PD.

Another potential mechanism accounting for the association between PD and RA is the possibility that oral microbiota might end up in the synovium, triggering a local inflammatory process. For example, Reichert et al. found genetic material from *P. gingivalis* in the synovium of 7/42 (16.7%) of RA patients vs 4/114 (3.5%) of HC, $p = 0.009$ [34]. However, this does not appear to be a specific finding, as similar organisms were also observed in the synovium of subjects with OA [35], and others have found that bacterial DNA as a whole is present in subjects with a variety of disorders [36–39]. It was suggested that this finding reflects non-specific trapping of killed bacteria by inflamed joints [40].

A third potential mechanism is that the arthritic process, and its therapy, may contribute to PD. That is, the immunosuppressive therapy of RA might predispose to the bacterial overgrowth that defines PD, or the decreased mobility of the hand and wrist resulting from the disease process in RA could impair oral hygiene, thus contributing to PD. This explanation would not entirely account for the findings of severe PD in patients with NORA [26, 31], nor for data showing that antibodies again *P. gingivalis* develop prior to the development of symptoms associated with RA [41]. More importantly, the possibility that active RA results in PD would not account for the findings reported in several prospective studies, in which periodontal therapy consisting of SRP has been shown to be therapeutic for RA [42–45]. In open-label studies, Erciyas et al. reported improved Disease Activity Score (DAS) levels and inflammatory markers among 60 subjects with mild or moderate RA who underwent SRP [42]; Biyikoglu et al. reported improved DAS and inflammatory markers among the 10 of 15 RA patients who underwent SRP and completed the study [43]; and Ribeiro et al. observed improved ESR among 22 subjects with RA who underwent SRP, but not in a parallel albeit not evidently randomized group of 16 subjects who underwent dental cleaning alone [44]. Although these open-label studies were not without biases in their design and analysis, similar findings were reported in a randomized study published by Ortiz et al. [45]. In this study, 40 subjects with active RA on stable therapy and severe PD were randomized to receive treatment for the latter versus no additional care, stratifying for baseline use of tumor necrosis factor inhibitor (TNFi) therapy in 20 of the subjects. They found substantial improvements in multiple clinical and laboratory markers of RA regardless of background TNFi use in the SRP arm.

A fourth potential mechanism accounting for the link between PD and RA is that as PD is an inflammatory process, PD and RA may reflect similar immunoregulatory environments that therefore might tend to co-occur in the same population, not unlike the associations between spondyloarthritis and inflammatory bowel disease or psoriasis. This possibility is supported by shared genetics between RA and PD, particularly among HLA-DRB1 alleles containing the SE [46]. There are multiple schema for classifying HLA-DRB1 risk alleles in RA but studies have largely shifted to analysis of amino acid residues rather than alleles. Amino acid residues encoded at positions 11, 71, and 74 in HLA-DRB1 are thought to be most important in RA risk [47]. To our knowledge, the association between PD and the SE at the amino acid level has yet to be explored. Additional evidence for shared pathophysiologic mechanisms between RA and PD includes other genetic susceptibility factors [48], as well as findings that inflammation in periodontal tissue is mediated at least in part by cytokines such as interleukin (IL)-1, IL-6, and TNF, that have become therapeutic targets in RA [49]. However, the possibility that these shared mechanisms account for the association between PD and RA ultimately fail to account for the findings discussed above that treatment of PD results in improved clinical parameters in RA.

A fifth mechanism is that *P. gingivalis* may itself be the target of the immune system in RA. Several studies in patients with RA have shown elevated IgG antibodies directed against *P. gingivalis* [50–54]. However, other studies have reported contradictory findings [26, 55, 56], and the presence of these antibodies may reflect that this organism is present in the context of an inflammatory milieu without necessarily being pathogenic. Thus, although it is certainly plausible that there may be heterogeneity in the disease, with such antibodies contributing to the disease process in a subset of patients, the role of these antibodies in the pathogenesis of RA requires further study.

Finally, the association between PD and RA may be mediated by *P. gingivalis*, (the "2-hit" model of RA pathogenesis). According to this model, *P. gingivalis* contributes to RA through citrullination of proteins via its peptidylarginine deiminase (PAD) enzyme, resulting in the development of ACPAs [57]. ACPAs serve as diagnostic markers for RA, and third-generation ACPA assays have sensitivity ranging from 61.3 to 82.9 and specificity ranging from 93 to 97.6 for the diagnosis of RA [58]. Human proteins are not typically citrullinated. However, the PAD enzyme in humans and *P. gingivalis* converts the amino acid arginine into citrulline residues. Humans encode five PAD isotypes (PAD1-PAD4, and PAD6), of which PAD2 and PAD4 have been found in the synovial tissue and fluid of persons with RA, which may be a site where the citrullination occurs [59–61]. The significance of PAD in RA is underscored by studies showing that the PAD4 locus is associated with a ~ 2-fold risk of RA in a variety of populations [62–65]. *P. gingivalis* carries its own version of PAD (known as *P. gingivalis* PAD, or PPAD), possibly the only bacterial species that does so [66]. PPAD is capable of citrullinating human proteins [57]. There are several lines of evidence that this citrullination process may be directly pathogenic for the disease, rather than a bystander phenomenon. One is that in the collagen-induced arthritis model of RA, infection with *P. gingivalis* results in earlier onset and increased severity of the disease, findings that are abrogated if the *P. gingivalis* lacks PPAD [67]. Also, in the same model, tolerization with citrulline-containing peptides prior to induction of arthritis resulted in less disease severity and lower production of anti-CCP antibodies [68]. It is therefore of particular interest that cigarette smoking is associated only with anti-CCP+ RA [32], consistent with the possibility that cigarette smoking contributes to RA by inducing periodontitis. Of note, this association between *P. gingivalis* and RA may be limited to CCP+ disease, which is strongly associated with the major histocompatibility complex, particularly the SE [69, 70]. In contrast, *P. copri* appears to be more strongly linked to RA patients lacking the SE [11], who are often CCP-. *Thus, the pathophysiology of these two subsets of RA may be different, which clearly could have implications with respect to diagnosis and treatment.*

To summarize, multiple explanations for the association between PD and RA have been proposed. The model that arguably is best supported by the data is that PD is mediated in large part by a limited set of organisms, one of which is *P. gingivalis*. This species has the unique capacity to citrullinate human proteins, which when modified are targeted by the immune system to form ACPAs, the hallmark antibody of RA. Cigarette smoking may play into this association largely by increasing the risk of PD, thus accounting for its association with anti-CCP+, but not anti-CCP-, RA. The most important clinical implication of this theory is that treatment of PD appears to result in improvement in the RA disease process. This model is shown in Fig. 15.1.

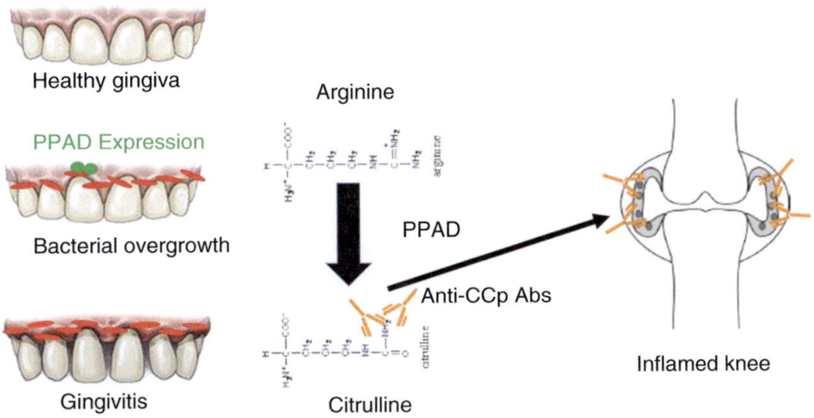

Fig. 15.1 Overgrowth of pathogenic bacteria such as *P. gingivalis* (red) occurs in the gingiva, resulting in inflamed tissue. This bacterial overgrowth is associated with expression of PPAD, which converts the amino acid arginine into citrulline. Antibodies against citrulline (anti-CCPs) then deposit in synovial tissue, resulting in arthritis

Additional Microbiomes in RA

As detailed above, much of the literature on the microbiota in RA has centered on the enteric or gingival microbiota. One other habitat that may be relevant is the lung. Interstitial lung disease is common in RA patients [71], indicating that the lungs may be a source of inflammation. Perhaps due to relative inaccessibility, the microbiota of the lungs has not been studied extensively. Recently, Scher and colleagues performed bronchial alveolar lavage on 20 patients with NORA, 12 healthy controls, and 10 patients with sarcoidosis [72]. The RA patients demonstrated decreased alpha diversity and depletion of several families, such as Burkholderiaceae, Actinomycetaceae, and Spirochaetaceae. However, similar findings were seen in the patients with sarcoidosis, and principal coordinates analysis showed that the sarcoidosis and RA patients clustered together, apart from the controls. Thus, Scher concluded that these findings may reflect an inflammatory lung, rather than a specific RA, phenotype. This stands in contrast to the gut microbiota studies, where several of the findings—particularly the outgrowth of *P. copri*—appear to be unique to RA [11].

One final habitat that was evaluated in a single study is the salivary microbiota. Note that these results cannot be compared with those of the gingival microbiota, as these are two fairly distinct habitats [73]. Counterintuitively, Zhang et al. found *P. gingivalis* among multiple other organisms to be depleted in the saliva of NORA patients, while several species of *Prevotella* were elevated in the RA saliva [15]. Interestingly, the same study also found several species of *Prevotella* to be elevated in the control gingival plaques. Partial normalization of the oral microbiota was observed following introduction of immunosuppressive therapy.

Therapeutic Alterations of the Microbiota

Antibiotics

There have been numerous controlled studies of antibiotics as potential therapeutic agents in RA. As summarized in Table 15.1, this benefit was seen in multiple different classes of antibiotics, including fluoroquinolones, tetracyclines (minocycline > doxycycline, tetracycline), and sulfa antibiotics, including but not limited to sulfasalazine. The effectiveness of antibiotics may not necessarily be attributable to their antimicrobial activity, as many of them particularly the tetracyclines may contain intrinsic anti-inflammatory activity, such as inhibition of matrix metalloproteinases (MMPs) [74]. Indeed,

O'Dell and colleagues suggested that the effectiveness of low-dose doxycycline in one study proved that the mechanism was through inhibition of MMPs [75], although none of these studies included an assessment of the microbiota. It has also been proposed that the effectiveness of tetracyclines and sulfa drugs is due to their ability to eradicate oral pathogens [40]. As we learn more about potential microbial contributing factors to RA, the possibility that antibiotics were effective due at least in part to antimicrobial activity becomes increasingly plausible. Whatever the mechanism of effectiveness, antibiotics are generally not considered optimal long-term therapy, due to risks such as resistance to antibiotics and development of *Clostridium difficile* colitis. The key perhaps is to find means of altering the microbiota that do not carry the risks associated with antibiotics. For example, as discussed above, specific therapy of periodontal disease appears to be effective therapy for RA [45] perhaps by eradicating *P. gingivalis*, an approach that has a better safety profile than long-term use of antibiotics.

Probiotics

There have been four small sample size RCTs of probiotics in RA (Table 15.3). A fifth study was published [76] but appears to be duplicative of one of the other four [77]. Although two of them reported positive findings, these effects were minimal. For example, Mandel et al. [78] reported efficacy on the basis of small effect sizes and non-statistically significant findings such as improved patient-reported ability to participate in daily activities in 4/22 (18%) in the probiotic arm as compared to 2/22 (9.1%) in the placebo arm, $p = 0.53$. Likewise, after excluding 14 of 60 subjects from the analysis due to failure to follow the protocol, Alipour et al. [77] reported that the swollen joint count decreased from a mean (25th–75th percentiles) of 0 (0–2) to 0 (0–1) in the intervention group, compared to a decrease in the placebo group from 1 (0–1.75) to 1 (0–1.75); the between-group p-value was not reported. They did, however, report that patients given the probiotic were more likely to have a EULAR response (8/22 [36%] vs 1/24 [4.2%], $p = 0.007$) as well as significantly lower inflammatory cytokine levels in the probiotic group. Overall, however, the effects of probiotics in RA appear to be small at best. As will be discussed in the individualized medicine chapter (Chap. 35), there are multiple reasons for this lack of substantial effects, including failure of the probiotic to alter the microbiota or the selection of the wrong probiotic.

Diet

Although dietary therapies can rapidly alter the microbiota [79, 80] dietary therapy has also not been found to be a successful therapeutic approach for RA. A Cochrane review evaluated

Table 15.3 Probiotic trials in RA

Study	*n*	Probiotic	Duration	Outcome
Hatakka et al. [110]	21	LGG	12 months	No statistically significant differences in a variety of clinical and immunologic parameters
Mandel et al. [78]	45	BC	60 days	ACR20 attained by 8/22 (36%) completers of BC vs 6/22 (27%) completers of placebo, *p*-value not provided. No statistically significant differences in a variety of patient-reported outcomes or laboratory values
Pineda et al. [111]	29	LR	90 days	ACR20 attained by 3/15 (20%) probiotic vs 1/14 (14%) placebo ($p = 0.33$)
Alipour et al. [77]	60[a]	LC	8 weeks	Very minimal improvements favoring probiotic

[a]Out of 60 initial participants, only 46 were analyzed; the other 14 were excluded due to not following the protocol
BC Bacillus coagulans, *LC Lactobacillus casei*, *LGG Lactobacillus rhamnosus* GG, *LR Lactobacillus reuteri* RC-14 and *Lactobacillus rhamnosus* GR-1 (both administered)

15 controlled dietary intervention studies in RA, including vegetarian, elemental, vegan, and Mediterranean diets [81]. There were no consistent benefits observed. The vegetarian and Mediterranean diets resulted in decreased pain, but no improvements in function or objective findings. Other interventions likewise failed to show substantial effects. The authors also noted substantial dropout in the treatment arms, which they attributed to diet unpalatability. The failure of some of these studies may pertain to some of them evidently being carbohydrate-rich diets, which might have the effect of increasing the abundance of *Prevotella* [79], which as noted above may not be optimal in patients with RA. Clearly, future interventions must be targeted towards eradicating known dysbiosis. An additional factor to consider is that a patient's baseline microbiota may influence response to dietary therapy [82] and thus may need to be assessed as part of the intervention.

Concluding Remarks

Over 100 years ago, RA was considered to be an infectious disease. By the late twentieth century, this hypothesis had fallen out of favor, even though some clinical trials of antibiotics showed effectiveness. Currently, there is accumulating evidence that there are infectious triggers to RA. That two geographically distinct studies of newly diagnosed subjects with RA have both shown an abundance of *P. copri* in their intestines [11, 13], particularly in light of the data showing the same organism to be an immunologic target in RA [21], is highly suggestive that this organism may be part of the pathogenesis of the disease. Given that its abundance appears to be normal in established disease [11, 14], it remains to be seen whether attempts to target this organism therapeutically might bear fruit. In contrast, the gingival microbiota, particularly in patients with severe periodontal disease, appears to be a worthwhile therapeutic target. Whether antibiotics are effective due to their ability to eradicate oral pathogens is unclear, and few would advocate chronic use of antibiotics in light of the array of medications available today. However, just as routine screening of the eyes is part of the management of children with JIA, perhaps routine screening of the gingiva should be part of the care of RA patients, with appropriate local therapy as needed.

References

1. Bailey CF. The treatment of chronic rheumatic and rheumatoid arthritis by radiant heat and cataphoresis. Br Med J. 1909;1:13–5.
2. Mayberry J. The history of 5-ASA compounds and their use in ulcerative colitis--trailblazing discoveries in gastroenterology. J Gastrointestin Liver Dis. 2013;22:375–7.
3. Vaahtovuo J, Munukka E, Korkeamaki M, Luukkainen R, Toivanen P. Fecal microbiota in early rheumatoid arthritis. J Rheumatol. 2008;35:1500–5.
4. Shinebaum R, Neumann VC, Cooke EM, Wright V. Comparison of faecal florae in patients with rheumatoid arthritis and controls. Br J Rheumatol. 1987;26:329–33.
5. Severijnen AJ, Kool J, Swaak AJ, Hazenberg MP. Intestinal flora of patients with rheumatoid arthritis: induction of chronic arthritis in rats by cell wall fragments from isolated Eubacterium aerofaciens strains. Br J Rheumatol. 1990;29:433–9.
6. Dearlove SM, Barr K, Neumann V, Isdale A, Bird HA, Gooi HC, et al. The effect of non-steroidal anti-inflammatory drugs on faecal flora and bacterial antibody levels in rheumatoid arthritis. Br J Rheumatol. 1992;31(7):443.
7. Eckburg PB, Bik EM, Bernstein CN, Purdom E, Dethlefsen L, Sargent M, et al. Diversity of the human intestinal microbial flora. Science. 2005;308:1635–8.
8. Goodman AL, Kallstrom G, Faith JJ, Reyes A, Moore A, Dantas G, et al. Extensive personal human gut microbiota culture collections characterized and manipulated in gnotobiotic mice. Proc Natl Acad Sci U S A. 2011;108:6252–7.
9. Toivanen P. Normal intestinal microbiota in the aetiopathogenesis of rheumatoid arthritis. Ann Rheum Dis. 2003;62:807–11.
10. Arumugam M, Raes J, Pelletier E, Le Paslier D, Yamada T, Mende DR, et al. Enterotypes of the human gut microbiome. Nature. 2011;473:174–80.
11. Scher JU, Sczesnak A, Longman RS, Segata N, Ubeda C, Bielski C, et al. Expansion of intestinal Prevotella copri correlates with enhanced susceptibility to arthritis. Elife. 2013;2:e01202.
12. Gregersen PK, Silver J, Winchester RJ. The shared epitope hypothesis. An approach to understanding the molecular genetics of susceptibility to rheumatoid arthritis. Arthritis Rheum. 1987;30:1205–13.

13. Maeda Y, Kurakawa T, Umemoto E, Motooka D, Ito Y, Gotoh K, et al. Dysbiosis contributes to arthritis development via activation of autoreactive T cells in the intestine. Arthritis Rheumatol. 2016;68(11):2646–61.
14. Chen J, Wright K, Davis JM, Jeraldo P, Marietta EV, Murray J, et al. An expansion of rare lineage intestinal microbes characterizes rheumatoid arthritis. Genome Med. 2016;8:43.
15. Zhang X, Zhang D, Jia H, Feng Q, Wang D, Liang D, et al. The oral and gut microbiomes are perturbed in rheumatoid arthritis and partly normalized after treatment. Nat Med. 2015;21:895–905.
16. Cao Y, Shen J, Ran ZH. Association between Faecalibacterium prausnitzii reduction and inflammatory bowel disease: a meta-analysis and systematic review of the literature. Gastroenterol Res Pract. 2014;2014:872725.
17. Stoll ML, Kumar R, Morrow CD, Lefkowitz EJ, Cui X, Genin A, et al. Altered microbiota associated with abnormal humoral immune responses to commensal organisms in enthesitis-related arthritis. Arthritis Res Ther. 2014;16:486.
18. Di Paola M, Cavalieri D, Albanese D, Sordo M, Pindo M, Donati C, et al. Alteration of Fecal Microbiota profiles in juvenile idiopathic arthritis. Associations with HLA-B27 allele and disease status. Front Microbiol. 2016;7:1703.
19. Smith PM, Howitt MR, Panikov N, Michaud M, Gallini CA, Bohlooly YM, et al. The microbial metabolites, short-chain fatty acids, regulate colonic Treg cell homeostasis. Science. 2013;341:569–73.
20. Hamer HM, Jonkers D, Venema K, Vanhoutvin S, Troost FJ, Brummer RJ. Review article: the role of butyrate on colonic function. Aliment Pharmacol Ther. 2008;27:104–19.
21. Pianta A, Arvikar S, Strle K, Drouin EE, Wang Q, Costello CE, et al. Evidence for immune relevance of Prevotella copri, a gut microbe, in patients with rheumatoid arthritis. Arthritis Rheumatol. 2016;69(5):964–75.
22. Cuvelier C, Barbatis C, Mielants H, De Vos M, Roels H, Veys E. Histopathology of intestinal inflammation related to reactive arthritis. Gut. 1987;28:394–401.
23. Hindryckx P, Laukens D, Serry G, Van Praet L, Cuvelier C, Mielants H, et al. Subclinical gut inflammation in spondyloarthritis is associated with a pro-angiogenic intestinal mucosal phenotype. Ann Rheum Dis. 2011;70:2044–8.
24. Cekici A, Kantarci A, Hasturk H, Van Dyke TE. Inflammatory and immune pathways in the pathogenesis of periodontal disease. Periodontology 2000. 2014;64:57–80.
25. Bingham CO 3rd, Moni M. Periodontal disease and rheumatoid arthritis: the evidence accumulates for complex pathobiologic interactions. Curr Opin Rheumatol. 2013;25:345–53.
26. Scher JU, Ubeda C, Equinda M, Khanin R, Buischi Y, Viale A, et al. Periodontal disease and the oral microbiota in new-onset rheumatoid arthritis. Arthritis Rheum. 2012;64(10):3083–94.
27. Scaling HD. Root planning is recommended in the nonsurgical treatment of chronic periodontitis. J Evid Based Dent Pract. 2016;16:56–8.
28. de Pablo P, Dietrich T, McAlindon TE. Association of periodontal disease and tooth loss with rheumatoid arthritis in the US population. J Rheumatol. 2008;35:70–6.
29. Dev YP, Khuller N, Basavaraj P, Suresh G. Rheumatoid Arthritis among periodontitis patients in Baddi industrial Estate of Himachal Pradesh, India: a cross sectional study. J Clin Diagnos Res. 2013;7:2334–7.
30. Joseph R, Rajappan S, Nath SG, Paul BJ. Association between chronic periodontitis and rheumatoid arthritis: a hospital-based case-control study. Rheumatol Int. 2013;33:103–9.
31. Wolff B, Berger T, Frese C, Max R, Blank N, Lorenz HM, et al. Oral status in patients with early rheumatoid arthritis: a prospective, case-control study. Rheumatology (Oxford). 2014;53:526–31.
32. Klareskog L, Stolt P, Lundberg K, Kallberg H, Bengtsson C, Grunewald J, et al. A new model for an etiology of rheumatoid arthritis: smoking may trigger HLA-DR (shared epitope)-restricted immune reactions to autoantigens modified by citrullination. Arthritis Rheum. 2006;54:38–46.
33. Kinane DF, Chestnutt IG. Smoking and periodontal disease. Crit Rev Oral Biol Med. 2000;11:356–65.
34. Reichert S, Haffner M, Keysser G, Schafer C, Stein JM, Schaller HG, et al. Detection of oral bacterial DNA in synovial fluid. J Clin Periodontol. 2013;40:591–8.
35. Temoin S, Chakaki A, Askari A, El-Halaby A, Fitzgerald S, Marcus RE, et al. Identification of oral bacterial DNA in synovial fluid of patients with arthritis with native and failed prosthetic joints. J Clin Rheumatol. 2012;18:117–21.
36. Johnson S, Sidebottom D, Bruckner F, Collins D. Identification of mycoplasma fermentans in synovial fluid samples from arthritis patients with inflammatory disease. J Clin Microbiol. 2000;38:90–3.
37. Johnson SM, Bruckner F, Collins D. Distribution of mycoplasma pneumoniae and mycoplasma salivarium in the synovial fluid of arthritis patients. J Clin Microbiol. 2007;45:953–7.
38. Wilkinson NZ, Kingsley GH, Jones HW, Sieper J, Braun J, Ward ME. The detection of DNA from a range of bacterial species in the joints of patients with a variety of arthritides using a nested, broad-range polymerase chain reaction. Rheumatology (Oxford). 1999;38:260–6.
39. van der Heijden IM, Wilbrink B, Tchetverikov I, Schrijver IA, Schouls LM, Hazenberg MP, et al. Presence of bacterial DNA and bacterial peptidoglycans in joints of patients with rheumatoid arthritis and other arthritides. Arthritis Rheum. 2000;43:593–8.

40. Sandhya P, Danda D, Sharma D, Scaria V. Does the buck stop with the bugs?: an overview of microbial dysbiosis in rheumatoid arthritis. Int J Rheum Dis. 2016;19:8–20.
41. Johansson L, Sherina N, Kharlamova N, Potempa B, Larsson B, Israelsson L, et al. Concentration of antibodies against Porphyromonas gingivalis is increased before the onset of symptoms of rheumatoid arthritis. Arthritis Res Ther. 2016;18:201.
42. Erciyas K, Sezer U, Ustun K, Pehlivan Y, Kisacik B, Senyurt SZ, et al. Effects of periodontal therapy on disease activity and systemic inflammation in rheumatoid arthritis patients. Oral Dis. 2013;19:394–400.
43. Biyikoglu B, Buduneli N, Aksu K, Nalbantsoy A, Lappin DF, Evrenosoglu E, et al. Periodontal therapy in chronic periodontitis lowers gingival crevicular fluid interleukin-1beta and DAS28 in rheumatoid arthritis patients. Rheumatol Int. 2013;33:2607–16.
44. Ribeiro J, Leao A, Novaes AB. Periodontal infection as a possible severity factor for rheumatoid arthritis. J Clin Periodontol. 2005;32:412–6.
45. Ortiz P, Bissada NF, Palomo L, Han YW, Al-Zahrani MS, Panneerselvam A, et al. Periodontal therapy reduces the severity of active rheumatoid arthritis in patients treated with or without tumor necrosis factor inhibitors. J Periodontol. 2009;80:535–40.
46. Bonfil JJ, Dillier FL, Mercier P, Reviron D, Foti B, Sambuc R, et al. A "case control" study on the role of HLA DR4 in severe periodontitis and rapidly progressive periodontitis. Identification of types and subtypes using molecular biology (PCR.SSO). J Clin Periodontol. 1999;26:77–84.
47. Raychaudhuri S, Sandor C, Stahl EA, Freudenberg J, Lee HS, Jia X, et al. Five amino acids in three HLA proteins explain most of the association between MHC and seropositive rheumatoid arthritis. Nat Genet. 2012;44:291–6.
48. Schaefer AS, Jochens A, Dommisch H, Graetz C, Jockel-Schneider Y, Harks I, et al. A large candidate-gene association study suggests genetic variants at IRF5 and PRDM1 to be associated with aggressive periodontitis. J Clin Periodontol. 2014;41:1122–31.
49. Preshaw PM, Taylor JJ. How has research into cytokine interactions and their role in driving immune responses impacted our understanding of periodontitis? J Clin Periodontol. 2011;38(Suppl 11):60–84.
50. Okada M, Kobayashi T, Ito S, Yokoyama T, Komatsu Y, Abe A, et al. Antibody responses to periodontopathic bacteria in relation to rheumatoid arthritis in Japanese adults. J Periodontol. 2011;82:1433–41.
51. Ogrendik M, Kokino S, Ozdemir F, Bird PS, Hamlet S. Serum antibodies to oral anaerobic bacteria in patients with rheumatoid arthritis. MedGenMed. 2005;7:2.
52. Mikuls TR, Payne JB, Reinhardt RA, Thiele GM, Maziarz E, Cannella AC, et al. Antibody responses to Porphyromonas gingivalis (P. Gingivalis) in subjects with rheumatoid arthritis and periodontitis. Int Immunopharmacol. 2009;9:38–42.
53. Kharlamova N, Jiang X, Sherina N, Potempa B, Israelsson L, Quirke AM, et al. Antibodies to Porphyromonas gingivalis indicate interaction between oral infection, smoking, and risk genes in rheumatoid arthritis Etiology. Arthritis Rheumatol. 2016;68:604–13.
54. Hitchon CA, Chandad F, Ferucci ED, Willemze A, Ioan-Facsinay A, van der Woude D, et al. Antibodies to porphyromonas gingivalis are associated with anticitrullinated protein antibodies in patients with rheumatoid arthritis and their relatives. J Rheumatol. 2010;37:1105–12.
55. Mikuls TR, Payne JB, Yu F, Thiele GM, Reynolds RJ, Cannon GW, et al. Periodontitis and Porphyromonas gingivalis in patients with rheumatoid arthritis. Arthritis Rheumatol. 2014;66:1090–100.
56. Seror R, Le Gall-David S, Bonnaure-Mallet M, Schaeverbeke T, Cantagrel A, Minet J, et al. Association of anti-porphyromonas gingivalis antibody Titers with Nonsmoking status in early rheumatoid arthritis: results from the prospective French cohort of patients with early rheumatoid arthritis. Arthritis Rheumatol. 2015;67:1729–37.
57. Wegner N, Wait R, Sroka A, Eick S, Nguyen KA, Lundberg K, et al. Peptidylarginine deiminase from Porphyromonas gingivalis citrullinates human fibrinogen and alpha-enolase: implications for autoimmunity in rheumatoid arthritis. Arthritis Rheum. 2010;62:2662–72.
58. Taylor P, Gartemann J, Hsieh J, Creeden J. A systematic review of serum biomarkers anti-cyclic citrullinated peptide and rheumatoid factor as tests for rheumatoid arthritis. Autoimmune Dis. 2011;2011:815038.
59. Foulquier C, Sebbag M, Clavel C, Chapuy-Regaud S, Al Badine R, Mechin MC, et al. Peptidyl arginine deiminase type 2 (PAD-2) and PAD-4 but not PAD-1, PAD-3, and PAD-6 are expressed in rheumatoid arthritis synovium in close association with tissue inflammation. Arthritis Rheum. 2007;56:3541–53.
60. Chang X, Yamada R, Suzuki A, Sawada T, Yoshino S, Tokuhiro S, et al. Localization of peptidylarginine deiminase 4 (PADI4) and citrullinated protein in synovial tissue of rheumatoid arthritis. Rheumatology (Oxford). 2005;44:40–50.
61. Kinloch A, Lundberg K, Wait R, Wegner N, Lim NH, Zendman AJ, et al. Synovial fluid is a site of citrullination of autoantigens in inflammatory arthritis. Arthritis Rheum. 2008;58:2287–95.
62. Suzuki A, Yamada R, Chang X, Tokuhiro S, Sawada T, Suzuki M, et al. Functional haplotypes of PADI4, encoding citrullinating enzyme peptidylarginine deiminase 4, are associated with rheumatoid arthritis. Nat Genet. 2003;34:395–402.
63. Poor G, Nagy ZB, Schmidt Z, Brozik M, Meretey K, Gergely P Jr. Genetic background of anticyclic citrullinated peptide autoantibody production in Hungarian patients with rheumatoid arthritis. Ann N Y Acad Sci. 2007;1110:23–32.

64. Du Y, Liu X, Guo JP, Liu X, Li R, Zhao Y, et al. Association between PADI4 gene polymorphisms and anti-cyclic citrullinated peptide antibody positive rheumatoid arthritis in a large Chinese Han cohort. Clin Exp Rheumatol. 2014;32:377–82.
65. Yamamoto K, Yamada R. Genome-wide single nucleotide polymorphism analyses of rheumatoid arthritis. J Autoimmun. 2005;25(Suppl):12–5.
66. Gabarrini G, de Smit M, Westra J, Brouwer E, Vissink A, Zhou K, et al. The peptidylarginine deiminase gene is a conserved feature of Porphyromonas gingivalis. Sci Rep. 2015;5:13936.
67. Maresz KJ, Hellvard A, Sroka A, Adamowicz K, Bielecka E, Koziel J, et al. Porphyromonas gingivalis facilitates the development and progression of destructive arthritis through its unique bacterial peptidylarginine deiminase (PAD). PLoS Pathog. 2013;9:e1003627.
68. Kuhn KA, Kulik L, Tomooka B, Braschler KJ, Arend WP, Robinson WH, et al. Antibodies against citrullinated proteins enhance tissue injury in experimental autoimmune arthritis. J Clin Investig. 2006;116:961–73.
69. Cui J, Taylor KE, Destefano AL, Criswell LA, Izmailova ES, Parker A, et al. Genome-wide association study of determinants of anti-cyclic citrullinated peptide antibody titer in adults with rheumatoid arthritis. Mol Med. 2009;15:136–43.
70. Kokkonen H, Brink M, Hansson M, Lassen E, Mathsson-Alm L, Holmdahl R, et al. Associations of antibodies against citrullinated peptides with human leukocyte antigen-shared epitope and smoking prior to the development of rheumatoid arthritis. Arthritis Res Ther. 2015;17:125.
71. Doyle TJ, Dellaripa PF, Batra K, Frits ML, Iannaccone CK, Hatabu H, et al. Functional impact of a spectrum of interstitial lung abnormalities in rheumatoid arthritis. Chest. 2014;146:41–50.
72. Scher JU, Joshua V, Artacho A, Abdollahi-Roodsaz S, Ockinger J, Kullberg S, et al. The lung microbiota in early rheumatoid arthritis and autoimmunity. Microbiome. 2016;4:60.
73. Segata N, Haake SK, Mannon P, Lemon KP, Waldron L, Gevers D, et al. Composition of the adult digestive tract bacterial microbiome based on seven mouth surfaces, tonsils, throat and stool samples. Genome Biol. 2012;13:R42.
74. Nordstrom D, Lindy O, Lauhio A, Sorsa T, Santavirta S, Konttinen YT. Anti-collagenolytic mechanism of action of doxycycline treatment in rheumatoid arthritis. Rheumatol Int. 1998;17:175–80.
75. O'Dell JR, Elliott JR, Mallek JA, Mikuls TR, Weaver CA, Glickstein S, et al. Treatment of early seropositive rheumatoid arthritis: doxycycline plus methotrexate versus methotrexate alone. Arthritis Rheum. 2006;54:621–7.
76. Vaghef-Mehrabany E, Alipour B, Homayouni-Rad A, Sharif SK, Asghari-Jafarabadi M, Zavvari S. Probiotic supplementation improves inflammatory status in patients with rheumatoid arthritis. Nutrition. 2014;30:430–5.
77. Alipour B, Homayouni-Rad A, Vaghef-Mehrabany E, Sharif SK, Vaghef-Mehrabany L, Asghari-Jafarabadi M, et al. Effects of lactobacillus casei supplementation on disease activity and inflammatory cytokines in rheumatoid arthritis patients: a randomized double-blind clinical trial. Int J Rheum Dis. 2014;17:519–27.
78. Mandel DR, Eichas K, Holmes J. Bacillus coagulans: a viable adjunct therapy for relieving symptoms of rheumatoid arthritis according to a randomized, controlled trial. BMC Complement Altern Med. 2010;10(1):1.
79. Wu GD, Chen J, Hoffmann C, Bittinger K, Chen YY, Keilbaugh SA, et al. Linking long-term dietary patterns with gut microbial enterotypes. Science. 2011;334:105–8.
80. David LA, Maurice CF, Carmody RN, Gootenberg DB, Button JE, Wolfe BE, et al. Diet rapidly and reproducibly alters the human gut microbiome. Nature. 2014;505:559–63.
81. Hagen KB, Byfuglien MG, Falzon L, Olsen SU, Smedslund G. Dietary interventions for rheumatoid arthritis. Cochrane Database Syst Rev. 2009;1:CD006400.
82. Kang C, Zhang Y, Zhu X, Liu K, Wang X, Chen M, et al. Healthy subjects differentially respond to dietary capsaicin correlating with the specific gut enterotypes. J Clin Endocrinol Metab. 2016;101(12):4681–9. jc20162786.
83. Borg AA, Davis MJ, Fowler PD, Shadforth MF, Dawes PT. Rifampicin in early rheumatoid arthritis. Scand J Rheumatol. 1993;22:39–42.
84. Ogrendik M. Levofloxacin treatment in patients with rheumatoid arthritis receiving methotrexate. South Med J. 2007;100:135–9.
85. Ogrendik M. Effects of clarithromycin in patients with active rheumatoid arthritis. Curr Med Res Opin. 2007;23:515–22.
86. Saviola G, Abdi-Ali L, Campostrini L, Sacco S, Baiardi P, Manfredi M, et al. Clarithromycin in rheumatoid arthritis: the addition to methotrexate and low-dose methylprednisolone induces a significant additive value--a 24-month single-blind pilot study. Rheumatol Int. 2013;33:2833–8.
87. Ogrendik M. Efficacy of roxithromycin in adult patients with rheumatoid arthritis who had not received disease-modifying antirheumatic drugs: a 3-month, randomized, double-blind, placebo-controlled trial. Clin Ther. 2009;31:1754–64.
88. Ogrendik M, Karagoz N. Treatment of rheumatoid arthritis with roxithromycin: a randomized trial. Postgrad Med. 2011;123:220–7.
89. Sreekanth VR, Handa R, Wali JP, Aggarwal P, Dwivedi SN. Doxycycline in the treatment of rheumatoid arthritis--a pilot study. J Assoc Physicians India. 2000;48:804–7.
90. St Clair EW, Wilkinson WE, Pisetsky DS, Sexton DJ, Drew R, Kraus VB, et al. The effects of intravenous doxycycline therapy for rheumatoid arthritis: a randomized, double-blind, placebo-controlled trial. Arthritis Rheum. 2001;44:1043–7.

91. van der Laan W, Molenaar E, Ronday K, Verheijen J, Breedveld F, Greenwald R, et al. Lack of effect of doxycycline on disease activity and joint damage in patients with rheumatoid arthritis. A double blind, placebo controlled trial. J Rheumatol. 2001;28:1967–74.
92. Pillemer S, Gulko P, Ligier S, Yarboro C, Gourley M, Goldbach-Mansky R, et al. Pilot clinical trial of intravenous doxycycline versus placebo for rheumatoid arthritis. J Rheumatol. 2003;30:41–3.
93. Kloppenburg M, Breedveld FC, Terwiel JP, Mallee C, Dijkmans BA. Minocycline in active rheumatoid arthritis. A double-blind, placebo-controlled trial. Arthritis Rheum. 1994;37:629–36.
94. Tilley BC, Alarcon GS, Heyse SP, Trentham DE, Neuner R, Kaplan DA, et al. Minocycline in rheumatoid arthritis. A 48-week, double-blind, placebo-controlled trial. MIRA trial group. Ann Intern Med. 1995;122:81–9.
95. O'Dell JR, Haire CE, Palmer W, Drymalski W, Wees S, Blakely K, et al. Treatment of early rheumatoid arthritis with minocycline or placebo: results of a randomized, double-blind, placebo-controlled trial. Arthritis Rheum. 1997;40:842–8.
96. O'Dell JR, Blakely KW, Mallek JA, Eckhoff PJ, Leff RD, Wees SJ, et al. Treatment of early seropositive rheumatoid arthritis: a two-year, double-blind comparison of minocycline and hydroxychloroquine. Arthritis Rheum. 2001;44:2235–41.
97. Skinner M, Cathcart ES, Mills JA, Pinals RS. Tetracycline in the treatment of rheumatoid arthritis. A double blind controlled study. Arthritis Rheum. 1971;14:727–32.
98. Gompels LL, Smith A, Charles PJ, Rogers W, Soon-Shiong J, Mitchell A, et al. Single-blind randomized trial of combination antibiotic therapy in rheumatoid arthritis. J Rheumatol. 2006;33:224–7.
99. Smith A, Dore C, Charles P, Vallance A, Potier T, Mackworth-Young C. Randomised double-blind trial of combination antibiotic therapy in rheumatoid arthritis. Int J Rheumatol. 2011;2011:585497.
100. Harkness JA, Griffin AJ, Heinrich I, Gibson T, Grahame R. A double-blind comparative study of metronidazole and placebo in rheumatoid arthritis. Rheumatol Rehabil. 1982;21:231–4.
101. Marshall DA, Hunter JA, Capell HA. Double blind, placebo controlled study of metronidazole as a disease modifying agent in the treatment of rheumatoid arthritis. Ann Rheum Dis. 1992;51:758–60.
102. Ogrendik M, Hakguder A, Keser N. Treatment of rheumatoid arthritis with ornidazole. A randomized, double-blind, placebo-controlled study. Rheumatology (Oxford). 2006;45:636–7.
103. Ash G, Baker R, Rajapakse C, Swinson DR. Study of sulphamethoxazole in rheumatoid arthritis. Br J Rheumatol. 1986;25:285–7.
104. Wojtulewski JA, Gow PJ, Walter J, Grahame R, Gibson T, Panayi GS, et al. Clotrimazole in rheumatoid arthritis. Ann Rheum Dis. 1980;39:469–72.
105. Neumann VC, Grindulis KA, Hubball S, McConkey B, Wright V. Comparison between penicillamine and sulphasalazine in rheumatoid arthritis: Leeds-Birmingham trial. Br Med J. 1983;287:1099–102.
106. Pullar T, Hunter JA, Capell HA. Sulphasalazine in rheumatoid arthritis: a double blind comparison of sulphasalazine with placebo and sodium aurothiomalate. Br Med J. 1983;287:1102–4.
107. Pinals RS, Kaplan SB, Lawson JG, Hepburn B. Sulfasalazine in rheumatoid arthritis. A double-blind, placebo-controlled trial. Arthritis Rheum. 1986;29:1427–34.
108. Williams HJ, Ward JR, Dahl SL, Clegg DO, Willkens RF, Oglesby T, et al. A controlled trial comparing sulfasalazine, gold sodium thiomalate, and placebo in rheumatoid arthritis. Arthritis Rheum. 1988;31:702–13.
109. Hannonen P, Mottonen T, Hakola M, Oka M. Sulfasalazine in early rheumatoid arthritis. A 48-week double-blind, prospective, placebo-controlled study. Arthritis Rheum. 1993;36:1501–9.
110. Hatakka K, Martio J, Korpela M, Herranen M, Poussa T, Laasanen T, et al. Effects of probiotic therapy on the activity and activation of mild rheumatoid arthritis--a pilot study. Scand J Rheumatol. 2003;32:211–5.
111. Pineda Mde L, Thompson SF, Summers K, de Leon F, Pope J, Reid G. A randomized, double-blinded, placebo-controlled pilot study of probiotics in active rheumatoid arthritis. Med Sci Monit. 2011;17:CR347–54.

Spondyloarthritis

16

Heleen Cypers, S. Louis Bridges Jr.,
and Dirk Elewaut

Abbreviations

ANKENT	Ankylosing enthesopathy mouse model
AS	Ankylosing spondylitis
ASCA	Anti-saccharomyces antibody
ASDAS	Ankylosing spondylitis disease activity scale
ATG16L1	Autophagy-related 16-like 1
CD	Crohn's disease
CTLA-4	Cytotoxic T lymphocyte antigen 4
DC	Dendritic cell
DGGE	Denaturing gradient gel electrophoresis
ER	Endoplasmic reticulum
ERA	Enthesitis-related arthritis
ERAP	Endoplasmic receptor aminopeptidase
FISH	Fluorescent in situ hybridization
FMT	Fecal microbial transplantation
HLA	Human leukocyte antigen
IBD	Inflammatory bowel disease
IL	Interleukin
IL-23R	Interleukin 23 receptor
ILC	Innate lymphoid cell
LPS	Lipopolysaccharide
MAIT	Mucosal-associated invariant T (cell)
MHC	Major histocompatibility complex
mNY	Modified New York
MRI	Magnetic resonance imaging
NF-κB	Nuclear factor-κB
NOD	Nucleotide oligomerization domain
Nr-axSpA	Non-radiographic axial spondyloarthritis
OMP	Outer membrane protein
PAMP	Pathogen-associated molecular pattern
pANCA	Peripheral antineutrophil cytoplasmic antibody
PBMC	Peripheral blood mononuclear cell
PRR	Pattern recognition receptor
PsA	Psoriatic arthritis
RA	Rheumatoid arthritis
ReA	Reactive arthritis
rRNA	Ribosomal ribonucleic acid
SCFA	Short-chain fatty acids
SF	Synovial fluid
SFB	Segmented filamentous bacteria
SFMC	Synovial fluid mononuclear cell
sIgA	Secretory immunoglobulin A

H. Cypers (✉)
Department of Rheumatology, Ghent University Hospital, Ghent, Belgium
e-mail: heleen.cypers@ugent.be

S. L. Bridges Jr.
Division of Clinical Immunology and Rheumatology, Comprehensive Arthritis, Musculoskeletal, Bone and Autoimmunity Center, University of Alabama at Birmingham, Birmingham, AL, USA
e-mail: LBridges@uab.edu

D. Elewaut
Department of Rheumatology, Ghent University Hospital, Ghent, Belgium

Unit for Molecular Immunology and Inflammation, VIB Inflammation Research Center, Ghent University, Ghent, Belgium
e-mail: dirk.elewaut@ugent.be

G. Ragab et al. (eds.), *The Microbiome in Rheumatic Diseases and Infection*,
https://doi.org/10.1007/978-3-319-79026-8_16

SpA	Spondyloarthritis
SPF	Specific pathogen-free
Spp	Subspecies
STAT3	Signal transducer and activator of transcription 3
TGF	Transforming growth factor
TLR	Toll-like receptor
Treg	Regulatory T cell
UPR	Unfolded protein response

Introduction

Spondyloarthritis (SpA) indicates a group of clinically and genetically related disorders characterized by chronic inflammation of the axial skeleton (sacroiliitis and spondylitis), the peripheral joints, and/or the entheses. SpA comprises different subtypes, including ankylosing spondylitis (AS), psoriatic arthritis (PsA), juvenile-onset SpA (enthesitis-related arthritis, ERA), reactive arthritis (ReA), and inflammatory bowel disease (IBD)-related arthritis. These are the initially described clinical phenotypes. Over time it became apparent that these diseases are interrelated with regard to clinical characteristics, familial clustering, and genetic susceptibility. It is generally accepted that SpA is due to a chronic inflammatory response that develops in genetically predisposed people, but the underlying cause of the inflammation is not known. The most important genetic susceptibility factor in SpA is the major histocompatibility complex (MHC) class I surface antigen HLA-B27 (human leukocyte antigen B27) [1]. However, environmental factors also contribute to SpA pathogenesis, and multiple lines of reasoning indicate an important role for microorganisms in triggering disease. Specific gastrointestinal or urogenital pathogens have been linked with ReA, but in other SpA subtypes, no specific causative microorganism has been identified. Rather, inappropriate immune responses to commensal bacteria or alterations in resident microbial communities (dysbiosis) are proposed to be factors in SpA development. Indeed, several genetic susceptibility factors linked with SpA may impact the handling, processing, and response to microbial antigens.

Ankylosing Spondylitis/Axial SpA

Ankylosing spondylitis (AS) is the prototype example of SpA. It is characterized by inflammation of the axial skeleton, that is, the sacroiliac joints (usually the first to be involved) and the spine (spondylitis), with or without peripheral arthritis or enthesitis. Typical for SpA is that inflammation coincides with pathological new bone formation. In AS this causes fusion (ankylosis) of sacroiliac joints and vertebrae, which may lead to development of so-called bamboo spine (fusion of consecutive vertebrae), with significant reduction of axial mobility [2]. The modified New York (mNY) criteria were specifically developed for diagnosis of AS. They are dependent on the presence of characteristic radiographic lesions (erosions, sclerosis, ankylosis, joint space changes) in the sacroiliac joints. The availability of magnetic resonance imaging (MRI), which can detect active inflammation before structural lesions are seen on plain radiographs, has led to the identification of non-radiographic axial SpA (nr-axSpA), which can be regarded as an earlier form of AS. Multiple studies have found that AS and nr-axSpA, when carefully selected on the basis of objective signs of inflammation, are similar with regard to symptoms, disease impact, and therapy response [3]. Hence, the division between these two is rather arbitrary, as it is based on scoring of sacroiliac radiographs, which is subjective and shows considerable inter-reader variability [4]. Both of these clinical entities can in fact be seen as part of a disease continuum [1]. In 2009 ASAS proposed new classification criteria for axial and peripheral SpA. Axial SpA encompasses both the radiographic (AS) and non-radiographic forms. Peripheral SpA includes ReA, the SpA-like PsA subtype, IBD-associated arthritis, and other forms of arthritis fitting the SpA criteria (previously often called undifferentiated SpA).

Intestinal Inflammation in SpA

There is a close relationship between gut and joint inflammation in SpA. This is most obvious in reactive arthritis (ReA), where disease is known to be triggered by gastrointestinal infections with *Salmonella*, *Shigella*, *Yersinia*, or *Campylobacter* subspecies (spp.). The risk of developing ReA is increased by carriage of HLA-B27; the pattern of joint involvement is typical for SpA. Hence, ReA can be considered a subtype of SpA. Moreover, up to 20% of patients with ReA eventually develop AS within 10–20 years, especially if they are HLA-B27 positive [5]. In addition, a reciprocal overlap exists between IBD and SpA: about 5–10% of SpA patients develop IBD. Conversely, up to 30% of IBD patients may develop SpA-like articular inflammation.

Multiple genetic susceptibility factors have also been found to be shared between IBD and SpA patients. Furthermore, by performing systematic ileocolonoscopies, it was demonstrated that ~50% of all SpA patients have microscopic signs of bowel inflammation, without associated gastrointestinal symptoms [6]. These studies involved patients with AS, ReA, and undifferentiated SpA, as well as healthy controls and patients with other rheumatic diseases, such as rheumatoid arthritis (RA). None of the control patients and only one RA patient showed gut lesions. Later, these lesions were also described in PsA but only in the oligoarticular (SpA-like) subgroup [7]. Similar findings have also been reported in juvenile SpA [8]. Gut inflammation in SpA can affect the ileum as well as the colon but is most common in the terminal ileum and ileocecal valve. Two types of inflammation can be distinguished based on histopathological characteristics (not on disease duration): an acute type resembling infectious enterocolitis (granulocytic infiltration with normal mucosal architecture) and a chronic type with disturbance of mucosal architecture and a chronic lymphoplasmacytic cellular infiltrate in the lamina propria (Fig. 16.1) [9]. Some of these histological changes (e.g., sarcoid granulomas, aphthoid ulcers, microgranulomas) are particularly similar to those seen in Crohn's disease (CD), suggesting that this microscopic inflammation may represent an early, subclinical form of CD. This is further strengthened by the fact that SpA patients with chronic microscopic gut inflammation have an increased risk (up to 20%) of developing overt CD [10]. Follow-up studies showed that gut and joint inflammation was clearly linked, with remission of joint inflammation coinciding with disappearance of gut inflammation and vice versa; all patients in articular remission had normal gut histology on reexamination (despite previous or current use of NSAIDs).

Interestingly, chronic gut inflammation in SpA is also linked to more extensive bone marrow edema of the sacroiliac joints and a higher rate of evolution to AS [10, 11]. This suggests an important influence of intestinal inflammation on disease extent and prognosis in SpA. The presence of microscopic gut inflammation in SpA has since been confirmed by several other investigators [12–17].

Normal histology:

- Slender villi and straight crypts
- Absence of inflammatory cell infiltrates in epithelium

Acute inflammation:

- Increased amount of granulocytes in villus and crypt epithelium (focal inflammation)
- Preserved architecture of villi and crypts

Chronic inflammation:

- Crypt and villus distortion
- Chronic lymphoplasmacytic cellular infiltrate in the lamina propria (and in this case active granulocytic infiltration of villus epithelium)

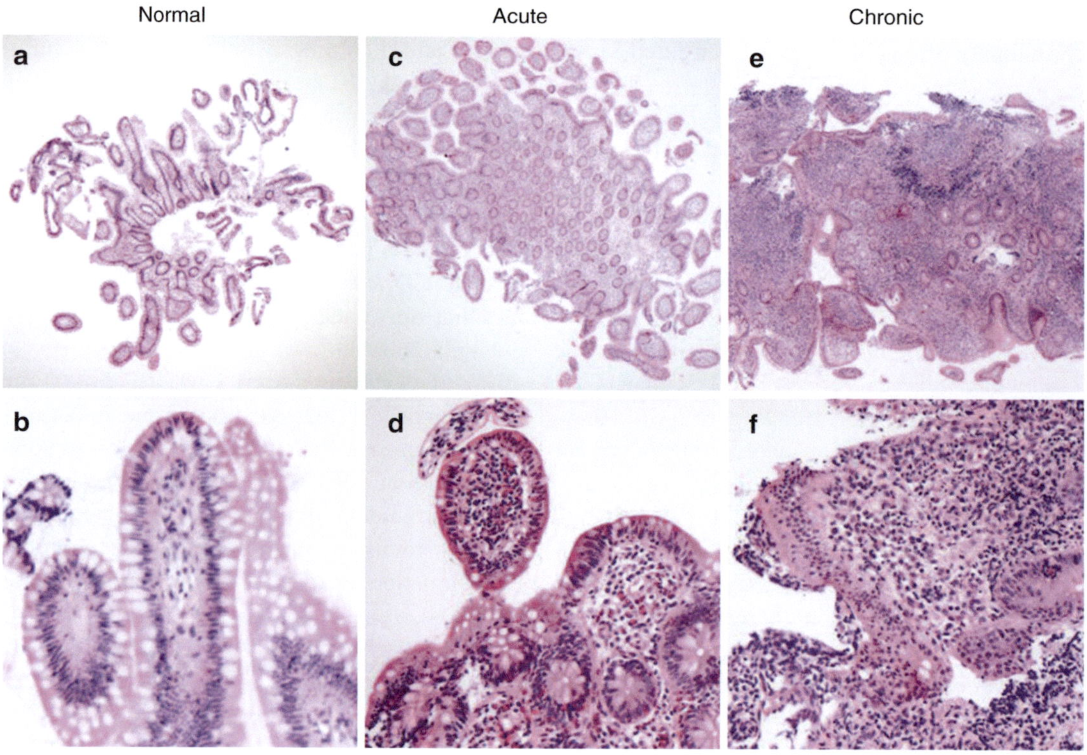

Fig. 16.1 Different patterns of ileal biopsy findings in SpA patients. (**a**) Normal histology of ileal mucosa featuring slender villi and straight crypts; absence of inflammatory cell infiltrates (H&E; original magnification ×4). (**b**) Higher magnification emphasizing lack of inflammatory cell infiltration in villus epithelium (H&E; original magnification ×20). (**c**) Focal active inflammation in mucosa with preserved architecture of villi and crypts (H&E; original magnification ×4). (**d**) Increased amount of granulocytes in villus and crypt epithelium with well-preserved epithelium (H&E; original magnification ×20). (**e**) Chronic dense inflammatory cell infiltration of lamina propria with crypt and villus alterations (H&E; original magnification ×4). (**f**) Active granulocytic infiltration of villus epithelium and chronic dense lymphoplasmacytic cellular infiltrate in the lamina propria (H&E; original magnification ×20). Reproduced from "Microscopic gut inflammation in axial spondyloarthritis: a multiparametric predictive model. Van Praet L, Van den Bosch FE, Jacques P, Carron P, Jans L, Colman R, Glorieus E, Peeters H, Mielants H, De Vos M, Cuvelier C, Elewaut D. Ann Rheum Dis. 2013 Mar;72 (3):414–7. doi: https://doi.org/10.1136/annrheumdis-2012-202,135. Epub 2012 Nov 8. Copyright © 2013 with permission from BMJ Publishing Group Ltd."

The Microbiota in SpA

Dysbiosis of the intestinal microbiota, with decreased diversity, has consistently been found in IBD, where the most common hypothesis for pathogenesis involves an exaggerated immune response to commensal gut bacteria (see also Chap. 19 in this book) [18]. Based on the links between gut and joint inflammation in SpA and the overlap with IBD, it is reasonable to presume that intestinal microorganisms play a role in SpA pathogenesis as well. This is most obvious in the ReA subtype, where arthritis is triggered by specific gastrointestinal infections. In addition, in three animal models for SpA, disease is abrogated when the animals are raised in germ-free conditions [19–21].

Microbiota Studies in SpA

The first comprehensive analysis of the intestinal microbiota in SpA was a 2002 study comparing fecal samples of AS patients and controls by denaturing gradient gel electrophoresis (DGGE) and fluorescence in situ hybridization (FISH) for specific bacterial groups. This study showed high interindividual variability and no specific differences in colonization profiles between patients and controls. However, there was a higher prevalence of sulfate-reducing bacteria in patients with AS. There were no differences in fecal colonization with *Klebsiella pneumoniae* or *Bacteroides vulgatus* (implicated in AS, see below) [22].

More recently, studies have been performed using next-generation sequencing of 16S ribosomal RNA (rRNA) gene amplicons. Table 16.1 summarizes microbiota studies in SpA in humans and animal models for SpA. In children with SpA (enthesitis-related arthritis, ERA), decreased fecal *Faecalibacterium prausnitzii* was observed compared to healthy controls [26]. *Faecalibacterium prausnitzii* has anti-inflammatory properties

Table 16.1 Microbiome studies in SpA in humans and animal models for SpA

Disease	Technology	Sample	Microbiota changes (versus healthy controls)	Ref.
Ankylosing spondylitis	DGGE + FISH	Feces	↑ Sulfate-reducing bacteria N.B. No difference in *Klebsiella pneumoniae* or *Bacteroides vulgatus*	[22]
Ankylosing spondylitis	16S rRNA amplicon seq.	Ileal biopsies	↑ *Lachnospiraceae*, *Veillonellaceae*, *Prevotellaceae*, *Porphyromonadaceae*, and *Bacteroidaceae* ↓ *Ruminococcaceae* and *Rikenellaceae* N.B. No difference in *Klebsiella* spp. or ReA-associated bacteria	[23]
Axial SpA ± gut inflammation	16S rRNA amplicon seq.	Ileal + colonic biopsies	*Dialister* (part of *Veillonellaceae*) ~ gut inflammation and ASDAS	[24]
Axial SpA	16S rRNA amplicon seq.	Subgingival plaques	No difference versus HCs despite more periodontitis in SpA	[25]
Enthesitis-related arthritis (juvenile SpA)	16S rRNA amplicon seq.	Feces	↓ *Faecalibacterium prausnitzii* (part of *Clostridiaceae*) and *Lachnospiraceae* ↑ *Bifidobacterium* ↑ *Akkermansia muciniphila* (*Verrucomicrobiaceae*) in subgroup ↑ *Bacteroides* in (another) subgroup	[26]
HLA-B27 tg rats Fisher 344 background F33-3 line	16S rRNA amplicon seq.	Feces	↓ *Firmicutes* spp. ↑ *Proteobacteria* spp. ↑ *Akkermansia muciniphila* (also linked with arthritis development) N.B. Changes present by 10 weeks of age ~ development of intestinal inflammation	[27]
HLA-B27 tg rats. Lewis background F1 21-3 × 283-2 males (no intestinal inflammation)	16S rRNA amplicon seq.	Feces	↑ *Prevotella* spp. (part of *Prevotellaceae*) ↑ *Bacteroides vulgatus* ↓ *Rikenellaceae*	[28]

Bacterial families are given in parentheses if applicable
The phylum *Firmicutes* includes i.a. the *Clostridiaceae*, *Lachnospiraceae*, *Ruminococcaceae*, and *Veillonellaceae* families
The phylum *Bacteroidetes* includes i.a. the *Prevotellaceae*, *Porphyromonadaceae*, *Bacteroidaceae*, and *Rikenellaceae* families
The phylum *Proteobacteria* includes i.a. the *Campylobacteraceae* and the *Enterobacteriaceae* families
The phylum *Verrucomicrobia* includes i.a. the *Verrucomicrobiaceae* family
The phylum *Actinobacteria* includes i.a. the *Bifidobacteriaceae* family
DGGE denaturing gradient gel electrophoresis, *FISH* fluorescence in situ hybridization, *Seq.* sequencing, *HCs* healthy controls, *ReA* reactive arthritis, *ASDAS* ankylosing spondylitis disease activity score, *tg* transgenic, *spp.* subspecies

through production of butyrate, and a decrease in its abundance as well as in its enzymes (involved in butyrate pathways) has been found in IBD [29]. In addition, a subgroup of these ERA patients fell into a distinct cluster characterized by an increase in *Bacteroides* species, while another subgroup showed elevations in *Akkermansia muciniphila*, a mucus-degrading species. A relatively lower diversity of the intestinal microbiota was found in PsA patients who showed lower *Akkermansia* and *Ruminococcus* spp., which have also been shown to be reduced in IBD [30]. In contrast, increased microbial diversity (without an overall change in microbial load) was seen in the terminal ileum of AS patients compared to healthy controls, with a higher abundance of *Lachnospiraceae*, *Veillonellaceae*, *Prevotellaceae*, *Porphyromonadaceae*, and *Bacteroidaceae* and a decrease in *Ruminococcaceae* and *Rikenellaceae* [23]. A trend for increased microbial diversity in inflamed versus non-inflamed SpA and healthy control samples was also found in a 2016 study [24]. Here, ileum and colon biopsies from SpA patients with and without microscopic gut inflammation and from healthy controls were compared. In this study a specific genus was also linked with disease activity and inflammation: *Dialister* was significantly correlated with the ankylosing spondylitis disease activity score (ASDAS), and a higher abundance of *Dialister* was seen in inflamed versus non-inflamed or healthy control biopsies [24]. *Dialister* is part of the *Veillonellaceae* family of the *Firmicutes* phylum. Biochemically *Dialister* appears to be largely unreactive and asaccharolytic [31]. However, *Dialister* spp. are reported to produce propionate (a short-chain fatty acid) out of succinate [32]. Its possible pathogenetic role in SpA awaits further clarification.

The finding of increased diversity in the latter two studies is remarkable considering the reduced diversity found in IBD. A possible explanation for this could be the absence of substantial mucosal damage in SpA in contrast to full-blown IBD. It is possible that intestinal inflammation in SpA represents an earlier stage of inflammation compared to IBD and therefore harbors a different microbiota profile. In IBD cases with higher epithelial damage, more extreme dysbiosis and a more reduced species diversity are indeed seen [33]. Alternatively, genetic differences between IBD and SpA could be the basis of this discrepancy. In support of this hypothesis, a difference in microbial composition has been shown between CD patients with and without *ATG16L1* (autophagy-related 16-like 1) and *NOD2* (nucleotide oligomerization domain 2) risk alleles [34]. Also, different sample types (e.g., analysis of stool versus biopsies) could explain discrepancies between various studies.

Another microbial site that is interesting to investigate is the oral cavity. Associations between periodontal infections/the oral microbiota and RA have been extensively studied (see Chap. 15.) In a recent paper, the oral microbiota composition of axial SpA patients versus healthy controls was compared by 16S rRNA sequencing. Axial SpA patients showed a significantly greater prevalence of periodontitis versus healthy controls. However no significant difference in bacterial community structure or diversity was shown. Also, no specific bacterial taxa associated with SpA could be identified, although due to small sample size in this study, false negative results are a possibility [25].

Specific Bacterial Species Triggering SpA

Some specific bacteria, particularly *Klebsiella pneumoniae*, have been suggested to play a role in AS pathogenesis. This hypothesis is based on antigenic similarities between HLA-B27 and *Klebsiella* (see below) and on increased levels of anti-*Klebsiella* IgA antibodies found in the serum of SpA patients [35, 36]. However, these results have not consistently been reproduced [22]. A 2004 study found no significant differences with respect to cellular or humoral immune responses to *Klebsiella pneumoniae* in AS patients versus healthy controls [37]. In a 1978 study in AS, an association between active inflammatory disease and fecal *Klebsiella pneumoniae* was described. However, in the 2002 DGGE study mentioned earlier, no differences were found in fecal colonization with *Klebsiella pneumonia* between AS patients and healthy controls [22]. Also, in the recent 16S rRNA study on ileum biopsies, no association between *Klebsiella* spp. and AS was seen [23]. In conclusion, at this moment, a definite role for a specific triggering species in SpA (except for ReA) has not consistently been proven.

Antimicrobial Antibodies in SpA

Several antibodies to commensal bacteria have been found in the serum of IBD patients, supporting the hypothesis of an increased responsiveness to commensal bacteria underlying disease. These include antibodies against CBir1 flagellin, IgA and IgG anti-*Saccharomyces cerevisiae* antibodies (ASCAs), IgA antibodies against *E. coli* outer membrane protein (OMP) C, and IgA antibodies against I2 derived from *Pseudomonas fluorescens*. In UC there is also a link with peripheral antineutrophil cytoplasmic antibodies (pANCA) [38, 39]. Based on the overlap between IBD and SpA, these antibodies have also been investigated in patients with SpA, with varying results. At this moment it appears that these antibodies are rather nonspecific. Also, no correlation with the presence of subclinical gut inflammation has been found [40–46].

The Role of the Microbiota in Animal Models for SpA

The HLAB27 Transgenic Rat Model

Rats overexpressing HLA-B27 develop intestinal inflammation and SpA-like joint disease (peripheral arthritis, sacroiliitis, and sometimes spondylitis of tail vertebrae) [47]. Interestingly, these animals do not develop disease when raised in germ-free conditions, providing convincing evidence for implicating the microbiota in SpA pathogenesis [19]. Reintroduction of bacteria (especially *Bacteroides* spp.) reestablished inflammation [48]. Moreover, intestinal dysbiosis was shown in these rats, with higher abundance of *Prevotella* spp. and *Bacteroides vulgatus* and lower *Rikenellaceae* spp. compared to wild-type animals [28]. This study was performed in a HLA-B27 transgenic rat line that does not develop gastrointestinal inflammation (so local inflammation could not be a confounding factor). A recent study described the intestinal immune response in HLA-B27 transgenic rats more in detail [27]. Early activation of innate immunity (increased expression of TNFα and interleukin (IL)-1β), an increase in antimicrobial peptides (S100A8 and RegIIIγ), and expansion of mucosal Th17 cells were seen. Interestingly, these changes, which indicate an immunological hyperresponsiveness in the gut, occurred prior to the onset of dysbiosis and clinical inflammation. In addition, increased secretory IgA (sIgA) coating of intestinal bacteria and increased *Akkermansia muciniphila* colonization were linked with HLA-B27 expression and with arthritis development. As mentioned earlier, *Akkermansia muciniphila* was also overrepresented in fecal samples of a subset of ERA patients [26]. Exposure of wild-type animals to dysbiotic feces from HLA-B27 animals does not induce disease, indicating that dysbiosis alone, in the absence of HLA-B27 expression, is not sufficient to trigger disease in this model [27].

SKG Mice Injected with Curdlan

SKG mice spontaneously develop autoimmune arthritis resembling RA under conventional microbial conditions. This is due to a mutation in ZAP-70, which leads to an increase of autoreactive T cells. Under specific pathogen-free (SPF) conditions, SKG mice remain healthy. However if, under these conditions, they are injected with curdlan (β-1,3-glucan aggregates), they develop an Th17/IL-23-dependent SpA-like disease with enthesitis, sacroiliitis, peripheral arthritis, dactylitis, plantar fasciitis, vertebral inflammation, ileitis resembling CD, and unilateral uveitis [21, 49]. Beta-glucan is a major component of bacterial and fungal cell walls; hence this indicates that interactions between the host's immune system and microorganisms affect the development of specific disease phenotypes [21]. In subsequent experiments, the impact of genetic background and the microbiota on specific disease characteristics (arthritis versus ileitis) was further elucidated. Ileitis (and concurrent ileal IL-23 expression, endoplasmic reticulum (ER) stress, and IL-17 production) was dependent on the host's microbiota, Toll-like receptor 4 (TLR4) signaling, and SKG allele presence; ileitis was absent in curdlan-treated germ-free SKG mice and significantly attenuated in mice with limited microbiota exposure or in $TLR4^{-/-}$ mice. Wild-type mice injected with curdlan developed arthritis (albeit milder), but not ileitis. Also gut microbiota profiles differed significantly between wild-type and SKG mice, and curdlan injection further shifted these profiles. Ileitis, but not arthritis, was suppressed by microbiota transfer upon co-housing SKG mice with wild-type mice. Arthritis and spondylitis still developed after curdlan injection in germ-free SKG mice, or in those with limited microbiota exposure, but with a low incidence, indicating that the diversity of the microbiota also influenced articular symptoms. Histological joint scores, however, did not differ between $TLR\text{-}4^{+/+}$ and $TLR4^{-/-}$ mice [50]. Interestingly, when these mice are infected with *Chlamydia muridarum*, they develop characteristic features of reactive arthritis, including asymmetric arthritis, enthesitis, spondylitis, sacroiliitis, conjunctivitis, and psoriasis-like skin disease; this was associated with impaired *Chlamydia muridarum* clearance and elevated TNF levels [51].

The Ankylosing Enthesopathy (ANKENT) Mouse Model

ANKENT is an inflammatory disease characterized by enthesitis and ankylosis of the ankle and tarsal joints. It develops spontaneously (albeit in rather low frequency, ~10%) in some inbred strains of normal mice. It occurs almost exclusively in males, and its frequency varies among strains, whereby the highest frequency is found in B10.BR (H-2κ haplotype) male mice. Its incidence is also significantly increased in HLA-B27 transgene mice [52]. As in the two previous models, ANKENT does not develop when animals are held in germ-free conditions [20]. Disease is reestablished after recolonization with a mixture of common intestinal bacteria (*Bacteroides* spp. and *Enterococcus* spp. and/or *Veillonella* spp. and *Staphylococcus* spp.), whereas this is not the case in mice recolonized with *Lactobacillus* spp. [53]. Repeated intraperitoneal lipopolysaccharide (LPS) injection before disease development, however, leads to a decrease in ANKENT incidence, possibly through upregulation of negative immunoregulatory pathways (higher serum levels of IL-10 were seen in LPS-treated mice) [54].

Mechanisms Linking the Intestinal Microbiota with SpA Pathogenesis

In SpA, genetic susceptibility factors may influence the response to bacteria and may eventually lead to dysbiosis and inflammation. Conversely, the composition and metabolic activity of the intestinal microbiota can affect the host's immune response, thereby possibly triggering or aggravating inflammation.

Factors Involved in the Response to Intestinal Microorganisms

The Intestinal Epithelial Barrier

Under normal circumstances, unwanted immune responses toward commensal gut bacteria are avoided by two main mechanisms. Firstly, exposure of microorganisms to the immune system is limited by the physical barrier that is the intestinal epithelium and its associated mucus layer. Secondly, immune responses that do develop are kept in check due to a tolerogenic microenvironment in the lamina propria, which is characterized by the presence of specialized dendritic cells (DCs) and macrophages, and high levels of anti-inflammatory mediators. Additional help in maintaining intestinal barrier function is provided by Paneth cells, which produce antimicrobial peptides, and by secretory IgA (sIgA), which binds and neutralizes toxins and pathogens in the gut lumen [55, 56]. An overexpression of Paneth cell-derived antimicrobial peptides was seen in the ileum of patients with AS and subclinical gut inflammation, as well as in CD patients with a low degree of inflammation, whereas a reduced number of Paneth cells were seen in CD patients with a high degree of gut inflammation [57]. In HLA-B27 transgenic rats, increased sIgA coating of intestinal bacteria was seen [27], and in some studies increased sIgA was demonstrated in serum of AS patients [58, 59]. Whether these changes represent compensatory mechanisms for increased bacterial exposure or are in themselves the cause of dysbiosis (loss of protective commensal organisms) is not known [60].

Innate Immunity

Bacterial Sensing by Innate Immune Cells

Innate immune cells sense antigens through a limited number of germ line-encoded invariant receptors, capable of recognizing conserved patterns of microbial structures known as pathogen-associated molecular patterns (PAMPs). These receptors are called pattern recognition receptors (PRRs) and recognize a broad class of pathogens. Examples of these are transmembrane Toll-like receptors (TLRs) and cytosolic nucleotide oligomerization domain receptors (NODs).

TLR4 binds LPS, a component of Gram-negative bacteria. This binding leads to activation of the nuclear factor-κB (NF-κB) signaling pathway and a pro-inflammatory response (e.g., IL-23 secretion). Two mutations in *TLR4* (Asp299Gly and Thr399Ile) have been associated with IBD susceptibility, but no link with AS was found [61]. Also, in the SKG mouse model, the induction of ileitis (but not arthritis) was TLR4 dependent. On the other hand, the expression of TLR2 and TLR4 was shown to be higher in inflamed synovium of SpA versus RA patients [62].

It is well established that certain polymorphisms in *NOD2/CARD15* are associated with CD susceptibility. In SpA patients, their overall frequency appears not to be increased, although they were found to be associated with a higher risk of chronic microscopic gut inflammation [63, 64]. Polymorphisms in *CARD9* (caspase recruitment domain family member 9) are associated with both SpA and IBD [65, 66]. *CARD9* codes for a protein essential for signaling downstream of the PRRs dectin-1 and dectin-2. These receptors recognize beta-glucan, a component of bacterial and fungal cell walls. CARD9 deficiency in mice leads to impaired intestinal epithelial repair [67]. On the other hand, beta-glucan administration to SKG mice leads to a SpA-like disease in these animals [21].

Processing of Microorganisms

Macrophages in SpA patients may respond aberrantly to microorganisms on the one hand by increased pro-inflammatory cytokine secretion and, on the other, by diminished clearance of intracellular bacteria (leading to dissemination of the organisms and systemic inflammation). Macrophages positive for CD163, a marker of alternative (M2) activation, were found to be increased in SpA versus RA synovium. CD163+ macrophages were also increased in colon mucosa of SpA and CD (but not UC) patients [68]. Additionally, CD163 was shown to be associated with impaired lymphocyte activation in SpA synovium, possibly leading to defective clearance of intracellular bacteria [69]. On the other hand, peripheral blood macrophages from AS patients showed higher IL-23 production in response to LPS compared to healthy controls [70]. Also, reduced IL-10 production was seen in peripheral blood mononuclear cells (PBMCs) from AS patients in response to autologous *Bacteroides*, and HLA-B27 transgenic rats also show an intrinsic defect in IL-10 production in response to TLR ligands [71, 72]. Similarly, mice with myeloid-specific deficiency in A20 (also called TNFAIP3), a protein involved in negative feedback of NF-κB signaling, spontaneously develop enthesitis [73].

Innate Lymphoid Cells (ILCs)

ILCs are a recently described type of cells that are capable of rapidly secreting large amounts of cytokines when stimulated by stress signals, microbial compounds, or cytokines [74]. ILC type 3 appears to be very important for gut immunity. They secrete IL-22 and IL-17 and express the Th17-associated transcription factor RORγt (retinoic-acid-receptor-related orphan nuclear receptor γt). Intestinal IL-22 is essential for epithelial integrity and repair [75]. ILC3s have also been shown to directly induce cell death of commensal bacteria-specific CD4 T cells in a MHC class II-dependent manner [76].

The role of intestinal ILCs has not been extensively investigated in SpA. A recent study described an increase of ILC3-like cells (although RORγt negative) in gut, synovial fluid, and bone marrow of patients with AS that had the capacity to produce IL-17 and IL-22 and expressed α4β7 [77].

Adaptive Immunity

HLA-B27

HLA-B27 is the most important genetic susceptibility factor in SpA [78]. As a MHC class I molecule, the physiological role of HLA-B27 is antigen presentation to CD8 T cells. Hence, it was speculated that certain B27 alleles might bind specific bacterial peptides and present them to cytotoxic T cells, which would then cross-react with endogenous antigens causing chronic inflammation (*the arthritogenic peptide theory*). Several reports indeed described the presence of HLA-B27-restricted CD8 T cells to bacterial peptides in HLA-B27-positive patients with ReA [79–81]. Also, HLA-B27-restricted autoreactive CD8 T cells specific for cartilage-derived peptides were found in synovial fluid (SF) of patients with AS [82]. However, two animal models for SpA, SKG mice injected with curdlan and HLA-B27 transgenic rats, are not dependent on CD8 T cells but are dependent on CD4 T cells (which interact with MHC class II molecules) [83]. Bacterial antigen-specific T cells in ReA have also found to be CD4+. Furthermore, they showed signs of impaired Th1 responses, possibly inhibiting effective clearance of bacteria [84]. Moreover, these CD4+ T cells reacted not only to bacterial antigens but also to HLA-B27 itself, possibly through cross-reactivity: HLA-B27 contains amino acid sequences that are identical to those found in Gram-negative bacterial proteins [85, 86]. Also, anti-HLA-B27 monoclonal antibodies were found to bind *Klebsiella*, *Shigella*, and *Yersinia* antigens [87–89].

Few studies have examined bacteria-specific CD4 T cell responses in non-ReA SpA patients. A 2012 study found higher frequencies of *E. coli*-specific Th1 cells in SF and peripheral blood of patients with AS compared to patients with RA [90]. An antigen-specific proliferative response of SF mononuclear cells (SFMCs) and PBMCs to the outer membrane protein (OMP) of *Salmonella typhimurium* was found in enthesitis-related JIA [91]. Impaired Th1 responses, characterized by lower IFNγ and IL-2 production, have been described in peripheral blood, synovium, and gut mucosa of non-ReA SpA patients, and this was restored after anti-TNFα therapy, suggesting that chronic TNF exposure might be the cause of this impairment [92].

Nevertheless, no specific arthritogenic peptide nor specific autoantibodies have been identified in SpA, so that alternative hypotheses linking HLA-B27 to SpA have been postulated. One possibility is that aberrant intracellular peptide processing combined with altered peptide presentation by HLA-B27 plays a role. This is supported by the discovery of ERAP-1 (endoplasmic reticulum aminopeptidase 1) polymorphisms, associated with HLA-B27-positive SpA patients. ERAP-1 encodes a peptidase involved in peptide trimming before MHC class I presentation [93, 94].

HLA-B27 may also contribute to SpA pathogenesis through triggering of local innate immunity. Two hypotheses have been proposed for this: HLA-B27 may form heavy chain dimers, which activate NK-type receptors [95]. However, monodimer formation is also seen in other HLA-B molecules not associated with SpA [95]. Secondly, HLA-B27 may misfold in the ER, activating the unfolded protein response (UPR), which leads to a pro-inflammatory reaction (i.e., IL-23 secretion) [96]. However, the increased LPS-induced IL-23 secretion seen in PBMCs from AS patients versus healthy controls (see above) was not associated with the induction of an UPR, even after upregulation of expression of HLA-B27 [70]. In line with this, another study found no increased activation of the UPR in synovial tissue and PBMCs from HLA-B27-positive AS patients versus those with other inflammatory joint diseases and healthy controls [97].

There is also evidence that HLA-B27 may affect dendritic cell and macrophage function. For instance, aberrant activity of DCs, including preferential induction of Th17 cells, was shown in DCs derived from HLA-B27 transgenic rats [98]. Enhanced intracellular replication/impaired elimination of *Salmonella enteritidis* has been seen in HLA-B27-transfected monocytes through modulation of Salmonella genes [99, 100]. This suggests that HLA-B27 might contribute to disease by increasing translocation of certain enteric bacteria.

The IL-23 Receptor (IL-23R)

The IL-17/IL-23 pathway has emerged as a crucial factor in SpA pathogenesis, as illustrated by increased IL-23 and IL-17 expression in SpA joints and the effectiveness of IL-17 or IL-23 blocking therapy. Moreover, certain polymorphisms in the IL-23R gene are associated with SpA, psoriasis, and IBD [66, 101]. Intestinal IL-23 is produced by macrophages, DCs, Paneth cells, and epithelial cells in response to microbial stimuli or after activation of the UPR. IL-23 supports the survival of effector Th17 cells, stimulating their expression of IL-17 and IL-22, and inhibits differentiation to T regulatory (Treg) cells [102–104]. Besides Th17 cells, IL-23R is expressed by many innate immune cell populations, e.g., ILC3s, γδ T cells, and mucosal-associated invariant T (MAIT) cells, all of which are characterized by IL-17 secretion and expression of RORγt [105, 106]. IL-23 expression in DCs has been shown to be induced by infection with *Chlamydia trachomatis*, a ReA-associated microorganism [107]. The triggering of arthritis and ileitis in SKG mice by microbial-derived curdlan (see above) is also IL-23 dependent.

Immunoregulation

Tregs in the gut are crucial for counterbalancing inflammatory responses to commensal bacteria. Tregs suppress inflammation by producing IL-10 and transforming growth factor (TGF) β and by expressing cytotoxic T lymphocyte antigen 4 (CTLA-4). They also induce class switching of B cells to produce IgA antibodies against commensal organisms [108, 109]. Treg cells have not been extensively studied in SpA. Alterations in Treg cell frequencies have not consistently been found in peripheral blood of SpA patients, but in SF, an increased number of Treg cells was described in peripheral SpA patients compared to AS and RA patients [110]. An increase in IL-10-producing Treg cells was found in the ileum of AS patients with chronic gut inflammation [111].

Some genetic polymorphisms associated with SpA may influence Treg cell function. For example, polymorphisms in *STAT3* (signal transducer and activator of transcription 3) are associated with both IBD and AS [66, 112]. STAT3 activation by IL-6 and IL-23, in combination with IL-1β, TGFβ, and RORγt, is associated with Th17 formation. On the other hand, STAT3 activation by IL-10 in Treg cells is crucial for their ability to suppress these pathogenic Th17 responses [113].

Microbial Factors Influencing Immunity in SpA

Data from animal studies have given us insight into how intestinal microorganisms or their metabolites can influence the intestinal, and subsequently systemic, immune system.

As mentioned above, the IL-17/IL-23 pathway plays an important role in SpA development. In mice, segmented filamentous bacteria (SFB) have been shown to induce Th17 cell differentiation, possibly by stimulating DCs to produce IL-23 and IL-6 [114]. Indole-3-aldehyde, a tryptophan metabolite produced by certain microbiota such as *Lactobacillus*, can drive IL-22 expression in group 3 ILCs [115], which in turn limits the expansion of SFB, inhibiting Th17 cell development [116].

Colonization of mice with *Clostridia* species (clusters IV and XIVa) induces Treg cell development by providing an environment rich in transforming growth factor-β [117]. Polysaccharide A, expressed by *Bacteroides fragilis* also modulates DCs to induce Tregs [118]. On the other hand, certain *bacteroides* species have been shown to mediate chronic colitis and arthritis in HLA-B27 transgenic rats [48].

An increase in sulfate-reducing bacteria has been described in fecal samples of AS patients (see above [22]). These bacteria produce hydrogen sulfide (H_2S) as a by-product, which can disrupt the epithelial barrier. Associations between these bacteria and IBD have also been described [119].

Short-chain fatty acids (SCFAs), such as butyrate, are produced by several commensal bacteria (e.g., *Bacteroides*, *Clostridia* species) as a result of carbohydrate fermentation. They are an important nutritional source for enterocytes and have immunomodulatory properties. Low doses of butyrate were shown to enhance epithelial barrier function, whereas high doses increased intestinal permeability due to epithelial cell apoptosis [120]. SCFAs induce the differentiation of colonic Treg cells in mice, at least partly through stimulation of IL-10 and retinoic acid production by intestinal DCs and macrophages [121, 122]. Butyrate has also been shown to decrease pro-inflammatory cytokine expression in vitro in human lamina propria mononuclear cells [123]. A reduction in butyrate-producing bacteria has been described in IBD as well as in ERA patients [26, 124]. Figure 16.2 summarizes the interactions between intestinal microorganisms and intestinal immune cells that are thought to play a role in SpA pathogenesis.

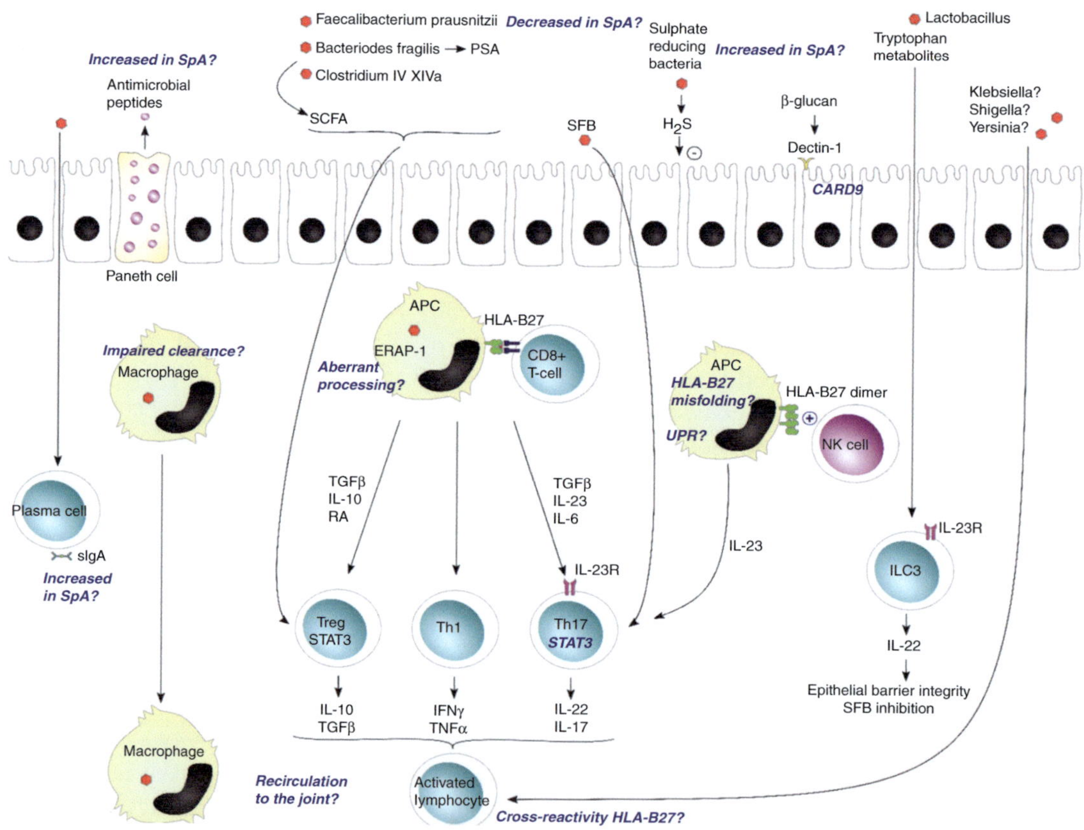

Fig. 16.2 Interactions between intestinal microorganisms and intestinal immune cells that are thought to play a role in SpA pathogenesis. The main hypotheses with regard to HLA-B27 and SpA development are depicted: presentation of an arthritogenic peptide to CD8+ T cells, misfolding in the ER causing ER stress and the UPR, and/or recognition of HLA-B27 heavy chain dimers by NK-type receptors. *H_2S* hydrogen sulfide, *SFB* segmented filamentous bacteria, *PSA* polysaccharide A, *SFCA* short-chain fatty acid, *RA* retinoic acid, *HLA-B27* human leukocyte antigen B27, *STAT* signal transducer and activator of transcription, *ERAP* endoplasmic reticulum aminopeptidase, *UPR* unfolded protein response, *CARD* caspase recruitment domain-containing protein, *TLR* Toll-like receptor, *IL* interleukin, *IL-23R* IL-23 receptor, *sIgA* secretory IgA, *TGF* transforming growth factor, *TNF* tumor necrosis factor

Trafficking of Bacterial Antigens From Gut to Joint

The exact mechanisms linking gut and joint inflammation in SpA have not been elucidated. One hypothesis is that intestinal bacteria or fragments thereof traffic to the joints and cause inflammation locally. Evidence supporting this hypothesis has mainly been found in ReA. Indeed, antigens or nucleic acids from ReA-associated microorganisms as well as T cells specific for these bacteria have consistently been detected in SF of ReA patients [79–81, 125–128]. More direct proof came from the discovery of identical T cell expansions in the colon and synovium of a patient with enterogenic ReA [129]. However, materials from skin or gut commensals are also found in the SF of ReA patients [130, 131]. Also, bacterial nucleic acids have been detected in various forms of arthritis, such as RA, so their pathogenic relevance is unclear [132–135]. Furthermore, long-term antibiotics have no proven benefit in the treatment of ReA (at least not when triggered by enteric infections) nor in peripheral SpA [136, 137].

An alternative hypothesis is that bacterial antigens prime intestinal T cells and macrophages, which then preferentially travel to the joints possibly due to aberrant expression of adhesion molecules, aberrant neovascularization, or local factors within the synovium. In the joint lymphocytes might be reactivated by cross-reacting with self-peptides (such as HLA-B27 itself, given its shared amino acid sequences with Gram-negative bacteria). Gut leukocytes indeed appear to have the capacity to interact with synovial vessels and enter the joint [138, 139]. Moreover, gut-derived Th17 cells were demonstrated in the spleen of K/BxN TCR transgenic mice at the onset of their genetically determined arthritis, and the frequency of these cells correlated with the titer of autoantibodies. Hence, this study provided a link between the intestinal Th17 pool (induction of which is influenced by gut microbiota such as SFB) and the development of arthritis. Of note, there was minimal emigration of Th17 cells from the gut in mice without arthritis [140].

Alternatively (or simultaneously), aberrant interaction with intestinal bacteria and/or intestinal inflammation could lead to increased systemic inflammation, which ultimately would affect the joints or entheses (which might show hyperresponsiveness to inflammatory stimuli due to genetic characteristics of SpA). A proposed mechanism for SpA pathogenesis and how intestinal inflammation or the microbiota might play a role in this is illustrated in Fig. 16.3.

Possible Therapeutic Implications

Given the evidence described above, therapeutic interventions to manipulate the gut microbiota in SpA are interesting to consider. On the one hand, an individual's global microbiota composition, once established, appears to be quite stable over time, highlighting the importance of early life colonization and exposure [141]. Also, short-term diet-induced changes in the microbiota composition appear to return quickly to the pre-intervention stage [142]. On the other hand, long-term studies looking at dietary interventions have not yet been performed. Also, antibiotics have been shown to have not only short-term but also long-term (years) impact on microbial composition, suggesting that there is some plasticity and hence room for interventional changes [143]. This has been illustrated by the success of treating persistent *Clostridium difficile* infection via fecal microbial transplants (FMT), where the composition of the recipient becomes highly similar to that of the donor [144]. Successful case reports have also been described for FMT in IBD (see Chap. 19.) A perhaps more appealing alternative for FMT are "synthetic stools," currently being developed and containing key species derived from the stool of healthy people [145]. Probiotic bacteria were shown to be protective in experimental models of colitis, including in HLA-B27 transgenic rats (*Lactobacillus rhamnosus GG*) [146, 147]. Also, consumption of *Lactobacillus casei* prior to infection abolished gut and joint inflammation triggered by *Salmonella* in mice, and this coincided with decreased expression of TNFα, IL-17, IL-23, IL-1β, and IL-6 in the gut [148]. Prebiotics containing chicory-derived long-chain inulin and oligofructose reduced colitis and prevented arthritis in

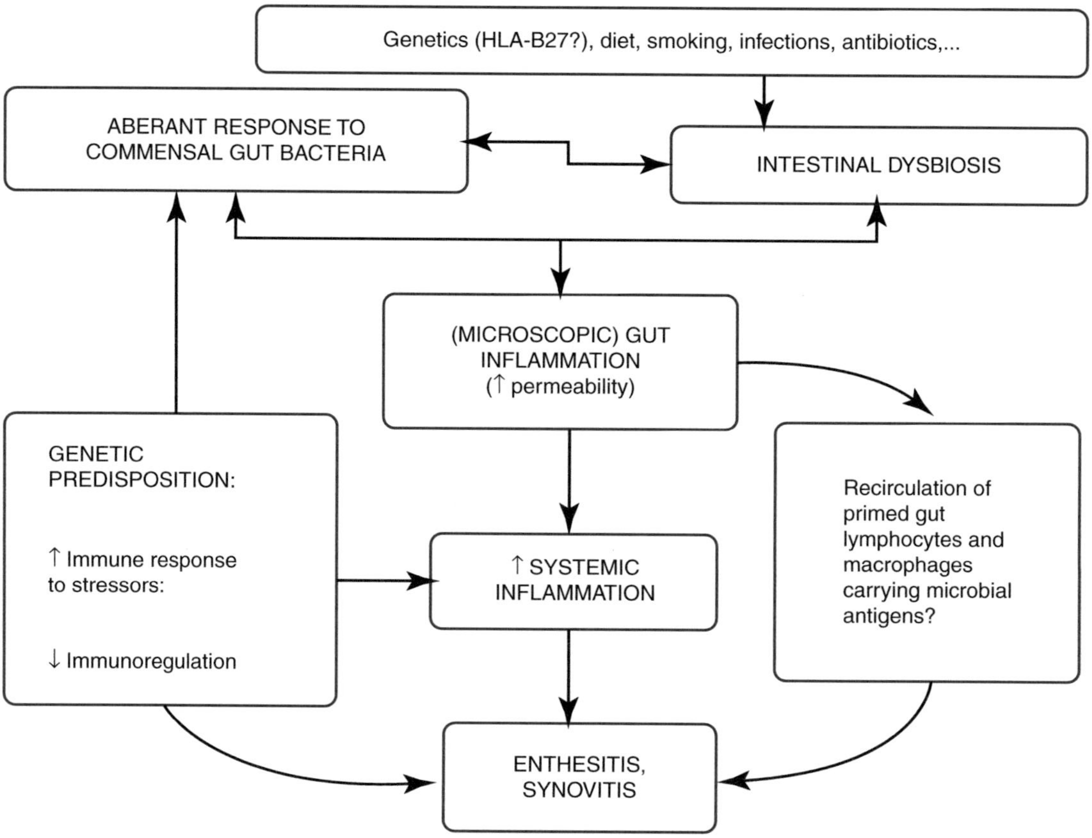

Fig. 16.3 Hypothesis for SpA pathogenesis involving intestinal inflammation and the gut microbiota. Genetic predisposition causes hyperresponsiveness to acute triggers in certain sites such as the gut (bacterial stress) or the entheses/joints (mechanical stress). This hyperresponsiveness leads to increased innate and adaptive immunity with a Th1/Th17 polarization. In the gut there is an altered responsiveness to commensal bacteria, e.g., altered recognition/processing, impaired clearance, exaggerated pro-inflammatory responses, etc. Characteristics of the host's immune system (PRRs, MHC proteins) and/or environmental factors might cause intestinal dysbiosis. Conversely, intestinal microorganisms influence the development and activation of the immune system; hence dysbiosis may cause gut inflammation. On the other hand, mucosal inflammation in itself can alter the gut microbiota, and it is difficult to ascertain which comes first. Loss of epithelial barrier integrity and increased permeability as a result of mucosal damage further increases exposure (and response) to mucosal bacteria. Ongoing acute insults/deficient immune regulation/failure to reestablish a normal gut ecosystem eventually lead to chronic systemic inflammation

the HLA-B27 transgenic rat model. This beneficial effect was associated with alterations to the gut microbiota (increased endogenous *Bifidobacteria* and *Lactobacilli)*, as well as a decrease in pro-inflammatory cytokines and an increase in immunoregulatory cytokines [149]. One RCT in 63 active SpA patients with probiotics containing *Streptococcus salivarius*, *Bifidobacterium lactis*, and *Lactobacillus acidophilus*, however, did not demonstrate a benefit over placebo [150]. Likewise, a pediatric study of ERA patients failed to identify any benefit to probiotics [151]. On the other hand, these interventions in SpA are not yet fine-tuned regarding microbiota composition and function. Perhaps if pre-/probiotic interventions become more specific and are able to fill in specific (bacterial/functional) niches, a therapeutic effect might be possible.

References

1. Rudwaleit M, Sieper J. Referral strategies for early diagnosis of axial spondyloarthritis. Nat Rev Rheumatol. 2012;8(5):262–8.
2. Poddubnyy D, Rudwaleit M. Early spondyloarthritis. Rheum Dis Clin N Am. 2012;38(2):387.

3. Sieper J, van der Heijde D. Review: nonradiographic axial spondyloarthritis: new definition of an old disease? Arthritis Rheum. 2013;65(3):543–51.
4. van Tubergen A, Heuft-Dorenbosch L, Schulpen G, Landewe R, Wijers R, van der Heijde D, et al. Radiographic assessment of sacroiliitis by radiologists and rheumatologists: does training improve quality? Ann Rheum Dis. 2003;62(6):519–25.
5. Leirisalo-Repo M. Prognosis, course of disease, and treatment of the spondyloarthropathies. Rheum Dis Clin N Am. 1998;24(4):737.
6. Cuvelier C, Barbatis C, Mielants H, De Vos M, Roels H, Veys E. Histopathology of intestinal inflammation related to reactive arthritis. Gut. 1987;28(4):394–401.
7. Schatteman L, Mielants H, Veys EM, Cuvelier C, De Vos M, Gyselbrecht L, et al. Gut inflammation in psoriatic arthritis: a prospective ileocolonoscopic study. J Rheumatol. 1995;22(4):680–3.
8. Mielants H, Veys EM, Cuvelier C, De Vos M, Goemaere S, Maertens M, et al. Gut inflammation in children with late onset pauciarticular juvenile chronic arthritis and evolution to adult spondyloarthropathy – a prospective study. J Rheumatol. 1993;20(9):1567–72.
9. Van Praet L, Van den Bosch FE, Jacques P, Carron P, Jans L, Colman R, et al. Microscopic gut inflammation in axial spondyloarthritis: a multiparametric predictive model. Ann Rheum Dis. 2013;72(3):414–7.
10. DeVos M, Mielants H, Cuvelier C, Elewaut A, Veys E. Long-term evolution of gut inflammation in patients with spondyloarthropathy. Gastroenterology. 1996;110(6):1696–703.
11. Van Praet L, Jans L, Carron P, Jacques P, Glorieus E, Colman R, et al. Degree of bone marrow oedema in sacroiliac joints of patients with axial spondyloarthritis is linked to gut inflammation and male sex: results from the GIANT cohort. Ann Rheum Dis. 2014;73(6):1186–9.
12. Grillet B, de Clerck L, Dequeker J, Rutgeerts P, Geboes K. Systematic ileocolonoscopy and bowel biopsy study in spondylarthropathy. Br J Rheumatol. 1987;26(5):338–40.
13. Lee YH, Ji JD, Kim JS, Bak YT, Lee CH, Kim CH, et al. Ileocolonoscopic and histologic studies of Korean patients with ankylosing spondylitis. Scand J Rheumatol. 1997;26(6):473–6.
14. Leirisalo-Repo M, Turunen U, Stenman S, Helenius P, Seppala K. High frequency of silent inflammatory bowel disease in spondylarthropathy. Arthritis Rheum. 1994;37(1):23–31.
15. Porzio V, Biasi G, Corrado A, De Santi M, Vindigni C, Viti S, et al. Intestinal histological and ultrastructural inflammatory changes in spondyloarthropathy and rheumatoid arthritis. Scand J Rheumatol. 1997;26(2):92–8.
16. Simenon G, Van Gossum A, Adler M, Rickaert F, Appelboom T. Macroscopic and microscopic gut lesions in seronegative spondyloarthropathies. J Rheumatol. 1990;17(11):1491–4.
17. Smale S, Natt RS, Orchard TR, Russell AS, Bjarnason I. Inflammatory bowel disease and spondylarthropathy. Arthritis Rheum. 2001;44(12):2728–36.
18. Nagalingam NA, Lynch SV. Role of the microbiota in inflammatory bowel diseases. Inflamm Bowel Dis. 2012;18(5):968–84.
19. Taurog JD, Richardson JA, Croft JT, Simmons WA, Zhou M, Fernandez-Sueiro JL, et al. The germfree state prevents development of gut and joint inflammatory disease in HLA-B27 transgenic rats. J Exp Med. 1994;180(6):2359–64.
20. Rehakova Z, Capkova J, Stepankova R, Sinkora J, Louzecka A, Ivanyi P, et al. Germ-free mice do not develop ankylosing enthesopathy, a spontaneous joint disease. Hum Immunol. 2000;61(6):555–8.
21. Ruutu M, Thomas G, Steck R, Degli-Esposti MA, Zinkernagel MS, Alexander K, et al. β-glucan triggers spondylarthritis and Crohn's disease-like ileitis in SKG mice. Arthritis Rheum. 2012;64(7):2211–22.
22. Stebbings S, Munro K, Simon MA, Tannock G, Highton J, Harmsen H, et al. Comparison of the faecal microflora of patients with ankylosing spondylitis and controls using molecular methods of analysis. Rheumatology. 2002;41(12):1395–401.
23. Costello ME, Ciccia F, Willner D, Warrington N, Robinson PC, Gardiner B, et al. Intestinal dysbiosis in ankylosing spondylitis. Arthritis Rheumatol. 2014;67(3):686–91.
24. Tito RY, Cypers H, Joossens M, Varkas G, Van Praet L, Glorieus E, et al. Dialister as microbial marker of disease activity in spondyloarthritis. Arthritis Rheumatol. 2016;69(1):114–21.
25. Bisanz JE, Suppiah P, Thomson WM, Milne T, Yeoh N, Nolan A, et al. The oral microbiome of patients with axial spondyloarthritis compared to healthy individuals. PeerJ. 2016;4:e2095.
26. Stoll ML, Kumar R, Morrow CD, Lefkowitz EJ, Cui X, Genin A, et al. Altered microbiota associated with abnormal humoral immune responses to commensal organisms in enthesitis-related arthritis. Arthritis Res Ther. 2014;16(6):486.
27. Asquith M, Stauffer P, Davin S, Mitchell C, Lin MP, Rosenbaum JT. Perturbed mucosal immunity and dysbiosis accompany clinical disease in a rat model of spondyloarthritis. Arthritis Rheumatol. 2016;68(9):2151–62.
28. Lin P, Bach M, Asquith M, Lee AY, Akileswaran L, Stauffer P, et al. HLA-B27 and human beta2-microglobulin affect the gut microbiota of transgenic rats. PLoS One. 2014;9(8):e105684.
29. Erickson AR, Cantarel BL, Lamendella R, Darzi Y, Mongodin EF, Pan C, et al. Integrated metagenomics/metaproteomics reveals human host-microbiota signatures of Crohn's disease. PLoS One. 2012;7(11):e49138.
30. Scher JU, Ubeda C, Artacho A, Attur M, Isaac S, Reddy SM, et al. Decreased bacterial diversity characterizes the altered gut microbiota in patients with psoriatic arthritis, resembling dysbiosis in inflammatory bowel disease. Arthritis Rheumatol. 2015;67(1):128–39.
31. Rocas IN, Siqueira JF Jr. Characterization of dialister species in infected root canals. J Endod. 2006;32(11):1057–61.
32. Morotomi M, Nagai F, Sakon H, Tanaka R. Dialister succinatiphilus sp. nov. and Barnesiella intestini-

hominis sp. nov., isolated from human faeces. Int J Syst Evol Microbiol. 2008;58(Pt 12):2716–20.
33. Gevers D, Kugathasan S, Denson LA, Vazquez-Baeza Y, Van Treuren W, Ren B, et al. The treatment-naive microbiome in new-onset Crohn's disease. Cell Host Microbe. 2014;15(3):382–92.
34. Frank DN, Robertson CE, Hamm CM, Kpadeh Z, Zhang T, Chen H, et al. Disease phenotype and genotype are associated with shifts in intestinal-associated microbiota in inflammatory bowel diseases. Inflamm Bowel Dis. 2011;17(1):179–84.
35. Ahmadi K, Wilson C, Tiwana H, Binder A, Ebringer A. Antibodies to Klebsiella pneumoniae lipopolysaccharide in patients with ankylosing spondylitis. Br J Rheumatol. 1998;37(12):1330–3.
36. Maki-Ikola O, Lehtinen K, Nissila M, Granfors K. IgM, IgA and IgG class serum antibodies against Klebsiella pneumoniae and Escherichia coli lipopolysaccharides in patients with ankylosing spondylitis. Br J Rheumatol. 1994;33(11):1025–9.
37. Stone MA, Payne U, Schentag C, Rahman P, Pacheco-Tena C, Inman RD. Comparative immune responses to candidate arthritogenic bacteria do not confirm a dominant role for Klebsiella pneumonia in the pathogenesis of familial ankylosing spondylitis. Rheumatology (Oxford). 2004;43(2):148–55.
38. Landers CJ, Cohavy O, Misra R, Yang H, Lin YC, Braun J, et al. Selected loss of tolerance evidenced by Crohn's disease-associated immune responses to auto- and microbial antigens. Gastroenterology. 2002;123(3):689–99.
39. Targan SR, Landers CJ, Yang H, Lodes MJ, Cong Y, Papadakis KA, et al. Antibodies to CBir1 flagellin define a unique response that is associated independently with complicated Crohn's disease. Gastroenterology. 2005;128(7):2020–8.
40. Hoffman IEA, Demetter P, Peeters M, De Vos M, Mielants H, Veys EM, et al. Anti-Saccharomyces cerevisiae IgA antibodies are raised in ankylosing spondylitis and undifferentiated spondyloarthropathy. Ann Rheum Dis. 2003;62(5):455–9.
41. Aydin SZ, Atagunduz P, Temel M, Bicakcigil M, Tasan D, Direskeneli H. Anti-Saccharomyces cerevisiae antibodies (ASCA) in spondyloarthropathies: a reassessment. Rheumatology (Oxford). 2008;47(2):142–4.
42. de Vries M, van der Horst-Bruinsma I, van Hoogstraten I, van Bodegraven A, von Blomberg BM, Ratnawati H, et al. pANCA, ASCA, and OmpC antibodies in patients with ankylosing spondylitis without inflammatory bowel disease. J Rheumatol. 2010;37(11):2340–4.
43. Mundwiler ML, Mei L, Landers CJ, Reveille JD, Targan S, Weisman MH. Inflammatory bowel disease serologies in ankylosing spondylitis patients: a pilot study. Arthritis Res Ther. 2009;11(6):R177.
44. Torok HP, Glas J, Gruber R, Brumberger V, Strasser C, Kellner H, et al. Inflammatory bowel disease-specific autoantibodies in HLA-B27-associated spondyloarthropathies: increased prevalence of ASCA and pANCA. Digestion. 2004;70(1):49–54.
45. Wallis D, Asaduzzaman A, Weisman M, Haroon N, Anton A, McGovern D, et al. Elevated serum anti-flagellin antibodies implicate subclinical bowel inflammation in ankylosing spondylitis: an observational study. Arthritis Res Ther. 2013;15(5):R166.
46. Riente L, Chimenti D, Pratesi F, Delle Sedie A, Tommasi S, Tommasi C, et al. Antibodies to tissue transglutaminase and Saccharomyces cerevisiae in ankylosing spondylitis and psoriatic arthritis. J Rheumatol. 2004;31(5):920–4.
47. Hammer RE, Maika SD, Richardson JA, Tang JP, Taurog JD. Spontaneous inflammatory disease in transgenic rats expressing HLA-B27 and human beta 2m: an animal model of HLA-B27-associated human disorders. Cell. 1990;63(5):1099–112.
48. Rath HC, Herfarth HH, Ikeda JS, Grenther WB, Hamm TE Jr, Balish E, et al. Normal luminal bacteria, especially Bacteroides species, mediate chronic colitis, gastritis, and arthritis in HLA-B27/human beta2 microglobulin transgenic rats. J Clin Invest. 1996;98(4):945–53.
49. Benham H, Rehaume LM, Hasnain SZ, Velasco J, Baillet AC, Ruutu M, et al. Interleukin-23 mediates the intestinal response to microbial beta-1,3-glucan and the development of spondyloarthritis pathology in SKG mice. Arthritis Rheumatol. 2014;66(7):1755–67.
50. Rehaume LM, Mondot S, Aguirre de Carcer D, Velasco J, Benham H, Hasnain SZ, et al. ZAP-70 genotype disrupts the relationship between microbiota and host, leading to spondyloarthritis and ileitis in SKG mice. Arthritis Rheumatol. 2014;66(10):2780–92.
51. Baillet AC, Rehaume LM, Benham H, O'Meara CP, Armitage CW, Ruscher R, et al. High Chlamydia burden promotes tumor necrosis factor-dependent reactive arthritis in SKG mice. Arthritis Rheumatol. 2015;67(6):1535–47.
52. Weinreich S, Eulderink F, Capkova J, Pla M, Gaede K, Heesemann J, et al. HLA-B27 as a relative risk factor in ankylosing enthesopathy in transgenic mice. Hum Immunol. 1995;42(2):103–15.
53. Sinkorova Z, Capkova J, Niederlova J, Stepankova R, Sinkora J. Commensal intestinal bacterial strains trigger ankylosing enthesopathy of the ankle in inbred B10.BR (H-2(k)) male mice. Hum Immunol. 2008;69(12):845–50.
54. Capkova J, Hrncir T, Kubatova A, Tlaskalova-Hogenova H. Lipopolysaccharide treatment suppresses spontaneously developing ankylosing enthesopathy in B10.BR male mice: the potential role of interleukin-10. BMC Musculoskelet Disord. 2012;13:110.
55. Abraham C, Medzhitov R. Interactions between the host innate immune system and microbes in inflammatory bowel disease. Gastroenterology. 2011;140(6):1729–37.
56. Sun M, He C, Cong Y, Liu Z. Regulatory immune cells in regulation of intestinal inflammatory response to microbiota. Mucosal Immunol. 2015;8(5):969–78.
57. Ciccia F, Bombardieri M, Rizzo A, Principato A, Giardina AR, Raiata F, et al. Over-expression of paneth cell-derived anti-microbial peptides in the

gut of patients with ankylosing spondylitis and subclinical intestinal inflammation. Rheumatology. 2010;49(11):2076–83.
58. Collado A, Sanmarti R, Serra C, Gallart T, Canete JD, Gratacos J, et al. Serum levels of secretory IgA in ankylosing spondylitis. Scand J Rheumatol. 1991;20(3):153–8.
59. Wendling D, Didier JM, Seilles E. Serum secretory immunoglobulins in ankylosing spondylitis. Clin Rheumatol. 1996;15(6):590–3.
60. Asquith M, Elewaut D, Lin P, Rosenbaum JT. The role of the gut and microbes in the pathogenesis of spondyloarthritis. Best Pract Res Clin Rheumatol. 2014;28(5):687–702.
61. Adam R, Sturrock RD, Gracie JA. TLR4 mutations (Asp299Gly and Thr399Ile) are not associated with ankylosing spondylitis. Ann Rheum Dis. 2006;65(8):1099–101.
62. De Rycke L, Vandooren B, Kruithof E, De Keyser F, Veys EM, Baeten D. Tumor necrosis factor alpha blockade treatment down-modulates the increased systemic and local expression of toll-like receptor 2 and toll-like receptor 4 in spondylarthropathy. Arthritis Rheum. 2005;52(7):2146–58.
63. Crane AM, Bradbury L, van Heel DA, McGovern DP, Brophy S, Rubin L, et al. Role of NOD2 variants in spondylarthritis. Arthritis Rheum. 2002;46(6):1629–33.
64. Laukens D, Georges M, Libioulle C, Sandor C, Mni M, Vander Cruyssen B, et al. Evidence for significant overlap between common risk variants for Crohn's disease and Ankylosing spondylitis. PLoS One. 2010;5(11):e13795.
65. Cortes A, Hadler J, Pointon JP, Robinson PC, Karaderi T, Leo P, et al. Identification of multiple risk variants for ankylosing spondylitis through high-density genotyping of immune-related loci. Nat Genet. 2013;45(7):730–8.
66. Lees CW, Barrett JC, Parkes M, Satsangi J. New IBD genetics: common pathways with other diseases. Gut. 2011;60(12):1739–53.
67. Sokol H, Conway KL, Zhang M, Choi M, Morin B, Cao Z, et al. Card9 mediates intestinal epithelial cell restitution, T-helper 17 responses, and control of bacterial infection in mice. Gastroenterology. 2013;145(3):591–601 e3.
68. Baeten D, Demetter P, Cuvelier CA, Kruithof E, Van Damme N, De Vos M, et al. Macrophages expressing the scavenger receptor CD163: a link between immune alterations of the gut and synovial inflammation in spondyloarthropathy. J Pathol. 2002;196(3):343–50.
69. Baeten D, Moller HJ, Delanghe J, Veys EM, Moestrup SK, De Keyser F. Association of CD163+ macrophages and local production of soluble CD163 with decreased lymphocyte activation in spondylarthropathy synovitis. Arthritis Rheum. 2004;50(5):1611–23.
70. Zeng L, Lindstrom MJ, Smith JA. Ankylosing spondylitis macrophage production of higher levels of interleukin-23 in response to lipopolysaccharide without induction of a significant unfolded protein response. Arthritis Rheum. 2011;63(12):3807–17.
71. Qian BF, Tonkonogy SL, Sartor RB. Aberrant innate immune responses in TLR-ligand activated HLA-B27 transgenic rat cells. Inflamm Bowel Dis. 2008;14(10):1358–65.
72. Stebbings SM, Taylor C, Tannock GW, Baird MA, Highton J. The immune response to autologous bacteroides in ankylosing spondylitis is characterized by reduced interleukin 10 production. J Rheumatol. 2009;36(4):797–800.
73. De Wilde K, Martens A, Lambrecht S, Jacques P, Drennan MB, Debusschere K, et al. A20 inhibition of STAT1 expression in myeloid cells: a novel endogenous regulatory mechanism preventing development of enthesitis. Ann Rheum Dis. 2017;76(3):585–92.
74. Eberl G, Colonna M, Di Santo JP, McKenzie AN. Innate lymphoid cells. Innate lymphoid cells: a new paradigm in immunology. Science. 2015;348(6237):aaa6566.
75. Murphy KP. The mucosal immune system. In: Janeway's immunobiology. 8th ed. London: Garland Science; 2012. p. 465–508.
76. Hepworth MR, Fung TC, Masur SH, Kelsen JR, McConnell FM, Dubrot J, et al. Immune tolerance. Group 3 innate lymphoid cells mediate intestinal selection of commensal bacteria-specific CD4(+) T cells. Science. 2015;348(6238):1031–5.
77. Ciccia F, Guggino G, Rizzo A, Saieva L, Peralta S, Giardina A, et al. Type 3 innate lymphoid cells producing IL-17 and IL-22 are expanded in the gut, in the peripheral blood, synovial fluid and bone marrow of patients with ankylosing spondylitis. Ann Rheum Dis. 2015;74(9):1739–47.
78. Brewerton DA, Hart FD, Nicholls A, Caffrey M, James DC, Sturrock RD. Ankylosing spondylitis and HL-A 27. Lancet. 1973;1(7809):904–7.
79. Hermann E, Yu DT, Meyer zum Buschenfelde KH, Fleischer B. HLA-B27-restricted CD8 T cells derived from synovial fluids of patients with reactive arthritis and ankylosing spondylitis. Lancet. 1993;342(8872):646–50.
80. Kuon W, Holzhutter HG, Appel H, Grolms M, Kollnberger S, Traeder A, et al. Identification of HLA-B27-restricted peptides from the Chlamydia trachomatis proteome with possible relevance to HLA-B27-associated diseases. J Immunol. 2001;167(8):4738–46.
81. Ugrinovic S, Mertz A, Wu P, Braun J, Sieper JA. Single nonamer from the Yersinia 60-kDa heat shock protein is the target of HLA-B27-restricted CTL response in Yersinia-induced reactive arthritis. J Immunol. 1997;159(11):5715–23.
82. Atagunduz P, Appel H, Kuon W, Wu P, Thiel A, Kloetzel PM, et al. HLA-B27-restricted CD8+ T cell response to cartilage-derived self peptides in ankylosing spondylitis. Arthritis Rheum. 2005;52(3):892–901.
83. May E, Dorris ML, Satumtira N, Iqbal I, Rehman MI, Lightfoot E, et al. CD8 alpha beta T cells are not essential to the pathogenesis of arthritis or

colitis in HLA-B27 transgenic rats. J Immunol. 2003;170(2):1099–105.
84. Thiel A, Wu P, Lauster R, Braun J, Radbruch A, Sieper J. Analysis of the antigen-specific T cell response in reactive arthritis by flow cytometry. Arthritis Rheum. 2000;43(12):2834–42.
85. Frauendorf E, von Goessel H, May E, Marker-Hermann E. HLA-B27-restricted T cells from patients with ankylosing spondylitis recognize peptides from B*2705 that are similar to bacteria-derived peptides. Clin Exp Immunol. 2003;134(2):351–9.
86. Boyle LH, Goodall JC, Opat SS, Gaston JS. The recognition of HLA-B27 by human CD4(+) T lymphocytes. J Immunol. 2001;167(5):2619–24.
87. Alvarez-Navarro C, Cragnolini JJ, Dos Santos HG, Barnea E, Admon A, Morreale A, et al. Novel HLA-B27-restricted epitopes from Chlamydia trachomatis generated upon endogenous processing of bacterial proteins suggest a role of molecular mimicry in reactive arthritis. J Biol Chem. 2013;288(36):25810–25.
88. Scofield RH, Warren WL, Koelsch G, Harley JB. A hypothesis for the HLA-B27 immune dysregulation in spondyloarthropathy: contributions from enteric organisms, B27 structure, peptides bound by B27, and convergent evolution. Proc Natl Acad Sci U S A. 1993;90(20):9330–4.
89. Huang F, Hermann E, Wang J, Cheng XK, Tsai WC, Wen J, et al. A patient-derived cytotoxic T-lymphocyte clone and two peptide-dependent monoclonal antibodies recognize HLA-B27-peptide complexes with low stringency for peptide sequences. Infect Immun. 1996;64(1):120–7.
90. Syrbe U, Scheer R, Wu P, Sieper J. Differential synovial Th1 cell reactivity towards Escherichia coli antigens in patients with ankylosing spondylitis and rheumatoid arthritis. Ann Rheum Dis. 2012;71(9):1573–6.
91. Singh YP, Singh AK, Aggarwal A, Misra R. Evidence of cellular immune response to outer membrane protein of Salmonella typhimurium in patients with enthesitis-related arthritis subtype of juvenile idiopathic arthritis. J Rheumatol. 2011;38(1):161–6.
92. Baeten D, Van Damme N, Van den Bosch F, Kruithof E, De Vos M, Mielants H, et al. Impaired Th1 cytokine production in spondyloarthropathy is restored by anti-TNFalpha. Ann Rheum Dis. 2001;60(8):750–5.
93. Evans DM, Spencer CC, Pointon JJ, Su Z, Harvey D, Kochan G, et al. Interaction between ERAP1 and HLA-B27 in ankylosing spondylitis implicates peptide handling in the mechanism for HLA-B27 in disease susceptibility. Nat Genet. 2011;43(8):761–7.
94. Reveille JD. Genetics of spondyloarthritis – beyond the MHC. Nat Rev Rheumatol. 2012;8(5):296–304.
95. Ambarus C, Yeremenko N, Tak PP, Baeten D. Pathogenesis of spondyloarthritis: autoimmune or autoinflammatory? Curr Opin Rheumatol. 2012;24(4):351–8.
96. Colbert RA, Tran TM, Layh-Schmitt G. HLA-B27 misfolding and ankylosing spondylitis. Mol Immunol. 2014;57(1):44–51.
97. Neerinckx B, Carter S, Lories RJ. No evidence for a critical role of the unfolded protein response in synovium and blood of patients with ankylosing spondylitis. Ann Rheum Dis. 2014;73(3):629–30.
98. Glatigny S, Fert I, Blaton MA, Lories RJ, Araujo LM, Chiocchia G, et al. Proinflammatory Th17 cells are expanded and induced by dendritic cells in spondylarthritis-prone HLA-B27-transgenic rats. Arthritis Rheum. 2012;64(1):110–20.
99. Penttinen MA, Heiskanen KM, Mohapatra R, DeLay ML, Colbert RA, Sistonen L, et al. Enhanced intracellular replication of Salmonella enteritidis in HLA-B27-expressing human monocytic cells: dependency on glutamic acid at position 45 in the B pocket of HLA-B27. Arthritis Rheum. 2004;50(7):2255–63.
100. Ge S, Danino V, He Q, Hinton JC, Granfors K. Microarray analysis of response of Salmonella during infection of HLA-B27- transfected human macrophage-like U937 cells. BMC Genomics. 2010;11:456.
101. Rahman P, Inman RD, Gladman DD, Reeve JP, Peddle L, Maksymowych WP. Association of interleukin-23 receptor variants with ankylosing spondylitis. Arthritis Rheum. 2008;58(4):1020–5.
102. Langrish CL, McKenzie BS, Wilson NJ, de Waal Malefyt R, Kastelein RA, Cua DJ. IL-12 and IL-23: master regulators of innate and adaptive immunity. Immunol Rev. 2004;202:96–105.
103. Abraham C, Cho J. Interleukin-23/Th17 pathways and inflammatory bowel disease. Inflamm Bowel Dis. 2009;15(7):1090–100.
104. Gaffen SL, Jain R, Garg AV, Cua DJ. The IL-23-IL-17 immune axis: from mechanisms to therapeutic testing. Nat Rev Immunol. 2014;14(9):585–600.
105. Sutton CE, Mielke LA, Mills KH. IL-17-producing gammadelta T cells and innate lymphoid cells. Eur J Immunol. 2012;42(9):2221–31.
106. Treiner E. Mucosal-associated invariant T cells in inflammatory bowel diseases: bystanders, defenders, or offenders? Front Immunol. 2015;6:27.
107. Goodall JC, Wu C, Zhang Y, McNeill L, Ellis L, Saudek V, et al. Endoplasmic reticulum stress-induced transcription factor, CHOP, is crucial for dendritic cell IL-23 expression. Proc Natl Acad Sci U S A. 2010;107(41):17698–703.
108. Cerutti A, Rescigno M. The biology of intestinal immunoglobulin A responses. Immunity. 2008;28(6):740–50.
109. Cong Y, Feng T, Fujihashi K, Schoeb TR, Elson CO. A dominant, coordinated T regulatory cell-IgA response to the intestinal microbiota. Proc Natl Acad Sci U S A. 2009;106(46):19256–61.
110. Appel H, Wu P, Scheer R, Kedor C, Sawitzki B, Thiel A, et al. Synovial and peripheral blood CD4+FoxP3+ T cells in spondyloarthritis. J Rheumatol. 2011;38(11):2445–51.
111. Ciccia F, Accardo-Palumbo A, Giardina A, Di Maggio P, Principato A, Bombardieri M, et al. Expansion of intestinal CD4+CD25(high) Treg cells in patients with ankylosing spondylitis a putative role for Interleukin-10 in prevent-

ing intestinal Th17 response. Arthritis Rheum. 2010;62(12):3625–34.
112. Danoy P, Pryce K, Hadler J, Bradbury LA, Farrar C, Pointon J, et al. Association of variants at 1q32 and STAT3 with ankylosing spondylitis suggests genetic overlap with Crohn's disease. PLoS Genet. 2010;6(12):e1001195.
113. Chaudhry A, Rudra D, Treuting P, Samstein RM, Liang Y, Kas A, et al. CD4+ regulatory T cells control TH17 responses in a Stat3-dependent manner. Science. 2009;326(5955):986–91.
114. Ivanov II, Atarashi K, Manel N, Brodie EL, Shima T, Karaoz U, et al. Induction of intestinal Th17 cells by segmented filamentous bacteria. Cell. 2009;139(3):485–98.
115. Zelante T, Iannitti RG, Cunha C, De Luca A, Giovannini G, Pieraccini G, et al. Tryptophan catabolites from microbiota engage aryl hydrocarbon receptor and balance mucosal reactivity via Interleukin-22. Immunity. 2013;39(2):372–85.
116. Qiu J, Guo X, Chen ZM, He L, Sonnenberg GF, Artis D, et al. Group 3 innate lymphoid cells inhibit T-cell-mediated intestinal inflammation through aryl hydrocarbon receptor signaling and regulation of microflora. Immunity. 2013;39(2):386–99.
117. Atarashi K, Tanoue T, Shima T, Imaoka A, Kuwahara T, Momose Y, et al. Induction of colonic regulatory T cells by indigenous Clostridium species. Science. 2011;331(6015):337–41.
118. Round JL, Mazmanian SK. Inducible Foxp3+ regulatory T-cell development by a commensal bacterium of the intestinal microbiota. Proc Natl Acad Sci U S A. 2010;107(27):12204–9.
119. Rowan FE, Docherty NG, Coffey JC, O'Connell PR. Sulphate-reducing bacteria and hydrogen sulphide in the aetiology of ulcerative colitis. Br J Surg. 2009;96(2):151–8.
120. Peng L, He Z, Chen W, Holzman IR, Lin J. Effects of butyrate on intestinal barrier function in a Caco-2 cell monolayer model of intestinal barrier. Pediatr Res. 2007;61(1):37–41.
121. Furusawa Y, Obata Y, Fukuda S, Endo TA, Nakato G, Takahashi D, et al. Commensal microbe-derived butyrate induces the differentiation of colonic regulatory T cells. Nature. 2013;504(7480):446–50.
122. Singh N, Gurav A, Sivaprakasam S, Brady E, Padia R, Shi H, et al. Activation of Gpr109a, receptor for niacin and the commensal metabolite butyrate, suppresses colonic inflammation and carcinogenesis. Immunity. 2014;40(1):128–39.
123. Segain JP, Raingeard de la Bletiere D, Bourreille A, Leray V, Gervois N, Rosales C, et al. Butyrate inhibits inflammatory responses through NFkappaB inhibition: implications for Crohn's disease. Gut. 2000;47(3):397–403.
124. Huttenhower C, Kostic AD, Xavier RJ. Inflammatory bowel disease as a model for translating the Microbiome. Immunity. 2014;40(6):843–54.
125. Gaston JS, Cox C, Granfors K. Clinical and experimental evidence for persistent Yersinia infection in reactive arthritis. Arthritis Rheum. 1999;42(10):2239–42.
126. Gerard HC, Branigan PJ, Schumacher HR Jr, Hudson AP. Synovial chlamydia trachomatis in patients with reactive arthritis/Reiter's syndrome are viable but show aberrant gene expression. J Rheumatol. 1998;25(4):734–42.
127. Granfors K, Jalkanen S, Lindberg AA, Maki-Ikola O, von Essen R, Lahesmaa-Rantala R, et al. Salmonella lipopolysaccharide in synovial cells from patients with reactive arthritis. Lancet. 1990;335(8691):685–8.
128. Granfors K, Jalkanen S, von Essen R, Lahesmaa-Rantala R, Isomaki O, Pekkola-Heino K, et al. Yersinia antigens in synovial-fluid cells from patients with reactive arthritis. N Engl J Med. 1989;320(4):216–21.
129. May E, Marker-Hermann E, Wittig BM, Zeitz M, Meyer zum Buschenfelde KH, Duchmann R. Identical T-cell expansions in the colon mucosa and the synovium of a patient with enterogenic spondyloarthropathy. Gastroenterology. 2000;119(6):1745–55.
130. Cox CJ, Kempsell KE, Gaston JS. Investigation of infectious agents associated with arthritis by reverse transcription PCR of bacterial rRNA. Arthritis Res Ther. 2003;5(1):R1–8.
131. Siala M, Jaulhac B, Gdoura R, Sibilia J, Fourati H, Younes M, et al. Analysis of bacterial DNA in synovial tissue of Tunisian patients with reactive and undifferentiated arthritis by broad-range PCR, cloning and sequencing. Arthritis Res Ther. 2008;10(2):R40.
132. Gerard HC, Wang Z, Wang GF, El-Gabalawy H, Goldbach-Mansky R, Li Y, et al. Chromosomal DNA from a variety of bacterial species is present in synovial tissue from patients with various forms of arthritis. Arthritis Rheum. 2001;44(7):1689–97.
133. Olmez N, Wang GF, Li Y, Zhang H, Schumacher HR. Chlamydial nucleic acids in synovium in osteoarthritis: what are the implications? J Rheumatol. 2001;28(8):1874–80.
134. Pacheco-Tena C, Alvarado De La Barrera C, Lopez-Vidal Y, Vazquez-Mellado J, Richaud-Patin Y, Amieva RI, et al. Bacterial DNA in synovial fluid cells of patients with juvenile onset spondyloarthropathies. Rheumatology (Oxford). 2001;40(8):920–7.
135. van der Heijden IM, Wilbrink B, Tchetverikov I, Schrijver IA, Schouls LM, Hazenberg MP, et al. Presence of bacterial DNA and bacterial peptidoglycans in joints of patients with rheumatoid arthritis and other arthritides. Arthritis Rheum. 2000;43(3):593–8.
136. Sieper J, Fendler C, Laitko S, Sorensen H, Gripenberg-Lerche C, Hiepe F, et al. No benefit of long-term ciprofloxacin treatment in patients with reactive arthritis and undifferentiated oligoarthritis: a three-month, multicenter, double-blind, randomized, placebo-controlled study. Arthritis Rheum. 1999;42(7):1386–96.

137. Smieja M, MacPherson DW, Kean W, Schmuck ML, Goldsmith CH, Buchanan W, et al. Randomised, blinded, placebo controlled trial of doxycycline for chronic seronegative arthritis. Ann Rheum Dis. 2001;60(12):1088–94.
138. Salmi M, Andrew DP, Butcher EC, Jalkanen S. Dual binding capacity of mucosal immunoblasts to mucosal and synovial endothelium in humans: dissection of the molecular mechanisms. J Exp Med. 1995;181(1):137–49.
139. Salmi M, Jalkanen S. Human leukocyte subpopulations from inflamed gut bind to joint vasculature using distinct sets of adhesion molecules. J Immunol. 2001;166(7):4650–7.
140. Morton AM, Sefik E, Upadhyay R, Weissleder R, Benoist C, Mathis D. Endoscopic photoconversion reveals unexpectedly broad leukocyte trafficking to and from the gut. Proc Natl Acad Sci U S A. 2014;111(18):6696–701.
141. Faith JJ, Guruge JL, Charbonneau M, Subramanian S, Seedorf H, Goodman AL, et al. The long-term stability of the human gut microbiota. Science. 2013;341(6141):1237439.
142. Walker AW, Ince J, Duncan SH, Webster LM, Holtrop G, Ze X, et al. Dominant and diet-responsive groups of bacteria within the human colonic microbiota. ISME J. 2011;5(2):220–30.
143. Jernberg C, Lofmark S, Edlund C, Jansson JK. Long-term ecological impacts of antibiotic administration on the human intestinal microbiota. ISME J. 2007;1(1):56–66.
144. Khoruts A, Dicksved J, Jansson JK, Sadowsky MJ. Changes in the composition of the human fecal microbiome after bacteriotherapy for recurrent Clostridium difficile-associated diarrhea. J Clin Gastroenterol. 2010;44(5):354–60.
145. Wang ZK, Yang YS, Chen Y, Yuan J, Sun G, Peng LH. Intestinal microbiota pathogenesis and fecal microbiota transplantation for inflammatory bowel disease. World J Gastroenterol. 2014;20(40):14805–20.
146. Dieleman LA, Goerres MS, Arends A, Sprengers D, Torrice C, Hoentjen F, et al. Lactobacillus GG prevents recurrence of colitis in HLA-B27 transgenic rats after antibiotic treatment. Gut. 2003;52(3):370–6.
147. Schultz M, Veltkamp C, Dieleman LA, Grenther WB, Wyrick PB, Tonkonogy SL, et al. Lactobacillus plantarum 299V in the treatment and prevention of spontaneous colitis in interleukin-10-deficient mice. Inflamm Bowel Dis. 2002;8(2):71–80.
148. Noto Llana M, Sarnacki SH, Aya Castaneda Mdel R, Bernal MI, Giacomodonato MN, Cerquetti MC. Consumption of lactobacillus casei fermented milk prevents Salmonella reactive arthritis by modulating IL-23/IL-17 expression. PLoS One. 2013;8(12):e82588.
149. Hoentjen F, Welling GW, Harmsen HJ, Zhang X, Snart J, Tannock GW, et al. Reduction of colitis by prebiotics in HLA-B27 transgenic rats is associated with microflora changes and immunomodulation. Inflamm Bowel Dis. 2005;11(11):977–85.
150. Jenks K, Stebbings S, Burton J, Schultz M, Herbison P, Highton J. Probiotic therapy for the treatment of spondyloarthritis: a randomized controlled trial. J Rheumatol. 2010;37(10):2118–25.
151. Shukla A, Gaur P, Aggarwal A. Double blind placebo controlled randomized trial of probiotics in Enthesitis-related-arthritis category of JIA: effect on clinical and immunological parameters. Arthritis Rheum. 2015;67:S10.

Juvenile Idiopathic Arthritis 17

Miika Arvonen and Matthew L. Stoll

Abbreviations

ANA	Antinuclear antibody
CCP	Cyclic citrullinated peptide antibody
EBV	Epstein-Barr virus
EEN	Exclusive enteral nutrition
ERA	Enthesitis-related arthritis
FMT	Fecal microbiota transplantation
HLA	Human leukocyte antigen
JADAS	Juvenile arthritis disease activity score
PSRA	Post-streptococcal reactive arthritis
ReA	Reactive arthritis
SpA	Spondyloarthritis

Introduction of the JIA Categories

JIA is a heterogeneous condition, consisting of several categories with distinct clinical, pathophysiological, and genetic features [1]. It is not a single disease but a heterogeneous collection of conditions involving a spectrum of clinical findings [2]. About 20% of the risk for JIA may come from genetic factors [3], indicating a strong role for environmental factors, including the human intestinal microbiota. The International League of Associations for Rheumatology criteria divide JIA into seven categories of which oligoarthritis and seronegative polyarthritis are the most common ones in Western nations [4] and are well-represented in microbiota studies. Many children in these categories are diagnosed in early childhood, before age 5 [4]. Rheumatoid factor-positive polyarthritis and enthesitis-related arthritis (ERA) are usually diagnosed in older children and are roughly described as juvenile counterparts of the classical forms of adult rheumatoid arthritis and adult spondyloarthritis (SpA), respectively [5]; the microbiota in juvenile SpA has been investigated as well. The role of the microbiota in juvenile psoriatic arthritis has yet to be studied. Finally, undifferentiated arthritis is a variable condition with overlapping features shared by several of the preceding categories. However, at least the JIA categories of polyarticular and oligoarticular arthritis are believed to be antigen-driven lymphocyte-mediated autoimmune diseases with abnormalities in the adaptive immune system [6]. In contrast, systemic JIA appears to be an autoinflammatory syndrome, which shows no consistent associations with autoantibodies or human leukocyte antigen types (HLA) [6, 7]. There have not been any studies evaluating the gut microbiota in this category either.

M. Arvonen (✉)
Department of Pediatrics, Kuopio University Hospital, Kuopio, Finland
e-mail: Miika.Arvonen@kuh.fi

M. L. Stoll
Department of Pediatrics/Division of Rheumatology, University of Alabama at Birmingham, Birmingham, AL, USA

G. Ragab et al. (eds.), *The Microbiome in Rheumatic Diseases and Infection*, https://doi.org/10.1007/978-3-319-79026-8_17

Early-Life Events Which Are Associated with the Risk of JIA

Overview

Increased incidence of autoimmune diseases in Western countries has been linked with changes in early colonization of indigenous microbes, which educate the immune system [8]. For proper health, human mucosal immunity needs to maintain tolerance toward nutrients and beneficial microbes but simultaneously suppress any invasive pathogens without excess injury to the host mucosal barrier. Inappropriate colonization of beneficial microbes may result in perturbations of mucosal and peripheral immune maturation, which in turn can result in a higher risk of chronic autoimmune diseases in later life. The maturation process seems to start during pregnancy, since maternal health has been shown to impact the meconium microbiota composition and inflammatory disease susceptibility of the offspring [9]. For example, a recent Israeli study observed a distinctive pattern of month of birth in JIA patients compared to the healthy population; one interpretation of this finding is that seasonal environmental pathogens or alterations in maternal vitamin D levels may influence the risk of subsequent autoimmunity [10]. Additionally, a cluster of JIA cases that occurred following the influenza A H3N2 outbreak in 1977 was linked to prenatal sensitization to the H2N2 strain that may have occurred in 1963 [11]. However, for the most part, the association of prenatal events and subsequent risk of JIA is largely unknown. What has been studied in greater detail as risk factors for JIA are early-life events, such as mode of delivery, feeding practice, and exposure to systemic antimicrobial agents. All of these affect the development of the microbiota and consequently may have profound effects on immune maturation [12–14].

Mode of Delivery

Two Scandinavian registry-based studies [15, 16] have investigated the mode of delivery and future risk of JIA. In the Danish epidemiological study, children delivered by elective Caesarean section had an increased risk of JIA compared to vaginally delivered children [16]. Of note, this protective benefit did not extend to children with emergent Caesarean sections. This finding is supported by a Swedish study showing a tendency toward higher Caesarean section rates among children with JIA compared to controls (OR 1.1, 95% CI 1.0–1.3) although this study did not assess the differences between elective and unplanned sections. It should be noted that elective Caesarean sections are generally characterized by absence of stress signals induced by childbirth, whereas this is not the case with unplanned sections [17]. In addition, the amniotic sac will be frequently ruptured in emergent sections, thus exposing the fetus to maternal microbiota, while infants born by elective sections typically have no exposure to the maternal microbiota. Instead, such infants are colonized by skin bacteria such as *Staphylococcus*, *Corynebacterium*, and *Propionibacterium* spp. In contrast, vaginal delivery promotes the colonization of *Bifidobacteria* and *Bacteroides* [18, 19] as well as *Lactobacilli* and *Streptococci.* The microbial alteration and reduction of the microbial diversity in infants born by Caesarean section are reported to persist at least until 2 years of age [20–22], although there is contradictory data [3]. Besides the disturbed bacterial colonization of the mucosa, the mode of delivery imprints epigenetic regulation of gene expression, the long-term consequences of which are unknown [17]. Caesarean sections reduce the infant's early immune activation, as measured by leukocyte counts, and the secretion of proinflammatory cytokines, such as IL-1β, IL-6, and TNFα, and also delay the achievement of the humoral immune tolerance during the first year of life as measured by higher counts of food antigen-specific IgA, IgG, and IgM secreting B cells in peripheral blood, at least in infants who are at risk for allergic disease [17, 23–25].

Infant Feeding Practices

A second early-life event that appears to impact future risk of JIA is mode of feeding. Unlike mode of delivery, this information is more challenging to study, as feeding practices are not captured in insurance-based registries and thus generally rely on recall. In the first study evaluating the risk of JIA in breastfed compared with bottle-fed infants [26], breastfeeding was shown to have a protective effect on the development of JIA. Subsequent studies have supported this finding, although breastfeeding seemed to reduce the risk of developing certain JIA subtypes more than others. Specifacally, a shorter duration [27] or less frequent [26] breastfeeding was associated with development of oligoarticular JIA [28], but there was no protective effect of breastfeeding on polyarticular JIA [28]. In a large British registry study [29], breastfeeding seemed to decrease susceptibility to ERA and juvenile psoriatic arthritis more so than other forms of JIA [29]. Breastfeeding was also protective against the adult counterpart of ERA, spondyloarthropathy [30]. In the British study [29], breastfeeding influenced also the severity of JIA at presentation. Breastfed infants had younger age but milder symptoms during the onset of the disease as measured with lower scores on the childhood health assessment questionnaire, a marker of functional limitations. In recent Swedish prospective population-based study [31], parents filled out questionnaires on breastfeeding and introduction of solid foods ($n = 10{,}565$ completed questionnaires). This data was coupled 16 years later with the Swedish National Patient Register to identify children diagnosed with JIA ($n = 32$). Children who had been breastfed for less than 4 months had 3.5 increased risk of JIA compared to those breastfed more than 4 months. The patient sample in the study was too small to analyze the risk in different JIA categories, but the biggest category of the sample of the study was oligoarthritis (44%, 14/32). The study also evaluated potential confounding factors such as family history, parental education, and cigarette smoking, concluding that these factors did not affect the final outcome.

Mechanistically, the association between feeding practice and future risk of JIA may be due to altered microbial populations or to altered mucosal immunity. Breastfed infants have higher abundance of *Bifidobacterium*, *Lactobacilli*, and *Streptococci* than their bottle-fed counterparts [32] supporting dominance of the microbes already colonized during vaginal delivery [18]. Breastfeeding seems to influence not only the colonization of fecal microbiota but also imprinting of mucosal immunity [33]. Specifically, based upon studies in humans and mice, Perez et al. [33] postulated that breast milk includes mononuclear cells containing bacterial DNA, which the infant uses to train the immune system to recognize these foreign DNA fragments and thus to respond appropriately to microbial challenge [33].

The mechanism by which bottle-feeding was associated with an increased risk of JIA may differ based upon the subtype. As summarized above, bottle-feeding may be associated with both increased risks of oligoarticular JIA and SpA. Patients with ERA and ankylosing spondylitis show antibodies against commensal microbiota [34, 35]. In contrast, the predominant antibody in oligoarticular JIA is the antinuclear antibody (ANA) [36]. Of potential relevance, neonatal mice raised in germ-free conditions do not develop secondary lymphoid tissue in their intestinal mucosa and yet produce ANAs when exposed to segmented filamentous bacteria [37]. Van Dijkhuizen et al. presented data at Pediatric Rheumatology European conference [38] that the intestinal microbial composition was different in ANA-positive patients with respect to ANA-negative patients, suggesting that early-life events affecting the intestinal microbiota may be specifically associated with arthritis associated with a positive ANA.

Early Antibiotic Exposure

A third early-life factor that can influence the microbiota is exposure to antibiotics. Antibiotic use during infancy was recently shown to reverse the beneficial effects of breastfeeding with respect to development of a normal microbiota [39]. Two separate registry-based studies demonstrated that early-life exposure to antibiotics was associated with a higher risk of development of JIA later in life, even exposure that took place years before the onset of the disease [40, 41]. Both studies also showed a dose-dependent relationship between the use of antibiotics and JIA, and one study showed that those children exposed to antibiotics with wider total microbial coverage [41] appeared to have a higher risk of JIA than children exposed to a limited repertoire of antibiotics, even after adjusting for a total number of courses [42]. The study by Horton et al. [40] did not detect any obvious differences among classes of antibiotics, although it may not have been powered to see such an effect. Of note, broad-spectrum antibiotics have been associated with loss of intestinal microbial diversity [43, 44], which has been observed in children with JIA [45]. Neither studies evaluating antibiotic exposure and subsequent risk of JIA could fully exclude the possibilities that either children who develop JIA are more prone to developing infections early in life or that the infections themselves contributed to the risk. Indeed, a previous study conducted in Sweden showed that hospitalization in the first year of life was associated with risk of later JIA [15] raising the need to dissect whether the infection itself or antibiotics directed against the infection play a role in this finding. Along those lines, Horton et al. [40] concluded in their study that the relationship between exposure to antibiotics and JIA held even after adjusting for infections, although in their study based on primary health care, it was impossible to assess whether upper respiratory tract infections treated with antibiotics were intrinsically different than those not associated with antibiotic therapy.

Immunologic Maturation and JIA

A question that arises from the above studies is what are the potential mechanisms by which early colonization patterns might influence subsequent risk of JIA? Differences in the colonization pattern of mucosal microbes in different populations have been suspected to contribute to the innate immunity maturation and future incidence of autoimmune disease in the population level [8]. Vatanen et al. [8] studied the differences in the infant fecal microbiota in countries with high (Finland and Estonia) compared to low (Russia) incidence of childhood type 1 diabetes and likely JIA [46–49]. Interestingly, the Vatanen study showed that infants in countries with high incidence type 1 diabetes had an elevated fecal abundance of *Bacteroides* with a lower fecal abundance of *E. coli* compared to the Russian children. The potential significance of these findings was demonstrated in both mice and humans, where the lipopolysaccharide (LPS) from *E. coli* compared to that of *Bactroides dorei* demonstrated increased capacity both to engender inflammatory cytokine production from human peripheral blood cells and mouse splenocytes and also to induce tolerance to endotoxin in both humans and mice. Vatanen et al. concluded that the pattern of high *Bacteroides* compared to *E. coli* colonizing the infant gut could cause a reduced immune education of the mucosal innate immunity. This conclusion is in accordance with the extended version of hygiene hypothesis that the increased risk of autoimmunity could be due to deficient triggering of mucosal immunity in infancy [50]. It is therefore potentially highly significant that several studies have shown elevated fecal abundance of *Bacteroides* in children with type 1 diabetes and JIA. Specifically, this finding has been reported in separate studies in Finnish children with both type 1 diabetes and new-onset oligoarticular and seronegative polyarticular JIA, although these studies also showed a decreased fecal abundance of one species within the *Bacteroides* genus, *B. fragilis* [51, 52], possibly reflecting the ability of its polysaccharide tail to promote development of regulatory T cells [53]. The latter finding in particular indicates that specialized symbiont-derived molecules can promote tolerance toward commensals. In fact, mediators of intestinal mucosal tolerance mediated by innate and adaptive immune pathways have been studied from mucosal biopsies of JIA patients suffering from gastrointestinal symptoms [54]. This study showed that JIA patients in remission displayed higher intestinal messenger RNA levels of Toll-like receptor 4 together with higher expression of the anti-inflammatory mediators IL10, TGFβ, and FOXP3 compared with expression in patients with active JIA [54]. In accordance with this finding, stimulation of the Toll-like receptor 9 on apical mucosa by selected microbial conserved structures was shown to induce regulatory T-cell responses and confer protection against experimental arthritis [55] but induced proinflammatory cascades on basolateral side [56]. Therefore, altered mucosal innate immunity, potentially influenced by early development of the fecal microbiota, may affect the subsequent risk of JIA (Fig. 17.1).

Another illustration of mucosal immunity affecting systemic disease risk comes from findings from helminth parasites. Helminths ensure their survival through regulating immune pathways, thereby shielding themselves from an inflammatory process [57]. Many helminth infections can induce regulatory T-cell responses, which in mouse models of arthritis have translated to reduction of disease severity during helminth infection [58]. A potential therapeutic benefit of one helminth parasite, *Trichuris suis*, was also demonstrated in humans with IBD [59, 60], although this therapy has not been evaluated in children with JIA. However, there are data from studies in humans that parasites may affect the pathways associated with arthritis: an inverse relationship was detected between helminth exposure and presence of ANAs, and furthermore ANA titers increased following eradication of the parasite [61]. These findings are of particular interest in light of the studies summarized above that the microbiota may contribute to the development of ANAs [37, 38].

Alteration of Fecal Microbial Profiles in JIA Compared with Controls

Five studies and one congress abstract have been published so far evaluating changes in the fecal microbiota in children with JIA [34, 38, 45, 52, 62]. All of these studies evaluated the fecal microbiota, rather than intestinal biopsy specimens. This may be an important limitation, as the microbiota varies greatly along the length of the

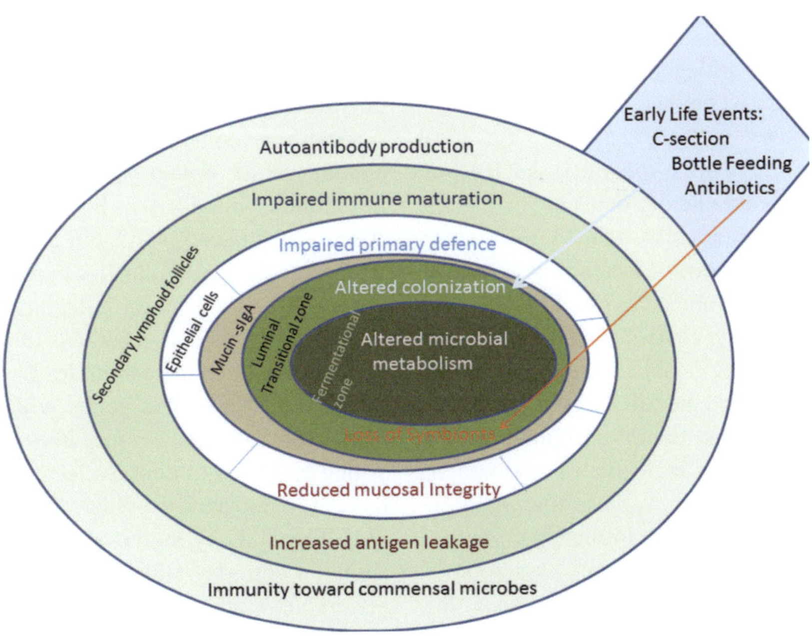

Fig. 17.1 Schematic presentation of the potential effect of altered intestinal microbiome in JIA. Early life factors, such as Caesarean section, bottle feeding and early exposure to antibiotics, can impair colonization of the commensal microbiota (blue square in the right corner). The commensal microbiota can induce mucosal immune maturation and development of adequate mucosal integrity (innermost circles). Impaired maturation and integrity of mucosal immune system predisposes host to humoral immune responses toward commensal microbiota and self-antigens (outer circle)

gastrointestinal tract [63] and fecal microbiota differs from that of the mucosa [64]. Another potential limitation of these studies is failure to take into account all of the medications that could impact the microbiota. While all of them excluded children with recent exposure to antibiotics, other medications that can impact the fecal microbiota, such as laxatives and proton pump inhibitors [44, 65, 66], were not consistently assessed. This limitation is not unique to studies in JIA but appears to be fairly widespread among studies evaluating patients with inflammatory disorders in general. All of the studies in children with JIA published to date involved PCR amplification of the hypervariable 16S ribosomal DNA regions but differ to some extent in the specific hypervariable region studied; one of them also included whole genome shotgun metagenomics (Table 17.1). Thus, these studies may not be directly comparable, as choice of hypervariable region can impact the findings [67]. One study querying the fecal microbiota used liquid chromatography and mass spectrometry to identify fecal water metabolites in ERA patients and controls [68]. Table 17.1 summarizes the study methods and populations, and Table 17.2 lists the critical findings therein, which are also summarized below.

Two of those studies evaluated the fecal microbiota profile in oligo-/polyarticular JIA [45, 52], with some contradictory data observed at the phylum level. Specifically, the Finnish study demonstrated in newly diagnosed subjects decreased *Firmicutes* and increased *Bacteroidetes* compared to healthy controls, while an Italian study in children with established ERA and polyarticular JIA [45] revealed that *Firmicutes* were more abundant in JIA. Since the Italian but not the Finnish study was inclusive of children on immunosuppressive therapy, these findings raise the question as to whether immunosuppressive therapies might affect the microbiota. Sulfasalazine undoubtedly does, as it is an antibiotic. Most of the ERA patients in the study of Di Paola et al. were exposed to sulfasalazine [45], but none in the Indian or North American studies were [34, 62]. There are very little data on the extent to which other medications might impact the microbiota. A study in mice presented at the 2016 American College of Rheumatology annual conference demonstrated that *Firmicutes* were more resistant to methotrexate than were *Bacteroidetes* [69], a finding which could potentially result in the loss of *Bacteroidetes* in JIA reported by Di Paola et al. [45], although the dose of methotrexate used in the study by Nayak et al. [70] was not reflective of that used in clinical practice to treat rheumatic diseases. Still different phylum-level findings were reported in a study inclusive of children from Italy and the Netherlands presented at the Pediatric Rheumatology European Society Meeting 2016, with this study reporting increased *Proteobacteria* and decreased *Actinobacteria* in children with JIA compared to controls [38]. Interestingly, despite differences at the phylum level, some consistent findings have been seen at the genus/species level. Specifically, decreased *Faecalibacterium prausnitzii* was reported among both polyarticular JIA patients in the Italian study [45] and ERA patients in the North American study [34]. Likewise, a nonsignificant underrepresentation of different species belonging to *Clostridium* cluster IV, which includes *F. prausnitzii*, was found in the Finnish study of polyarticular and oligoarticular JIA subjects [52].

Another consistent finding is increased abundance of *Bacteroides*, a finding reported in children with ERA in both Indian and North American studies [34, 62, 69] as well as children with oligo-/polyarticular JIA in the Finnish study [52]. These findings may reflect immune priming associated with *Bacteroides*, as discussed above, and this might be the case at least with respect to the association of this genus with development of oligoarthritis and seronegative polyarthritis in young children. In contrast, *Bacteroides* may be directly pathogenic in older children with ERA [34]. The study by Stoll et al. [34] showed expansion of mucin-degrading organisms *Akkermansia muciniphila* and *Bacteroides* in children with ERA accompanied by loss of *F. prausnitzii* [34]. This injury to the mucin layer combined with loss of *F. prausnitzii* might enable *Bacteroides* to be located closer to epithelial cells than it normally is [71], permitting it to be targeted by the mucosal immune system. Indeed, Stoll et al. [34]

Table 17.1 Studies on fecal microbiota in juvenile idiopathic arthritis

Study	Number of patients	Number of controls	Nation	Disease category	Patient characteristics	Hypervariable region
Stoll et al. [34]	25	13	USA	ERA	DMARD-naive and on DMARD	V4
Tejesvi et al. [52]	31	29	Finland	Seroneg. poly, oligo	Newly onset, DMARD-naive,	V4–V5
Aggarwal et al. [62]	33	14	India	ERA	Established disease, on DMARD	V3
Di Paola et al. [45]	29	29	Italy	Seroneg. poly, ERA	Established disease, on DMARD	V5–V6
Stoll et al. [68]	24	19	USA	ERA	DMARD-naive and on DMARD	NA
Stoll et al. [69]	30	19	USA	ERA	Newly onset, DMARD-naïve	V4

DMARD disease-modifying antirheumatic drugs, *ERA* enthesitis-related arthritis, *seroneg. poly* seronegative polyarthritihs, *oligo* oligoarthritis, *NA* not applicable

demonstrated that children with ERA had altered humoral immunity toward commensal microbes including *Bacteroides* [34]. Animal data also show that *Bacteroides* may be directly pathogenic in models of HLA-B27-associated arthritis [72, 73]. Thus, the mechanism by which Bacteroides is associated with JIA awaits further clarification.

One other finding that emerges from this research is that the functional potential of the microbiota might be essential with respect to disease pathogenesis. The decreased abundance of *F. prausnitzii* and other species belonging to beneficial *Clostridium* cluster IV may result in reduced production of butyrate, an important substrate for epithelial cell proliferation and maintenance of the intestinal integrity [74, 75]. Of note, increased intestinal permeability has been identified in children with JIA [76]. The synergistic effect of these symbionts is also important for induction of regulatory T cell [77]. Indeed, Stoll et al. showed, in ERA, decreased content of fecal water metabolites involved in the butanoate pathway, which makes butyrate [78], which is a key metabolite in the induction of regulatory T cells [79]. Additionally, the study by Stoll et al. [68] showed reduced diversity of fecal metabolites, particularly those within the tryptophan pathway, in children with ERA as compared to healthy controls. The authors argued that these alterations may affect the selection between regulatory and effector T cells [68]. Thus, bacterial metabolites may themselves affect mucosal immune function, contributing to the pathogenesis of ERA (Fig. 17.1).

Spreading of the Mucosal Inflammation to the Target Organ, Synovial Membranes

How do altered microbial populations and immunity to the microbiota translate into arthritis? Presumably, an initial step is development of intestinal inflammation. Studies in children with ERA have demonstrated increased intestinal inflammation by colonoscopy [80], leukocyte scintigraphy [81], and fecal calprotectin [82]. Since mucosal inflammation exacerbates antigen leakage and consequently antigen-mediated immune activation, this could trigger humoral immune responses. For example, Fotis et al. demonstrated increased humoral reactivity toward LPS from different aerobic gram-negative rods in JIA patients compared with controls [83]. The LPS reactivity correlated with juvenile arthritis disease activity scores (JADAS) in 27 patients. In addition, Stoll et al. [34] reported that among children with ERA, serum IgA levels against commensal microbiota (*B. fragilis*) were directly proportional to the fecal abundance of the *Bacteroides* genus.

Intestinal dendritic cells can steer T cell activation status, and in addition, intestinal dendritic cells activate T cells to express gut-associated

Table 17.2 Fecal microbial taxonomic and functional alterations in JIA

	Disease category
Microbial alteration "loss of symbionts"	
Reduction of *Faecalibacterium prausnitzii* [34]	ERA
Reduction of *Faecalibacterium prausnitzii* [45]	Seronegative polyarticular JIA
Underrepresentation of members of *Clostridium* cluster IV (a trend) [52]	Oligoarthritis, seronegative polyarthritis
Microbial alteration substituting Microbiota	
Increase of *Bacteroides or B. fragilis* [34, 62, 69]	ERA
Increase of *Bacteroides* [34, 52, 62]	Oligoarthritis, seronegative polyarthritis
Increase of *Enterococcus* [62]	ERA
Microbial functional alteration	
Decreased genetic potential of the butanoate pathway [69]	ERA
Decreased content of butanoate pathway [68]	ERA
Decreased content of tryptophan pathway [68]	ERA
Immune response toward microbiota/related to microbial alteration	
Divergent relationship between *B. fragilis* antibody and abundance of *Bacteroides* in JIA and control group [34]	ERA
Divergent relationship between *F. prausnitzii* antibody and abundance of *F. prausnitzii* in JIA and control group [34]	ERA
ANA positivity related to microbial alteration (abstract) [38]	Different JIA categories

ERA enthesitis-related arthritis, JIA juvenile idiopathic arthritis

homing receptors like α4β7 integrin and CCR9, which guide activated T cells circulating through the blood to migrate back to the bowel in normal situation [84]. During natural cell death, dendritic cells inactivate T cells, which recognize autoantigens, ensuring central tolerance. An opposite interaction occurs between dendritic and T cells during bacterial invasion. Since a heterogeneous expression of adhesion molecules is found in synovial endothelial cells during synovitis [85, 86], mucosal T cells can circulate through the blood and home into the inflamed joints. This theory is supported by the finding that leukocytes expressing gut-specific homing receptors have been found in inflamed synovial fluid from patients with ERA and adult SpA [87, 88]. Likewise, intestinal secretory antibodies directed against enteropathogenic microbes could be transferred into the joint spaces and be able to bind to cross-reactive self-antigens [89].

Another possibility was proposed by Saxena et al. [90], who suggested that ERA might be a continuum of adult reactive arthritis (ReA). In the latter condition, triggering microbes have been identified in synovial tissue [91]. Specifically, the Indian group has argued that *Salmonella* may be a triggering organism for ERA, as it is in some cases of reactive arthritis in adults [92]. They reported increased T-cell responses toward *Salmonella* outer membrane protein in ERA patients compared to controls. Although *Salmonella* is not a common cause of ReA in developed nations, it is plausible that other organisms might likewise be the target of aberrant immunity, as recently suggested [93]. It should be noted that these two alternative theories linking gut and synovial inflammation—migration of gut-derived T cells into joints versus disease caused by pathologic T cell or humoral immunity against specific enteric organisms—are not necessarily mutually exclusive possibilities.

Finally, it bears mention that the fecal microbiota may not be the only relevant microbial habitat in JIA. As discussed elsewhere in this text (Chap. 15), the oral microbiota has been a subject of interest in adults with RA, particularly with respect to an association between RA and gingivitis. The category of JIA that is most similar to RA is RF+ polyarticular JIA. Consistent with the data in adults with RA, children with anti-cyclic citrullinated peptide antibody (CCP)-positive JIA demonstrated increased antibodies toward oral microbiota associated with gingivitis as well as poorer oral health, compared to children with anti-CCP-negative JIA [94].

Infections in Context of JIA Pathogenesis

So far, the discussion has been on the association of the microbiota as a whole with JIA. However, specific viral and bacterial infections have been linked to the development of JIA as well. Such studies have been limited to children with established JIA; longitudinal studies following previously healthy children before the onset of JIA have not been conducted. Several alphaviruses have been linked to arthritis in adults, with less convincing associations reported in the pediatric population [95]. In addition, hepatitis B and C viruses, human T-lymphotropic virus, human immunodeficiency virus, mumps, and rubella have been linked to the development of chronic arthritis, although again not JIA [96]. One of the common features in the many arthrogenic viruses is their ability to cause long-standing infection in the host and to induce autoantibody production [97–99] and T-cell-mediated autoimmunity. Most studies evaluating the role of infectious agents as a trigger of JIA have used microbial-specific antibodies to look for evidence of exposure [100–102]. Along those lines, a British uncontrolled study [100] showed that 50% of JIA subjects had antibodies against *Chlamydia pneumoniae*, while none had antibodies against *C. trachomatis*, suggesting possible pathogenicity of the former. A subsequent Turkish study [101] provided contradictory data, showing no difference in *C. pneumoniae* seropositivity between JIA patients and controls. In a Polish study [102], IgG seropositivity toward *Mycoplasma pneumoniae* was more common in JIA than in control children. In addition, a Canadian study demonstrated a significant correlation of new diagnoses of JIA (other than ERA) with four epidemics of *Mycoplasma pneumoniae* between 1975 and 1992 in the province of Manitoba [103].

Two specific viruses warrant further attention: parvovirus B19 and the Epstein-Barr virus (EBV), which have been associated with clinical disease resembling JIA and are suspected to contribute to the onset of JIA [104, 105]. Infection by parvovirus causes both asymptomatic and symptomatic clinical diseases with wide spectrum of manifestations including arthritis. Typically, parvovirus viremia resolves in 1 week. Persistent parvovirus viremia together with symmetric arthritis has been reported in children with generalized antibody deficiency or a specific inability to produce antibody against capsid protein [106, 107]. A unique region in capsid protein VP1 of parvovirus B19 possesses phospholipase A2 activity [108]. Interestingly, parvovirus infection has also been associated with the development of antiphospholipid antibodies [109]. Although such antibodies are not typically reported in JIA, they have been observed in children with JIA who have persistent infection with parvovirus B19 [110, 111]. Antibodies toward parvovirus have also been detected in ocular fluid of JIA patients with uveitis [112]. Several studies have shown increased exposure to parvovirus B19 among children with JIA compared to controls [113–116], although this finding is not universally seen [117].

The role of EBV in the pathogenesis of JIA has been investigated only in small studies. In an Iranian uncontrolled study, EBV seropositivity was a common feature in hospitalized JIA patients, and the authors suggested that EBV infection could be linked with a refractory disease course of JIA [105]. In contrast, a Taiwanese study did not find differences in EBV or cytomegalovirus positivity in JIA patients compared with controls [118]. Massa et al. reported T-cell cytotoxic responses including increased IFN-γ directed against self-derived HLA epitopes in EBV-positive oligoarticular JIA patients but not with EBV-positive healthy controls [119]. In contrast, Kawada et al. reported a remission in three patients with refractory JIA after EBV infection associated with an increase in IFN-γ production [120], which the authors suggested to indicate that increased IFN-γ could resolve the autoimmunity by controlling TH17-mediated immunity [121]. Taken together, studies on the association of viral infections and JIA are inconclusive but intriguing. Since viruses can contribute to effector T-cell homeostasis [122, 123] and effector T cells play a critical role in the course of JIA [124, 125], future studies assessing the role of viral pathogens in JIA are warranted.

There are several mechanisms by which an infectious organism could predispose to arthritis. One is molecular mimicry. A classic example of molecular mimicry resulting in an autoimmune disease is acute rheumatic fever following infection with *Streptococcus pyogenes*, in which T cells against the streptococcal M protein cross-react with human cardiac myosin [126]. A

Norwegian study [127] compared the characteristics of post-streptococcal reactive arthritis (PSRA) with other forms of juvenile arthritis. Healthy controls were not involved in the study. Recent streptococcal infection was identified in 9% of new-onset JIA patients (3/33). Arthritis due to PSRA was still present 6 weeks and 6 months after admission in 33% (7/21) and 10% (2/21), respectively. Another organism that has been linked to chronic arthritis potentially via the molecular mimicry route is *Klebsiella pneumoniae*, with one group showing elevated fecal carriage in ankylosing spondylitis [128]. Similarly, the Indian pediatric study showed that the fecal abundance of *Klebsiella pneumoniae* was higher in ERA than in healthy controls [62]. However, other studies in adult and pediatric SpA have not seen such an association [34, 45, 129]. *K. pneumoniae* is postulated to be one of the candidates in the pathogenesis of spondyloarthritis via molecular mimicry mechanism, since bacterial antigens of *K. pneumoniae*, nitrogenase and pullulanase, share molecular features with self-antigens HLA-B27 and collagens I, III, and IV [130].

Alternatively, infections can have a nonspecific bystander effect on T cells via co-stimulatory signals [123] and bystander [131–134] and polyclonal lymphocyte activation [135]. Finally, posttranscriptional modification of host peptides, such as citrullination and glycation, is linked to development of various autoimmune diseases via generation of remnant epitopes [136]. T lymphocytes with weak reactivity against native host peptides can develop much stronger reactivity following posttranslational modification [137]. As discussed in depth in the RA chapter [Chap. 15], pathogenesis of seropositive polyarticular JIA is linked with gingival inflammation by *Porphyromonas gingivalis* [138, 139], which is able to convert arginine residues in proteins to citrulline, a candidate autoantigen in this JIA category. A recent study showed that children with antibodies against citrullinated peptides, compared to those lacking such antibodies, also carried elevated titers of antibodies against oral microbiota associated with gingivitis [94]; similar findings have been reported in adults with RA [140]. Thus, to the extent that microbial agents themselves can modify host proteins, as *P. gingivalis* can do [141], they can contribute directly to the pathogenesis of JIA.

Therapeutic Potential of the Microbial Alteration

The promise of the microbiota lies in studies designed to improve the disease state through alterations in the microbiota. The consistency of studies showing alterations in the microbiota yields hope that such efforts to treat the disease state through alterations in the microbiota will yield fruit, although optimism should be tempered by the possibility that altered immunologic maturation, even if induced by early-life shifts in the microbiota, may not easily be reversible. In addition, the methods used to induce alterations in the microbiota must be carefully considered to ensure that the new microbiota is less likely to be associated with the disease state as compared to the current.

There are several tools that can used to alter the microbiota, including diet, probiotics, and fecal transplant (FMT). FMT will only be mentioned briefly, as this has not been studied in JIA. It may be effective in patients with IBD, perhaps more so in young versus older subjects [142], so it may be worthy of consideration as a therapeutic tool in JIA.

There was one pediatric study of probiotics, which was conducted in India. In this study, patients with long-standing ERA with average disease duration of 3 years were randomized to placebo or probiotic therapy. The probiotic VSL3 contained *Streptococcus thermophilus*, *Bifidobacterium breve*, *B. longum*, *B. infantis*, *Lactobacillus acidophilus*, *L. plantarum*, *L. paracasei*, and *L. delbrueckii*; both groups were also treated with nonsteroidal anti-inflammatory drugs for the duration of the 12-week study, but no patients were on immunosuppressive therapy. Clinical response was seen in both groups ($p < 0.01$ compared to their respective baselines), but no between-group differences were observed in disease activity at the end of the trial ($p = 0.16$).

The failure of this particular probiotic therapy, even with the failed trial of probiotics in ankylosing spondylitis [143], should not necessarily be taken as evidence that probiotics in general would not work for children with ERA. Future probiotic studies should be informed by the specific deficiencies that have been identified in the patient population under question, with the intent of replacing deficient bacteria. This was not the case herein; none of the bacteria provided in this trial were differentially abundant between patients and controls. It would be of greater interest to treat with *Faecalibacterium prausnitzii* or other *Clostridium* cluster IV members, although logistically, this might be challenging due to these species being obligate anaerobic bacteria. Another potential approach might be to treat with butyrate, an important metabolic product of *Faecalibacterium prausnitzii* or other *Clostridium* cluster IV members [144, 145]. This has not been studied in humans but was successful in reducing disease activity in a mouse model of colitis, with the improvement attributed to induction of regulatory T cells [79, 145, 146].

Finally, exclusive enteral nutrition (EEN) is an established treatment option in pediatric Crohn's disease, and its anti-inflammatory effect is postulated to be caused by modification of the intestinal microbiota [147]. Children treated with EEN need to be supervised closely by a nutritionist to ensure that they are meeting all of their daily requirements, and it can be challenging to maintain adherence with long-term use of EEN. Nevertheless, this has been studied in JIA. In uncontrolled studies, a group from Sweden has reported use of EEN in a total of seven patients with JIA (three ERA, three seronegative polyarthritis, and one oligoarthritis) spanning two studies [148, 149]. EEN had a significant beneficial effect on active joint count ($p = 0.031$), the JADAS27 disease activity index ($p = 0.016$), and morning stiffness ($p = 0.031$). Additionally, in a child with seronegative polyarticular JIA, EEN treatment resulted in a shift in the *Bacteroidetes*/*Firmicutes* ratio increased toward increased abundance of *Firmicutes* [150]. This may be a particularly promising result in light of the findings of decreased *Firmicutes* in children with polyarticular JIA [52], although it is not clear that the change in the microbiota was the reason for the clinical response to EEN. Other dietary approaches that might favorably alter the microbiota include cutting back on meat intake and increased consumption of vegetables, with both changes potentially driving down the abundance of *Bacteroides* [151, 152], which as discussed above are elevated in children with JIA [34, 52, 62].

Conclusions Maturation of mucosal immunity to defend against microbes and tolerate different environmental antigens is a fundamental process and dependent on the early colonization of the commensal microbiota [153, 154]. Environmental factors such as Caesarean section, bottle-feeding, and early exposure to antibiotics can result in altered microbiota, which in turn may result in impaired development of the immune system, since our microbiota play such an important role in immune maturation [18, 155]. Impaired maturation of mucosal immunity predisposes to both microbial infections and aberrant immunologic responses toward commensal microbiota as well as toward self-antigens [37, 153, 154]. This may account for findings that children with JIA are more likely to have been exposed to C-section, bottle-feeding, hospitalization for infection, and courses of antibiotics [15, 16, 26–29, 31, 40, 41]. Additionally, they have altered humoral and cellular responses to infectious organisms and increased production of antinuclear antibodies [34, 36], all of which changes can be related to the contents and function of the intestinal microbiota.

While the mucosal maturation process can be addressed only through preventive rather than therapeutic measures by the time a child has developed JIA, taxonomic and functional alterations found in JIA [34, 38, 45, 52, 62, 69] may suggest potential avenues for therapeutic interventions. As studies show that JIA patients lack normal symbionts and metabolites, these could potentially be replaced directly, or their abundance might be adjusted with dietary therapy. In addition, the microbial habitants in the oral cavity of seropositive JIA are associated with gingivitis and formation of citrullinated peptides, which are known autoantigens of that JIA category [94], and therapy of gingivitis appears to be effective at reducing disease severity in RA [72]. There are several new approaches to modify the mucosal microbiota toward one that might be less conducive to disease [142, 144, 145, 151, 152, 156, 157]. These therapies may open a new paradigm of therapy for children with JIA.

References

1. Petty RE, Southwood TR, Manners P, Baum J, Glass DN, Goldenberg J, et al. International League of Associations for Rheumatology classification of juvenile idiopathic arthritis: second revision, Edmonton, 2001. J Rheumatol. 2004;31:390–2.
2. Martini A, Lovell DJ. Juvenile idiopathic arthritis: state of the art and future perspectives. Ann Rheum Dis. 2010;69:1260–3.
3. Hinks A, Cobb J, Marion MC, Prahalad S, Sudman M, Bowes J, et al. Dense genotyping of immune-related disease regions identifies 14 new susceptibility loci for juvenile idiopathic arthritis. Nat Genet. 2013;45:664–9.
4. Nordal E, Zak M, Aalto K, Berntson L, Fasth A, Herlin T, et al. Ongoing disease activity and changing categories in a long-term nordic cohort study of juvenile idiopathic arthritis. Arthritis Rheum. 2011;63:2809–18.
5. van Rossum M, van Soesbergen R, de Kort S, ten Cate R, Zwinderman AH, de Jong B, et al. Anti-cyclic citrullinated peptide (anti-CCP) antibodies in children with juvenile idiopathic arthritis. J Rheumatol. 2003;30:825–8.
6. Lin YT, Wang CT, Gershwin ME, Chiang BL. The pathogenesis of oligoarticular/polyarticular vs systemic juvenile idiopathic arthritis. Autoimmun Rev. 2011;10:482–9.
7. Prakken B, Albani S, Martini A. Juvenile idiopathic arthritis. Lancet. 2011;377:2138–49.
8. Vatanen T, Kostic AD, d'Hennezel E, Siljander H, Franzosa EA, Yassour M, et al. Variation in microbiome LPS immunogenicity contributes to autoimmunity in humans. Cell. 2016;165:842–53.
9. Gosalbes MJ, Llop S, Valles Y, Moya A, Ballester F, Francino MP. Meconium microbiota types dominated by lactic acid or enteric bacteria are differentially associated with maternal eczema and respiratory problems in infants. Clin Exp Allergy. 2013;43:198–211.
10. Berkun Y, Lewy H, Padeh S, Laron Z. Seasonality of birth of patients with juvenile idiopathic arthritis. Clin Exp Rheumatol. 2015;33:122–6.
11. Pritchard MH, Matthews N, Munro J. Antibodies to influenza A in a cluster of children with juvenile chronic arthritis. Br J Rheumatol. 1988;27:176–80.
12. Koenig JE, Spor A, Scalfone N, Fricker AD, Stombaugh J, Knight R, et al. Succession of microbial consortia in the developing infant gut microbiome. Proc Natl Acad Sci U S A. 2011;108(Suppl 1):4578–85.
13. Bates JM, Mittge E, Kuhlman J, Baden KN, Cheesman SE, Guillemin K. Distinct signals from the microbiota promote different aspects of zebrafish gut differentiation. Dev Biol. 2006;297:374–86.
14. Hooper LV, Wong MH, Thelin A, Hansson L, Falk PG, Gordon JI. Molecular analysis of commensal host-microbial relationships in the intestine. Science. 2001;291:881–4.
15. Carlens C, Jacobsson L, Brandt L, Cnattingius S, Stephansson O, Askling J. Perinatal characteristics, early life infections and later risk of rheumatoid arthritis and juvenile idiopathic arthritis. Ann Rheum Dis. 2009;68:1159–64.
16. Kristensen K, Henriksen L. Cesarean section and disease associated with immune function. J Allergy Clin Immunol. 2016;137:587–90.
17. Cho CE, Norman M. Cesarean section and development of the immune system in the offspring. Am J Obstet Gynecol. 2013;208:249–54.
18. Rautava S, Luoto R, Salminen S, Isolauri E. Microbial contact during pregnancy, intestinal colonization and human disease. Nat Rev Gastroenterol Hepatol. 2012;9:565–76.
19. Biasucci G, Rubini M, Riboni S, Morelli L, Bessi E, Retetangos C. Mode of delivery affects the bacterial community in the newborn gut. Early Hum Dev. 2010;86(Suppl 1):13–5.
20. Jakobsson HE, Abrahamsson TR, Jenmalm MC, Harris K, Quince C, Jernberg C, et al. Decreased gut microbiota diversity, delayed Bacteroidetes colonisation and reduced Th1 responses in infants delivered by caesarean section. Gut. 2014;63:559–66.
21. Rutayisire E, Huang K, Liu Y, Tao F. The mode of delivery affects the diversity and colonization pattern of the gut microbiota during the first year of infants' life: a systematic review. BMC Gastroenterol. 2016;16:86. https://doi.org/10.1186/s12876,016-0498-0.
22. Chu D, Ma J, Prince A, Antony K, Seferovic M, Aagaard K. Maturation of the infant microbiome community structure and function across multiple body sites and in relation to mode of delivery. Nat Med. 2017;23:314–28.
23. Huurre A, Kalliomaki M, Rautava S, Rinne M, Salminen S, Isolauri E. Mode of delivery – effects on gut microbiota and humoral immunity. Neonatology. 2008;93:236–40.
24. Salminen S, Gibson GR, McCartney AL, Isolauri E. Influence of mode of delivery on gut microbiota composition in seven year old children. Gut. 2004;53(9):1388.

25. Dominguez-Bello MG, Costello EK, Contreras M, Magris M, Hidalgo G, Fierer N, et al. Delivery mode shapes the acquisition and structure of the initial microbiota across multiple body habitats in newborns. Proc Natl Acad Sci U S A. 2010;107: 11971–5.
26. Mason T, Rabinovich CE, Fredrickson DD, Amoroso K, Reed AM, Stein LD, et al. Breast feeding and the development of juvenile rheumatoid arthritis. J Rheumatol. 1995;22:1166–70.
27. Kasapcopur O, Tasdan Y, Apelyan M, Akkus S, Caliskan S, Sever L, et al. Does breast feeding prevent the development of juvenile rheumatoid arthritis? J Rheumatol. 1998;25:2286–7.
28. Rosenberg AM. Evaluation of associations between breast feeding and subsequent development of juvenile rheumatoid arthritis. J Rheumatol. 1996;23:1080–2.
29. Hyrich KL, Baildam E, Pickford H, Chieng A, Davidson JE, Foster H, et al. Influence of past breast feeding on pattern and severity of presentation of juvenile idiopathic arthritis. Arch Dis Child. 2016;101:348–51.
30. Montoya J, Matta NB, Suchon P, Guzian MC, Lambert NC, Mattei JP, et al. Patients with ankylosing spondylitis have been breast fed less often than healthy controls: a case-control retrospective study. Ann Rheum Dis. 2016;75:879–82.
31. Kindgren E, Fredrikson M, Ludvigsson J. Early feeding and risk of Juvenile idiopathic arthritis: a case control study in a prospective birth cohort. Pediatr Rheumatol Online J. 2017;15:46,017-0175-z.
32. Harmsen HJ, Wildeboer-Veloo AC, Raangs GC, Wagendorp AA, Klijn N, Bindels JG, et al. Analysis of intestinal flora development in breast-fed and formula-fed infants by using molecular identification and detection methods. J Pediatr Gastroenterol Nutr. 2000;30:61–7.
33. Perez PF, Dore J, Leclerc M, Levenez F, Benyacoub J, Serrant P, et al. Bacterial imprinting of the neonatal immune system: lessons from maternal cells? Pediatrics. 2007;119:e724–32.
34. Stoll ML, Kumar R, Morrow CD, Lefkowitz EJ, Cui X, Genin A, et al. Altered microbiota associated with abnormal humoral immune responses to commensal organisms in enthesitis-related arthritis. Arthritis Res Ther. 2014;16:486,014-0486-0.
35. Wallis D, Asaduzzaman A, Weisman M, Haroon N, Anton A, McGovern D, et al. Elevated serum anti-flagellin antibodies implicate subclinical bowel inflammation in ankylosing spondylitis: an observational study. Arthritis Res Ther. 2013;15:R166.
36. Ravelli A, Felici E, Magni-Manzoni S, Pistorio A, Novarini C, Bozzola E, et al. Patients with antinuclear antibody-positive juvenile idiopathic arthritis constitute a homogeneous subgroup irrespective of the course of joint disease. Arthritis Rheum. 2005;52:826–32.
37. Van Praet JT, Donovan E, Vanassche I, Drennan MB, Windels F, Dendooven A, et al. Commensal microbiota influence systemic autoimmune responses. EMBO J. 2015;34:466–74.
38. Van Dijkhuizen P, Del Chierico F, Malattia C, Russo A, Marafon DP, ter Haar NM, et al. The composition of the gut microbiota differs between children with JIA and healthy controls. 2016.
39. Korpela K, Salonen A, Virta LJ, Kekkonen RA, de Vos WM. Association of early-life antibiotic use and protective effects of breastfeeding: role of the intestinal microbiota. JAMA Pediatr. 2016;170:750–7.
40. Horton DB, Scott FI, Haynes K, Putt ME, Rose CD, Lewis JD, et al. Antibiotic exposure and juvenile idiopathic arthritis: a case-control study. Pediatrics. 2015;136:e333–43.
41. Arvonen M, Virta LJ, Pokka T, Kroger L, Vahasalo P. Repeated exposure to antibiotics in infancy: a predisposing factor for juvenile idiopathic arthritis or a sign of this group's greater susceptibility to infections? J Rheumatol. 2015;42(3):521–6.
42. Arvonen M, Berntson L, Pokka T, Karttunen TJ, Vahasalo P, Stoll ML. Gut microbiota-host interactions and juvenile idiopathic arthritis. Pediatr Rheumatol Online J. 2016;14:44,016-0104-6.
43. Panda S, El khader I, Casellas F, Lopez Vivancos J, Garcia Cors M, Santiago A, et al. Short-term effect of antibiotics on human gut microbiota. PLoS One. 2014;9:e95476.
44. Jernberg C, Lofmark S, Edlund C, Jansson JK. Long-term ecological impacts of antibiotic administration on the human intestinal microbiota. ISME J. 2007;1:56–66.
45. Di Paola M, Cavalieri D, Albanese D, Sordo M, Pindo M, Donati C, et al. Alteration of fecal microbiota profiles in juvenile idiopathic arthritis. Associations with HLA-B27 allele and disease status. Front Microbiol. 2016;7:1703.
46. Malievskiy V. Prevalence and incidence of juvenile idiopathic arthritis in children in the republic of Bashkortostan: the epidemiological study. Pediatr Rheumatol. 2011;9(Suppl 1):145.
47. Berntson L, Andersson Gare B, Fasth A, Herlin T, Kristinsson J, Lahdenne P, et al. Incidence of juvenile idiopathic arthritis in the Nordic countries. A population based study with special reference to the validity of the ILAR and EULAR criteria. J Rheumatol. 2003;30:2275–82.
48. Pruunsild C, Uibo K, Liivamagi H, Tarraste S, Talvik T, Pelkonen P. Incidence of juvenile idiopathic arthritis in children in Estonia: a prospective population-based study. Scand J Rheumatol. 2007;36: 7–13.
49. Virta L, Helenius H, Klaukka T. Incidence of Juvenile idiopathic arthritis is increasing in Finland [in Finnish]. Suom Laakaril. 2008;35:2806–9.
50. Rautava S, Ruuskanen O, Ouwehand A, Salminen S, Isolauri E. The hygiene hypothesis of atopic disease – an extended version. J Pediatr Gastroenterol Nutr. 2004;38:378–88.
51. Giongo A, Gano KA, Crabb DB, Mukherjee N, Novelo LL, Casella G, et al. Toward defining the

autoimmune microbiome for type 1 diabetes. ISME J. 2011;5:82–91.
52. Tejesvi MV, Arvonen M, Kangas SM, Keskitalo PL, Pirttila AM, Karttunen TJ, et al. Faecal microbiome in new-onset juvenile idiopathic arthritis. Eur J Clin Microbiol Infect Dis. 2016;35(3):363–70.
53. Round JL, Lee SM, Li J, Tran G, Jabri B, Chatila TA, et al. The toll-like receptor 2 pathway establishes colonization by a commensal of the human microbiota. Science. 2011;332:974–7.
54. Arvonen M, Vahasalo P, Turunen S, Salo HM, Maki M, Laurila K, et al. Altered expression of intestinal human leucocyte antigen D-related and immune signalling molecules in juvenile idiopathic arthritis. Clin Exp Immunol. 2012;170:266–73.
55. Zonneveld-Huijssoon E, van Wijk F, Roord S, Delemarre E, Meerding J, de Jager W, et al. TLR9 agonist CpG enhances protective nasal HSP60 peptide vaccine efficacy in experimental autoimmune arthritis. Ann Rheum Dis. 2012;71(10): 1706–15.
56. Lee J, Gonzales-Navajas JM, Raz E. The "polarizing-tolerizing" mechanism of intestinal epithelium: its relevance to colonic homeostasis. Semin Immunopathol. 2008;30:3–9.
57. McSorley HJ, Maizels RM. Helminth infections and host immune regulation. Clin Microbiol Rev. 2012;25:585–608.
58. Eissa MM, Mostafa DK, Ghazy AA, El Azzouni MZ, Boulos LM, Younis LK. Anti-arthritic activity of Schistosoma mansoni and Trichinella spiralis derived-antigens in adjuvant arthritis in rats: role of FOXP3+ Treg cells. PLoS One. 2016;11:e0165916.
59. Summers RW, Elliott DE, Qadir K, Urban JF Jr, Thompson R, Weinstock JV. Trichuris suis seems to be safe and possibly effective in the treatment of inflammatory bowel disease. Am J Gastroenterol. 2003;98:2034–41.
60. Summers RW, Elliott DE, Urban JF Jr, Thompson RA, Weinstock JV. Trichuris suis therapy for active ulcerative colitis: a randomized controlled trial. Gastroenterology. 2005;128:825–32.
61. Mutapi F, Imai N, Nausch N, Bourke CD, Rujeni N, Mitchell KM, et al. Schistosome infection intensity is inversely related to auto-reactive antibody levels. PLoS One. 2011;6:e19149.
62. Aggarwal A, Sarangi AN, Gaur P, Shukla A, Aggarwal R. Gut microbiome in children with enthesitis-related arthritis in a developing country, and the effect of probiotic administration. Clin Exp Immunol. 2016;187(3):480–9.
63. Stearns JC, Lynch MD, Senadheera DB, Tenenbaum HC, Goldberg MB, Cvitkovitch DG, et al. Bacterial biogeography of the human digestive tract. Sci Rep. 2011;1:170.
64. Momozawa Y, Deffontaine V, Louis E, Medrano JF. Characterization of bacteria in biopsies of colon and stools by high throughput sequencing of the V2 region of bacterial 16S rRNA gene in human. PLoS One. 2011;6:e16952. https://doi.org/10.1371/journal.pone.0016952.
65. Imhann F, Bonder MJ, Vich Vila A, Fu J, Mujagic Z, Vork L, et al. Proton pump inhibitors affect the gut microbiome. Gut. 2016;65:740–8.
66. van der Wulp MY, Derrien M, Stellaard F, Wolters H, Kleerebezem M, Dekker J, et al. Laxative treatment with polyethylene glycol decreases microbial primary bile salt dehydroxylation and lipid metabolism in the intestine of rats. Am J Physiol Gastrointest Liver Physiol. 2013;305:G474–82.
67. Schloss PD, Gevers D, Westcott SL. Reducing the effects of PCR amplification and sequencing artifacts on 16S rRNA-based studies. PLoS One. 2011;6:e27310. https://doi.org/10.1371/journal.pone.0027310.
68. Stoll ML, Kumar R, Lefkowitz EJ, Cron RQ, Morrow CD, Barnes S. Fecal metabolomics in pediatric spondyloarthritis implicate decreased metabolic diversity and altered tryptophan metabolism as pathogenic factors. Genes Immun. 2016;17: 400–5.
69. Stoll M, Weiss P, Weiss J, Nigrovic P, Edelheit B, Bridges S, et al. Age and fecal microbial strain-specific differences in patients with spondyloarthritis. Arth Res Ther. 2018;20:14.
70. Nayak RR, Loughlin CO, Fischbach M, Turnbaugh PJ. Methotrexate is an antibacterial drug metabolized by human gut bacteria. In: 2016 ACR/ARHP annual meeting. 2016.
71. Swidsinski A, Loening-Baucke V, Schulz S, Manowsky J, Verstraelen H, Swidsinski S. Functional anatomy of the colonic bioreactor: impact of antibiotics and Saccharomyces boulardii on bacterial composition in human fecal cylinders. Syst Appl Microbiol. 2016;39:67–75.
72. Ortiz P, Bissada NF, Palomo L, Han YW, Al-Zahrani MS, Panneerselvam A, et al. Periodontal therapy reduces the severity of active rheumatoid arthritis in patients treated with or without tumor necrosis factor inhibitors. J Periodontol. 2009;80:535–40.
73. Dieleman LA, Goerres MS, Arends A, Sprengers D, Torrice C, Hoentjen F, et al. Lactobacillus GG prevents recurrence of colitis in HLA-B27 transgenic rats after antibiotic treatment. Gut. 2003;52:370–6.
74. Segain JP, Raingeard de la Bletiere D, Bourreille A, Leray V, Gervois N, Rosales C, et al. Butyrate inhibits inflammatory responses through NFkappaB inhibition: implications for Crohn's disease. Gut. 2000;47:397–403.
75. Sokol H, Pigneur B, Watterlot L, Lakhdari O, Bermudez-Humaran LG, Gratadoux JJ, et al. Faecalibacterium prausnitzii is an anti-inflammatory commensal bacterium identified by gut microbiota analysis of Crohn disease patients. Proc Natl Acad Sci U S A. 2008;105:16731–6.
76. Picco P, Gattorno M, Marchese N, Vignola S, Sormani MP, Barabino A, et al. Increased gut permeability in juvenile chronic arthritides. A multivariate analysis of the diagnostic parameters. Clin Exp Rheumatol. 2000;18:773–8.
77. Atarashi K, Tanoue T, Oshima K, Suda W, Nagano Y, Nishikawa H, et al. Treg induction by a rationally

selected mixture of clostridia strains from the human microbiota. Nature. 2013;500:232–6.

78. Stoll ML, Wilson L, Barnes S, Kumar R, Genin A, Cron RQ, et al. Multiomics study of gut microbiota in enthesitis-related arthritis identify diminished microbial diversity and altered typtophan metabolism as potential factors in disease pathogenesis. Arthritis Rheum. 2015;67:S10.
79. Smith PM, Howitt MR, Panikov N, Michaud M, Gallini CA, Bohlooly-y M, et al. The microbial metabolites, short-chain fatty acids, regulate colonic Treg cell homeostasis. Science. 2013;341:569–73.
80. Mielants H, Veys EM, Cuvelier C, De Vos M, Goemaere S, Maertens M, et al. Gut inflammation in children with late onset pauciarticular juvenile chronic arthritis and evolution to adult spondyloarthropathy – a prospective study. J Rheumatol. 1993;20:1567–72.
81. Lionetti P, Pupi A, Veltroni M, Fonda C, Cavicchi MC, Azzari C, et al. Evidence of subclinical intestinal inflammation by 99m technetium leukocyte scintigraphy in patients with HLA-B27 positive juvenile onset active spondyloarthropathy. J Rheumatol. 2000;27:1538–41.
82. Stoll ML, Punaro M, Patel AS. Fecal calprotectin in children with the enthesitis-related arthritis subtype of juvenile idiopathic arthritis. J Rheumatol. 2011;38:2274–5.
83. Fotis L, Shaikh N, Baszis KW, Samson CM, Lev-Tzion R, French AR, et al. Serologic evidence of gut-driven systemic inflammation in juvenile idiopathic arthritis. J Rheumatol. 2017;44:1624–31.
84. McGhee JR, Kunisawa J, Kiyono H. Gut lymphocyte migration: we are halfway 'home'. Trends Immunol. 2007;28:150–3.
85. Salmi M, Andrew DP, Butcher EC, Jalkanen S. Dual binding capacity of mucosal immunoblasts to mucosal and synovial endothelium in humans: dissection of the molecular mechanisms. J Exp Med. 1995;181:137–49.
86. Fantini MC, Pallone F, Monteleone G. Common immunologic mechanisms in inflammatory bowel disease and spondylarthropathies. World J Gastroenterol. 2009;15:2472–8.
87. Black AP, Bhayani H, Ryder CA, Pugh MT, Gardner-Medwin JM, Southwood TR. An association between the acute phase response and patterns of antigen induced T cell proliferation in juvenile idiopathic arthritis. Arthritis Res Ther. 2003;5:R277–84.
88. Elewaut D, De Keyser F, Van Den Bosch F, Lazarovits AI, De Vos M, Cuvelier C, et al. Enrichment of T cells carrying beta7 integrins in inflamed synovial tissue from patients with early spondyloarthropathy, compared to rheumatoid arthritis. J Rheumatol. 1998;25:1932–7.
89. Wilson C, Rashid T, Tiwana H, Beyan H, Hughes L, Bansal S, et al. Cytotoxicity responses to peptide antigens in rheumatoid arthritis and ankylosing spondylitis. J Rheumatol. 2003;30:972–8.
90. Saxena N, Misra R, Aggarwal A. Is the enthesitis-related arthritis subtype of juvenile idiopathic arthritis a form of chronic reactive arthritis? Rheumatology. 2006;45:1129.
91. Granfors K, Jalkanen S, von Essen R, Lahesmaa-Rantala R, Isomaki O, Pekkola-Heino K, et al. Yersinia antigens in synovial-fluid cells from patients with reactive arthritis. N Engl J Med. 1989;320:216–21.
92. Singh YP, Singh AK, Aggarwal A, Misra R. Evidence of cellular immune response to outer membrane protein of Salmonella typhimurium in patients with enthesitis-related arthritis subtype of juvenile idiopathic arthritis. J Rheumatol. 2011;38:161–6.
93. Stoll ML, Duck LW, Cron RQ, Elson CO. Identification of a potential commensal immunologic target in enthesitis-related arthritis. Arthritis Rheumatol. 2016;68(Suppl 10:1):4550.
94. Lange L, Thiele GM, McCracken C, Wang G, Ponder LA, Angeles-Han ST, et al. Symptoms of periodontitis and antibody responses to Porphyromonas gingivalis in juvenile idiopathic arthritis. Pediatr Rheumatol Online J. 2016;14:8,016-0068-6.
95. Turunen M, Kuusisto P, Uggeldahl PE, Toivanen A. Pogosta disease: clinical observations during an outbreak in the province of North Karelia, Finland. Br J Rheumatol. 1998;37:1177–80.
96. Marks M, Marks JL. Viral arthritis. Clin Med (Lond). 2016;16:129–34.
97. Page C, Francois C, Goeb V, Duverlie G. Human parvovirus B19 and autoimmune diseases. Review of the literature and pathophysiological hypotheses. J Clin Virol. 2015;72:69–74.
98. Lei Y, Hu T, Song X, Nie H, Chen M, Chen W, et al. Production of autoantibodies in chronic hepatitis B virus infection is associated with the augmented function of blood CXCR5+CD4+ T cells. PLoS One. 2016;11:e0162241.
99. Cornillet M, Verrouil E, Cantagrel A, Serre G, Nogueira L. In ACPA-positive RA patients, antibodies to EBNA35-58Cit, a citrullinated peptide from the Epstein-Barr nuclear antigen-1, strongly cross-react with the peptide beta60-74Cit which bears the immunodominant epitope of citrullinated fibrin. Immunol Res. 2015;61:117–25.
100. Taylor-Robinson D, Thomas B, Rooney M. Association of Chlamydia pneumoniae with chronic juvenile arthritis. Eur J Clin Microbiol Infect Dis. 1998;17:211–2.
101. Altun S, Kasapcopur O, Aslan M, Karaarslan S, Koksal V, Saribas S, et al. Is there any relationship between Chlamydophila pneumoniae infection and juvenile idiopathic arthritis? J Med Microbiol. 2004;53:787–90.
102. Postepski J, Opoka-Winiarska V, Koziol-Montewka M, Korobowicz A, Tuszkiewicz-Misztal E. Role of mycoplasma pneumoniae infection in aetiopathogenesis of juvenile idiopatic arthritis. Med Wieku Rozwoj. 2003;7:271–7.
103. Oen K, Fast M, Postl B. Epidemiology of juvenile rheumatoid arthritis in Manitoba, Canada, 1975-92: cycles in incidence. J Rheumatol. 1995;22: 745–50.

104. Nocton JJ, Miller LC, Tucker LB, Schaller JG. Human parvovirus B19-associated arthritis in children. J Pediatr. 1993;122:186–90.
105. Aghighi Y, Gilani Sh M, Razavi M, Zamani A, Daneshjoo K. Juvenile rheumatoid arthritis in children with Epstein Barr virus infection. Pak J Biol Sci. 2007;10:3638–43.
106. Adams ST, Schmidt KM, Cost KM, Marshall GS. Common variable immunodeficiency presenting with persistent parvovirus B19 infection. Pediatrics. 2012;130:e1711–5.
107. Kurtzman GJ, Cohen BJ, Field AM, Oseas R, Blaese RM, Young NS. Immune response to B19 parvovirus and an antibody defect in persistent viral infection. J Clin Invest. 1989;84:1114–23.
108. Deng X, Dong Y, Yi Q, Huang Y, Zhao D, Yang Y, et al. The determinants for the enzyme activity of human parvovirus B19 phospholipase A2 (PLA2) and its influence on cultured cells. PLoS One. 2013;8:e61440.
109. Chen DY, Tzang BS, Chen YM, Lan JL, Tsai CC, Hsu TC. The association of anti-parvovirus B19-VP1 unique region antibodies with antiphospholipid antibodies in patients with antiphospholipid syndrome. Clin Chim Acta. 2010;411:1084–9.
110. Von Landenberg P, Lehmann HW, Knoll A, Dorsch S, Modrow S. Antiphospholipid antibodies in pediatric and adult patients with rheumatic disease are associated with parvovirus B19 infection. Arthritis Rheum. 2003;48:1939–47.
111. Lehmann HW, Plentz A, von Landenberg P, Kuster RM, Modrow S. Different patterns of disease manifestations of parvovirus B19-associated reactive juvenile arthritis and the induction of antiphospholipid-antibodies. Clin Rheumatol. 2008;27:333–8.
112. de Groot-Mijnes JD, Dekkers J, de Visser L, Rothova A, van Loon AM, de Boer JH. Antibody production against B19 virus in ocular fluid of JIA-associated uveitis patients. Ophthalmology. 2015;122:1270,1272.e1.
113. Oguz F, Akdeniz C, Unuvar E, Kucukbasmaci O, Sidal M. Parvovirus B19 in the acute arthropathies and juvenile rheumatoid arthritis. J Paediatr Child Health. 2002;38:358–62.
114. Lehmann HW, Knoll A, Kuster RM, Modrow S. Frequent infection with a viral pathogen, parvovirus B19, in rheumatic diseases of childhood. Arthritis Rheum. 2003;48:1631–8.
115. Angelini F, Cancrini C, Colavita M, Panei P, Concato C, Romiti ML, et al. Role of parvovirus B19 infection in juvenile chronic arthritis. Is more investigation needed? Clin Exp Rheumatol. 2003;21:684.
116. Gonzalez B, Larranaga C, Leon O, Diaz P, Miranda M, Barria M, et al. Parvovirus B19 may have a role in the pathogenesis of juvenile idiopathic arthritis. J Rheumatol. 2007;34:1336–40.
117. Weissbrich B, Suss-Frohlich Y, Girschick HJ. Seroprevalence of parvovirus B19 IgG in children affected by juvenile idiopathic arthritis. Arthritis Res Ther. 2007;9:R82.
118. Tsai YT, Chiang BL, Kao YF, Hsieh KH. Detection of Epstein-Barr virus and cytomegalovirus genome in white blood cells from patients with juvenile rheumatoid arthritis and childhood systemic lupus erythematosus. Int Arch Allergy Immunol. 1995;106:235–40.
119. Massa M, Mazzoli F, Pignatti P, De Benedetti F, Passalia M, Viola S, et al. Proinflammatory responses to self HLA epitopes are triggered by molecular mimicry to Epstein-Barr virus proteins in oligoarticular juvenile idiopathic arthritis. Arthritis Rheum. 2002;46:2721–9.
120. Kawada J, Ito Y, Torii Y, Kimura H, Iwata N. Remission of juvenile idiopathic arthritis with primary Epstein-Barr virus infection. Rheumatology (Oxford). 2013;52:956–8.
121. Damsker JM, Hansen AM, Caspi RR. Th1 and Th17 cells: adversaries and collaborators. Ann N Y Acad Sci. 2010;1183:211–21.
122. Rothe K, Quandt D, Schubert K, Rossol M, Klingner M, Jasinski-Bergner S, et al. Latent cytomegalovirus infection in rheumatoid arthritis and increased frequencies of cytolytic LIR-1+CD8+ T cells. Arthritis Rheumatol. 2016;68:337–46.
123. Petrelli A, van Wijk F. CD8(+) T cells in human autoimmune arthritis: the unusual suspects. Nat Rev Rheumatol. 2016;12:421–8.
124. Hunter PJ, Nistala K, Jina N, Eddaoudi A, Thomson W, Hubank M, et al. Biologic predictors of extension of oligoarticular juvenile idiopathic arthritis as determined from synovial fluid cellular composition and gene expression. Arthritis Rheum. 2010;62:896–907.
125. Wehrens EJ, Mijnheer G, Duurland CL, Klein M, Meerding J, van Loosdregt J, et al. Functional human regulatory T cells fail to control autoimmune inflammation due to PKB/c-akt hyperactivation in effector cells. Blood. 2011;118:3538–48.
126. Cunningham MW. Rheumatic fever, autoimmunity and molecular mimicry: the streptococcal connection. Int Rev Immunol. 2014;33:314–29.
127. Riise OR, Lee A, Cvancarova M, Handeland KS, Wathne KO, Nakstad B, et al. Recent-onset childhood arthritis – association with Streptococcus pyogenes in a population-based study. Rheumatology (Oxford). 2008;47:1006–11.
128. Eastmond CJ, Calguner M, Shinebaum R, Cooke EM, Wright V. A sequential study of the relationship between faecal Klebsiella aerogenes and the common clinical manifestations of ankylosing spondylitis. Ann Rheum Dis. 1982;41:15–20.
129. Hunter T, Harding GK, Kaprove RE, Schroeder ML. Fecal carriage of various Klebsiella and Enterobacter species in patients with active ankylosing spondylitis. Arthritis Rheum. 1981;24:106–8.
130. Rashid T, Ebringer A. Autoimmunity in rheumatic diseases is induced by microbial infections via cross reactivity or molecular mimicry. Autoimmune Dis. 2012;2012:539282.

131. Puga Yung GL, Fidler M, Albani E, Spermon N, Teklenburg G, Newbury R, et al. Heat shock protein-derived T-cell epitopes contribute to autoimmune inflammation in pediatric Crohn's disease. PLoS One. 2009;4:e7714.
132. Ovelgonne JH, Koninkx JF, Pusztai A, Bardocz S, Kok W, Ewen SW, et al. Decreased levels of heat shock proteins in gut epithelial cells after exposure to plant lectins. Gut. 2000;46:679–87.
133. Arvans DL, Vavricka SR, Ren H, Musch MW, Kang L, Rocha FG, et al. Luminal bacterial flora determines physiological expression of intestinal epithelial cytoprotective heat shock proteins 25 and 72. Am J Physiol Gastrointest Liver Physiol. 2005;288:G696–704.
134. Tao Y, Drabik KA, Waypa TS, Musch MW, Alverdy JC, Schneewind O, et al. Soluble factors from Lactobacillus GG activate MAPKs and induce cytoprotective heat shock proteins in intestinal epithelial cells. Am J Physiol Cell Physiol. 2006;290:C1018–30.
135. Shiobara N, Suzuki Y, Aoki H, Gotoh A, Fujii Y, Hamada Y, et al. Bacterial superantigens and T cell receptor beta-chain-bearing T cells in the immunopathogenesis of ulcerative colitis. Clin Exp Immunol. 2007;150:13–21.
136. Hersh AO, Prahalad S. Immunogenetics of juvenile idiopathic arthritis: a comprehensive review. J Autoimmun. 2015;64:113–24.
137. Opdenakker G, Proost P, Van Damme J. Microbiomic and posttranslational modifications as preludes to autoimmune diseases. Trends Mol Med. 2016;22:746–57.
138. Yeoh N, Burton JP, Suppiah P, Reid G, Stebbings S. The role of the microbiome in rheumatic diseases. Curr Rheumatol Rep. 2013;15:314,012-0314-y.
139. Koziel J, Mydel P, Potempa J. The link between periodontal disease and rheumatoid arthritis: an updated review. Curr Rheumatol Rep. 2014;16:408,014-0408-9.
140. Hitchon CA, Chandad F, Ferucci ED, Willemze A, Ioan-Facsinay A, van der Woude D, et al. Antibodies to porphyromonas gingivalis are associated with anticitrullinated protein antibodies in patients with rheumatoid arthritis and their relatives. J Rheumatol. 2010;37:1105–12.
141. Wegner N, Wait R, Sroka A, Eick S, Nguyen KA, Lundberg K, et al. Peptidylarginine deiminase from Porphyromonas gingivalis citrullinates human fibrinogen and alpha-enolase: implications for autoimmunity in rheumatoid arthritis. Arthritis Rheum. 2010;62:2662–72.
142. Colman RJ, Rubin DT. Fecal microbiota transplantation as therapy for inflammatory bowel disease: a systematic review and meta-analysis. J Crohns Colitis. 2014;8:1569–81.
143. Jenks K, Stebbings S, Burton J, Schultz M, Herbison P, Highton J. Probiotic therapy for the treatment of spondyloarthritis: a randomized controlled trial. J Rheumatol. 2010;37:2118–25.
144. Hold GL, Schwiertz A, Aminov RI, Blaut M, Flint HJ. Oligonucleotide probes that detect quantitatively significant groups of butyrate-producing bacteria in human feces. Appl Environ Microbiol. 2003;69:4320–4.
145. Van den Abbeele P, Belzer C, Goossens M, Kleerebezem M, De Vos WM, Thas O, et al. Butyrate-producing Clostridium cluster XIVa species specifically colonize mucins in an in vitro gut model. ISME J. 2013;7:949–61.
146. Furusawa Y, Obata Y, Fukuda S, Endo TA, Nakato G, Takahashi D, et al. Commensal microbe-derived butyrate induces the differentiation of colonic regulatory T cells. Nature. 2013;504:446–50.
147. MacLellan A, Moore-Connors J, Grant S, Cahill L, Langille MGI, Van Limbergen J. The impact of exclusive enteral nutrition (EEN) on the gut microbiome in Crohn's disease: a review. Nutrients. 2017;9:0447. https://doi.org/10.3390/nu9050447.
148. Berntson L. Anti-inflammatory effect by exclusive enteral nutrition (EEN) in a patient with juvenile idiopathic arthritis (JIA): brief report. Clin Rheumatol. 2014;33(8):1173–5.
149. Berntson L, Hedlund-Treutiger I, Alving K. Anti-inflammatory effect of exclusive enteral nutrition in patients with juvenile idiopathic arthritis. Clin Exp Rheumatol. 2016;34:941–5.
150. Berntson L, Agback P, Dicksved J. Changes in fecal microbiota and metabolomics in a child with juvenile idiopathic arthritis (JIA) responding to two treatment periods with exclusive enteral nutrition (EEN). Clin Rheumatol. 2016;35(6):1501.
151. Wu GD, Chen J, Hoffmann C, Bittinger K, Chen YY, Keilbaugh SA, et al. Linking long-term dietary patterns with gut microbial enterotypes. Science. 2011;334:105–8.
152. Salonen A, de Vos WM. Impact of diet on human intestinal microbiota and health. Annu Rev Food Sci Technol. 2014;5:239–62.
153. Johansson ME, Gustafsson JK, Holmen-Larsson J, Jabbar KS, Xia L, Xu H, et al. Bacteria penetrate the normally impenetrable inner colon mucus layer in both murine colitis models and patients with ulcerative colitis. Gut. 2014;63:281–91.
154. Brandtzaeg P. Homeostatic impact of indigenous microbiota and secretory immunity. Benef Microbes. 2010;1:211–27.
155. Collado MC, Rautava S, Isolauri E, Salminen S. Gut microbiota: a source of novel tools to reduce the risk of human disease? Pediatr Res. 2015;77:182–8.
156. Ruemmele FM, Veres G, Kolho KL, Griffiths A, Levine A, Escher JC, et al. Consensus guidelines of ECCO/ESPGHAN on the medical management of pediatric Crohn's disease. J Crohns Colitis. 2014;8(10):1179–207.
157. Scher JU, Bretz WA, Abramson SB. Periodontal disease and subgingival microbiota as contributors for rheumatoid arthritis pathogenesis: modifiable risk factors? Curr Opin Rheumatol. 2014;26: 424–9.

18 Psoriasis and Psoriatic Arthritis

Madhura Castelino, Steve Eyre, and Anne Barton

Abbreviations

AMP	Antimicrobial peptide
AS	Ankylosing spondylitis
EA	Enteropathic arthritis
hBD	Human beta-defensin
HIV	Human immunodeficiency virus
HLA	Human leukocyte antigen
IBD	Inflammatory bowel disease
IL	Interleukin
PsA	Psoriatic arthritis
PsV	Psoriasis vulgaris
RA	Rheumatoid arthritis
ReA	Reactive arthritis
SpA	Spondyloarthritis
TLR	Toll-like receptor
uSpA	Undifferentiated spondyloarthritis

M. Castelino (✉)
Department of Rheumatology, NIHR Manchester Musculoskeletal Biomedical Research Unit, The University of Manchester, Manchester, UK
e-mail: madhura.castelino@manchester.ac.uk

S. Eyre · A. Barton
Division of Musculoskeletal and Dermatological Sciences, The University of Manchester, Manchester, UK
e-mail: steve.eyre@manchester.ac.uk; Anne.Barton@manchester.ac.uk

Psoriatic Arthritis (PsA)

The very first description of modern-day "psoriasis" in 1809 by Willan had connotations of an infective aetiology, as evidenced by the use of the term "lepra vulgaris"; differentiation of a separate entity was made by Hebra in 1841, who coined the term "psoriasis" [1]. During the same period, the association of psoriasis with arthritis was also reported by Baron Jean Luis Alibert (1818) [2]. In 1961, PsA was distinguished from rheumatoid arthritis (RA) based upon clinical, demographic, radiologic, and serologic findings [3]. In the early 1970s, PsA was classified [4] among the spondyloarthritides.

PsA has been defined as a chronic seronegative inflammatory arthritis usually negative for rheumatoid factor and occurring in the presence of psoriasis [4]. The so-named Classification Criteria for Psoriatic Arthritis (CASPAR) permit the diagnosis of PsA even in the absence of frank psoriasis [5]. As with any complex inflammatory condition, treatment and management of PsA require knowledge of the aetiology and pathogenesis of the condition. Pioneering work on the human genome has revolutionised the understanding of the influence of genetics in human health and disease [6, 7]. For complex diseases, even though the genetic make-up of an individual may increase the susceptibility of that individual to developing a condition, it does not necessarily result in disease. The development of complex diseases is multifactorial with environmental risk

G. Ragab et al. (eds.), *The Microbiome in Rheumatic Diseases and Infection*,
https://doi.org/10.1007/978-3-319-79026-8_18

factors contributing in addition to the host genetic susceptibility. Here we explore the evidence from genetic and epidemiological data that an interesting environmental factor, namely, the human microbiota, may play a role in the aetiopathogenesis of PsA.

Clinical Evidence for a Role of the Microbiota in Psoriatic Arthritis

PsA is included in the family of immune-mediated inflammatory disorders belonging to the spondyloarthritis (SpA) group, which also includes ankylosing spondylitis (AS), enteropathic arthritis (EA), reactive arthritis (ReA) and undifferentiated spondyloarthritis (uSpA). PsA shares several clinical manifestations with SpA including the pattern of articular manifestations, namely, the asymmetric polyarthritis, "ray" distribution of joint involvement, involvement of the axial skeleton and radiological changes such as periostitis, ankyloses and presence of "chunky" syndesmophytes [8, 9]. The synovium of PsA is also histologically similar to the synovium of SpA in general, characterised by increased vascularity and neutrophilic infiltration [10] which parallels the histologic findings in the skin of psoriatic lesion, where histologically increased vascularity and leukocyte infiltration have been noted in addition to the characteristic epidermal hyperplasia [11, 12]. In addition, increased vascularity observed in the synovial membrane of affected joints in PsA [10] is a feature that is also described in the synovial membrane of ReA patients [13] where an infective trigger has been established.

In the asymmetrical peripheral pauciarticular and axial subgroup of individuals within the heterogenic phenotype of PsA, both articular (large joint involvement) and extra-articular (enthesitis, dactylitis, iritis) clinical features are similar to the clinical features of enteropathic arthritis in patients with inflammatory bowel disease [14] where the gut is the primary site of inflammation. Furthermore, subclinical gastrointestinal inflammation has been reported [15, 16] in PsA. In addition, these features overlap those seen in ReA where there is a known microbial trigger and the portal of entry can be from the gastrointestinal, respiratory or genitourinary systems [17]. All this suggests that these microbial elements could be important environmental candidate susceptibility factors for PsA.

Infections Associated with Psoriasis and Psoriatic Arthritis

Skin psoriasis is a clinical feature of PsA, and in a subtype of psoriasis—guttate psoriasis—flares of skin lesions have a strong association with streptococcal infection, illustrating the potential of the microbiota to trigger skin disease [18]. Though studies exploring single organisms such as viruses [19–21] and bacteria [22–24] as causative risk factors for PsV and PsA have resulted in conflicting conclusions, the onset of the human immunodeficiency virus (HIV) epidemic in Africa was noted to be associated with increased incidence of PsV and PsA cases in HIV-positive individuals [25] and renewed interest in an infectious trigger for these conditions. The hypothesis of an infectious trigger was further strengthened by an observational study of incident cases of PsA which demonstrated that infections (skin, soft tissue and/or respiratory and urinary tract infections resulting in hospitalisation) requiring antibiotic treatment were correlated with a polyarticular pattern of PsA (OR 1.7, 95% CI 1.00–2.77) [26]. In addition, the same study noted a correlation with a history of infectious diarrhoea in the new-onset PsA group, although the association did not reach statistical significance. By contrast, a previous study exploring the precipitating events prior to the onset of PsA found no association with infectious diarrhoea; the authors speculated that true PsA incident cases may have been misclassified as reactive arthritis if diarrhoea was reported at presentation [27].

Evidence from Human Genetics to Support a Microbial Trigger

The genetic evidence to support the hypothesis that aberrant immune responses to antigenic peptides is important in the aetiology of PsA is provided by the association of several alleles in the human leukocyte antigen (HLA) Class 1 region of the major histocompatibility complex, including HLA-B27, HLA-B08, HLA-B38 and HLA-B39 [28–32], which have been reported to be associated with increased risk of PsA. The amino acid polymorphisms that these alleles encode for are similar to those implicated in susceptibility to SpA [33] and are hypothesised to recognise similar arthritogenic peptides at the binding groove (B pocket) of the HLA-B molecules resulting in an aberrant immune response through activation of memory T (CD8+) cells. The antigenic peptides, endogenous or exogenous, have not been identified for most cases of PsV or PsA; however, in the case of streptococcal-induced flares of guttate psoriasis, it is thought that homology of the M-protein of human keratin [34] drives the immune dysregulation. Other components of the streptococcus including streptococcal peptidoglycan (a component of Gram-positive bacterial cell walls) [35] and streptococcal CpG DNA [36] may also play the role of exogenous antigens in the pathogenesis of the psoriatic lesion through binding and activation of CD4+ and CD8+ T cells [37].

However, there may be several other mechanisms that drive the dysregulation by microbial triggers. For example, in HIV infection, enhanced secretion of type 1 cytokines by activated CD8+ T cells [38, 39]; structural homologies between HIV-1 env products and molecules involved in self-tolerance in the HLA and T-cell receptor chains [40]; superantigenic properties of HIV nef protein [41]; and the superimposed infections exacerbated by the viral-mediated destruction or the impairment of T helper 17 cells which are essential in host antimicrobial defences [42] have all been proposed as possible mechanisms that mediate the development of PsV and PsA in HIV-infected individuals.

There is histological evidence [43, 44] for the role of CD8+ T cells in the pathogenesis of PsA, which is in keeping with the hypothesis that psoriasis is a T-cell-mediated condition [37]. The role of CD8+ T cells is also supported by the association of non-HLA loci reported in genome-wide association studies of both PsV and PsA [45, 46] that map to loci containing genes affecting T helper 1 and T helper 17 cells including polymorphisms in the interleukin 1 (*IL1*), interleukin 21 (*IL21*) and interleukin 12B (*IL12B*) genes. Furthermore, variants associated with PsA but not PsV are enriched in enhancers in CD8 T cells [28]. The F-box and leucine-rich repeat protein 19 (*FBXL19*) gene associated with the nuclear factor kappa-light-chain-enhancer of activated B-cells (NF-κ*B*) pathway activation has also been reported to be associated with PsA [47]; the canonical pathway can be triggered by microbial products [48] and provides further support for the potential of microbial components to trigger inflammation in PsV and PsA.

Breach in the Barrier: Skin and Gut

The presence of microbes at all interfaces on the human host has led to various hypotheses about the effect that these elements have on immune homeostasis and development of immunological tolerance [49]. A disruption of this balance either due to a shift in the community composition of the microbiota [50] or the loss of integrity of the host/microbiota barrier [51, 52] has been postulated as the probable underlying mechanism of immunological disequilibrium.

In the context of PsV and PsA, there is evidence to support alteration of the barrier at sites of skin lesions. Psoriatic plaques demonstrate epidermal keratinocyte proliferation, leukocyte infiltration predominantly into the dermis and increased vascularity on histological examination [11]. It has been observed that even in normal skin the microbiota is not limited to the external surface or the epidermis of the skin and bacterial products including DNA containing 16S rRNA genes, bacteria-specific antigens and bacterial rRNA are ubiquitously detected throughout the subcutaneous regions of normal skin [53]. The histological abnormalities detected in psoriatic lesions may contribute to increased permeability of the skin barrier to commensals. In addition, there is genetic evidence implicating disruption of skin barrier integrity in disease aetiology as association of a deletion of two late cornified envelope genes (*LCE3C_LCE3B-del*) has been reported with PsA [54] and PsV [45]. It has been proposed that an altered repair response to physiological trauma causing barrier disruption may result in a leakier epidermal barrier that may allow for easier penetration by exogenous agents (such as allergens and/or micro-organisms) [55]. This barrier breach has been hypothesised to be due to stress to the keratinocytes through exposure to different environmental stimuli such as stress, local infection, drugs, trauma or ultraviolet skin damage. These triggers could further compromise the skin barrier integrity and initiate local pathological changes. In addition, an altered response to bacterial antigens such as lipopolysaccharides as a result of polymorphisms at the Toll-like receptor (TLR) 4 gene in chronic plaque psoriasis and PsA could drive the immune dysregulation [56]. In moderate-to-severe plaque psoriasis, LL-37-cathelicidin, an antimicrobial peptide (AMP), was demonstrated to be a T-cell autoantigen, and other AMPs such as human beta-defensin-2 (hBD2), hBD-3 (hBD3) and lysozyme have been reported to activate plasmacytoid dendritic cells [57], implicating cationic AMPs in innate immune activation in psoriatic plaques that may be linked to exposure to microbial elements.

Although the lesions in the skin are evident to the naked eye, there is epidemiological [58] and histological data [15, 16, 59] that suggest that there is also disruption to the gastrointestinal barrier both in PsV and PsA. A recent Danish cohort study [60] exploring the association between PsV and IBD observed a psoriasis-associated increased risk of Crohn disease (CD) and ulcerative colitis (UC), which was higher in severe psoriasis. This adds to the evidence from previous epidemiological studies [61–63] of an increased association of PsV and CD. Interestingly, an earlier study [64] from the USA also reported an increased risk of incident CD in women with PsV and PsA.

Both the skin and gastrointestinal tracts act as secondary lymphoid organs where immune surveillance occurs due to the presence of skin-associated lymphoid tissue [65] and gut-associated lymphoid tissue and provide, therefore, a portal for host-microbe interaction and immune activation. It has been demonstrated that commensals play an important role in the generation and maturation of lymphoid tissue as a part of the development of intestinal immune homeostasis [66] and specific gut commensals enhance the local gut mucosal immunity [67]. Similarly, skin commensals were found to have an autonomous role in cutaneous immune homeostasis [68]. Interestingly, a recent study has shown that intestinal microbiota promotes psoriasis-like skin inflammation because germ-free and antibiotic-treated mice had milder skin inflammation than conventional mice regardless of the genetic background of the animal [69]. In addition, using the K/BxN autoimmune arthritis mouse model, a regulatory role of the gut commensal- segmented filamentous bacteria, in the systemic manifestation of arthritis through the activation of the T follicular helper cells in the Peyer's patches has recently been demonstrated [70]. These studies suggest that in addition to the influence microbiota may have on the local immune components of the host at the site of interaction, communication between organs such as the skin and gut or gut and joint may also exist. Similarly, a skin-gut-joint axis is hypothesised but requires further exploration.

In summary, it is highly likely that breaches to the barriers through either physical measure (such as trauma, exposure to chemical or radiation stress) or local infections result in an altered repair mechanism that then allows for increased opportunistic interaction between the human host and the pathobionts/microbial elements that can trigger or drive a dysregulated immune system resulting in the development of inflammatory disease pathology.

Current Knowledge of the Microbiota in Psoriasis and PsA

Given the lessons learned in animal models and from genetic studies of disease in humans, attention has turned to investigating the microbiota in patients with PsV and PsA directly. With the advent of the next-generation sequencing techniques, the exploration of the microbial diversity and taxonomic identification in human health and disease can be conducted using a culture-independent, hypothesis-free method.

Dysbiosis in Psoriasis

Several culture-independent studies have explored the correlation between the skin microbiota and skin psoriasis, summarised in Table 18.1. A limitation of several of these studies is that patients and controls were not consistently sampled at the same locations, potentially introducing bias due to substantial differences in the microbiota in sebaceous, moist and dry areas of the skin [71].

Among the studies listed in Table 18.1, those exploring the bacterial microbiota have uniformly demonstrated a dysbiosis in psoriatic lesions when compared to normal skin. The largest such study [75] demonstrated decreased taxonomic diversity in the bacterial microbiota in psoriatic lesions when compared to unaffected skin. The dominant phyla observed in the skin were *Proteobacteria*, *Firmicutes* and *Actinobacteria*. Two distinct clusters were observed and labelled as cutaneotypes depending on the predominant phyla observed: cutaneotype 1 was predominantly *Proteobacteria*-associated, and cutaneotype 2 was *Firmicutes-/Actinobacteria*-associated. Of the two, the *Firmicutes-/Actinobacteria*-associated cluster was dominant in psoriatic plaques. These findings are consistent with two earlier studies. For example, at the phylum level, Gao et al. [73] reported the predominance of the *Firmicutes* phylum in both abundance and diversity in psoriatic lesions. However, the other two phyla, *Actinobacteria* and *Proteobacteria*, were found to be significantly lower in abundance in PsV skin compared to normal unaffected skin in that study. In a study by Fahlen et al. [74], skin microbiota from biopsies of psoriatic lesions also demonstrated an increase in *Firmicutes* and a significantly lower abundance of *Actinobacteria* when compared to normal skin. At the genus level too, the three studies report consistent findings: the major genera associated with the skin were *Corynebacterium*, *Staphylococcus*, *Streptococcus* and *Anaerococcus*. Both Gao et al. [73] and Fahlen et al. [74] reported an increased ratio of *Streptococcus/Propionibacteria* in PsV lesions, which was due to a relative reduction in abundance of the *Propionibacterium* species in psoriatic plaques.

Drago [77] investigated the bacterial skin microbiota in three conditions (psoriasis, atopic dermatitis and healthy individuals) using three related individuals (cousins) where lifestyle, gender and environmental factors were controlled. The reported differences in the taxonomic abundances at the level of the family were for the *Propionibacteriaceae* (increased in healthy and atopic dermatitis skin), *Streptococcaceae* (increased in psoriatic subject) and *Staphylococcaceae* (higher in atopic dermatitis subject and healthy control); however, the significance of these findings is limited due to the sample size.

The most recent study [78] explored community-wide, whole-genome metagenomics to characterise the microbiome in plaque psoriasis both taxonomically and functionally using whole-genome shotgun sequencing. They observed differences in microbial diversity with lower diversity in the plaques of the sebaceous (ear) sites compared with those from dry (elbow) microenvironment. The most abundant bacterial phyla belonged to the *Actinobacteria* and *Firmicutes* groups, and the most abundant bacterial species were noted to be *Staphylococcus epidermidis*, *Propionibacterium acnes*, *Staphylococcus caprae/capitis* and *Micrococcus luteus*. This was in addition to the fungus belonging to the *Malassezia* genus that has been observed in other studies exploring the fungal microbiota in psoriasis. There were two interesting observations reported, which are in keeping with current knowledge: first, the microbial composition is driven by individuality, i.e. the microbial signature is significantly more similar for an individual than for comparative sites between individuals. Second, the top five discriminatory features at the level of the genus

Table 18.1 Studies in psoriasis exploring the skin microbiota using culture-independent molecular techniques

Author/year	Aims/objectives of the study	Number of subjects	Site of sampling	Specimen collection	Platform used
Paulino et al. [72]	Identify the fungal species present in human skin, compare healthy with psoriatic lesions, understand specificity by host and time	$N = 3$ psoriasis; 5 healthy controls	At least three samples including unaffected skin from psoriasis individuals; forearms sampled from healthy controls	Skin swab	ABI3730
Gao et al. [73]	Compare bacterial populations in psoriatic lesions, from unaffected skin in subjects with psoriasis and from skin from healthy persons	$n = 12$; 6 healthy and 6 subjects with psoriasis	Psoriatic plaques and normal skin from forearm	Skin swab	Sanger sequencing
Fahlen et al. [74]	Comparison in microbiota between psoriatic and normal skin	$n = 10$ psoriatic patients and 12 control subjects	Unmatched skin sites (trunk and limbs)	Skin biopsy	Roche 454
Alekseyenko et al. [75]	Comparison of skin microbiota of psoriatic lesions, unaffected contralateral skin from psoriatic patients and similar skin loci in matched healthy controls	$n = 54$ psoriasis individuals $n = 37$ healthy controls Final analysis on set of 51 triplets	Matched skin sites for psoriatic plaques from psoriasis individuals with healthy controls and contralateral uninvolved skin from psoriasis individuals	Skin swabs	Roche 454
Takemoto et al. [76]	Characterisation of the skin fungal microbiome in subjects with psoriasis	$N = 12$ psoriatic patients and 12 healthy controls	Psoriatic scales and normal skin from the trunk	Psoriatic scales collected using tweezers and healthy skin sampled using OpSite transparent dressing	Roche 454
Drago et al. [77]	Comparison of skin microbiota between psoriasis, atopic dermatitis and healthy skin	Three male subjects (first cousins) $n = 1$ atopic dermatitis $n = 1$ psoriasis $n = 1$ healthy control Age, lifestyle, diet, clothing controlled	2 cm^2 retroauricular lesional skin and non-lesional skin (two samples each) of the left ear	Curette	Ion Torrent PGM
Tett et al. [78]	Shotgun metagenomic assessment of the skin microbiome in plaque psoriasis	$n = 28$ plaque psoriasis	Skin over the olecranon and retroauricular crease bilaterally with at least one unaffected site	Skin swab—premoistened	Illumina HiSeq 2000

between unaffected and psoriatic skin of the ear (sebaceous skin microenvironment) were *S. caprae/capitis*, *P. acnes*, *S. epidermidis*, *S. aureus* and *M. luteus*. The main difference between this observation when compared to the previous large psoriasis cohort study [75] is that *P. acnes* is found to be a significant differentiating feature between psoriatic and unaffected skin. This however may be due to the fact that the site that was evaluated for the discriminatory feature was limited to sebaceous skin microenvironment in the latest [78] study, whereas in the previous work [75], the samples were largely from the dry skin microenvironment.

Two studies [72, 76] explored the fungal microbiota in psoriatic lesions, and both reported the genus *Malassezia* to be the most abundant fungal organisms both in normal and psoriatic skin. Interestingly, Takemoto [76] reported a more diverse fungal microbiota in scales from psoriatic lesions and found discrete clustering of the fungal microbiota from psoriatic lesions when compared to healthy controls.

In addition to the skin microbiota, recently Eppinga et al. [79] explored the faecal abundances of *F. prausnitzii* and *E. coli*, organisms that have been noted to be altered in IBD patients. The stool samples of 29 psoriasis individuals, 13 individuals with IBD and psoriasis, 31 IBD subjects and 33 healthy controls were studied using quantitative PCR. A decrease in *F. prausnitzii* along with a concomitant increase in *E. coli* was reported in PsV; findings were consistent with those reported in IBD (Chap. 19).

Dysbiosis in PsA

As of this writing, there has only been one published study of the gut microbiota in PsA. Scher et al. [80] investigated the gut microbiota in treatment-naïve individuals with recent-onset PsA using faecal sampling and found a dysbiosis similar to that found in patients with IBD. Lower microbial diversity was found in the intestinal microbiota of individuals with PsA and PsC (individuals with cutaneous psoriasis without any clinical evidence of inflammatory arthritis) when compared to healthy controls. There was a relative decrease in the abundance of *Coprococcus* in both PsA and PsC cohorts when compared with healthy controls. However, a decrease in abundance of *Akkermansia*, *Ruminococcus* and *Pseudobutyrivibrio* was only observed in faecal samples from PsA patients. The study also reported a reduction in medium-chain fatty acids, hexanoate and heptanoate, similar to that in CD; interestingly hexanoate and heptanoate display antibacterial properties and have the ability to ameliorate colitis in animal models through the activation of peroxisome proliferator-activated receptor γ [81].

Implications of the Microbiota Studies in Psoriasis and PsA

In all the available studies, the *Firmicutes*- and *Actinobacteria*-associated phyla of bacteria appear to play a dominant role in the skin of psoriatic plaques of individuals with cutaneous psoriasis. Among these are well-known Gram-positive commensal bacteria such as *Propionibacterium*, *Corynebacterium*, *Staphylococcus* and *Streptococcus* that have been targeted to assess their discriminatory potential with mixed results. Interestingly, these bacteria have been described as mutualists, and their putative beneficial effects on host immunity have been extensively reviewed [82]: they are thought to influence host immunity through the secretion of toxins (such as bacteriocins); priming of adaptive and innate host immunity; prevention of oxidative damage to epidermal tissue; promotion of wound healing by stimulation of keratinocyte migration (in the case of *Streptococci* through the secretion of sublytic concentrations of streptolysin O) and enhancing the host cellular response (AMP induction) to pathogens. It is not clear why these predominantly beneficial skin bacteria are relatively increased in psoriatic plaques. It remains to be explored if the beneficial effects observed on the normal host still hold in the context of the psoriatic lesions (affected skin) in PsV and PsA. This may reflect a compensatory increase as a result of a pre-existing inflammatory process. Alternatively, the beneficial properties of these organisms may be attenuated by other factors that are not yet defined, or there may be species- or strain-level differences that have not been well-captured by existing studies.

While the changes in the skin demonstrate increased abundance of generally beneficial organisms, the findings in the gut have demonstrated the opposite. Specifically, studies [79] in PsV and PsA [80] have found a decreased abundance of the bacterial genera with anti-inflammatory effects, such as butyrate-producing *Faecalibacterium prausnitzii* and *Coprococcus* and *Akkermansia muciniphila*. This provides a basis for further hypothesis-driven studies in PsV and PsA to explore the link between the microbiome (microbial composition, host and bacterial—metabolomics, proteomics and transcriptomics) in its entirety and downstream anti/pro-inflammatory effects through the multitude of interactions with both the host and the external environment that drives or sustains disease states.

Summary

Clinical and epidemiological evidence support a role for the microbiota in both PsV and PsA susceptibility where, in a permissive environment of genetic susceptibility, an alteration in the microbial profile may provide the necessary trigger or provide the driving antigen for the development of inflammation (Fig. 18.1). The multifactorial risk factors associated with complex diseases such as PsV and PsA include genetics and non-genetic factors. Among the non-genetic factors, the human microbiota is a potentially modifiable risk factor and a future therapeutic target for prevention and control of PsV and PsA. Dissection of the underlying mechanism and exploration of the communication between organ systems such as gut-joint, gut-skin and possibly skin-gut-joint axes may provide a unique understanding of the disease pathogenesis and aid stratification based on the host-microbe interaction on the background of a susceptible genetic trait. This may also provide mechanistic insights into the aetiology and pathogenesis of the conditions which will aid development of treatment options. Currently the human studies into the microbiota in PsV and PsA have been cross-sectional; thus, it is difficult to ascertain the cause-effect relationship of the changes observed. Well-powered longitudinal studies are required that will help dissect the contribution and the effect of the microbiota in disease pathogenesis in these complex conditions. Such studies may pave the way for therapeutic trials involving modification of the cutaneous or intestinal microbiota as treatment for PsV or PsA.

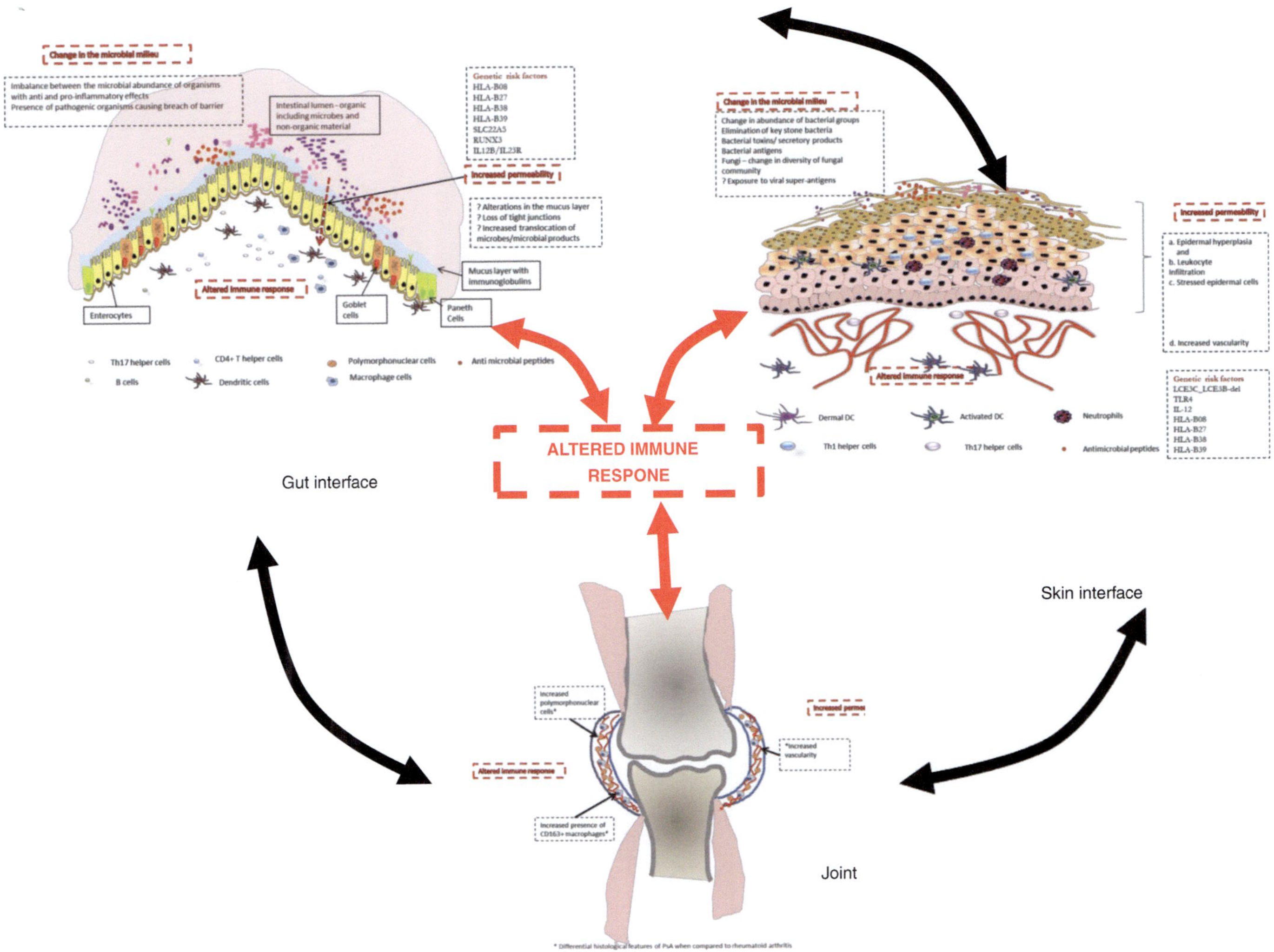

Fig. 18.1 Effect of the microbiota in the pathogenesis of PsV and PsA. The gut is characterised by an imbalance between microbial organisms with anti- and pro-inflammatory effects as well as by the presence of pathogenic organisms causing breach of barrier, resulting in loss of mucosal tight junctions and increased translocation of microbes and microbial products. The skin is also characterised by changes in the relative abundances of key bacterial groups, increased bacterial toxins and other secretory products and decreased fungal diversity. This results in epidermal hyperplasia, leukocyte infiltration, stressed epidermal cells and increased vascularity. The breach in the host-microbial barrier at both sites leads to increased or altered exposure of the host systemic immune system to microbes, which in turn triggers a dysregulated response in a susceptible host, resulting in local and distant organ involvement with migration of inflammatory cells from the skin and the gut to the skin, gut, and joint

References

1. Fry L. Psoriasis. Br J Dermatol. 1988;119(4):445–61.
2. O'Neill T, Silman AJ. Psoriatic arthritis. Historical background and epidemiology. Baillieres Clin Rheumatol. 1994;8(2):245–61.
3. Reed WB. Psoriatic arthritis. A complete clinical study of 86 patients. Acta Derm Venereol. 1961;41:396–403.
4. Moll JM, Wright V. Psoriatic arthritis. Semin Arthritis Rheum. 1973;3:55–78.
5. Taylor W, Gladman D, Helliwell P, Marchesoni A, Mease P, Mielants H. Classification criteria for psoriatic arthritis: development of new criteria from a large international study. Arthritis Rheum. 2006;54(8):2665–73.
6. Collins FS, Morgan M, Patrinos A. The human genome project: lessons from large-scale biology. Science. 2003;300(5617):286–90.
7. Lander ES, Linton LM, Birren B, Nusbaum C, Zody MC, Baldwin J, et al. Initial sequencing and analysis of the human genome. Nature. 2001;409(6822):860–921.
8. Gladman DD. Clinical, radiological, and functional assessment in psoriatic arthritis: is it different from other inflammatory joint diseases? Ann Rheum Dis. 2006;65(Suppl 3):iii22–4.
9. Helliwell PS, Hickling P, Wright V. Do the radiological changes of classic ankylosing spondylitis differ from the changes found in the spondylitis associated with inflammatory bowel disease, psoriasis, and reactive arthritis? Ann Rheum Dis. 1998;57(3):135–40.
10. Kruithof E, Baeten D, De Rycke L, Vandooren B, Foell D, Roth J, et al. Synovial histopathology of psoriatic arthritis, both oligo- and polyarticular, resembles spondyloarthropathy more than it does rheumatoid arthritis. Arthritis Res Ther. 2005;7(3):R569–80.
11. Griffiths CEM, Barker JN. Pathogenesis and clinical features of psoriasis. Lancet. 2007;370(9583):263–71.
12. Nestle FO, Kaplan DH, Barker J. Psoriasis. N Engl J Med. 2009;361(5):496–509.
13. Reece RJ, Canete JD, Parsons WJ, Emery P, Veale DJ. Distinct vascular patterns of early synovitis in psoriatic, reactive, and rheumatoid arthritis. Arthritis Rheum. 1999;42(7):1481–4.
14. Levine JS, Burakoff R. Extraintestinal manifestations of inflammatory bowel disease. Gastroenterol Hepatol. 2011;7(4):235–41.
15. Lindqvist U, Kristjansson G, Pihl-Lundin I, Hagforsen E, Michaelsson G. Patients with psoriatic arthritis have an increased number of lymphocytes in the duodenal mucosa in comparison with patients with psoriasis vulgaris. J Rheumatol. 2006;33(5):924–7.
16. Scarpa R, Manguso F, D'Arienzo A, D'Armiento FP, Astarita C, Mazzacca G, et al. Microscopic inflammatory changes in colon of patients with both active psoriasis and psoriatic arthritis without bowel symptoms. J Rheumatol. 2000;27(5):1241–6.
17. Hannu T. Reactive arthritis. Best Pract Res Clin Rheumatol. 2011;25(3):347–57.
18. Telfer NR, Chalmers RJ, Whale K, Colman G. The role of streptococcal infection in the initiation of guttate psoriasis. Arch Dermatol. 1992;128(1):39–42.
19. Luxembourg A, Cailla H, Roux H, Roudier J. Do viruses play an etiologic role in ankylosing spondylitis or psoriatic arthritis? Clin Immunol Immunopathol. 1987;45(2):292–5.
20. Palazzi C, Olivieri I, D'Amico E, D'Agostino L, Nicolucci A, Pennese E, et al. Hepatitis C virus infection in psoriatic arthritis. Arthritis Rheum. 2005;53(2):223–5.
21. Taglione E, Vatteroni ML, Martini P, Galluzzo E, Lombardini F, Delle SA, et al. Hepatitis C virus infection: prevalence in psoriasis and psoriatic arthritis. J Rheumatol. 1999;26(2):370–2.
22. Rahman MU, Ahmed S, Schumacher HR, Zeiger AR. High levels of antipeptidoglycan antibodies in psoriatic and other seronegative arthritides. J Rheumatol. 1990;17(5):621–5.
23. Rantakokko K, Rimpilainen M, Uksila J, Jansen C, Luukkainen R, Toivanen P. Antibodies to streptococcal cell wall in psoriatic arthritis and cutaneous psoriasis. Clin Exp Rheumatol. 1997;15(4):399–404.
24. Vasey FB, Deitz C, Fenske NA, Germain BF, Espinoza LR. Possible involvement of group A streptococci in the pathogenesis of psoriatic arthritis. J Rheumatol. 1982;9(5):719–22.
25. Njobvu P, McGill P. Psoriatic arthritis and human immunodeficiency virus infection in Zambia. J Rheumatol. 2000;27(7):1699–702.
26. Eder L, Law T, Chandran V, Shanmugarajah S, Shen H, Rosen CF, et al. Association between environmental factors and onset of psoriatic arthritis in patients with psoriasis. Arthritis Care Res (Hoboken). 2011;63(8):1091–7.
27. Pattison E, Harrison BJ, Griffiths CEM, Silman AJ, Bruce IN. Environmental risk factors for the development of psoriatic arthritis: results from a case-control study. Ann Rheum Dis. 2008;67(5):672–6.
28. Bowes J, Budu-Aggrey A, Huffmeier U, Uebe S, Steel K, Hebert HL, et al. Dense genotyping of immune-related susceptibility loci reveals new insights into the genetics of psoriatic arthritis. Nat Commun. 2015;6:6046.
29. Eder L, Chandran V, Pellet F, Shanmugarajah S, Rosen CF, Bull SB, et al. Human leucocyte antigen risk alleles for psoriatic arthritis among patients with psoriasis. Ann Rheum Dis. 2012;71(1):50–5.
30. Fitzgerald O, Haroon M, Giles JT, Winchester R. Concepts of pathogenesis in psoriatic arthritis: genotype determines clinical phenotype. Arthritis Res Ther. 2015;17:115.
31. Okada Y, Han B, Tsoi LC, Stuart PE, Ellinghaus E, Tejasvi T, et al. Fine mapping major histocompatibility complex associations in psoriasis and its clinical subtypes. Am J Hum Genet. 2014;95(2):162–72.
32. Winchester R, Minevich G, Steshenko V, Kirby B, Kane D, Greenberg DA, et al. HLA associations reveal genetic heterogeneity in psoriatic arthritis and in the psoriasis phenotype. Arthritis Rheum. 2012;64(4):1134–44.

33. Sobao Y, Tsuchiya N, Takiguchi M, Tokunaga K. Overlapping peptide-binding specificities of HLA-B27 and B39: evidence for a role of peptide supermotif in the pathogenesis of spondylarthropathies. Arthritis Rheum. 1999;42(1):175–81.
34. McFadden J, Valdimarsson H, Fry L. Cross-reactivity between streptococcal M surface antigen and human skin. Br J Dermatol. 1991;125(5):443–7.
35. Baker BS, Powles A, Fry L. Peptidoglycan: a major aetiological factor for psoriasis? Trends Immunol. 2006;27(12):545–51.
36. Cai YH, Lu ZY, Shi RF, Xue F, Chen XY, Pan M, et al. Enhanced proliferation and activation of peripheral blood mononuclear cells in patients with psoriasis vulgaris mediated by streptococcal antigen with bacterial DNA. J Invest Dermatol. 2009;129(11):2653–60.
37. Tinazzi I, Adami S, Zanolin EM, Caimmi C, Confente S, Girolomoni G, et al. The early psoriatic arthritis screening questionnaire: a simple and fast method for the identification of arthritis in patients with psoriasis. Rheumatology (Oxford). 2012;51(11):2058–63.
38. Duvic M. Immunology of AIDS related to psoriasis. J Invest Dermatol. 1990;95(5 Suppl):38S–40S.
39. Fuchs D, Hausen A, Reibnegger G, Werner ER, Werner-Felmayer G, Dierich MP, et al. Interferon-gamma concentrations are increased in sera from individuals infected with human immunodeficiency virus type 1. J Acquir Immune Defic Syndr. 1989;2(2):158–62.
40. Silvestris F, Williams RC Jr, Dammacco F. Autoreactivity in HIV-1 infection: the role of molecular mimicry. Clin Immunol Immunopathol. 1995;75(3):197–205.
41. Torres BA, Johnson HM. Identification of an HIV-1 Nef peptide that binds to HLA class II antigens. Biochem Biophys Res Commun. 1994;200(2):1059–65.
42. Ndhlovu LC, Chapman JM, Jha AR, Snyder-Cappione JE, Pagan M, Leal FE, et al. Suppression of HIV-1 plasma viral load below detection preserves IL-17 producing T cells in HIV-1 infection. AIDS. 2008;22(8):990–2.
43. Costello P, Bresnihan B, O'Farrelly C, Fitzgerald O. Predominance of CD8+ T lymphocytes in psoriatic arthritis. J Rheumatol. 1999;26(5):1117–24.
44. Menon B, Gullick NJ, Walter GJ, Rajasekhar M, Garrood T, Evans HG, et al. Interleukin-17+CD8+ T cells are enriched in the joints of patients with psoriatic arthritis and correlate with disease activity and joint damage progression. Arthritis Rheumatol. 2014;66(5):1272–81.
45. Huffmeier U, Uebe S, Ekici AB, Bowes J, Giardina E, Korendowych E, et al. Common variants at TRAF3IP2 are associated with susceptibility to psoriatic arthritis and psoriasis. Nat Genet. 2010;42(11):996–9.
46. Liu Y, Helms C, Liao W, Zaba LC, Duan S, Gardner J, et al. A genome-wide association study of psoriasis and psoriatic arthritis identifies new disease loci. PLoS Genet. 2008;4(3):e1000041.
47. Stuart PE, Nair RP, Ellinghaus E, Ding J, Tejasvi T, Gudjonsson JE, et al. Genome-wide association analysis identifies three psoriasis susceptibility loci. Nat Genet. 2010;42:1000–4.
48. Lawrence T. The nuclear factor NF-kappaB pathway in inflammation. Cold Spring Harb Perspect Biol. 2009;1(6):a001651.
49. Hooper LV, Littman DR, Macpherson AJ. Interactions between the microbiota and the immune system. Science. 2012;336(6086):1268–73.
50. Round JL, Mazmanian SK. The gut microbiota shapes intestinal immune responses during health and disease. Nat Rev Immunol. 2009;9(5):313–23.
51. Bischoff SC, Barbara G, Buurman W, Ockhuizen T, Schulzke JD, Serino M, et al. Intestinal permeability – a new target for disease prevention and therapy. BMC Gastroenterol. 2014;14:189.
52. Lam YY, Ha CW, Campbell CR, Mitchell AJ, Dinudom A, Oscarsson J, et al. Increased gut permeability and microbiota change associate with mesenteric fat inflammation and metabolic dysfunction in diet-induced obese mice. PLoS One. 2012;7(3):e34233.
53. Nakatsuji T, Chiang HI, Jiang SB, Nagarajan H, Zengler K, Gallo RL. The microbiome extends to subepidermal compartments of normal skin. Nat Commun. 2013;4:1431.
54. Bowes J, Flynn E, Ho P, Aly B, Morgan AW, Marzo-Ortega H, et al. Variants in linkage disequilibrium with the late cornified envelope gene cluster deletion are associated with susceptibility to psoriatic arthritis. Ann Rheum Dis. 2010;69(12):2199–203.
55. de Cid CR, Riveira-Munoz E, Zeeuwen PL, Robarge J, Liao W, Dannhauser EN, et al. Deletion of the late cornified envelope LCE3B and LCE3C genes as a susceptibility factor for psoriasis. Nat Genet. 2009;41(2):211–5.
56. Smith RL, Hebert HL, Massey J, Bowes J, Marzo-Ortega H, Ho P, et al. Association of Toll-like receptor 4 (TLR4) with chronic plaque type psoriasis and psoriatic arthritis. Arch Dermatol Res. 2016;308(3):201–5.
57. Lande R, Botti E, Jandus C, Dojcinovic D, Fanelli G, Conrad C, et al. The antimicrobial peptide LL37 is a T-cell autoantigen in psoriasis. Nat Commun. 2014;5:5621.
58. Cohen AD, Dreiher J, Birkenfeld S. Psoriasis associated with ulcerative colitis and Crohn's disease. J Eur Acad Dermatol Venereol. 2009;23(5):561–5.
59. Schatteman L, Mielants H, Veys EM, Cuvelier C, De Vos M, Gyselbrecht L, et al. Gut inflammation in psoriatic arthritis: a prospective ileocolonoscopic study. J Rheumatol. 1995;22(4):680–3.
60. Egeberg A, Mallbris L, Warren RB, Bachelez H, Gislason GH, Hansen PR, et al. Association between psoriasis and inflammatory bowel disease: a Danish nationwide cohort study. Br J Dermatol. 2016;175(3):487–92.
61. Bernstein CN, Wajda A, Blanchard JF. The clustering of other chronic inflammatory diseases in inflammatory bowel disease: a population-based study. Gastroenterology. 2005;129(3):827–36.
62. Christophers E. Comorbidities in psoriasis. Clin Dermatol. 2007;25(6):529–34.

63. Lee FI, Bellary SV, Francis C. Increased occurrence of psoriasis in patients with Crohn's disease and their relatives. Am J Gastroenterol. 1990;85(8):962–3.
64. Li WQ, Han JL, Chan AT, Qureshi AA. Psoriasis, psoriatic arthritis and increased risk of incident Crohn's disease in US women. Ann Rheum Dis. 2013;72(7):1200–5.
65. Streilein JW. Skin-associated lymphoid tissues (SALT): origins and functions. J Invest Dermatol. 1983;80(Suppl):12s–6s.
66. Bouskra D, Brezillon C, Berard M, Werts C, Varona R, Boneca IG, et al. Lymphoid tissue genesis induced by commensals through NOD1 regulates intestinal homeostasis. Nature. 2008;456(7221):507–10.
67. Ivanov II, Atarashi K, Manel N, Brodie EL, Shima T, Karaoz U, et al. Induction of intestinal Th17 cells by segmented filamentous bacteria. Cell. 2009;139(3):485–98.
68. Naik S, Bouladoux N, Wilhelm C, Molloy MJ, Salcedo R, Kastenmuller W, et al. Compartmentalized control of skin immunity by resident commensals. Science. 2012;337(6098):1115–9.
69. Zakostelska Z, Malkova J, Klimesova K, Rossmann P, Hornova M, Novosadova I, et al. Intestinal microbiota promotes psoriasis-like skin inflammation by enhancing Th17 response. PLoS One. 2016;11(7):e0159539.
70. Teng F, Klinger CN, Felix KM, Bradley CP, Wu E, Tran NL, et al. Gut microbiota drive autoimmune arthritis by promoting differentiation and migration of Peyer's patch T follicular helper cells. Immunity. 2016;44(4):875–88.
71. Findley K, Oh J, Yang J, Conlan S, Deming C, Meyer JA, et al. Topographic diversity of fungal and bacterial communities in human skin. Nature. 2013;498(7454):367–70.
72. Paulino LC, Tseng CH, Strober BE, Blaser MJ. Molecular analysis of fungal microbiota in samples from healthy human skin and psoriatic lesions. J Clin Microbiol. 2006;44(8):2933–41.
73. Gao Z, Tseng CH, Strober BE, Pei Z, Blaser MJ. Substantial alterations of the cutaneous bacterial biota in psoriatic lesions. PLoS One. 2008;3:e2719.
74. Fahlen A, Engstrand L, Baker BS, Powles A, Fry L. Comparison of bacterial microbiota in skin biopsies from normal and psoriatic skin. Arch Dermatol Res. 2011;304(1):15–22.
75. Alekseyenko AV, Perez-Perez GI, De Souza A, Strober B, Gao Z, Bihan M, et al. Community differentiation of the cutaneous microbiota in psoriasis. Microbiome. 2013;1(1):31.
76. Takemoto A, Cho O, Morohoshi Y, Sugita T, Muto M. Molecular characterization of the skin fungal microbiome in patients with psoriasis. J Dermatol. 2015;42(2):166–70.
77. Drago L, De GR, Altomare G, Pigatto P, Rossi O, Toscano M. Skin microbiota of first cousins affected by psoriasis and atopic dermatitis. Clin Mol Allergy. 2016;14:2.
78. Tett A, Pasolli E, Farina S, Truong DT, Asnicar F, Zolfo M, et al. Unexplored diversity and strain-level structure of the skin microbiome associated with psoriasis. NPJ Biofilms Microbiomes. 2017;3:14.
79. Eppinga H, Sperna Weiland CJ, Thio HB, van der Woude CJ, Nijsten TE, Peppelenbosch MP, et al. Similar depletion of protective Faecalibacterium prausnitzii in psoriasis and inflammatory bowel disease, but not in hidradenitis suppurativa. J Crohns Colitis. 2016;10(9):1067–75.
80. Scher JU, Ubeda C, Artacho A, Attur M, Isaac S, Reddy SM, et al. Decreased bacterial diversity characterizes the altered gut microbiota in patients with psoriatic arthritis, resembling dysbiosis in inflammatory bowel disease. Arthritis Rheumatol. 2015;67(1):128–39.
81. Bassaganya-Riera J, Viladomiu M, Pedragosa M, De SC, Carbo A, Shaykhutdinov R, et al. Probiotic bacteria produce conjugated linoleic acid locally in the gut that targets macrophage PPAR gamma to suppress colitis. PLoS One. 2012;7(2):e31238.
82. Cogen AL, Nizet V, Gallo RL. Skin microbiota: a source of disease or defence? Br J Dermatol. 2008;158:442–55.

Inflammatory Bowel Disease 19

Wayne Young, Traci Jester, Matthew L. Stoll, and Ana Izcue

Abbreviations

Ahr	Aryl hydrocarbon receptor
ASCA	Anti-*Saccharomyces cerevisiae* antibodies
CD	Crohn disease
DSS	Dextran sulfate sodium
EEN	Exclusive enteral nutrition
FMT	Fecal microbial transplantation
FXR	Farnesoid X receptor
IBD	Inflammatory bowel disease
IL	Interleukin
ILC	Innate lymphoid cells
IPA	Indolepropionic acid
MyD88	Myeloid differentiation primary response 88
PSA	Polysaccharide A
SCFA	Short-chain fatty acids
SFB	Segmented filamentous bacteria
SpA	Spondyloarthritis
Treg	Regulatory T cells
TLR	Toll-like receptor
TNF	Tumor necrosis factor
UC	Ulcerative colitis

W. Young
Food Nutrition and Health Team, AgResearch, Palmerston North, New Zealand

Riddet Institute, Massey University, Palmerston North, New Zealand

High-Value Nutrition, National Science Challenge, Auckland, New Zealand

T. Jester
Department of Pediatrics, Division of Gastroenterology, University of Alabama at Birmingham, Birmingham, AL, USA

M. L. Stoll (✉)
Department of Pediatrics, Division of Rheumatology, University of Alabama at Birmingham, Birmingham, AL, USA
e-mail: mstoll@peds.uab.edu

A. Izcue
Institute of Molecular Medicine, RWTH Aachen University, Aachen, Germany

Microbiota and the Immune System in Intestinal Inflammation

IBD impacts approximately 200 per 100,000 individuals [1], depending on geographic location [2]. There are two major subtypes: Crohn Disease (CD) and ulcerative colitis (UC) (Table 19.1). IBD likely results from the combination of multiple factors. On the one hand, the increase in IBD prevalence in Western countries points to a role for environmental factors, and the microbiota is likely one of them [3, 4]. On the other hand, the genetic component of susceptibility to IBD includes numerous immune-related genes, underlining the role of genetically programmed immune factors in IBD pathogenesis [5]. Our understanding of the interactions between the intestinal immune system and the microbiota

G. Ragab et al. (eds.), *The Microbiome in Rheumatic Diseases and Infection*,
https://doi.org/10.1007/978-3-319-79026-8_19

Table 19.1 Comparison of features of CD and UC

Feature	Crohn disease	Ulcerative colitis
Location	Entire GI tract	Colon primarily
Continuity of inflammation	Skip lesions	Continuous
Depth of inflammation	Deep; can become transmural	Superficial
Pathology	Granulomas possible	Mucosal inflammation
Extraintestinal manifestations		
Arthritis	+	+
Cutaneous	+	+
Sclerosing cholangitis	+/–	+
Uveitis	+	+
Risk of colon cancer	Increased	Increased
Common symptoms	Diarrhea, weight loss, malabsorption, abdominal pain, growth failure	Bloody diarrhea, abdominal pain

Adapted from [162]

has greatly expanded over the last decade, aided by the mainstream adoption of new molecular tools allowing the molecular characterization of microbial communities. Early reports about gene mutations altering the microbiota in mouse models have to be assessed with caution, though, since the use of non-stringent controls in the early days introduced considerable errors into the system [6]. Still, the use of mice with genetic mutations has demonstrated that changes in the immune system suffice to alter the intestinal microbiota. Interestingly, the altered microbiota can then change the way the immune system responds to challenges. The pathways mediating the cross talk between the immune system and the microbiota are only beginning to be understood, and only a few specific mechanistic interactions have been demonstrated in patients or in preclinical models.

Immune Cells

Studies in recent years have highlighted the interplay between the microbiota, metabolism, and immune cells in intestinal inflammation. IBD is considered to arise from an imbalance between the inflammatory and the regulatory arms of the immune response. T cells and innate lymphoid cells (ILC) are some of the inflammatory cell types implicated in IBD, whereas FOXP3$^+$ regulatory T cells (Treg) dampen immune inflammation. Tregs could also affect intestinal immune responses by modulating IgA secretion into the intestine [7], since IgA has been shown to regulate the composition of the gut microbiota [8]. T cells and ILC do not act directly on the microbiota but appear to control it indirectly through intestinal epithelial cells and other mechanisms [9, 10]. Lymphocytes in the mucosa produce cytokines, such as IL-17 and IL-22, that act on epithelial cells enhancing their secretion of Reg3g and other antimicrobial peptides and thus altering the composition of the microbial community [11]. Intestinal myeloid immune cells, such as macrophages and dendritic cells, directly sense the microbiota but also react to changes in epithelial cells, such as increased cell death [10, 12]. They can instruct lymphocyte activity through antigen presentation and production of cytokines such as IL-23, a key player in intestinal inflammation in mice and humans, which enhances production of IL-17 and IL-22 by Th17 and ILC3 cells [13]. IL-23 mediates intestinal inflammation in animal models, and variants in *IL23R*, the gene coding the specific subunit of the IL-23 receptor, are associated with IBD susceptibility in patients [14]. Alterations in all these pathways can change the composition of the microbiota.

Intestinal Epithelial Cells

The intestinal epithelium also plays an active role in defense against pathogens and the interactions with the microbiota. It is a protective barrier as little as a single cell thick, which has a crucial role for excluding exogenous pathogens and antigens, but at the same time allowing water and nutrients to pass. Intestinal epithelial cells shape the microbial community by a variety of mechanisms including the secretion of antimicrobial peptides. It has been shown that several genes with variants associated with IBD susceptibility, including

NOD2, affect the secretion of antimicrobial peptides by epithelial cells [15]. Intestinal epithelial cells can sense the microbiota and respond to it, as seen in germ-free rats, which have reduced epithelial cell proliferation compared to conventionally raised rats [16]. Important regulators of bacteria and epithelial cell interactions are the toll-like receptors (TLRs), which recognize bacterial molecular motifs such as cell wall components and flagellin. These receptors are found on both immune and nonimmune cells, such as epithelial cells. Therefore, TLR signaling is a likely mechanism regulating bacteria-induced increases in cell proliferation. However, in the absence of intestinal injury, epithelial cell proliferation in mice deficient in either myeloid differentiation primary response 88 (MyD88, a transducer necessary for signaling by many TLRs) or TLR4-is similar to that in wild-type mice, suggesting the involvement of other bacterial signals [17].

In contrast, dextran sulfate sodium (DSS)-induced intestinal injury leads to decreased gut epithelial cell proliferation, acute inflammation, and increased mortality in MyD88-, TLR4-, or TLR2-deficient mice [18, 19]. This increased susceptibility to DSS-induced injury can be reproduced in wild-type mice by treating them with broad-spectrum antibiotics or antibodies targeting TLR2 or TLR4 [18, 19]. Administration of DSS to wild-type germ-free mice also produces greater colonic injury compared to mice that have a conventional microbiota [20, 21]. Initially, these results appear counterintuitive, as one might predict that mice that are unable to mount a TLR-dependent response against the microbiota would be less affected by DSS. However, these studies show that TLR signaling in epithelial cells is dispensable for intestinal epithelial cell proliferation under normal conditions, while in the presence of injury, both the intestinal microbiota and their interactions with TLRs are required for tissue repair.

Effects of the Microbiota on the Immune System

No longer viewed as merely passengers, the gut microbiota is widely thought to play a critical role in the development and progression of IBD. Experiments in mice show that mutations in genes associated with susceptibility to IBD, such as *Nod2*, can cause an imbalance in the microbial community (dysbiosis) that exacerbates colitis [22]. However, despite extensive investigation, no single microbial agent has been proven to cause IBD. Nevertheless, some broad patterns can be discerned across many studies. These include a loss of community diversity, increased representation of some Gammaproteobacteria, and decreased relative abundance of several taxa within the Firmicutes phylum [23]; see below.

Other groups of bacteria may protect against IBD through suppression or modulation of inflammatory responses. *Bacteroides thetaiotaomicron* has been shown to attenuate intestinal epithelial cell inflammation, suppress NF-κB activation [24], increase *Gata3* and *FoxP3* gene expression, and stimulate maturation of Treg [25], effects that could be common to humans and mice.

Bacteria in close proximity to epithelial cells may play an important role in gut immune responses. In mice, segmented filamentous bacteria (SFB), which are commensals in many different animal facilities, provide a striking example of the ability of the microbiota to alter the gut immune response. About a decade ago, it was shown that the presence of this commensal drastically increases the frequency of intestinal Th17 cells [26, 27]. SFB tightly adhere to intestinal epithelial cells, and this adhesion appears to be a strong inducer of Th17 responses across species [28]. Moreover, SFB also induce IgA production in the gut. Although SFB have been detected in human ileostomy samples [29], whether they play an equivalent role in humans is still subject of investigation.

Microbiota can also trigger systemic immune responses. Patients with CD have elevated levels of antibodies against flagellin antigens [30], which when present are associated with a more complicated disease course [31]. It is currently not known if these antibodies arise before the disease or after inflammation has exposed the intestinal contents directly to the immune system. Although these findings do not necessarily implicate the antibodies as being pathogenic, the T cells driving their production may be. Although microbiota-reactive CD4+ T cells are present in the gut of healthy individuals as well as IBD patients [32], adoptive transfer of flagellin-reactive T cells into T cell receptor-deficient mice results in colitis, particularly if the T cells have a Th17 phenotype [33].

Other bacteria, such as *Faecalibacterium prausnitzii*, *Bifidobacterium*, and *Lactobacillus* spp., protect the host through a variety of mechanisms, including modulation of cytokine production [34, 35] and strengthening of the gut barrier function [36]. The evidence for the efficacy of probiotic strains like *Bifidobacterium* and *Lactobacillus* in reducing the symptoms of CD in humans remains unclear, although some beneficial effects have been shown in patients with UC [37]. Additionally, the gut microbiota may protect the host by outcompeting pathogenic bacteria that drive gastrointestinal inflammation by preventing these pathogens from occupying niches [38].

Bacterial-Derived Metabolites

Aside from physical interactions between the microbiota and the host, the products of bacterial metabolism are important regulators of intestinal immunity. The most important metabolites are short-chain fatty acids (SCFA), including butyrate, which are primarily the products of nondigestible carbohydrate fermentation. In addition, bile acid metabolism and products of tryptophan metabolism also have a role.

Activation of the inflammasome can occur via microbiota-accessible carbohydrate (MAC) modulation of the gut microbiota as well as SCFA administration, which promotes IL-18-mediated epithelial repair following DSS-induced GI inflammation [39]. Butyrate produced by the gut microbiota, most prominently by members of the *Clostridia* class, has also been shown to induce the expansion of Tregs in mice, ameliorating intestinal inflammation in an adoptive T cell transfer model of colitis [40]. Several mechanisms have been suggested to explain the anti-inflammatory effect of SCFA. First, some SCFA such as butyrate and propionate alter the epigenetic status of the cells by inhibiting histone deacetylase activity [41]; the resulting changes could induce a regulatory state in both Tregs and innate cells [40, 42, 43]. Additionally, specific receptors on immune cells can recognize SCFA. Dendritic cells and macrophages acquire regulatory activity after recognition of butyrate through Gpr109a [44].

Bacteria can also affect the host by metabolizing bile acids. Bile acids are secreted into the small intestine to aid digestion, and they are toxic to bacteria and eukaryotic cells, modulating the composition of the microbiota. Many bacteria can deconjugate bile acids through removal of taurine or glycine, leading to secondary bile acids [45]. This microbial activity not only influences the rate of bile acid reabsorption through the intestine and subsequent recycling through the enterohepatic cycle, but it can also modulate lipid metabolism [46] and intestinal immunity [47]. Bile acids interact with the intracellular farnesoid X receptor (FXR) and transmembrane receptor Takeda G-protein-coupled receptor 5, which are specific bile acid receptors present in different cell types, including innate immune cells [48]. Inactivation of FXR increases the severity of trinitrobenzenesulfonic acid or DSS-induced colitis in mice, while expression of FXR mRNA was reported to be reduced in colon biopsies from areas of macroscopically inflamed mucosa in CD disease patients [47]. Activation of FXR regulates mechanisms that affect liver and intestinal homeostasis, including reducing the expression of key inflammatory cytokines such as IL-1β, TNF-α, and IFN-γ [47, 49].

Tryptophan metabolites derived from *Lactobacilli* and other microbes are recognized by the aryl hydrocarbon (Ahr) transcription factor and promote IL-22 production by T cells and ILC in preclinical mouse models [50]. IL-22 enhances secretion of antimicrobial peptides, epithelial cell regeneration, and barrier function, and the IL-22-mediated response increases resistance to colonization by the fungus *Candida albicans* in a mouse model and protects the mice from intestinal inflammation. It has also been shown that tryptophan deficiency, resulting either from the diet or from intestinal malabsorption, leads to dysbiosis and enhanced susceptibility to colitis [51]. Tryptophan deficiency is associated with decreased secretion of IL-22 and IL-17 by mucosal lymphocytes and lower production of intestinal antimicrobial peptides [51]. When these antimicrobial peptides are reduced, the composition of the microbiota is changed to a community that favors intestinal inflammation. More recently, activation of Ahr by kynurenine, a tryptophan metabolite that can be produced by both the microbiota and the host, was shown to increase expression of the IL10 receptor on intestinal epithelial cells [52]. Additionally, recent data have suggested that the IBD-associated polymorphism in caspase recruitment domain family member 9 (*CARD9*) functions by altering the microbiota and tryptophan metabolism [53]. *CARD9*-deficient mice harbor an altered microbiota with decreased capacity to produce Ahr ligands from tryptophan. This dysbiotic microbiota enhances intestinal inflammation in mice, an effect that can be counteracted by tryptophan-metabolizing *Lactobacillus* strains. Importantly, analysis of feces from IBD patients in remission and healthy patients showed that patients with IBD-associated polymorphisms in *CARD9* also have lower levels of Ahr ligands in their feces [53]. More recently, indolepropionic acid (IPA) and related compounds produced by microbial metabolism of tryptophan, tyrosine, and phenylalanine were shown to influence the innate and adaptive immune system in mice. Disruption of the microbial IPA pathway led to increased intestinal permeability and higher frequencies of circulating neutrophils, monocytes, and effector/memory T cells [54]. These data underline the interdependence in the immune/microbiota dynamics. Changes in the immune system, like CARD9 dysfunction, may alter the composition of the microbiota. This altered microbiota affects then the immune response, increasing the severity of colitis.

The Contents of the Microbiota in IBD

From 2010 to the time of this writing, 44 studies using next-generation sequencing methods evaluating the microbiota or metagenome in IBD have been published (Table 19.2). The majority of the studies evaluated the bacterial populations through 16S amplicon sequencing, with a smaller number looking at the fungome or the full metagenome. There is substantial heterogeneity in the study designs, with respect to the disease under study (CD, UC, or both), subject age (pediatrics or adult), disease status (treatment-naïve, long-standing disease, remission), and sample sites (fecal or mucosal). Despite this heterogeneity in study design, several bacteria and one fungus emerged as being consistently negatively or positively associated with IBD, by appearing either over- or underrepresented in patients.

Differences in the Structure of the Microbiota

Structural differences are generally assessed through measures of alpha (within sample) or beta (between samples) diversity. Patients with CD are typically found to have diminished alpha diversity, that is, their microbiota is less diverse, as assessed by either the richness or evenness of the samples [55–71]; this is a less consistent finding in UC (e.g., [56]), although has been reported as well [72]. As discussed previously, the loss of fecal community diversity is often manifested as a decreased abundance of some members of the Firmicutes phylum, including *F. prausnitzii*, a prominent member of the healthy microbiota with significant anti-inflammatory effects [34]. Other species that appear to decrease in relative abundance in IBD include *Bacteroides fragilis*, *B. vulgatus*, *Ruminococcus albus*, Ruminococcus *callidus*, and *Ruminococcus bromii* [73].

While the focus of most studies has been on changes in taxonomic diversity and composition, more recent metagenomic studies indicate that

Table 19.2 Microbiota in IBD

Study	Subjects (n)	Prior abx	Site	Age (years)	Tx	Increased organisms/functions	Decreased organisms/functions	Comments
Bacterial populations								
Willing et al. [78]	CD, UC	OK	Mostly fecal; some mucosal	Groups ranged from mean 47 to 55 years	N/A	*Bifidobacteriaceae* (CD), *Coriobacteriaceae* (CD), *Ruminococcaceae* (CD), *Anaeroplasmataceae* (CD)	*Ruminococcaceae incertae sedis* (CD), *F. prausnitzii* (CD)	No differences were noted between HC and UC
Lepage et al. [101]	UC	OK	Sigmoid colon	18–52	Yes	*Actinobacteria*	Subset with lower *Bacteroides* and *Prevotella*	
Walker et al. [55]	CD (6), UC (6), HC (5)	2 months	Colon	IBD: 24–73 (mean 34); HC: 45–73 (mean 57)	N/A	*Bacteroidetes* (CD, UC), *Enterobacteriaceae* (CD)	*Firmicutes* (UC)	Decreased AD (CD)
Hansen et al. [56]	CD (11), UC (11), HC (12)	3 months	Distal colon	6–16	None	*Faecalibacterium* (CD)	*Actinobacteria* (CD,UC), *Parabacteroides* (UC), *Burkholderiales* (UC), *Coriobacteriaceae* (CD)	Decreased AD in CD only
Kellermayer et al. [88]	CD (15), HC (26)	6 months	TV colon	7–17 (CD), 3–17 (HC)	None	*Sutterella*	*Roseburia*, *Eubacterium*, *Subdoligranulum*	
Michail et al. [72]	Severe UC (27), HC (26)	1 month	Fecal	13 (mean)	Yes	*Proteobacteria*, *Fusobacteria*, *Spirochaetes*	*Firmicutes*, *Lentisphaerae*, *Verrucomicrobia*	Lower AD in UC
Morgan et al. [23]	CD (121), IC (8), UC (75), HC (27)	OK	TI, colon, feces	Median 27–41	Yes	*Clostridium* (CD,UC), *Enterobacteriaceae* (CD)—especially *Escherichia/Shigella*	Butyrate-producing organisms: *Roseburia* (CD,UC), *Phascolarctobacterium* (CD,UC), *Ruminococcaceae* (CD), *Leuconostocaceae* (UC)	Among IBD patients, treatments, particularly abx, were associated with alterations in the microbiota Biopsy and fecal samples differed while showing similar trends
Papa et al. [117]	CD (23), UC (43), HC (24)	N/A	Feces	3–24	Yes	*Escherichia/Shigella*	Multiple rare bacteria from *Rikenellaceae*, *Porphyromonadaceae*, *Peptococcaceae*, and *Akkermansia*	Decreased AD with active disease

Study	Subjects (n)	Prior abx	Site	Age (years)	Tx	Increased organisms/functions	Decreased organisms/functions	Comments
Prideaux et al. [57]	CD (22), UC (30), HC (35)	OK	TI, cecum, rectum	20–63	Yes	*Bacteroidetes* (UC)	*F. prausnitzii* (CD), *Roseburia* (CD), *Firmicutes* (UC), *Coprococcus* (UC), *Dorea* (UC)	Decreased AD (CD)
Tong et al. [58]	CD (16), UC (16), HC (32)	N/A	Multiple biopsy sites	UC 36 years, CD 41 years, HC 60 years	Yes	*Actinobacteria* (IBD as a whole), *Escherichia* (CD)	*Firmicutes* (IBD as a whole), *Faecalibacterium* (CD)	Decreased AD (UC, CD)
Tyler et al. [89]	UC (34), FAP (18)	OK	Pouch and afferent limb	38 (FAP), 52 (UC without pouchitis), 41 (UC with pouchitis)	Yes	*Bacteroidetes*, *Proteobacteria*	*Blautia*, *Bacteroides*, *Parabacteroides*, *Sutterella*	Study compared fecal microbiota in UC versus FAP patients with a pouch 1 year post-IPAA
Chen et al. [59]	CD (26), UC (41), HC (21)	2 months	TI, cecum, rectum, feces	18–70	Yes	Feces: *Fusobacteria* (CD), *Proteobacteria* (CD, UC). Cecum: *Firmicutes* (UC). Rectum: *Proteobacteria* (CD)	Feces: *Faecalibacterium* (CD) TI: *Proteobacteria* (CD) Cecum: *Prevotellaceae* (CD). Rectum: *Prevotella* (UC)	Lower AD in both IBD groups in feces and mucosa Mostly reported changes in rare bacteria
Davenport et al. [163]	CD (13), UC (14), HC (27)	N/A	Multiple biopsy sites	38 ± 11 (CD), 41 ± 11 (UC), 61 ± 7 (HC)	Yes	*Bacteroidetes* (CD)		PICRUsT showed that UC and CD clustered apart, while HC clustered with both
Gevers et al. [79]	CD (468), HC (229)	N/A	Rectal, TI, feces	<17	No	*Enterobacteriaceae*, *Fusobacteriaceae*, *Neisseriaceae*	*Erysipelotrichaceae*, *Bifidobacteriaceae*, *Bacteroides*, *Faecalibacterium*, *Roseburia*, *Blautia*	Most of the findings were seen in the biopsy specimens; not stool *Enterobacteriaceae* predicted poor response to therapy, while *Fusobacterium* and *Haemophilus* predicted good response to therapy

(continued)

Table 19.2 (continued)

Study	Subjects (n)	Prior abx	Site	Age (years)	Tx	Increased organisms/functions	Decreased organisms/functions	Comments
Kolho et al. [80]	CD (36), UC (26), HC (8), JIA (18)	OK	Fecal	9–18	Yes	*B. fragilis* (CD), *Sutterella wadsworthia* (UC), organisms related to *C. difficile*	*F. prausnitzii* (CD)	Some bacteria predicted response to TNFi, particularly *C. sphenoides* and *Haemophilus* species
								Partial normalization seen among responder to TNFi, compared to non-responders
Lavelle et al. [118]	UC (5), HC (4)	3 months	Cecum, TV colon, DC, rectum	21–58	Yes	*Clostridiaceae*, *Peptostreptococcaceae*, *Enterobacteriaceae*, *Ruminococcaceae*, *Bifidobacteriaceae*, *Actinomycetaceae*	*Bacteroidaceae*, *Akkermansia*	Only the controls underwent bowel preparation
								Within the colon, there was more variability among pts and then within sites, so the authors concluded that stool sampling likely captures a patient's microbiota
Perez-Brocal et al. [60]	CD (20), HC (20)	OK	Feces	14–72	Yes	*Actinomyces*, *P. acnes*, some *Enterobacteriaceae*, *Fusobacterium*	*Roseburia*, *F. prausnitzii*, *Ruminococcus bromii*	Lower AD
Quince et al. [61]	CD (23), HC (21)	3 months	Feces	6–15	Yes	*Peptostreptococcus*, *Escheriia/Shigella*, *Atopobium*, *E. faecalis*	*Faecalibacterium*, *Bifidobacterium adolescentis*, *Ruminococcus bromii*	Lower AD in CD. EEN further lowered AD and dropped abundance of organisms already depleted in CD, such as *F. prausnitzii*
Reshef et al. [164]	UC (131), FAP (9)	1 month	Feces	45 (UC), 57 (FAP)	Yes	Minimal differences	Minimal differences	Study compared fecal microbiota in UC versus FAP patients with a pouch
								No differences in AD

Study	Subjects (n)	Prior abx	Site	Age (years)	Tx	Increased organisms/ functions	Decreased organisms/functions	Comments
Wang et al. [128]	IBD (10), HC (5)	OK	Colon	IBD 10–80. No info on the 5 HC	Yes	*Bradyrhizobiaceae*, *Enterobacteriaceae*, *Comamonadaceae*, *Moraxellaceae*		UC and CD samples were pooled for the analysis
Assa et al. [83]	CD (10), HC (15)	3 months	TI	11–16	None	*F. prausnitzii*	None	No differences in AD
Dunn et al. [62]	CD (10), HC (5)	OK	Fecal	9–16		*Bacteroidetes*, *Proteobacteria*	*Firmicutes*	Decreased AD Multiple organisms were predictive of therapeutic response to EEN
Forbes et al. [165]	CD (15), UC (21), HC (7)	OK	Multiple biopsy sites	Probably adults	N/A	*Firmicutes*, *Proteobacteria* (UC)	*Bacteroidetes* (UC)	Increased AD in IBD
Hasler et al. [166]	CD (19), UC (17), HC (27)	OK	TI, sigmoid	18–72	Yes	N/A	N/A	No differences in AD
Hedin et al. [63]	Inactive CD (21), HC (46)	N/A	Rectal	16–35	Yes		*F. prausnitzii*	Decreased AD in CD
Hoarau et al. [64]	CD (20), HC (49)	OK	Fecal	Children and adults	Yes	*E. coli*, *Serratia marcescens*, *Ruminococcus gnavus*	*F. prausnitzii*	Decreased AD in CD
Liguori et al. [65]	CD (23), HC (10)	2 months	Colon	Mean 38–48	Yes	*Enterococcus*, *Alicyclobacillus*, *Lactobacillus*	*Faecalibacterium*, *Blautia*, *Dorea*, *Coprococcus*, *Roseburia*, *Parabacteroides*	Decreased AD in CD
Mar et al. [66]	UC (30), HC (13)	OK	Fecal	22–76	Yes	*Streptococcus*, *Bifidobacterium*, *Enterococcus*	*Bacteroides*, *Prevotella*, *Lachnospiraceae*, *Ruminococcaceae*	Decreased AD in UC
Naftali et al. [81]	CD (31), HC (5)	1 month	Colon, TI	40 (mean)	Yes		*Faecalibacterium*	
Shaw et al. [67]	CD (15), UC (4), HC (10)	OK	Fecal	≤17	No	Positive dysbiosis index in both UC, CD[a]		Decreased AD (both CD, UC)

(continued)

Table 19.2 (continued)

Study	Subjects (n)	Prior abx	Site	Age (years)	Tx	Increased organisms/ functions	Decreased organisms/functions	Comments
Shah et al. [90]	UC (10), HC (13)	N/A	DC, sigmoid	UC: 5–17, HC 11–16	No	*Haemophilus*	*Verrucomicrobia*, *Roseburia*	No differences in AD
Sokol et al. [68]	CD (149), UC (86), HC (38)	2 months	Fecal	40 (mean)	Yes	*Streptococcus anginosus* (IBD as a whole)	*Ruminococcus*, *Coprococcus*, *Blautia*, *Eubacterium Dorea* (IBD as a whole)	Decreased AD (UC, CD)
Takahashi et al. [102]	CD (10), HC (10)	OK	Fecal	Adults	Yes	*Actinomyces*, *Bifidobacterium*	*Bacteroides*, *Eubacterium*, *Faecalibacterium*, *Ruminococcus*	
Tyler et al. [167]	UC (184), FAP (≥30)	OK	TI, sigmoid, pouch	Mean 45	Off at time of surgery	No differences after controlling for antibiotic exposure	No differences after controlling for antibiotic exposure	Study compared fecal microbiota in UC versus FAP patients with a pouch 1 year post-IPAA
He et al. [82]	CD 49, HC 54	OK	Fecal	CD mean 29, HC mean 21	Not stated	*Clostridium symbiosum*, *E. coli*, *Klebsiella pneumoniae*, *Streptococcus salivarius*, and *Clostridium bolteae*	*Bifidobacterium* species, *F. prausnitzii*, *Alistipes shahii*, and *Roseburia* species	Decreased AD
Ijaz et al. [69]	CD 19, HC 31	2 months	Fecal	CD: 10–13. Ctrl: 36–50	Yes	*Enterobacteriaceae*, *Pasteurellaceae*, *Veillonella*, *Dorea*, *Anaerostipes*, *Clostridium* XVIII, *Clostridium* XIVa	*Ruminococcaceae*, *Lachnospiraceae*, *Parabacteroides*, *Akkermansia*, *Methanobrevibacter*	Lower AD in CD Lower genetic functional capacity in CD No differences in fecal SCFA
Knoll et al. [70]	CD (6), UC (6), HC (12)	2 months	Fecal	8–20	Yes	*E. coli* (CD, UC), *Ruminococcus* (CD, UC)	*E. rectale* (UC) and *F. prausnitzii* (UC)	Lower AD in IBD Similar trends were observed in both disease groups, with the findings more pronounced in UC patients
Pascal et al. [71]	IBD in remission: CD (34), UC (33), HC (111)	4 weeks	Fecal	18–58	Yes	*Streptococcus* (UC), *Collinsella* (CD,UC), *Dialister* (CD), *Sutterella* (CD)	*Sutterella* (UC), *Anaerostipes* (CD), *Methanobrevibacter* (CD), Coriobacteriaceae (CD), *Erysipelotrichaceae* (CD), *Peptostreptococcaceae* (CD), *Faecalibacterium* (CD)	Lower AD in CD

Fungal populations								
Kellermayer et al. [88]	CD (15), HC (26)	6 months	TV colon	7–17 (CD), 3–17 (HC)	None	*Malassezia* was associated with granulomatous CD		
Chehoud et al. [135]	CD (26), UC (6), HC (90)	2 weeks	Fecal	IBD: 3–21; controls were pediatric and adult	Yes	*Candida*	*Cladosporium cladosporioides*	IBD patients (CD, UC) were analyzed together Decreased AD
Mukhopadhya et al. [168]	IBD (25), HC (14)	3 months	Sigmoid/rectum	Mostly children, although some adults	None	*Basidiomycota*	*Ascomycota*	
Hoarau et al. [64]	CD (20), HC (49)	OK	Fecal	Children and adults	Yes	*Candida*		Increased AD in CD
Liguori et al. [65]	CD (23), HC (10)	2 months	Colon	Mean 38–48	Yes	*Saccharomycetes*, *Exobasidiomycetes*, *Sordariomycetes*, *Cystofilobasidiaceae* *Dioszegia*, *Candida glabrata*	*Leptosphaeria* and *Trichosporon*	No differences in AD
Mar et al. [66]	UC (30), HC (13)	OK	Fecal	22–76	Yes	*C. albicans*, *Debaryomyces*	*Alternaria*, *Aspergillus flavus*, *Aspergillus*, *Cibarius*, *Candida sojae*	
Sokol et al. [68]	CD (149), UC (86), HC (38)	2 months	Fecal	40 (mean)	Yes	*Basidiomycota* (IBD)	*Ascomycota*	
El Mouzan et al. [169]	CD (15), HC (20)	6 months, except for one patient with CD	Fecal and biopsy	4–18	N/A	Biopsy: *Psathyrellaceae*, *Cortinariaceae*, *Psathyrella*, *Gymnopilus*. Fecal: *Cortinariaceae*, *Hymenochaete*, and *Gymnopilus*	Fecal: *Monilinia*	No differences in AD

(continued)

Table 19.2 (continued)

Study	Subjects (n)	Prior abx	Site	Age (years)	Tx	Increased organisms/functions	Decreased organisms/functions	Comments
Metagenome								
Erickson et al. [74]	Inactive or mild CD (8), HC (4)	1 year	Fecal	Approx. 50	N/A	Replication, recombination, and repair	COH transport and metabolism, energy production and conversion, amino acid transport and metabolism, transcription, intracellular trafficking, defense mechanisms, butyrate production	Six of eight had prior major bowel surgery Decreased functional richness in CD
Greenblum et al. [170]	IBD in remission (25), HC (99)	N/A	Fecal	Adults	N/A	Enzyme transport, phosphotransferase		
Dunn et al. [100]	CD (15), HC (5)	OK	Fecal	9–16	Yes	Butanoate, fatty acid metabolism, glyoxylate metabolism, nitrotoluene degradation	NOD-like receptor signaling, polycyclic aromatic hydrocarbon degradation, sphingolipid metabolism	Patients who went into remission following EEN were more similar at baseline to the controls, as compared to patients who did not go into remission
He et al. [82]	CD 49, HC 54	OK	Fecal	CD mean 29, HC mean 21	Not stated	Xenobiotic degradation	SCFA production, carbohydrate metabolism	

AD alpha diversity, *CD* Crohn disease, *DC* descending colon, *DMARD* disease-modifying antirheumatic drugs, *EEN* exclusive enteral nutrition, *FAP* familial adenomatous polyposis, *HC* healthy control, *IBD* inflammatory bowel disease, *IC* indeterminate colitis, *IPAA* ileal pouch-anal anastomosis, *N/A* not available, *PICRUsT* Phylogenetic Investigation of Communities by Reconstruction of Unobserved States, *SCFA* short-chain fatty acids, *TI* terminal ileum, *TV* transverse, *UC* ulcerative colitis

[a]Dysbiosis index in the Shaw study was based upon the Gevers 2014 study: the increased in CD taxa comprise *Enterobacteriaceae*, *Pasteurellaceae*, *Fusobacteriaceae*, *Neisseriaceae*, *Veillonellaceae*, and *Gemellaceae*. Decreased-in-CD taxa are *Bacteroidales*, *Clostridiales* (excluding *Veillonellaceae*), *Erysipelotrichaceae*, and *Bifidobacteriaceae*

the overall quantity of bacteria is also reduced in IBD. In patients with IBD, the fecal metagenome has been shown to possess up to 25% fewer microbial genes, suggesting a lower functional diversity [74]. Metagenomic changes include a loss of genes encoding amino acid and carbohydrate metabolism in IBD compared to healthy controls, while genes involved in transport, secretion, and virulence factors were increased [23]. This raises the possibility that the key factor in IBD is a loss of metabolic pathways, rather than differences in actual taxonomic abundances [23]. Indeed, diminished diversity of fecal metabolomics has also been observed in IBD [75]. A feature of a healthy, diverse microbiome is a high degree of functional redundancy [76]. It is conceivable that a loss of functional redundancy could render the microbiome less able to adapt to adverse perturbations and/or allow potentially pathogenic bacteria to take over previously occupied niches. The concept of protection through niche occupation has been demonstrated in mouse studies in which disruption of the microbiota using oral antibiotics enabled the expansion of pathogenic *Salmonella enterica* serovar *Typhimurium* and *Clostridium difficile*, which are able to utilize host-derived sugars that were previously monopolized by commensal bacteria [38]. In line with this experimental result, infection with opportunistic pathogens such as *C. difficile* is a significant cause of morbidity in IBD patients [77], indicating that they may present an unoccupied niche in their intestinal environment. The *Enterobacteriaceae*, members of the Proteobacteria phylum, have a remarkably diverse pan-genome, and, therefore, they may be well placed to take advantage of any newly vacated niches [76].

Faecalibacterium prausnitzii (Depleted in CD)

Of the 38 studies in CD that included assessments of the bacterial populations, 15 of them reported depletion of *F. prausnitzii* [57–61, 63–65, 70, 71, 78–82], with only two showing the opposite result [56, 83]. This has been observed in both fecal and biopsy specimens, in recent-onset and long-standing disease. Abundance of *F. prausnitzii* also appears to be higher in CD patients in remission versus those with active disease [84], and low abundance of *F. prausnitzii* is predictive of future flares among CD patients undergoing surgical resection [85]. This depletion of *F. prausnitzii* is thus among the most consistent findings of any bacterial species in any disease state. *F. prausnitzii* may have direct regulatory properties; when added to cultures of human peripheral blood mononuclear cells, it upregulated the generation of Tregs and interleukin (IL)-10 [34, 86, 87].

Another mechanism by which *F. prausnitzii* may protect against gut inflammation is through generation of SCFA, including but not limited to butyrate. Indeed, another five studies that did not report depletion of *F. prausnitzii* in IBD patients did identify depletion of other butyrate-producing organisms, such as *Roseburia* and *Blautia* [23, 68, 88–90]. Notably, some of these organisms were also depleted in UC [23, 89, 90]. As reviewed [91], the generation of SCFAs occurs through the metabolism of so-called nondigestible carbohydrates. Branched-chain carbohydrates, which constitute nondigestible fiber, can in fact be metabolized by certain bacteria, constituting their energy source. The breakdown product is the SCFA, which act as proton sinks for the regeneration of NAD+ from NADH during glycolysis [92]. Because bacteria lack mitochondria, they are largely unable to metabolize SCFA any further, thus leaving them to the human host. However, it is important to note that while certain SCFAs may be the metabolic endpoint for some bacteria, SCFAs can act as a substrate for others. For example, acetate and lactate produced by lactic acid bacteria, such as *Bifidobacterium* and *Lactobacillus* spp., can be used as a carbon and energy source by bacteria such as *Eubacterium rectale*, *Roseburia faecis*, and *Faecalibacterium prausnitzii*, which in turn produce butyrate as their metabolic by-product [93–95]. Beneficial properties of SCFAs include inhibition of enteropathogens, increased intestinal epithelial cell health, increased mucin production, and induction of regulatory T cells [96, 97]. It is thus not surprising that fecal metabolomics studies have also shown diminished production of SCFAs in patients compared to controls [98, 99]. Additionally, two studies looking at the IBD metagenome showed decreased genetic potential for butyrate or other SCFA production [74, 82], although another study reported the reverse [100].

Bacteroides (Depleted in CD, UC)

Several studies have demonstrated that the *Bacteroides* genus is depleted in both CD and UC [66, 79, 89, 101, 102]. This conclusion was also reached by a review article that, despite being published in 2016, was limited to studies using older technologies such as culture and restriction-length fragment polymorphism and thus has no overlapping studies with the present chapter [103]. A limitation of some of the widely used sequencing technologies is the inability to identify organisms at the species level. However, it is plausible that the depleted organism is *B. fragilis*. This organism prevents intestinal inflammation in mouse models of colitis, mostly through its component polysaccharide A (PSA) [104]. PSA has been reported to induce Foxp3+ Tregs that suppress Th17-mediated intestinal inflammation [105, 106]. In humans, PSA also enhances in vitro Treg induction [107]. A beneficial effect of *Bacteroides* may not be limited to IBD; diminished fecal abundance of *Bacteroides* has also been observed in rheumatoid arthritis [108, 109] and spondyloarthritis (SpA) [110].

A protective effect of *Bacteroides* may be limited to adults. While virtually all studies in adults with IBD that reported differential abundance of *Bacteroides* found it to be protective ([103] and Table 19.2), the pediatrics data are mixed. Of the two studies in pediatric CD that reported differential abundance, one found it to be depleted [79], and the other elevated [80]. Consistent with this observation is that a study that was limited to specific bacteria, including *Bacteroides*, reported decreased abundance in older as compared to younger subjects with CD [111]. Interestingly, studies in juvenile idiopathic arthritis have also shown elevated abundance of fecal *Bacteroides* [112–114], and an increase in *B. ovatus* may precede the onset of type I diabetes in high-risk children [115]. The implications of these findings are not clear. However, an explanation may have been provided by Vatanen et al., who compared the ability of *B. dorei* and *Escherichia coli* to induce endotoxin tolerance, which refers to diminished immunologic response to endotoxin following initial exposure. The authors showed that *B. dorei* had diminished ability to induce endotoxin tolerance, and showed as well that injection of this organism, as compared to injection of *E. coli*, failed to delay the onset of diabetes in a mouse model of the disease [116]. Thus, *Bacteroides* in children may be a two-edged sword, both providing benefit through the PSA tail of *B. fragilis* but also providing increased risk of autoimmunity through altered immunologic maturation.

Akkermansia muciniphila (Depleted in CD, UC)

The third and final organism consistently depleted in IBD is *A. muciniphila*, which was found to be depleted in four studies [69, 72, 117, 118]. This organism was isolated in 2004 and given its name based upon its ability to thrive on intestinal mucins [119]. Most of the literature on this organism focuses on a potentially beneficial role in obesity and metabolic syndrome (e.g., [120]); there is very little literature on its role in inflammatory disease. Asquith et al. demonstrated that in the HLA-B27+ rat model of SpA and IBD, *A. muciniphila* emerges at onset of clinical disease [121], and Stoll et al. reported increased abundance of *A. muciniphila* in a subset of pediatric SpA patients [112]. As patients with SpA and IBD have altered intestinal permeability [122, 123], it is possible that by increasing intestinal permeability, *A. muciniphila* results in increased bacterial invasiveness, which in turn promotes intestinal inflammation. These authors speculate that the decreased abundance of *A. muciniphila* in patients with IBD may be an epiphenomenon reflecting loss of substrate, as previously suggested [90]. That is, as the inflammatory process progresses, the mucin content is lost as has been reported [124], resulting in depletion of *A. muciniphila*.

Other mucus-associated bacteria that may have a role in IBD are sulfate-reducing bacteria such as *Desulfovibrio piger* [125]. Sulfate-reducing bacteria compete with acetogens and methanogens for hydrogen to produce energy by reducing sulfated mucus glycans, leaving H_2S as a by-product [126]. H_2S has genotoxic properties and can disrupt the mucus structure, as sulfides are potent reducers of disulfide bonds [127].

Enterobacteriaceae, Especially *E. coli/Shigella* (Increased in CD, UC)

Thirteen studies have reported increased abundance of the *Enterobacteriaceae* family or specifically of *E. coli/Shigella* (which often cannot be distinguished by 16S sequencing), in patients with CD or UC [23, 55, 58, 60, 61, 64, 69, 70, 79, 82, 117, 118, 128]; none have revealed depletion of this organism. The increased *Enterobacteriaceae* abundance may stem from their capacity to use sialic acid and fucose liberated from mucus [38]. Among this family, adherent-invasive *E. coli* (AIEC) has gained particular interest [118]. Pathogenic bacteria such as AIEC may have virulence factors allowing them to interact with M cells, specialized epithelial cells on the surface of Peyer's patches. AIEC could use this interaction to translocate across the epithelial cell barrier into the mucosa [129]. In support of the hypothesis that AIEC contributes to disease by translocating through the intestinal wall barrier, Knoll et al. reported that abundance of *E. coli* correlated with genes implicated in bacterial adhesion to the intestinal mucosa [70]. Additionally, AIEC contains virulence factors such as α-hemolysins that can contribute to impairment of the intestinal wall barrier function, in essence by punching holes in the wall [130]; colonization of colitis-prone IL-10 deficient mice with *E. coli* containing α-hemolysin induced active disease, significantly less so if the bacteria lacked this virulence factor [130]. As reviewed [118], other mechanisms by which AIEC has been linked to IBD include impairment of autophagy as well as of the ubiquitin proteasome activity, the latter resulting in increased activation of NF-κB. Importantly, it has also been proposed that the inflammatory process itself promotes the growth of *Enterobacteriaceae* and thus that the increased abundance of this family may be the consequence not the cause of the underlying disease process [131].

Bifidobacteriaceae (Increased in CD, UC)

Four studies reported increased abundance of the *Bifidobacteriaceae* family in IBD [66, 78, 102, 118], with two reporting it to be depleted [79, 82]. This finding of increased abundance of the *Bifidobacteriaceae* family in IBD, particularly in UC, appears to be a counterintuitive finding, as several species of *Bifidobacterium* are widely incorporated into probiotics, including VSL # 3, which is widely used as therapy for UC (see treatment, below). Indeed, the possibility that these findings reflected prior use of probiotics cannot be entirely excluded. However, in some model systems, *Bifidobacterium* can demonstrate proinflammatory effects in vitro, with variation at the species or even the strain level. Specifically, He et al. noted variations among *Bifidobacteria* species to induce IL-12 and tumor necrosis factor (TNF) production from a cell line [132], while Medina et al. demonstrated differences among strains within the *Bifidobacterium longum* species in their ability to induce production of TNF by human peripheral blood mononuclear cells [133]. Conversely, a protective role for *Bifidobacterium longum* in murine colitis has been demonstrated [134]. In light of this contradictory information, there are insufficient data upon which to draw firm conclusions regarding the role of the *Bifidobacteriaceae* family in IBD.

Candida (Increased in CD, UC)

As shown in Table 19.2, most of the studies focused on bacteria. However, just as bacteria can be amplified through sequencing of the 16S ribosomal DNA, so can fungi through their counterpart, the 18S ribosomal DNA. Of the eight studies that evaluated the fungome in patients with IBD, only one consistent result has been reported: increased abundance of *Candida* in patients with CD and to a lesser extent UC; this has been reported in four studies [64–66, 135]. In addition to demonstrating increased fecal abundance of *Candida*, Hoarau et al., also reported an association between abundance of *C. tropicalis* and presence of anti-*Saccharomyces cerevisiae* antibodies (ASCA), which they stated could be triggered by *Candida* as well as by *Saccharomyces cerevisiae*. Despite this finding, the role of fungal organisms in the pathogenesis of IBD is yet unknown. It is possible that they reflect fungal overgrowth secondary to antibiotics, although findings that ASCA appear prior to development of symptoms suggest that the fungal dysbiosis may be upstream of clinical disease [136]. In addition, mice deficient in dectin-1, a pattern recognition receptor specific for fungi, developed a more severe form of chemical colitis, and polymorphisms in the dectin-1 gene were likewise associated with increased severity of UC in humans [137], suggesting an important role for fungi in the pathogenesis of IBD.

In summary, numerous studies have identified abnormalities in the contents of the human intestinal microbiota in patients with IBD. That the same microbiota are consistently identified as being present in abnormal quantities, either high or low, and are often observed at disease onset, gives credence to the possibility that some of these abnormalities may contribute to the pathogenesis of the disease. Even within the disease, the extent of the microbiota-based abnormalities often correlates with disease severity [84] and can be used to predict response to therapy [85], underscoring a potential pathogenic role. The potential for microbiota-based therapy will be discussed below.

Therapeutic Manipulation of the Microbiota

In practice, there are four ways that the microbiota can be therapeutically altered: diet, antibiotics, probiotics, and fecal microbial transplant. Each of those modalities has been reviewed in depth elsewhere [138–141] and will be summarized briefly below and in Table 19.3.

Table 19.3 Microbial interventions in IBD

	Crohn disease		Ulcerative colitis	
Intervention	Pediatric	Adult	Pediatric	Adult
Antibiotics	+	+	+/−	+/−
Probiotics, e.g., VSL # 3	−	−	+	+
EEN	+	+/−	−	−
FMT	+	+	+	+

Adapted from [153]

Diet

One dietary intervention that has a clearly established place in the treatment of IBD is exclusive enteral nutrition (EEN), which consists of a complete replacement of typical solid foods with liquid nutritional supplements for a period of 4–12 weeks, either orally or via nasogastric tube [142]. EEN appears to be more effective in CD as compared to UC and possibly more effective in children than adults [143]. In children with CD, EEN is as effective as are corticosteroids at inducing remission [144], is thus standard of care for induction therapy in Europe [145], and is increasingly being offered or recommended to patients in the United States in lieu of corticosteroids. The mechanism by which EEN is effective is unclear. While it has striking effects on the microbiota, the net effect is seemingly to make the microbiota even more dysbiotic than its baseline state, with lower alpha diversity and even lower abundance of *F. prausnitzii* [146].

Other dietary approaches have been considered, although most were not necessarily designed with a specific intent of altering the microbiota, so will not be discussed herein. One exception is a diet high in nonabsorbable carbohydrates, such as fructo-oligosaccharides. The rationale behind such a diet is that it may result in increased abundance of butyrate-producing organisms, such as *F. prausnitzii*, which are capable of digesting fiber. In practice, however, studies have not supported this approach [147].

Antibiotics

Antibiotics are a double-edged sword in IBD. Epidemiologic data indicate that early-childhood exposure to antibiotics is associated with an increased risk of acquiring the disease [148], and antibiotics are a risk factor for development of *Clostridium difficile* infection, an important cause of morbidity in patients with IBD [149]. However, there is also an important role for antibiotics as induction and maintenance therapy, particularly in CD, where several studies have demonstrated an important role as induction therapy as well as postoperative management [150]. They are also used to treat pouchitis, which consists of an inflammatory process of the ileal pouch that occurs with colectomy followed by ileal pouch-anal anastomosis [150]. In UC, antibiotics are less effective, although they may have benefit as add-on therapy to standard treatments [151]. In addition to their therapeutic role, antibiotics are often required to treat infectious complications, including but not limited to abscess development in CD and *C. difficile* infections.

Probiotics

Probiotics are defined as live organisms that are administered in order to have a therapeutic effect on a disease state. In addition to altering the contents of the microbiota, they are postulated to have beneficial effects on gut barrier wall function, immunity, and production of antimicrobial metabolites, among others [152, 153]. A widely used probiotic in patients with UC is VSL # 3, which is a mixture of eight bacterial strains including four species within the *Lactobacillus* genus, three within the *Bifidobacterium* genus, and *Streptococcus thermophilus*. As reviewed [152], randomized and open-label studies in both children and adults with UC have generally found that addition of VSL # 3 to standard treatment reduces disease activity. These findings are not generalizable to all probiotics, as the same review reported that *E. coli Nissle* 1917 was generally ineffective [152]. In addition, while probiotics may be beneficial in the management of pouchitis, they are not otherwise considered to be beneficial in the treatment of CD [153]. While generally considered safe, serious infectious events associated with probiotic strains have been reported [154].

Fecal Microbial Transplantation (FMT)

Although it has been reported that the idea behind FMT dates to nearly two millennia ago [155], this is a relatively recent development in IBD. The initial purpose behind FMT was as a therapeutic alternative to subjects with recurrent *C. difficile* infections [156], although improvements were subsequently noted in the underlying bowel disease of subjects who had both IBD and *C. difficile* [157]. Thus, subsequent studies were geared toward using FMT as a therapy for IBD itself. After some positive case reports [158, 159], randomized trials were conducted, with mixed results [160]. However, studies that used multiple donors and also that involved pretreatment with antibiotics, presumably to clear out the existing microbiota to allow the normal microbiota to take root, appeared to have shown particular benefit [141, 160]. In the United States, the Food and Drug Administration has deemed FMT to be experimental for any purpose other than treatment of recurrent *C. difficile* infection, so this procedure is only available in the context of a clinical trial. Multiple parameters, including whether the transplants should consist of donor samples or defined consortium of microbiota, and whether they should be administered via upper (e.g., by gavage) or lower (endoscopy) delivery, have yet to be definitively established. In addition, as with probiotic therapy, this treatment carries with it a rare but non-zero risk of serious infections caused by the introduced bacteria [161]. Thus, the precise role of FMT in the management of CD and UC has yet to be fully defined.

Conclusions

In this chapter, we have presented compelling evidence that the microbiota is altered in patients with IBD, particularly CD. It is likely that at least some of these changes, such as increased abundance of pathogenic bacteria including adherent-invasive *E. coli* and depletion of butyrate-producing organisms such as *F. prausnitzii*, contribute to the disease. The microbiota has a profound impact on intestinal immune responses, which drive intestinal inflammation. In turn, the immune system can impact the microbiota and cause dysbiosis. This resulting dysbiosis could lead to exacerbation of inflammation in IBD. Therapeutic manipulation of the microbiota through EEN, antibiotics, and probiotics is a routine part of clinical care for both CD and UC. We hope that the future holds in store more targeted means of altering the microbiota that can safely and effectively restore a more normal state.

References

1. Kappelman MD, Rifas-Shiman SL, Kleinman K, Ollendorf D, Bousvaros A, Grand RJ, et al. The prevalence and geographic distribution of Crohn's disease and ulcerative colitis in the United States. Clin Gastroenterol Hepatol. 2007;5(12):1424–9.
2. de Mesquita MB, Civitelli F, Levine A. Epidemiology, genes and inflammatory bowel diseases in childhood. Dig Liver Dis. 2008;40(1):3–11.
3. Seneca H, Henderson E. Normal intestinal bacteria in ulcerative colitis. Gastroenterology. 1950;15(1 1):34–9.
4. Thorburn AN, Macia L, Mackay CR. Diet, metabolites, and "western-lifestyle" inflammatory diseases. Immunity. 2014;40(6):833–42.
5. Jostins L, Ripke S, Weersma RK, Duerr RH, McGovern DP, Hui KY, et al. Host-microbe interactions have shaped the genetic architecture of inflammatory bowel disease. Nature. 2012;491(7422):119–24.
6. Ubeda C, Lipuma L, Gobourne A, Viale A, Leiner I, Equinda M, et al. Familial transmission rather than defective innate immunity shapes the distinct intestinal microbiota of TLR-deficient mice. J Exp Med. 2012;209(8):1445–56.
7. Kawamoto S, Maruya M, Kato LM, Suda W, Atarashi K, Doi Y, et al. Foxp3(+) T cells regulate immunoglobulin a selection and facilitate diversification of bacterial species responsible for immune homeostasis. Immunity. 2014;41(1):152–65.
8. Kawamoto S, Tran TH, Maruya M, Suzuki K, Doi Y, Tsutsui Y, et al. The inhibitory receptor PD-1 regulates IgA selection and bacterial composition in the gut. Science. 2012;336(6080):485–9.
9. Rankin LC, Girard-Madoux MJ, Seillet C, Mielke LA, Kerdiles Y, Fenis A, et al. Complementarity and redundancy of IL-22-producing innate lymphoid cells. Nat Immunol. 2016;17(2):179–86.
10. Thaiss CA, Zmora N, Levy M, Elinav E. The microbiome and innate immunity. Nature. 2016;535(7610):65–74.
11. Vaishnava S, Yamamoto M, Severson KM, Ruhn KA, Yu X, Koren O, et al. The antibacterial lectin RegIIIgamma promotes the spatial segregation of microbiota and host in the intestine. Science. 2011;334(6053):255–8.
12. Nakahashi-Oda C, Udayanga KG, Nakamura Y, Nakazawa Y, Totsuka N, Miki H, et al. Apoptotic epithelial cells control the abundance of Treg cells at barrier surfaces. Nat Immunol. 2016;17(4):441–50.
13. Ahern PP, Izcue A, Maloy KJ, Powrie F. The interleukin-23 axis in intestinal inflammation. Immunol Rev. 2008;226:147–59.
14. Abraham C, Cho JH. IL-23 and autoimmunity: new insights into the pathogenesis of inflammatory bowel disease. Annu Rev Med. 2009;60:97–110.
15. Mukherjee S, Hooper LV. Antimicrobial defense of the intestine. Immunity. 2015;42(1):28–39.
16. Goodlad RA, Ratcliffe B, Fordham JP, Wright NA. Does dietary fibre stimulate intestinal epithelial cell proliferation in germ free rats? Gut. 1989;30(6):820–5.
17. Fukata M, Michelsen KS, Eri R, Thomas LS, Hu B, Lukasek K, et al. Toll-like receptor-4 is required for intestinal response to epithelial injury and limiting bacterial translocation in a murine model of acute colitis. Am J Physiol Gastrointest Liver Physiol. 2005;288(5):G1055–65.
18. Rakoff-Nahoum S, Paglino J, Eslami-Varzaneh F, Edberg S, Medzhitov R. Recognition of commensal microflora by toll-like receptors is required for intestinal homeostasis. Cell. 2004;118(2):229–41.
19. Silva MA, Jury J, Porras M, Vergara P, Perdue MH. Intestinal epithelial barrier dysfunction and dendritic cell redistribution during early stages of inflammation in the rat: role for TLR-2 and -4 blockage. Inflamm Bowel Dis. 2008;14(5):632–44.
20. Maslowski KM, Vieira AT, Ng A, Kranich J, Sierro F, Yu D, et al. Regulation of inflammatory responses by gut microbiota and chemoattractant receptor GPR43. Nature. 2009;461(7268):1282–6.
21. Hernández-Chirlaque C, Aranda CJ, Ocón B, Capitán-Cañadas F, Ortega-González M, Carrero JJ, et al. Germ-free and antibiotic-treated mice are highly susceptible to epithelial injury in DSS colitis. J Crohn's Colitis. 2016;10(11):1324–35.
22. Couturier-Maillard A, Secher T, Rehman A, Normand S, De Arcangelis A, Haesler R, et al. NOD2-mediated dysbiosis predisposes mice to transmissible colitis and colorectal cancer. J Clin Investig. 2013;123(2):700–11.
23. Morgan XC, Tickle TL, Sokol H, Gevers D, Devaney KL, Ward DV, et al. Dysfunction of the intestinal microbiome in inflammatory bowel disease and treatment. Genome Biol. 2012;13(9):R79.
24. Kelly D, Campbell JI, King TP, Grant G, Jansson EA, Coutts AG, et al. Commensal anaerobic gut bacteria attenuate inflammation by regulating nuclear-cytoplasmic shuttling of PPAR-gamma and RelA. Nat Immunol. 2004;5(1):104–12.
25. Hoffmann TW, Pham H-P, Bridonneau C, Aubry C, Lamas B, Martin-Gallausiaux C, et al. Microorganisms linked to inflammatory bowel disease-associated dysbiosis differentially impact host physiology in gnotobiotic mice. ISME J. 2016;10(2):460–77.
26. Gaboriau-Routhiau V, Rakotobe S, Lecuyer E, Mulder I, Lan A, Bridonneau C, et al. The key role of segmented filamentous bacteria in the coordinated

maturation of gut helper T cell responses. Immunity. 2009;31(4):677–89.
27. Lecuyer E, Rakotobe S, Lengline-Garnier H, Lebreton C, Picard M, Juste C, et al. Segmented filamentous bacterium uses secondary and tertiary lymphoid tissues to induce gut IgA and specific T helper 17 cell responses. Immunity. 2014;40(4):608–20.
28. Atarashi K, Tanoue T, Ando M, Kamada N, Nagano Y, Narushima S, et al. Th17 cell induction by adhesion of microbes to intestinal epithelial cells. Cell. 2015;163(2):367–80.
29. Jonsson H. Segmented filamentous bacteria in human ileostomy samples after high-fiber intake. FEMS Microbiol Lett. 2013;342(1):24–9.
30. Lodes MJ, Cong Y, Elson CO, Mohamath R, Landers CJ, Targan SR, et al. Bacterial flagellin is a dominant antigen in Crohn disease. J Clin Investig. 2004;113(9):1296–306.
31. Targan SR, Landers CJ, Yang H, Lodes MJ, Cong Y, Papadakis KA, et al. Antibodies to CBir1 flagellin define a unique response that is associated independently with complicated Crohn's disease. Gastroenterology. 2005;128(7):2020–8.
32. Hegazy AN, West NR, Stubbington MJT, Wendt E, Suijker KIM, Datsi A, et al. Circulating and tissue-resident CD4(+) T cells with reactivity to intestinal Microbiota are abundant in healthy individuals and function is altered during inflammation. Gastroenterology. 2017;153(5):1320–37.e16.
33. Feng T, Qin H, Wang L, Benveniste EN, Elson CO, Cong Y. Th17 cells induce colitis and promote Th1 cell responses through IL-17 induction of innate IL-12 and IL-23 production. J Immunol. 2011;186(11):6313–8.
34. Sokol H, Pigneur B, Watterlot L, Lakhdari O, Bermudez-Humaran LG, Gratadoux JJ, et al. Faecalibacterium prausnitzii is an anti-inflammatory commensal bacterium identified by gut microbiota analysis of Crohn disease patients. Proc Natl Acad Sci U S A. 2008;105(43):16731–6.
35. Smelt MJ, de Haan BJ, Bron PA, van Swam I, Meijerink M, Wells JM, et al. The impact of lactobacillus plantarum WCFS1 teichoic acid D-alanylation on the generation of effector and regulatory T-cells in healthy mice. PLoS One. 2013;8(4):e63099.
36. Zakostelska Z, Kverka M, Klimesova K, Rossmann P, Mrazek J, Kopecny J, et al. Lysate of probiotic Lactobacillus casei DN-114 001 ameliorates colitis by strengthening the gut barrier function and changing the gut microenvironment. PLoS One. 2011;6(11):e27961.
37. Shen J, Zuo ZX, Mao AP. Effect of probiotics on inducing remission and maintaining therapy in ulcerative colitis, Crohn's disease, and pouchitis: meta-analysis of randomized controlled trials. Inflamm Bowel Dis. 2014;20(1):21–35.
38. Ng KM, Ferreyra JA, Higginbottom SK, Lynch JB, Kashyap PC, Gopinath S, et al. Microbiota-liberated host sugars facilitate post-antibiotic expansion of enteric pathogens. Nature. 2013;502(7469):96–9.
39. Macia L, Tan J, Vieira AT, Leach K, Stanley D, Luong S, et al. Metabolite-sensing receptors GPR43 and GPR109A facilitate dietary fibre-induced gut homeostasis through regulation of the inflammasome. Nat Commun. 2015;6:6734.
40. Furusawa Y, Obata Y, Fukuda S, Endo TA, Nakato G, Takahashi D, et al. Commensal microbe-derived butyrate induces the differentiation of colonic regulatory T cells. Nature. 2013;504(7480):446–50.
41. Donohoe DR, Collins LB, Wali A, Bigler R, Sun W, Bultman SJ. The Warburg effect dictates the mechanism of butyrate-mediated histone acetylation and cell proliferation. Mol Cell. 2012;48(4):612–26.
42. Arpaia N, Campbell C, Fan X, Dikiy S, van der Veeken J, de Roos P, et al. Metabolites produced by commensal bacteria promote peripheral regulatory T-cell generation. Nature. 2013;504(7480):451–5.
43. Chang PV, Hao L, Offermanns S, Medzhitov R. The microbial metabolite butyrate regulates intestinal macrophage function via histone deacetylase inhibition. Proc Natl Acad Sci U S A. 2014;111(6):2247–52.
44. Singh N, Gurav A, Sivaprakasam S, Brady E, Padia R, Shi H, et al. Activation of Gpr109a, receptor for niacin and the commensal metabolite butyrate, suppresses colonic inflammation and carcinogenesis. Immunity. 2014;40(1):128–39.
45. Sayin SI, Wahlstrom A, Felin J, Jantti S, Marschall HU, Bamberg K, et al. Gut microbiota regulates bile acid metabolism by reducing the levels of tauro-beta-muricholic acid, a naturally occurring FXR antagonist. Cell Metab. 2013;17(2):225–35.
46. Joyce SA, MacSharry J, Casey PG, Kinsella M, Murphy EF, Shanahan F, et al. Regulation of host weight gain and lipid metabolism by bacterial bile acid modification in the gut. Proc Natl Acad Sci U S A. 2014;111(20):7421–6.
47. Vavassori P, Mencarelli A, Renga B, Distrutti E, Fiorucci S. The bile acid receptor FXR is a modulator of intestinal innate immunity. J Immunol. 2009;183(10):6251–61.
48. Schubert K, Olde Damink SWM, von Bergen M, Schaap FG. Interactions between bile salts, gut microbiota, and hepatic innate immunity. Immunol Rev. 2017;279(1):23–35.
49. Gadaleta RM, van Erpecum KJ, Oldenburg B, Willemsen EC, Renooij W, Murzilli S, et al. Farnesoid X receptor activation inhibits inflammation and preserves the intestinal barrier in inflammatory bowel disease. Gut. 2011;60(4):463–72.
50. Zelante T, Iannitti RG, Cunha C, De Luca A, Giovannini G, Pieraccini G, et al. Tryptophan Catabolites from Microbiota engage aryl hydrocarbon receptor and balance mucosal reactivity via Interleukin-22. Immunity. 2013;39(2):372–85.
51. Hashimoto T, Perlot T, Rehman A, Trichereau J, Ishiguro H, Paolino M, et al. ACE2 links amino acid malnutrition to microbial ecology and intestinal inflammation. Nature. 2012;487(7408):477–81.

52. Lanis JM, Alexeev EE, Curtis VF, Kitzenberg DA, Kao DJ, Battista KD, et al. Tryptophan metabolite activation of the aryl hydrocarbon receptor regulates IL-10 receptor expression on intestinal epithelia. Mucosal Immunol. 2017;10(5):1133–44.
53. Lamas B, Richard ML, Leducq V, Pham HP, Michel ML, Da Costa G, et al. CARD9 impacts colitis by altering gut microbiota metabolism of tryptophan into aryl hydrocarbon receptor ligands. Nat Med. 2016;22(6):598–605.
54. Dodd D, Spitzer MH, Van Treuren W, Merrill BD, Hryckowian AJ, Higginbottom SK, et al. A gut bacterial pathway metabolizes aromatic amino acids into nine circulating metabolites. Nature. 2017;551(7682):648–52.
55. Walker AW, Sanderson JD, Churcher C, Parkes GC, Hudspith BN, Rayment N, et al. High-throughput clone library analysis of the mucosa-associated microbiota reveals dysbiosis and differences between inflamed and non-inflamed regions of the intestine in inflammatory bowel disease. BMC Microbiol. 2011;11:7.
56. Hansen R, Russell RK, Reiff C, Louis P, McIntosh F, Berry SH, et al. Microbiota of de-novo pediatric IBD: increased Faecalibacterium prausnitzii and reduced bacterial diversity in Crohn's but not in ulcerative colitis. Am J Gastroenterol. 2012;107(12):1913–22.
57. Prideaux L, Kang S, Wagner J, Buckley M, Mahar JE, De Cruz P, et al. Impact of ethnicity, geography, and disease on the microbiota in health and inflammatory bowel disease. Inflamm Bowel Dis. 2013;19(13):2906–18.
58. Tong M, Li X, Wegener Parfrey L, Roth B, Ippoliti A, Wei B, et al. A modular organization of the human intestinal mucosal microbiota and its association with inflammatory bowel disease. PLoS One. 2013;8(11):e80702.
59. Chen L, Wang W, Zhou R, Ng SC, Li J, Huang M, et al. Characteristics of fecal and mucosa-associated microbiota in Chinese patients with inflammatory bowel disease. Medicine (Baltimore). 2014;93(8):e51.
60. Perez-Brocal V, Garcia-Lopez R, Nos P, Beltran B, Moret I, Moya A. Metagenomic analysis of Crohn's disease patients identifies changes in the Virome and Microbiome related to disease status and therapy, and detects potential interactions and biomarkers. Inflamm Bowel Dis. 2015;21(11):2515–32.
61. Quince C, Ijaz UZ, Loman N, Eren AM, Saulnier D, Russell J, et al. Extensive modulation of the fecal Metagenome in children with Crohn's disease during exclusive enteral nutrition. Am J Gastroenterol. 2015;110(12):1718–29. quiz 30.
62. Dunn KA, Moore-Connors J, MacIntyre B, Stadnyk AW, Thomas NA, Noble A, et al. Early changes in microbial community structure are associated with sustained remission after nutritional treatment of pediatric Crohn's disease. Inflamm Bowel Dis. 2016;22(12):2853–62.
63. Hedin C, van der Gast CJ, Rogers GB, Cuthbertson L, McCartney S, Stagg AJ, et al. Siblings of patients with Crohn's disease exhibit a biologically relevant dysbiosis in mucosal microbial metacommunities. Gut. 2016;65(6):944–53.
64. Hoarau G, Mukherjee PK, Gower-Rousseau C, Hager C, Chandra J, Retuerto MA, et al. Bacteriome and mycobiome interactions underscore microbial dysbiosis in familial Crohn's disease. MBio. 2016;7(5):e01250–16.
65. Liguori G, Lamas B, Richard ML, Brandi G, da Costa G, Hoffmann TW, et al. Fungal dysbiosis in mucosa-associated microbiota of Crohn's disease patients. J Crohns Colitis. 2016;10(3):296–305.
66. Mar JS, LaMere BJ, Lin DL, Levan S, Nazareth M, Mahadevan U, et al. Disease severity and immune activity relate to distinct interkingdom gut microbiome states in ethnically distinct ulcerative colitis patients. MBio. 2016;7(4):e01072–16.
67. Shaw KA, Bertha M, Hofmekler T, Chopra P, Vatanen T, Srivatsa A, et al. Dysbiosis, inflammation, and response to treatment: a longitudinal study of pediatric subjects with newly diagnosed inflammatory bowel disease. Genome Med. 2016;8(1):75.
68. Sokol H, Leducq V, Aschard H, Pham HP, Jegou S, Landman C, et al. Fungal microbiota dysbiosis in IBD. Gut. 2016;66(6):1039–48.
69. Ijaz UZ, Quince C, Hanske L, Loman N, Calus ST, Bertz M, et al. The distinct features of microbial "dysbiosis" of Crohn's disease do not occur to the same extent in their unaffected, genetically-linked kindred. PLoS One. 2017;12(2):e0172605.
70. Knoll RL, Forslund K, Kultima JR, Meyer CU, Kullmer U, Sunagawa S, et al. Gut microbiota differs between children with Inflammatory Bowel Disease and healthy siblings in taxonomic and functional composition—a metagenomic analysis. Am J Physiol Gastrointest Liver Physiol. 2016;312(4):G327–39. ajpgi 00293 2016.
71. Pascal V, Pozuelo M, Borruel N, Casellas F, Campos D, Santiago A, et al. A microbial signature for Crohn's disease. Gut. 2017;66(5):813–22.
72. Michail S, Durbin M, Turner D, Griffiths AM, Mack DR, Hyams J, et al. Alterations in the gut microbiome of children with severe ulcerative colitis. Inflamm Bowel Dis. 2012;18(10):1799–808.
73. Kang S, Denman SE, Morrison M, Yu Z, Dore J, Leclerc M, et al. Dysbiosis of fecal microbiota in Crohn's disease patients as revealed by a custom phylogenetic microarray. Inflamm Bowel Dis. 2010;16(12):2034–42.
74. Erickson AR, Cantarel BL, Lamendella R, Darzi Y, Mongodin EF, Pan C, et al. Integrated metagenomics/metaproteomics reveals human host-microbiota signatures of Crohn's disease. PLoS One. 2012;7(11):e49138.
75. De Preter V, Machiels K, Joossens M, Arijs I, Matthys C, Vermeire S, et al. Faecal metabolite profiling identifies medium-chain fatty acids as discriminating compounds in IBD. Gut. 2015;64(3):447–58.

76. Bradley PH, Pollard KS. Proteobacteria explain significant functional variability in the human gut microbiome. Microbiome. 2017;5(1):36.
77. Nguyen GC, Kaplan GG, Harris ML, Brant SR. A national survey of the prevalence and impact of Clostridium difficile infection among hospitalized inflammatory bowel disease patients. Am J Gastroenterol. 2008;103(6):1443–50.
78. Willing BP, Dicksved J, Halfvarson J, Andersson AF, Lucio M, Zheng Z, et al. A pyrosequencing study in twins shows that gastrointestinal microbial profiles vary with inflammatory bowel disease phenotypes. Gastroenterology. 2010;139(6):1844–54.e1.
79. Gevers D, Kugathasan S, Denson LA, Vazquez-Baeza Y, Van Treuren W, Ren B, et al. The treatment-naive microbiome in new-onset Crohn's disease. Cell Host Microbe. 2014;15(3):382–92.
80. Kolho KL, Korpela K, Jaakkola T, Pichai MV, Zoetendal EG, Salonen A, et al. Fecal microbiota in pediatric inflammatory bowel disease and its relation to inflammation. Am J Gastroenterol. 2015;110(6):921–30.
81. Naftali T, Reshef L, Kovacs A, Porat R, Amir I, Konikoff FM, et al. Distinct microbiotas are associated with ileum-restricted and Colon-involving Crohn's disease. Inflamm Bowel Dis. 2016;22(2):293–302.
82. He Q, Gao Y, Jie Z, Yu X, Laursen JM, Xiao L, et al. Two distinct metacommunities characterize the gut microbiota in Crohn's disease patients. Gigascience. 2017;6(7):1–11.
83. Assa A, Butcher J, Li J, Elkadri A, Sherman PM, Muise AM, et al. Mucosa-associated ileal microbiota in new-onset pediatric Crohn's disease. Inflamm Bowel Dis. 2016;22(7):1533–9.
84. Tedjo DI, Smolinska A, Savelkoul PH, Masclee AA, van Schooten FJ, Pierik MJ, et al. The fecal microbiota as a biomarker for disease activity in Crohn's disease. Sci Rep. 2016;6:35216.
85. De Cruz P, Kang S, Wagner J, Buckley M, Sim WH, Prideaux L, et al. Association between specific mucosa-associated microbiota in Crohn's disease at the time of resection and subsequent disease recurrence: a pilot study. J Gastroenterol Hepatol. 2015;30(2):268–78.
86. Qiu X, Zhang M, Yang X, Hong N, Yu C. Faecalibacterium prausnitzii upregulates regulatory T cells and anti-inflammatory cytokines in treating TNBS-induced colitis. J Crohns Colitis. 2013;7(11):e558–68.
87. Rossi O, van Berkel LA, Chain F, Tanweer Khan M, Taverne N, Sokol H, et al. Faecalibacterium prausnitzii A2-165 has a high capacity to induce IL-10 in human and murine dendritic cells and modulates T cell responses. Sci Rep. 2016;6:18507.
88. Kellermayer R, Mir SA, Nagy-Szakal D, Cox SB, Dowd SE, Kaplan JL, et al. Microbiota separation and C-reactive protein elevation in treatment-naive pediatric granulomatous Crohn disease. J Pediatr Gastroenterol Nutr. 2012;55(3):243–50.
89. Tyler AD, Knox N, Kabakchiev B, Milgrom R, Kirsch R, Cohen Z, et al. Characterization of the gut-associated microbiome in inflammatory pouch complications following ileal pouch-anal anastomosis. PLoS One. 2013;8(9):e66934.
90. Shah R, Cope JL, Nagy-Szakal D, Dowd S, Versalovic J, Hollister EB, et al. Composition and function of the pediatric colonic mucosal microbiome in untreated patients with ulcerative colitis. Gut Microbes. 2016;7(5):384–96.
91. Koh A, De Vadder F, Kovatcheva-Datchary P, Backhed F. From dietary fiber to host physiology: short-chain fatty acids as key bacterial metabolites. Cell. 2016;165(6):1332–45.
92. den Besten G, van Eunen K, Groen AK, Venema K, Reijngoud DJ, Bakker BM. The role of short-chain fatty acids in the interplay between diet, gut microbiota, and host energy metabolism. J Lipid Res. 2013;54(9):2325–40.
93. Louis P, Young P, Holtrop G, Flint HJ. Diversity of human colonic butyrate-producing bacteria revealed by analysis of the butyryl-CoA:acetate CoA-transferase gene. Environ Microbiol. 2010;12(2):304–14.
94. Morrison DJ, Mackay WG, Edwards CA, Preston T, Dodson B, Weaver LT. Butyrate production from oligofructose fermentation by the human faecal flora: what is the contribution of extracellular acetate and lactate? Br J Nutr. 2006;96(3):570–7.
95. Scott KP, Martin JC, Duncan SH, Flint HJ. Prebiotic stimulation of human colonic butyrate-producing bacteria and bifidobacteria, in vitro. FEMS Microbiol Ecol. 2014;87(1):30–40.
96. Rios-Covian D, Ruas-Madiedo P, Margolles A, Gueimonde M, de Los Reyes-Gavilan CG, Salazar N. Intestinal short chain fatty acids and their link with diet and human health. Front Microbiol. 2016;7:185.
97. Smith PM, Howitt MR, Panikov N, Michaud M, Gallini CA, Bohlooly YM, et al. The microbial metabolites, short-chain fatty acids, regulate colonic Treg cell homeostasis. Science. 2013;341(6145):569–73.
98. Marchesi JR, Holmes E, Khan F, Kochhar S, Scanlan P, Shanahan F, et al. Rapid and noninvasive metabonomic characterization of inflammatory bowel disease. J Proteome Res. 2007;6(2):546–51.
99. Le Gall G, Noor SO, Ridgway K, Scovell L, Jamieson C, Johnson IT, et al. Metabolomics of fecal extracts detects altered metabolic activity of gut microbiota in ulcerative colitis and irritable bowel syndrome. J Proteome Res. 2011;10(9):4208–18.
100. Dunn KA, Moore-Connors J, MacIntyre B, Stadnyk A, Thomas NA, Noble A, et al. The gut microbiome of pediatric Crohn's disease patients differs from healthy controls in genes that can influence the balance between a healthy and dysregulated immune response. Inflamm Bowel Dis. 2016;22(11):2607–18.
101. Lepage P, Hasler R, Spehlmann ME, Rehman A, Zvirbliene A, Begun A, et al. Twin study indicates loss of interaction between microbiota and mucosa

of patients with ulcerative colitis. Gastroenterology. 2011;141(1):227–36.
102. Takahashi K, Nishida A, Fujimoto T, Fujii M, Shioya M, Imaeda H, et al. Reduced abundance of butyrate-producing bacteria species in the fecal microbial community in Crohn's disease. Digestion. 2016;93(1):59–65.
103. Zhou Y, Zhi F. Lower level of bacteroides in the gut microbiota is associated with inflammatory bowel disease: a meta-analysis. Biomed Res Int. 2016;2016:5828959.
104. Mazmanian SK, Round JL, Kasper DL. A microbial symbiosis factor prevents intestinal inflammatory disease. Nature. 2008;453(7195):620–5.
105. Round JL, Lee SM, Li J, Tran G, Jabri B, Chatila TA, et al. The Toll-like receptor 2 pathway establishes colonization by a commensal of the human microbiota. Science. 2011;332(6032):974–7.
106. Round JL, Mazmanian SK. Inducible Foxp3+ regulatory T-cell development by a commensal bacterium of the intestinal microbiota. Proc Natl Acad Sci U S A. 2010;107(27):12204–9.
107. Telesford KM, Yan W, Ochoa-Reparaz J, Pant A, Kircher C, Christy MA, et al. A commensal symbiotic factor derived from *Bacteroides fragilis* promotes human CD39(+)Foxp3(+) T cells and Treg function. Gut Microbes. 2015;6(4):234–42.
108. Scher JU, Sczesnak A, Longman RS, Segata N, Ubeda C, Bielski C, et al. Expansion of intestinal Prevotella copri correlates with enhanced susceptibility to arthritis. Elife. 2013;2:e01202.
109. Vaahtovuo J, Munukka E, Korkeamaki M, Luukkainen R, Toivanen P. Fecal microbiota in early rheumatoid arthritis. J Rheumatol. 2008;35(8):1500–5.
110. Tito RY, Cypers H, Joossens M, Varkas G, Van Praet L, Glorieus E, et al. Brief report: dialister as a microbial marker of disease activity in spondyloarthritis. Arthritis Rheumatol. 2017;69(1):114–21.
111. Nwosu FC, Thorkildsen LT, Avershina E, Ricanek P, Perminow G, Brackmann S, et al. Age-dependent fecal bacterial correlation to inflammatory bowel disease for newly diagnosed untreated children. Gastroenterol Res Pract. 2013;2013:302398.
112. Stoll ML, Kumar R, Morrow CD, Lefkowitz EJ, Cui X, Genin A, et al. Altered microbiota associated with abnormal humoral immune responses to commensal organisms in enthesitis-related arthritis. Arthritis Res Ther. 2014;16(6):486.
113. Tejesvi MV, Arvonen M, Kangas SM, Keskitalo PL, Pirttila AM, Karttunen TJ, et al. Faecal microbiome in new-onset juvenile idiopathic arthritis. Eur J Clin Microbiol Infect Dis. 2016;35(3):363–70.
114. Aggarwal A, Sarangi AN, Gaur P, Shukla A, Aggarwal R. Gut microbiome in children with enthesitis-related arthritis in a developing country and the effect of probiotic administration. Clin Exp Immunol. 2017;187(3):480–9.
115. Giongo A, Gano KA, Crabb DB, Mukherjee N, Novelo LL, Casella G, et al. Toward defining the autoimmune microbiome for type 1 diabetes. ISME J. 2011;5(1):82–91.
116. Vatanen T, Kostic AD, d'Hennezel E, Siljander H, Franzosa EA, Yassour M, et al. Variation in microbiome LPS immunogenicity contributes to autoimmunity in humans. Cell. 2016;165(4):842–53.
117. Papa E, Docktor M, Smillie C, Weber S, Preheim SP, Gevers D, et al. Non-invasive mapping of the gastrointestinal microbiota identifies children with inflammatory bowel disease. PLoS One. 2012;7(6):e39242.
118. Lavelle A, Lennon G, O'Sullivan O, Docherty N, Balfe A, Maguire A, et al. Spatial variation of the colonic microbiota in patients with ulcerative colitis and control volunteers. Gut. 2015;64(10):1553–61.
119. Derrien M, Vaughan EE, Plugge CM, de Vos WM. Akkermansia muciniphila gen. nov., sp. nov., a human intestinal mucin-degrading bacterium. Int J Syst Evol Microbiol. 2004;54(Pt 5):1469–76.
120. Woting A, Blaut M. The intestinal microbiota in metabolic disease. Forum Nutr. 2016;8(4):202.
121. Asquith MJ, Stauffer P, Davin S, Mitchell C, Lin P, Rosenbaum JT. Perturbed mucosal immunity and dysbiosis accompany clinical disease in a rat model of spondyloarthritis. Arthritis Rheumatol. 2016;68(9):2151–62.
122. Vaile JH, Meddings JB, Yacyshyn BR, Russell AS, Maksymowych WP. Bowel permeability and CD45RO expression on circulating CD20+ B cells in patients with ankylosing spondylitis and their relatives. J Rheumatol. 1999;26(1):128–35.
123. Munkholm P, Langholz E, Hollander D, Thornberg K, Orholm M, Katz KD, et al. Intestinal permeability in patients with Crohn's disease and ulcerative colitis and their first degree relatives. Gut. 1994;35(1):68–72.
124. Dorofeyev AE, Vasilenko IV, Rassokhina OA, Kondratiuk RB. Mucosal barrier in ulcerative colitis and Crohn's disease. Gastroenterol Res Pract. 2013;2013:431231.
125. Rey FE, Gonzalez MD, Cheng J, Wu M, Ahern PP, Gordon JI. Metabolic niche of a prominent sulfate-reducing human gut bacterium. Proc Natl Acad Sci U S A. 2013;110(33):13582–7.
126. Pitcher MC, Beatty ER, Harris RM, Waring RH, Cummings JH. Sulfur metabolism in ulcerative colitis: investigation of detoxification enzymes in peripheral blood. Dig Dis Sci. 1998;43(9):2080–5.
127. Ijssennagger N, Belzer C, Hooiveld GJ, Dekker J, van Mil SW, Muller M, et al. Gut microbiota facilitates dietary heme-induced epithelial hyperproliferation by opening the mucus barrier in colon. Proc Natl Acad Sci U S A. 2015;112(32):10038–43.
128. Wang W, Jovel J, Halloran B, Wine E, Patterson J, Ford G, et al. Metagenomic analysis of microbiome in colon tissue from subjects with inflammatory bowel diseases reveals interplay of viruses and bacteria. Inflamm Bowel Dis. 2015;21(6):1419–27.
129. Chassaing B, Rolhion N, de Vallee A, Salim SY, Prorok-Hamon M, Neut C, et al. Crohn disease—associated adherent-invasive E. coli bacteria target

mouse and human Peyer's patches via long polar fimbriae. J Clin Investig. 2011;121(3):966–75.
130. Bucker R, Schulz E, Gunzel D, Bojarski C, Lee IF, John LJ, et al. α-Haemolysin of *Escherichia coli* in IBD: a potentiator of inflammatory activity in the colon. Gut. 2014;63(12):1893–901.
131. Lupp C, Robertson ML, Wickham ME, Sekirov I, Champion OL, Gaynor EC, et al. Host-mediated inflammation disrupts the intestinal microbiota and promotes the overgrowth of Enterobacteriaceae. Cell Host Microbe. 2007;2(2):119–29.
132. He F, Morita H, Ouwehand AC, Hosoda M, Hiramatsu M, Kurisaki J, et al. Stimulation of the secretion of pro-inflammatory cytokines by Bifidobacterium strains. Microbiol Immunol. 2002;46(11):781–5.
133. Medina M, Izquierdo E, Ennahar S, Sanz Y. Differential immunomodulatory properties of Bifidobacterium logum strains: relevance to probiotic selection and clinical applications. Clin Exp Immunol. 2007;150(3):531–8.
134. Elian SD, Souza EL, Vieira AT, Teixeira MM, Arantes RM, Nicoli JR, et al. Bifidobacterium longum subsp. infantis BB-02 attenuates acute murine experimental model of inflammatory bowel disease. Benefic Microbes. 2015;6(3):277–86.
135. Chehoud C, Albenberg LG, Judge C, Hoffmann C, Grunberg S, Bittinger K, et al. Fungal signature in the gut microbiota of pediatric patients with inflammatory bowel disease. Inflamm Bowel Dis. 2015;21(8):1948–56.
136. Israeli E, Grotto I, Gilburd B, Balicer RD, Goldin E, Wiik A, et al. Anti-*Saccharomyces cerevisiae* and antineutrophil cytoplasmic antibodies as predictors of inflammatory bowel disease. Gut. 2005;54(9):1232–6.
137. Iliev ID, Funari VA, Taylor KD, Nguyen Q, Reyes CN, Strom SP, et al. Interactions between commensal fungi and the C-type lectin receptor Dectin-1 influence colitis. Science. 2012;336(6086):1314–7.
138. Hansen JJ, Sartor RB. Therapeutic manipulation of the microbiome in IBD: current results and future approaches. Curr Treat Options Gastroenterol. 2015;13(1):105–20.
139. Lewis JD, Abreu MT. Diet as a trigger or therapy for inflammatory bowel diseases. Gastroenterology. 2017;152(2):398–414.e6.
140. Nitzan O, Elias M, Peretz A, Saliba W. Role of antibiotics for treatment of inflammatory bowel disease. World J Gastroenterol. 2016;22(3):1078–87.
141. Reinisch W. Fecal microbiota transplantation in inflammatory bowel disease. Dig Dis. 2017;35(1–2):123–6.
142. MacLellan A, Moore-Connors J, Grant S, Cahill L, Langille MGI, Van Limbergen J. The impact of exclusive enteral nutrition (EEN) on the gut microbiome in Crohn's disease: a review. Nutrients. 2017;9(5):0447.
143. Richman E, Rhodes JM. Review article: evidence-based dietary advice for patients with inflammatory bowel disease. Aliment Pharmacol Ther. 2013;38(10):1156–71.
144. Dziechciarz P, Horvath A, Shamir R, Szajewska H. Meta-analysis: enteral nutrition in active Crohn's disease in children. Aliment Pharmacol Ther. 2007;26(6):795–806.
145. Ruemmele FM, Veres G, Kolho KL, Griffiths A, Levine A, Escher JC, et al. Consensus guidelines of ECCO/ESPGHAN on the medical management of pediatric Crohn's disease. J Crohns Colitis. 2014;8(10):1179–207.
146. Gerasimidis K, Bertz M, Hanske L, Junick J, Biskou O, Aguilera M, et al. Decline in presumptively protective gut bacterial species and metabolites are paradoxically associated with disease improvement in pediatric Crohn's disease during enteral nutrition. Inflamm Bowel Dis. 2014;20(5):861–71.
147. Benjamin JL, Hedin CR, Koutsoumpas A, Ng SC, McCarthy NE, Hart AL, et al. Randomised, double-blind, placebo-controlled trial of fructo-oligosaccharides in active Crohn's disease. Gut. 2011;60(7):923–9.
148. Kronman MP, Zaoutis TE, Haynes K, Feng R, Coffin SE. Antibiotic exposure and IBD development among children: a population-based cohort study. Pediatrics. 2012;130(4):e794–803.
149. Cojocariu C, Stanciu C, Stoica O, Singeap AM, Sfarti C, Girleanu I, et al. Clostridium difficile infection and inflammatory bowel disease. Turk J Gastroenterol. 2014;25(6):603–10.
150. Kerman DH, Deshpande AR. Gut microbiota and inflammatory bowel disease: the role of antibiotics in disease management. Postgrad Med. 2014;126(4):7–19.
151. Wang SL, Wang ZR, Yang CQ. Meta-analysis of broad-spectrum antibiotic therapy in patients with active inflammatory bowel disease. Exp Ther Med. 2012;4(6):1051–6.
152. Derikx LA, Dieleman LA, Hoentjen F. Probiotics and prebiotics in ulcerative colitis. Best Pract Res Clin Gastroenterol. 2016;30(1):55–71.
153. Durchschein F, Petritsch W, Hammer HF. Diet therapy for inflammatory bowel diseases: the established and the new. World J Gastroenterol. 2016;22(7):2179–94.
154. Doron S, Snydman DR. Risk and safety of probiotics. Clin Infect Dis. 2015;60(Suppl 2):S129–34.
155. Wang AY, Popov J, Pai N. Fecal microbial transplant for the treatment of pediatric inflammatory bowel disease. World J Gastroenterol. 2016;22(47):10304–15.
156. Eiseman B, Silen W, Bascom GS, Kauvar AJ. Fecal enema as an adjunct in the treatment of pseudomembranous enterocolitis. Surgery. 1958;44(5):854–9.
157. Fischer M, Kao D, Kelly C, Kuchipudi A, Jafri SM, Blumenkehl M, et al. Fecal microbiota transplantation is safe and efficacious for recurrent or refractory Clostridium difficile infection in patients with inflammatory bowel disease. Inflamm Bowel Dis. 2016;22(10):2402–9.
158. Zhang FM, Wang HG, Wang M, Cui BT, Fan ZN, Ji GZ. Fecal microbiota transplantation for severe

enterocolonic fistulizing Crohn's disease. World J Gastroenterol. 2013;19(41):7213–6.
159. Borody TJ, Warren EF, Leis S, Surace R, Ashman O. Treatment of ulcerative colitis using fecal bacteriotherapy. J Clin Gastroenterol. 2003;37(1):42–7.
160. Keshteli AH, Millan B, Madsen KL. Pretreatment with antibiotics may enhance the efficacy of fecal microbiota transplantation in ulcerative colitis: a meta-analysis. Mucosal Immunol. 2017;10(2):565–6.
161. Baxter M, Colville A. Adverse events in faecal microbiota transplant: a review of the literature. J Hosp Infect. 2016;92(2):117–27.
162. Wyllie R, Hyams J. Pediatric gastrointestinal and liver diseases. Philladelphia: Elsevier; 2015.
163. Davenport M, Poles J, Leung JM, Wolff MJ, Abidi WM, Ullman T, et al. Metabolic alterations to the mucosal microbiota in inflammatory bowel disease. Inflamm Bowel Dis. 2014;20(4):723–31.
164. Reshef L, Kovacs A, Ofer A, Yahav L, Maharshak N, Keren N, et al. Pouch inflammation is associated with a decrease in specific bacterial taxa. Gastroenterology. 2015;149(3):718–27.
165. Forbes JD, Van Domselaar G, Bernstein CN. Microbiome survey of the inflamed and noninflamed gut at different compartments within the gastrointestinal tract of inflammatory bowel disease patients. Inflamm Bowel Dis. 2016;22(4):817–25.
166. Hasler R, Sheibani-Tezerji R, Sinha A, Barann M, Rehman A, Esser D, et al. Uncoupling of mucosal gene regulation, mRNA splicing and adherent microbiota signatures in inflammatory bowel disease. Gut. 2016;66(12):2087–97.
167. Tyler AD, Kirsch R, Milgrom R, Stempak JM, Kabakchiev B, Silverberg MS. Microbiome heterogeneity characterizing intestinal tissue and inflammatory bowel disease phenotype. Inflamm Bowel Dis. 2016;22(4):807–16.
168. Mukhopadhya I, Hansen R, Meharg C, Thomson JM, Russell RK, Berry SH, et al. The fungal microbiota of de-novo paediatric inflammatory bowel disease. Microbes Infect. 2015;17(4):304–10.
169. El Mouzan M, Wang F, Al Mofarreh M, Menon R, Al Barrag A, Korolev KS, et al. Fungal Microbiota Profile in Newly Diagnosed Treatment-naïve Children with Crohn's Disease. J Crohns Colitis. 2017;11(5):586–592.
170. Greenblum S, Turnbaugh PJ, Borenstein E. Metagenomic systems biology of the human gut microbiome reveals topological shifts associated with obesity and inflammatory bowel disease. Proc Natl Acad Sci U S A. 2012;109(2):594–9.

20 Reactive Arthritis

Thomas Bardin

Abbreviations

ARA	American Rheumatism Association
DNA	Deoxyribonucleic acid
EB	Elementary body
HIV	Human immunodeficiency virus
HLA	Human leucocyte antigen
IL	Interleukin
INF-γ	Interferon gamma
RB	Reticular body
ReA	Reactive arthritis
RNA	Ribonucleic acid
SpA	Spondyloarthropathy
STI	Sextually transmitted infection
STReA	Sexually transmitted reactive arthritis
TH	T helper cell
TNF	Tumor necrosis factor

Definition

Reactive arthritis (ReA) is a form of spondyloarthropathy (SpA) which associates with the HLA-B27 antigen and can be defined as a sterile inflammatory arthritis triggered by an infection generally due to a limited number of strict or facultative intracellular pathogens. In 1976, Dumonde attempted to clarify the spectrum of infection-related joint diseases and characterized reactive arthritis by the lack of microorganism component in the affected joint(s), in opposition with post-infectious arthritis in which joints contained microorganism components (antigens at the time) but no viable microorganism by standard bacteriological techniques and to septic arthritis in which pathogens could be identified by microscopy examination or culture of joint materials [1]. Despite the later findings of antigens and nucleic acids in the synovial fluid and/or membrane of affected joints, the term reactive arthritis has been kept for HLA-B27-associated post-infectious arthritis. Reactive arthritis has also been called Reiter's syndrome to acknowledge the description by this German physician of an epidemics of post-*Shigella* arthritis during World War I, even though the condition was simultaneously recognized by the French physicians Fiessinger and Leroy on the French side. Following the discovery of the role that Reiter played in Nazi medicine, and of previous disease description, this eponym has now been abandoned [2].

Pathogens

ReA can be triggered by a limited number of pathogens, with distinct portals of entry, the main ones being venereal and digestive (Table 20.1).

T. Bardin
INSERM U1132, Rheumatology Department, Lariboisière Hospital Paris and University Paris Diderot, Paris, France
e-mail: thomas.bardin@aphp.fr

G. Ragab et al. (eds.), *The Microbiome in Rheumatic Diseases and Infection*, https://doi.org/10.1007/978-3-319-79026-8_20

Table 20.1 ReA-triggering infections

Sexually transmittable infections
Ureaplasma urealytica
Chlamydia trachomatis
Intestinal infections
Shigella flexneri and *S. sonnei*
Salmonella (non-typhoidal)
Y. enterocolitica and *Y. pseudotuberculosis*
Campylobacter jejuni and *C. coli*
Clostridium difficile
Other portals of entry
C. pneumoniae
Bacillus of Calmette and Guérin

Succeeding triggering infections by distinct pathogens have been observed to cause reactive joint inflammation in the same patient, highlighting the interplay of infectious triggers and genetic predisposition [3].

ReA and HLA-B27

Reactive arthritis is associated with the HLA-B27 gene, and this is one of the reasons to include ReA in the SpA spectrum. Overall, 40–60% of affected patients are HLA-B27 positive [4]. HLA-B27 seems to be associated with disease severity, and the proportion of B-27 carriers is increased in hospitalized patient series.

Microbiota and Reactive Arthritis

Only three studies have performed an evaluation of the fecal microbiota in ReA patients; Gupta et al. [5] used fecal culture to evaluate the microbiota of 30 rheumatoid arthritis patients, 34 healthy controls, and 60 subjects with either ReA or undifferentiated SpA. None of them grew pathogens typically associated with ReA. Thirty to forty percent of all groups grew *Klebsiella*, without any differences between the three groups, although higher carriage rates were noted in the SpA patients with active versus inactive disease. The authors concluded that *Klebsiella* may be a triggering agent. Likewise, Smith et al. [6] did not identify any differences between ReA patients or SpA patients as a whole compared to healthy controls, but they also used culture- rather than DNA-based methods. Recently, Manasson et al. [7] compared 32 adults with recent diagnoses of ReA with 32 healthy controls. Their study, although clouded by use of antibiotics to treat the ReA in 20 subjects in addition to three others who were treated with sulfasalazine, showed increased carriage of enteropathogens such as Pseudomonas and decreased carriage of butyrate-producing organisms such as Roseburia and Blautia, thus mimicing findings reported in patients with inflammatory bowel disease (Chap. 16). Therefore, the question as to whether the microbiota as a whole is altered in patients with ReA remains an understudied question.

Risk Factors

The main risk factors are infections with pathogens able to trigger ReA and genetic predisposition. Family studies have shown that ReA aggregated within families [8, 9]. HIV infection is an important risk factor, in particular in sub-Saharan Africa where ReA usually affects HLA-B27-negative patients infected by the virus [10].

Diagnosis

Preliminary classification criteria for ReA, then called Reiter's syndrome, were issued in 1981 by the American Rheumatism Association (now American College of Rheumatology). According to these, an episode of peripheral arthritis lasting more than 4 weeks occurring in association with urethritis or cervicitis could be classified as ReA [11]. The criteria most commonly used to diagnose ReA are those of the 1995 Berlin Third International Workshop: (1) the presence of a predominantly lower limb asymmetrical oligoarthritis and (2) clinical laboratory evidence of a preceding infection [12]. However, these are far from satisfactory as joint distribution is frequently atypical in enteric infection-related ReA, and the triggering infection is often difficult to demonstrate.

Sexually Transmitted Reactive Arthritis

Sexually transmitted reactive arthritis (STReA) is held as the most common form of ReA and follows a nongonococcal (or sometimes mixed) sextually transmitted infection (STI) mainly caused by *C. trachomatis*. Reported incidence after STI has varied from 3% to 8% and remains uncertain [13]. It appears to vary according to the genetic background and to the STI antibiotic treatment. In a 3-year study, we were able to compare the rates of arthritis in Greenland, after STIs which had or had not been treated by antibiotics active against *C. trachomatis*, in 103 patients with a previously established diagnostic of STReA, who therefore presumably carried the full genetic predisposition (including the B27 gene, which was present in all typed patients), and in 397 previously non-affected first-degree relatives. In the 4 weeks following STIs not treated or treated by penicillin only, the incidences of recurrences meeting the preliminary ARA criteria for ReA [11] were 37% in the patients with the full genetic predisposition and 4% in first-degree relatives. When STIs were treated by erythromycin or tetracycline, the rates of arthritis fell to 10% in STReA patients and 1% in family members, suggesting a preventive effect of anti-*Chlamydia* treatment of STIs [14]. These data also suggested that several genes and not solely HLA-B27 intervened in the predisposition to STReA.

The arthritis most frequently affects young men, a few weeks after the triggering infection [14, 15]. It is typically an asymmetrical inflammatory oligoarthritis involving the large joints of the lower limbs. Joint effusions are usually abundant and contain an inflammatory synovial fluid, with a high number of leucocytes and negative standard bacteriology. Enthesitis, including talalgias; axial involvement, responsible for sacroiliac and/or spine pain; and dactylitis can be observed. CRP and ESR are usually very elevated. Extra-articular features include conjunctivitis and urethritis and, less commonly, involvement of the heart (auriculoventricular block or aortitis) or skin (keratoderma blennorrhagica, circinate balanitis). Skin features can be indistinguishable from pustular psoriasis. The classical triad of arthritis, conjunctivitis, and urethritis is highly suggestive of the diagnosis but may be observed in ReA of other etiologies: it has been initially described in post-*Shigella* arthritis. Moreover, this triad is frequently incomplete. Conjunctivitis may be missing, and nongonococcal venereal infection is frequently asymptomatic, especially in women. A number of studies have shown that *Chlamydia* arthritis accounted for 15–30% of oligoarthritis of undetermined origin [15].

The course of STReA is severe in many patients, especially those tested HLA-B27 positive. Joint inflammation had to last for more than 4 weeks to meet the ARA preliminary criteria [11] and indeed has usually a prolonged course. Our Greenlandic cohort counted 153 nonselected patients seen through an epidemiological approach; 76 out of 79 tested patients were HLA-B27 positive. The mean duration of articular attacks was 11.4 weeks; arthritis was strikingly recurrent over the 15 years of mean follow-up, with the recurrence rate averaging 0.139 per patient year. Eighty percent of patients followed for at least 5 years experienced at least one arthritic recurrence. Of note, arthritis developed in the month following a diagnosis of urethritis or cervicitis in 62.6% of articular recurrences, whereas 37.4% of recurrences were not associated with a new symptomatic STI. The percentage of patients meeting the New York criteria for ankylosing spondylitis increased with follow-up to reach 40% after 15 years. Two patients were diagnosed with amyloid nephropathy following long-lasting inflammation. Recurrent uveitis flares frequently occurred during the course of the disease with no apparent temporal relationship with arthritis flares or STIs [14].

Role of *Chlamydia trachomatis*

The role of *C. trachomatis* in the development of STReA has been first supported by the frequent observation of genital chlamydial infection in the few weeks preceding articular features and by the epidemiological association of STReA with nongonococcal STI, of which *C. trachomatis* is a major agent. *C. trachomatis* is indeed the leading cause of bacterial STIs worldwide. Within the USA, 1,441,789 chlamydial infections were reported to CDC in 2014, most of which were either asymptomatic or minimally symptomatic and diagnosed after screening or because a contact was symptomatic [16]. Its implication in STReA has now been widely confirmed by a number of reports in which the presence of *Chlamydia* components within affected joints was characterized by transmission electron microscopy, immunofluorescence, and molecular biology techniques [15]. The latter techniques evidenced not only DNA but also short-lived RNA in synovial fluid and/or membrane, thus pleading in favor of viable *Chlamydiae* in affected joints.

C. trachomatis is a strict intracellular pathogen with a biphasic life cycle. Upon attachment, infectious elementary bodies (EBs) stimulate endocytosis by cells where they differentiate into vegetative reticulate bodies (RBs) to grow and divide within a membrane-bound vacuole called an inclusion. After 8–12 divisions, RBs differentiate into EBs, and the cell releases the contents of the inclusion to attach to adjacent cells and reinitiate the cycle. When appropriate factors are applied in vitro such as low-dose IFN-γ exposure, or improper antibiotic treatment, *Chlamydia* enters a non-replicative and uncultivable, yet viable, persistent state, a situation very similar to the one observed in STReA joints, where cultures are negative and nucleic acids are detected [15, 17]. The persistent state is characterized by a unique protein expression profile with, interestingly, increased expression of the pro-inflammatory lipopolysaccharide and heat-shock protein [15].

Even though underdiagnosis of chlamydial arthritis appears as highly probable, *Chlamydia* arthritis is likely to affect only a minority of infected patients. Factors intervening in the development of arthritis may be related to the virulence of the pathogen, and surprisingly one study has identified ocular strains in the joints of patients affected by STReA [18]. Host factors, presumably genetically determined, are also likely to play a role. The best described host factor, as indicated above, is HLA-B27. Potential mechanisms linking this molecule and SpA are discussed elsewhere in the textbook (Chap. 16). Additionally, type 1 cytokines, especially interferon-γ and TNFα, appear to play an important role in the defense against intracellular infections [19]. Studies of ReA patients performed in the 1980s have shown that they developed a predominantly TH2 cytokine pattern, which may favor intra-articular persistent infection. More recently one study found that *Chlamydia* arthritis patients frequently had a particular variant of the CCR5 chemokine receptor which could reduce the defense against *Chlamydiae* [20]. The way by which persistently infected cells end up in the joints is still unknown. Infected macrophages are likely to be responsible for the transportation of *Chlamydiae* to the joints, leading to the hypothesis that some macrophage defect may play a role, but the mechanism of their joint homing is still poorly understood.

Role of Other Sexually Transmitted Pathogens

Gonococci have been suspected to be involved in STReA. A more probable hypothesis is that they have been identified in ReA patients with mixed infections (both chlamydial and gonococcal), in which *C. trachomatis* and not *Gonococcus* was the ReA trigger. This conclusion was suggested by our findings that penicillin did not prevent post-urethritis articular flares, whereas antibiotics active against *C. trachomatis* did [21].

Mycoplasma have also been implicated following positive urethral cultures [22] and identification of DNA in the synovial fluid [23]. They are sensitive to the same antibiotics as *Chlamydiae*.

Reactive Arthritis Following Gastrointestinal Infections

The initial description of ReA has been made in the context of *Shigella* epidemics in a war context. Since then, ReA has been repeatedly described following small epidemics of *Yersinia*, *Salmonella*, and *Campylobacter* infections, with no sex predominance. The number of enteropathic pathogens associated with ReA is increasing. As for STReA, enteric infection-related ReA appears as a cause of undifferentiated arthritis [24].

Shigella

Shigella ReA is historically important as the first cases of the disease, later to be called ReA, were simultaneously reported in 1916 by French and German physicians during an epidemic of bacillary dysenteria during the World War I Somme battle [25, 26]. Since then, the occurrence of ReA after epidemics of *Shigella* dysenteria has been well documented, in particular by Paronen who reported 344 cases of ReA during an epidemic of *Shigella flexneri* dysentery affecting 150,000 people on the Karelian Isthmus in Finland during World War II, in 1944 [27, 28]. Disease had an incidence of 0.24% and affected mainly men (90%) but also some women (10%). As in STReA, arthritis involved primarily the lower limbs. It usually lasted for 2–4 months. Extra-articular features were common but more transient. The classical triad (arthritis, conjunctivitis, and sterile urethritis) was observed in 70% of affected people; 100 of these patients were seen 20 years after [28]. Only 20% were entirely asymptomatic after the first episode. The others had some disability of some degree; 32% had ankylosing spondylitis. Of 50 patients tested, 39 tested HLA-B27 positive. In 1966, Noer reported nine similar cases of ReA after an epidemic of *Shigella* dysentery developed in 602 crew members of a US navy ship, an incidence of 1.5% [29]. A 5-year follow-up study confirmed the chronicity of the disease [30].

In the civilian world, *Shigella*-reactive arthritis has also been reported, most often, in Western countries following imported infections. The incidence in Sweden after a documented *Shigella* stool infection has been estimated at 7% [31]. This nationwide study also showed that besides *S. flexneri*, *S. sonnei* and *S. dysenteriae* can also trigger ReA [31]. A more recent literature review gave a lower incidence estimate of 12 reactive arthritis cases per 1000 cases of *Shigella* infection [32].

Salmonella

Salmonella is one of the most frequent gastrointestinal infections and a well-established cause of ReA, which is mainly triggered by non-typhoidal *Salmonella* infections, including *S. Typhimurium* and *Enteritidis*, as established by several outbreak surveys [33, 34] or by population-based studies of patients with culture-confirmed infections [35, 36]. The incidence has been variously estimated. A recent study reported an incidence of 12 ReA cases per 1000 cases of *Salmonella* infection, very similar to the one after *Shigella* infection [32], but incidence varied according to clinical features taken into account. Clinical presentation is indeed very diverse ranging from arthralgias without joint swelling, low-back or heel pain, to true arthritis with joint swelling, which has been much less frequently observed than isolated arthralgias. Joint involvement most commonly does not follow the typical pattern of *Shigella*-induced ReA or *Shigella* arthritis. Arthritis does not predominate to large joints of the lower limbs, but frequently include small joints, particularly of the hands. Conjunctivitis and sterile urethritis can also be observed and are not always associated with arthritis [37]. Frequency of HLA-B27, which has been clearly associated with disease severity [37], varied widely across studies. Arthritis severity has also been shown to correlate with intestine infection severity and duration [33, 34]. Duration of arthritis symptoms frequently exceeds 3 months. Long-term follow-up shows that recurrences, uveitis, and axial symptoms including ankylosing spondylitis may develop in HLA-B27 patients [4]. However, the frequency of recurrences seems less than in post-STI ReA probably because re-infestations are less common.

Yersinia

Porcine animals are the main carriers of *Y. enterocolitica*. Human infection follows consumption of raw minced pork [38] or contaminated vegetable, e.g., iceberg lettuce or grated carrots [39]. As *Yersinia* is relatively cold-resistant, food contamination may occur in the refrigerator. ReA may follow infections by *Y. enterocolitica* or *Y. pseudotuberculosis*, which are fairly prevalent in Northern Europe and Germany. Infected patients may develop ReA or erythema nodosum in the weeks following diarrhea. ReA develops more commonly in adults and is associated with HLA-B27, whereas erythema nodosum is not associated with HLA-B27 and occurs mainly in children [39]. Initial symptoms of gastroenteritis such as diarrhea or abdominal pain are often mild but may also simulate acute appendicitis. Arthritis has been reported to develop in 12–21% of infected patients and to usually involve one or several joints, most commonly large joints of the lower limbs. Urethritis, conjunctivitis, atrioventricular block, and aortitis may be associated. Arthritis duration frequently exceeds 6 months [40]. In one study with a 10-year follow-up, recurrent or chronic arthritis appeared as rare, but bilateral sacroiliitis developed in one third of patients, all of whom tested positive for HLA-B27 [41].

Campylobacter jejuni and *C. coli*

Campylobacter jejuni accounts for 5–14% of all diarrheal disease worldwide and is the most common cause of human bacterial enteritis [42]. *C. jejuni* is the most common *Campylobacter* serotype, which accounts for 90–95% of positive stools. *C. coli* accounts for 5–10% of cases. ReA can develop after infection by both serotypes. The prevalence of ReA after *Campylobacter* infection has been estimated between 1% and 7% [43]. Symptoms include arthralgias to overt arthritis of small and large joints of the limbs and/or low-back pain. Sterile urethritis is rare. Patients with longer episodes of diarrhea seem particularly prone to develop ReA [44, 45]. Arthritis did not associate with the B-27 antigen in community-based series, in which the arthritis appeared mild, but frequency of the antigen has been found increased, up to 70%, in more severe hospitalized patients. Two to three percent of affected patients might develop a chronic arthritis course, but this point has been very little studied [46]. Antibiotic treatment of the initial gastrointestinal infection had no clear effect on the ReA incident rate; some studies even reporting that antibiotics may have favored ReA development [47].

Clostridium difficile

Clostridium difficile infection frequently complicates antibiotic treatment that allows unrestrained growth of the organism by disrupting the intestinal microbiota. It is responsible for 10–25% of antibiotic-associated diarrhea cases and may result in pseudomembranous colitis [48]. Most adult cases have delayed onset of symptoms that appear after the antibiotics have been discontinued and before the normal colonic microbiota has recovered. It is a rare cause of enteric infection-related ReA [49]. Affected patients are usually older than the other ReA patients and three quarters were tested HLA-B27 positive. There is no sex predominance. Fever is frequent; asymmetrical polyarthritis affecting the knees and ankles is the most frequent presentation and usually remits in a few weeks either spontaneously or after *C. difficile* infection treatment. Arthritis recurrences have been observed following reinfection. The disease has also been observed in children [50].

Pathophysiology of Enteric Infection-Related ReA

As for STReA, components of the culprit pathogens have been identified inside affected joints, particularly *Yersinia* and *Salmonella* antigens [51, 52]. *Yersinia* RNA has been identified in one patient [53], and, because of the short life of RNA, this finding suggested that living *Yersinia* could enter the joint. However, the finding of *Yersinia* nucleic acid in the joint appears as very rare [54], and *Yersinia* cannot be cultivated from ReA joint material suggesting the pathogen would rapidly die inside the joint in contrast to well-documented cases of *Yersinia* septic arthritis. Persistent infection by enteropathic pathogens is believed to play a key role in the development of ReA arthritis as suggested by the persistence of anti- *Yersinia* antibodies [55], and it is generally accepted that the microorganisms involved in enteric infection-related ReA persist either in the epithelium [56] or within associated lymphoid tissues. From these reservoirs, macrophages could bring pathogen components to joints where they would trigger inflammation. *Yersinia* lipopolysaccharide and heat shock protein have been detected in circulating phagocytes several years after the triggering infection [57]. As for STReA, patients with enteric infection-related ReA have been reported to develop an impaired Th1 response, favoring persistence of the infection through low levels of TNFα and interferon-γ secretion [58]. In addition, HLA-B27 has been implicated in the modulation of enteric pathogens and intestinal cell interaction [59, 60].

Reactive Arthritis Following Other Infections

C. pneumoniae is a common respiratory pathogen in humans, particularly in children. Several cases of arthritis following pulmonary infection by *C. pneumoniae* have been published, and nucleic acids of this pathogen have been identified in joint material of affected patients [61], so that *C. pneumoniae* has been included in the list of pathogens susceptible to trigger ReA, even if it seems to be involved less frequently than *C. trachomatis*.

Other pathogens, such as *Cryptosporidium enteritis* [62], *Giardia lamblia* [63], *E. coli* [64], and *Streptococcus* [65], have been reported in scattered case reports, but their involvement is not consensually accepted. ReA is an accepted, but rare, complication of intravesical instillation of Bacillus Calmette–Guérin vaccine to treat bladder cancer [66]. Aseptic reactive arthritis (Poncet's disease) has also been described during tuberculosis [67].

Management of Reactive Arthritis

Antibiotics

Treatment of the triggering infection is rarely needed in enteric infection-related ReA, as patients usually no longer have intestinal symptoms at the stage of arthritis. In STReA, management of the urethral chlamydia and/or *Mycoplasma* infection is important together with screening and management of other sexually transmitted diseases that can be associated (e.g., gonorrhea, syphilis, hepatitis C, HIV infection). Patient's partner(s) should also be screened and treated. Doxycycline should be given for 10 days or azithromycin as a single dose [16].

The effect of antibiotics on established ReA arthritis has been explored by several studies, as joint inflammation appears to be associated with persistent infection [68]. The course of *Chlamydia* arthritis does not seem to be influenced by antibiotic monotherapy, including long-term azithromycin [69]. However, one study concluded that a 9-month course of two antibiotics (rifampicin + doxycycline or azithromycin) was more effective than placebo on *C. trachomatis* or *C. pneumoniae* arthritis [70], so that these antibiotic regimens can be considered as therapy for *Chlamydia* arthritis patients. No effect of antibiotics has been demonstrated on the course of enteric infection-related ReA, and available data do not support the long-term use of antibiotics in these patients, even though a 3-month course of ciprofloxacin has been shown to eliminate *Yersinia* from sigmoid biopsies [71].

Other Drugs

NSAIDs and joint steroid injections are largely used as symptomatic treatments of ReA. Chronic arthritis can be treated by various disease-modifying antirheumatic drugs, including azathioprine [72], sulfasalazine [73], and methotrexate [74]. Despite the fear that they could worsen the causative infection, TNFα blockers appear as very efficient in refractory ReA [75, 76]. Tocilizumab has also been successfully used [77].

Preventive Measures

Patients with ReA should be educated to avoid new infestations, as these can trigger arthritis flares. Urethritis should be promptly treated with antibiotics active against *C. trachomatis* as this has been shown to significantly lower the risk of post-urethritis articular recurrence [21], whereas antibiotic treatment of intestinal infections does not seem to protect from ReA.

References

1. Dumonde CD. Introduction to part II: principal evidence associating rheumatic diseases with microbial infection. In: Dumonde CD, editor. Infection and immunology in the rheumatic diseases. Oxford: Blackwell; 1976. p. 95–6.
2. Panush RS, Wallace DJ, Dorff RE, Engleman EP. Retraction of the suggestion to use the term "Reiter's syndrome" sixty-five years later: the legacy of Reiter, a war criminal, should not be eponymic honor but rather condemnation. Arthritis Rheum. 2007;56(2):693–4.
3. Konttinen Y, Nordstrom D, Bergroth V, Leirisalo-Repo M, Santavirta S. Occurrence of different ensuing triggering infections preceding reactive arthritis: a follow up study. Br Med J (Clin Res Ed). 1988;296(6637):1644–5.
4. Leirisalo-Repo M, Helenius P, Hannu T, Lehtinen A, Kreula J, Taavitsainen M, Koskimies S. Long-term prognosis of reactive salmonella arthritis. Ann Rheum Dis. 1997;56(9):516–20.
5. Gupta NR, Malaviya A, Kaul R, Kumar A, Mehra NK, Shriniwas, Kumar R. Gut flora in HLA-B27 related reactive arthropathy. J Assoc Physicians India. 1986;34(9):634–6.
6. Smith GW, Blackwell CC, Nuki G. Faecal flora in spondyloarthropathy. Br J Rheumatol. 1997;36(8):850–4.
7. Manasson J, Shen N, Garcia Ferrer HR, Ubeda C, Iraheta I, Heguy A, Von Feldt JM, Espinoza LR, Garcia Kutzbach A, Segal LN, Ogdie A, Clemente JC, Scher JU. Gut Microbiota Perturbations in Reactive Arthritis and Postinfectious Spondyloarthritis. Arthritis Rheumatol. 2018;70:242–4.
8. Calin A, Marder A, Marks S, Burns T. Familial aggregation of Reiter's syndrome and ankylosing spondylitis: a comparative study. J Rheumatol. 1984;11(5):672–7.
9. Yunus M, Calabro JJ, Miller KA, Masi AT. Family studies with HLA typing in Reiter's syndrome. Am J Med. 1981;70(6):1210–4.
10. Adizie T, Moots RJ, Hodkinson B, French N, Adebajo AO. Inflammatory arthritis in HIV positive patients: a practical guide. BMC Infect Dis. 2016;16:100.
11. Willkens RF, Arnett FC, Bitter T, Calin A, Fisher L, Ford DK, Good AE, Masi AT. Reiter's syndrome. Evaluation of preliminary criteria for definite disease. Arthritis Rheum. 1981;24(6):844–9.
12. Kingsley G, Sieper J. Third international workshop on reactive arthritis. 23-26 September 1995, Berlin, Germany. Report and abstracts. Ann Rheum Dis. 1996;55(8):564–84.
13. Denison HJ, Curtis EM, Clynes MA, Bromhead C, Dennison EM, Grainger R. The incidence of sexually acquired reactive arthritis: a systematic literature review. Clin Rheumatol. 2016;35(11):2639–48.
14. Bardin T, Lathrop GM. Postvenereal Reiter's syndrome in Greenland. Rheum Dis Clin N Am. 1992;18(1):81–93.
15. Zeidler H, Hudson AP. New insights into *Chlamydia* and arthritis. Promise of a cure? Ann Rheum Dis. 2014;73(4):637–44.
16. O'Connell CM, Ferone ME. *Chlamydia* trachomatis genital infections. Microb Cell. 2016;3(9):390–403.
17. Gracey E, Inman RD. *Chlamydia*-induced ReA: immune imbalances and persistent pathogens. Nat Rev Rheumatol. 2011;8(1):55–9.
18. Gerard HC, Stanich JA, Whittum-Hudson JA, Schumacher HR, Carter JD, Hudson AP. Patients with *Chlamydia*-associated arthritis have ocular (trachoma), not genital, serovars of *C. Trachomatis* in synovial tissue. Microb Pathog. 2010;48(2):62–8.
19. Yin Z, Braun J, Neure L, Wu P, Eggens U, Krause A, Kamradt T, Sieper J. T cell cytokine pattern in the joints of patients with Lyme arthritis and its regulation by cytokines and anticytokines. Arthritis Rheum. 1997;40(1):69–79.
20. Gerard HC, Stanich JA, Oszust CE, Whittum-Hudson JA, Carter JD, Schumacher HR, Hudson AP. Functional CCR5 receptor protects patients with arthritis from high synovial burden of infecting *Chlamydia trachomatis*. Am J Med Sci. 2010;340(6):448–51.
21. Bardin T, Enel C, Cornelis F, Salski C, Jorgensen C, Ward R, Lathrop GM. Antibiotic treatment of venereal disease and Reiter's syndrome in a Greenland population. Arthritis Rheum. 1992;35(2):190–4.
22. Horowitz S, Horowitz J, Taylor-Robinson D, Sukenik S, Apte RN, Bar-David J, Thomas B, Gilroy C. *Ureaplasma urealyticum* in Reiter's syndrome. J Rheumatol. 1994;21(5):877–82.
23. Vittecoq O, Schaeverbeke T, Favre S, Daragon A, Biga N, Cambon-Michot C, Bebear C, Le Loet X. Molecular diagnosis of *Ureaplasma urealyticum* in an immunocompetent patient with destructive reactive polyarthritis. Arthritis Rheum. 1997;40(11):2084–9.
24. Fendler C, Laitko S, Sorensen H, Gripenberg-Lerche C, Groh A, Uksila J, Granfors K, Braun J, Sieper J. Frequency of triggering bacteria in patients with reactive arthritis and undifferentiated oligoarthritis and the relative importance of the tests used for diagnosis. Ann Rheum Dis. 2001;60(4):337–43.
25. Reiter H. Uber eine bisher unerkannte Spirochotinfektion (Spirochatosis arthritica). Deutsh Med Wschr. 1916;42:1535–6.
26. Fiessinger MN, Leroy EM. Contribution à l'étude d'une épidémie de dysenterie dans la Somme (Juillet-Octobre 1916). Bull Soc Med Paris. 1916;40:2030–69.
27. I P. Reiter's disease: a study of 344 cases observed in Finland. Acta Med Scand. 1948;131(Suppl 2012):1–114.
28. Sairanen E, Paronen I, Mahonen H. Reiter's syndrome: a follow-up study. Acta Med Scand. 1969;185(1–2):57–63.
29. Noer HR. An "experimental" epidemic of Reiter's syndrome. JAMA. 1966;198(7):693–8.

30. Calin A, Fries JF. An "experimental" epidemic of Reiter's syndrome revisited. Follow-up evidence on genetic and environmental factors. Ann Intern Med. 1976;84(5):564–6.
31. Hannu T, Mattila L, Siitonen A, Leirisalo-Repo M. Reactive arthritis attributable to *Shigella* infection: a clinical and epidemiological nationwide study. Ann Rheum Dis. 2005;64(4):594–8.
32. Ajene AN, Fischer Walker CL, Black RE. Enteric pathogens and reactive arthritis: a systematic review of *Campylobacter*, *Salmonella* and *Shigella*-associated reactive arthritis. J Health Popul Nutr. 2013;31(3):299–307.
33. Dworkin MS, Shoemaker PC, Goldoft MJ, Kobayashi JM. Reactive arthritis and Reiter's syndrome following an outbreak of gastroenteritis caused by *Salmonella* enteritidis. Clin Infect Dis. 2001;33(7):1010–4.
34. Locht H, Molbak K, Krogfelt KA. High frequency of reactive joint symptoms after an outbreak of *Salmonella* enteritidis. J Rheumatol. 2002;29(4):767–71.
35. Tuompo R, Hannu T, Mattila L, Siitonen A, Leirisalo-Repo M. Reactive arthritis following *Salmonella* infection: a population-based study. Scand J Rheumatol. 2013;42(3):196–202.
36. Townes JM, Deodhar AA, Laine ES, Smith K, Krug HE, Barkhuizen A, Thompson ME, Cieslak PR, Sobel J. Reactive arthritis following culture-confirmed infections with bacterial enteric pathogens in Minnesota and Oregon: a population-based study. Ann Rheum Dis. 2008;67(12):1689–96.
37. Ekman P, Kirveskari J, Granfors K. Modification of disease outcome in *Salmonella*-infected patients by HLA-B27. Arthritis Rheum. 2000;43(7):1527–34.
38. Rosner BM, Stark K, Hohle M, Werber D. Risk factors for sporadic *Yersinia enterocolitica* infections, Germany 2009-2010. Epidemiol Infect. 2012;140(10):1738–47.
39. Vasala M, Hallanvuo S, Ruuska P, Suokas R, Siitonen A, Hakala M. High frequency of reactive arthritis in adults after *Yersinia pseudotuberculosis* O:1 outbreak caused by contaminated grated carrots. Ann Rheum Dis. 2014;73(10):1793–6.
40. Hannu T, Mattila L, Nuorti JP, Ruutu P, Mikkola J, Siitonen A, Leirisalo-Repo M. Reactive arthritis after an outbreak of *Yersinia pseudotuberculosis* serotype O:3 infection. Ann Rheum Dis. 2003;62(9):866–9.
41. Leirisalo-Repo M, Suoranta H. Ten-year follow-up study of patients with *Yersinia* arthritis. Arthritis Rheum. 1988;31(4):533–7.
42. Rautelin H, Hanninen ML. *Campylobacters*: the most common bacterial enteropathogens in the Nordic countries. Ann Med. 2000;32(7):440–5.
43. Pope JE, Krizova A, Garg AX, Thiessen-Philbrook H, Ouimet JM. *Campylobacter* reactive arthritis: a systematic review. Semin Arthritis Rheum. 2007;37(1):48–55.
44. Hannu T, Mattila L, Rautelin H, Pelkonen P, Lahdenne P, Siitonen A, Leirisalo-Repo M. *Campylobacter*-triggered reactive arthritis: a population-based study. Rheumatology (Oxford). 2002;41(3):312–8.
45. Locht H, Krogfelt KA. Comparison of rheumatological and gastrointestinal symptoms after infection with *Campylobacter jejuni/coli* and enterotoxigenic *Escherichia coli*. Ann Rheum Dis. 2002;61(5):448–52.
46. Keithlin J, Sargeant J, Thomas MK, Fazil A. Systematic review and meta-analysis of the proportion of *Campylobacter* cases that develop chronic sequelae. BMC Public Health. 2014;14:1203.
47. Esan OB, Pearce M, van Hecke O, Roberts N, Collins DR, Violato M, McCarthy N, Perera R, Fanshawe TR. Factors associated with Sequelae of *Campylobacter* and non-typhoidal *Salmonella* infections: a systematic review. EBioMedicine. 2017;15:100–11.
48. Johanesen PA, Mackin KE, Hutton ML, Awad MM, Larcombe S, Amy JM, Lyras D. Disruption of the gut Microbiome: Clostridium difficile infection and the threat of antibiotic resistance. Genes (Basel). 2015;6(4):1347–60.
49. Prati C, Bertolini E, Toussirot E, Wendling D. Reactive arthritis due to Clostridium difficile. Joint Bone Spine. 2010;77(2):190–2.
50. Cappella M, Pugliese F, Zucchini A, Marchetti F. Clostridium difficile Enterocolitis and reactive arthritis: a case report and review of the literature. Case Rep Pediatr. 2016;2016:1591753.
51. Granfors K, Jalkanen S, Lindberg AA, Maki-Ikola O, von Essen R, Lahesmaa-Rantala R, Isomaki H, Saario R, Arnold WJ, Toivanen A. *Salmonella* lipopolysaccharide in synovial cells from patients with reactive arthritis. Lancet. 1990;335(8691):685–8.
52. Granfors K, Jalkanen S, von Essen R, Lahesmaa-Rantala R, Isomaki O, Pekkola-Heino K, Merilahti-Palo R, Saario R, Isomaki H, Toivanen A. *Yersinia* antigens in synovial-fluid cells from patients with reactive arthritis. N Engl J Med. 1989;320(4):216–21.
53. Gaston JS, Cox C, Granfors K. Clinical and experimental evidence for persistent *Yersinia* infection in reactive arthritis. Arthritis Rheum. 1999;42(10):2239–42.
54. Braun J, Tuszewski M, Ehlers S, Haberle J, Bollow M, Eggens U, Distler A, Sieper J. Nested polymerase chain reaction strategy simultaneously targeting DNA sequences of multiple bacterial species in inflammatory joint diseases. II. Examination of sacroiliac and knee joint biopsies of patients with spondyloarthropathies and other arthritides. J Rheumatol. 1997;24(6):1101–5.
55. Granfors K, Viljanen M, Tiilikainen A, Toivanen A. Persistence of IgM, IgG, and IgA antibodies to *Yersinia* in *Yersinia* arthritis. J Infect Dis. 1980;141(4):424–9.
56. de Koning J, Heesemann J, Hoogkamp-Korstanje JA, Festen JJ, Houtman PM, van Oijen PL. *Yersinia* in intestinal biopsy specimens from patients with seronegative spondyloarthropathy: correlation with specific serum IgA antibodies. J Infect Dis. 1989;159(1):109–12.
57. Granfors K, Merilahti-Palo R, Luukkainen R, Mottonen T, Lahesmaa R, Probst P, Marker-Hermann

E, Toivanen P. Persistence of *Yersinia* antigens in peripheral blood cells from patients with *Yersinia enterocolitica* O:3 infection with or without reactive arthritis. Arthritis Rheum. 1998;41(5):855–62.
58. Braun J, Yin Z, Spiller I, Siegert S, Rudwaleit M, Liu L, Radbruch A, Sieper J. Low secretion of tumor necrosis factor alpha, but no other Th1 or Th2 cytokines, by peripheral blood mononuclear cells correlates with chronicity in reactive arthritis. Arthritis Rheum. 1999;42(10):2039–44.
59. Saarinen M, Ekman P, Ikeda M, Virtala M, Gronberg A, Yu DT, Arvilommi H, Granfors K. Invasion of *Salmonella* into human intestinal epithelial cells is modulated by HLA-B27. Rheumatology (Oxford). 2002;41(6):651–7.
60. Granfors K. Host-microbe interaction in reactive arthritis: does HLA-B27 have a direct effect? J Rheumatol. 1998;25(9):1659–61.
61. Schumacher HR Jr, Gerard HC, Arayssi TK, Pando JA, Branigan PJ, Saaibi DL, Hudson AP. Lower prevalence of *Chlamydia* pneumoniae DNA compared with *Chlamydia* trachomatis DNA in synovial tissue of arthritis patients. Arthritis Rheum. 1999;42(9):1889–93.
62. Hay EM, Winfield J, McKendrick MW. Reactive arthritis associated with cryptosporidium enteritis. Br Med J (Clin Res Ed). 1987;295(6592):248.
63. Borman P, Seckin U, Ozoran K. Beaver fever--a rare cause of reactive arthritis. J Rheumatol. 2001;28(3):683.
64. Renou F, Wartel G, Raffray L, Kuli B, Fayeulle S, Yvin JL. Reactive arthritis due to *Escherichia coli* urinary tract infection. Rev Med Interne. 2011;32(1):e4–5.
65. Valtonen VV, Leirisalo M, Pentikainen PJ, Rasanen T, Seppala I, Larinkari U, Ranki M, Koskimies S, Malkamaki M, Makela PH. Triggering infections in reactive arthritis. Ann Rheum Dis. 1985;44(6):399–405.
66. Ben Abdelghani K, Fazaa A, Souabni L, Zakraoui L. Reactive arthritis induced by intravesical BCG therapy for bladder cancer. BMJ Case Rep. 2014;2014:bcr2013202741.
67. Kroot EJ, Hazes JM, Colin EM, Dolhain RJ. Poncet's disease: reactive arthritis accompanying tuberculosis. Two case reports and a review of the literature. Rheumatology (Oxford). 2007;46(3):484–9.
68. Barber CE, Kim J, Inman RD, Esdaile JM, James MT. Antibiotics for treatment of reactive arthritis: a systematic review and meta-analysis. J Rheumatol. 2013;40(6):916–28.
69. Kvien TK, Gaston JS, Bardin T, Butrimiene I, Dijkmans BA, Leirisalo-Repo M, Solakov P, Altwegg M, Mowinckel P, Plan PA, et al. Three month treatment of reactive arthritis with azithromycin: a EULAR double blind, placebo controlled study. Ann Rheum Dis. 2004;63(9):1113–9.
70. Carter JD, Espinoza LR, Inman RD, Sneed KB, Ricca LR, Vasey FB, Valeriano J, Stanich JA, Oszust C, Gerard HC, et al. Combination antibiotics as a treatment for chronic *Chlamydia*-induced reactive arthritis: a double-blind, placebo-controlled, prospective trial. Arthritis Rheum. 2010;62(5):1298–307.
71. Hoogkamp-Korstanje JA, Moesker H, Bruyn GA. Ciprofloxacin v placebo for treatment of *Yersinia enterocolitica* triggered reactive arthritis. Ann Rheum Dis. 2000;59(11):914–7.
72. Calin A. A placebo controlled, crossover study of azathioprine in Reiter's syndrome. Ann Rheum Dis. 1986;45(8):653–5.
73. Clegg DO, Reda DJ, Abdellatif M. Comparison of sulfasalazine and placebo for the treatment of axial and peripheral articular manifestations of the seronegative spondylarthropathies: a Department of Veterans Affairs cooperative study. Arthritis Rheum. 1999;42(11):2325–9.
74. Lally EV, Ho G Jr. A review of methotrexate therapy in Reiter syndrome. Semin Arthritis Rheum. 1985;15(2):139–45.
75. Brinster A, Guillot X, Prati C, Wendling D. Anti-TNF treatment of reactive arthritis. A monocentric experience. Joint Bone Spine. 2017;84(2):237–8.
76. Meyer A, Chatelus E, Wendling D, Berthelot JM, Dernis E, Houvenagel E, Morel J, Richer O, Schaeverbeke T, Gottenberg JE, et al. Safety and efficacy of anti-tumor necrosis factor alpha therapy in ten patients with recent-onset refractory reactive arthritis. Arthritis Rheum. 2011;63(5):1274–80.
77. Tanaka T, Kuwahara Y, Shima Y, Hirano T, Kawai M, Ogawa M, Arimitsu J, Hagihara K, Narazaki M, Ogata A, et al. Successful treatment of reactive arthritis with a humanized anti-interleukin-6 receptor antibody, tocilizumab. Arthritis Rheum. 2009;61(12):1762–4.

Systemic Lupus Erythematosus

21

Gaafar Ragab, Carina Dehner, Hazem Hamza, and Martin Kriegel

Abbreviations

AZA	Azathioprine
CCR6	Chemokine receptor 6
CMV	Cytomegalovirus
CRP	C-reactive protein
CSF	Cerebrospinal fluid
cSLE	Childhood systemic lupus erythematosus
CW	Cutaneous warts
ESRD	End stage renal disease
HAI	Hospital-acquired infection
HBV	Hepatitis B virus
HLA	Human leukocyte antigen
HPV	Human papillomavirus
HR	Hazard ratio
HZI	Herpes zoster infection
IBLs	Infected brain lesions
IFI	Invasive fungal infection
IFN	Interferon
JCV	John Cunningham virus
LMP1	Latent membrane protein
LN	Lupus nephritis
LPS	Lipopolysaccharides
MMF	Mycophenolate mofetil
NETs	Neutrophil extracellular traps
NKs	Natural killer cells
PCT	Procalcitonin
PDC	Plasmacytoid dendritic cells
PMNs	Polymorphonuclear cells
PRRs	Pattern recognition receptors
RA	Rheumatoid arthritis
ROS	Reactive oxygen species
SBE	Subacute bacterial endocarditis
SFB	Segmented filamentous bacteria
SLE	Systemic lupus erythematosus
SLEDAI	Systemic lupus erythematosus disease activity index
SMR	Standardized mortality ratio
SMRs	Standardized mortality ratios
TB	Tuberculosis
Tfh	Follicular helper T cells
TLR	Toll-like receptors
Tregs	Regulatory T cells
UTI	Urinary tract infections

G. Ragab (✉)
Rheumatology and Clinical Immunology Unit, Department of Internal Medicine, Faculty of Medicine, Cairo University, Cairo, Egypt
e-mail: gragab@kasralainy.edu.eg

C. Dehner
Department of Immunobiology, Yale School of Medicine, New Haven, CT, USA

H. Hamza
Virology Laboratory, National Research Centre, Cairo, Egypt

Department of Immunology, Interfaculty Institute of Cell Biology, Eberhard Karls University Tübingen, Tübingen, Germany

M. Kriegel
Department of Immunobiology, Yale School of Medicine, New Haven, CT, USA

G. Ragab et al. (eds.), *The Microbiome in Rheumatic Diseases and Infection*,
https://doi.org/10.1007/978-3-319-79026-8_21

Introduction

Systemic lupus erythematosus (SLE) is the epitome of autoimmune diseases. The pathogenesis, clinical manifestations, and management of SLE involve various aspects of microorganisms, either as potential triggers and perpetuators of disease, as infectious episodes, as complications from underlying immune dysregulation, or as adverse events from chronic immunosuppression. Despite significant progress that has been made in understanding the contributions of microorganisms to SLE, there are many questions that need to be answered.

Besides environmental factors, genetic risk factors have long been established to be important in the pathogenesis of autoimmune diseases including SLE. Several clinical case studies uncovered a family history of patients with either the same or closely related autoimmune diseases, which supports the possibility that a common genetic predisposition is at the core of autoimmune diseases [1]. Multiple genetic and genome-wide association studies have firmly established that HLA class II polymorphisms are a major genetic risk factor in many autoimmune diseases, as shown in detail for instance in rheumatoid arthritis (RA) [2, 3]. However, a genetically predisposed individual usually requires environmental exposures to initiate overt autoimmunity. With regard to potential triggers, infectious agents have long been implicated and are discussed herein.

The Role of Microorganisms in the Pathogenesis of SLE

The Microbiome

Chronic inflammatory disorders such as type 1 diabetes, Crohn's disease, or rheumatoid arthritis (RA) have been linked to gut microbial dysbiosis together with immune dysregulation. In addition, recent research suggests that early-life events and environmental factors play a significant role in the development of the adult immune system. In particular, diet and early-life exposures, e.g., infectious episodes or antibiotic exposures, influence immune cell numbers and functions. These factors are also influenced by the microbiota supporting an intricate interaction between environmental factors, the microbiota, and the host [4]. Additionally, the gut microbial communities change with increasing age, so another factor that contributes to dysbiosis is early-life perturbations [5]. Notably, several studies have shown that depletion of the gut microbiota in murine autoimmune models can affect autoantibody production as well as mortality [6]. Exact mechanisms through which the microbiota influences chronic immune-mediated diseases such as lupus remain to be established, but a multitude of effects on innate and adaptive immune cell functions are likely. In this chapter, we will focus on the effect of the microbiota on adaptive immune responses with implications for organ-specific and systemic autoimmunity and allude to potential roles in SLE.

Several groups have demonstrated in murine autoimmune models for multiple sclerosis or rheumatoid arthritis that Th17 cells, a subpopulation of CD4 T cells, are crucial in disease pathogenesis [7]. This subpopulation is characterized by expression of the chemokine receptor CCR6 as well as production of the inflammatory cytokine IL-17 [8, 9]. Th17 cells are, however, not the only cell type secreting IL-17. Voo et al. [10] have shown that there are a significant number of human $CD4^+$ $FOXP3^+$ regulatory T cells (Tregs) that have the capability to produce IL-17 upon activation, a subset that could not be found in the thymus. These are thought to be important in antimicrobial defense besides their regulatory function in autoimmunity and inflammation [10]. The differentiation of Tregs into an effector subset that is able to produce IL-17 may be mediated by epigenetic modifications [11]. This phenomenon may have evolved as a potent mechanism of the immune system to adapt to the vast variety of immune responses at different locations of the human body and at different stages of an immune response [12]. Th17 and Treg cells are the best-known counterparts in balancing the body's propensity to autoimmunity versus health and homeostasis.

Interestingly, both of the above CD4 helper subsets (Th17 and Tregs) are profoundly influenced by the microbiota. Induction of Tregs by certain microbiota has been reviewed in Chap. 5.

Herein, we summarize the role of gut commensals in the induction of Th17 cells. In mice, segmented filamentous bacteria (SFB), *Candidatus Arthromitus* or *Candidatus Savagella* are known as unique commensal bacteria that are able to stimulate maturation of the lymphoid cell compartments and to specifically induce Th17 cells in the small intestine [13]. Recently, a group in France succeeded for the first time in culturing SFB in vitro by mimicking their replicative niche, making it possible to study in detail its host interactions [13]. Importantly, SFB are capable of promoting pathogenic Th17 responses in mouse models of RA and multiple sclerosis. Thus, a possible influence of SFB on the pathogenesis of SLE seemed plausible, but studies using a lupus-prone mouse model suggest that SFB colonization might neither induce Th17 responses nor increase the incidence of disease [14].

Another important aspect of SFB biology is that these bacteria induce high levels of mucosal IgA and are highly IgA-coated. IgA is crucial for the homeostasis of the gut microbiota. Different levels of IgA coating of the microbiota have been exploited to identify pathogenic members of the human microbiota in inflammatory bowel disease [15]. It remains to be seen if extreme levels of IgA coating exist in non-gut diseases. An increased level of secretory IgA has been associated with intestinal dysbiosis in inflammatory bowel disease as well as psoriatic arthritis although the significance of this finding is unclear in the latter case [15, 16].

Production of high-affinity IgA is supported by a special subset of helper T cells, the T follicular helper (Tfh) cells, that have emerged as key players in the differentiation of memory B cells at several stages [17]. Interestingly, it has been suggested that Th17 cells act as progenitors for a subset of Tfh cells to promote the production of high-affinity IgA against commensal microbes [18]. This process is thought to occur via MyD88 signaling as loss of this pathway is accompanied by an inefficient IgA response as well as an altered commensal composition favoring a more inflammatory environment [19]. Several studies using lupus-prone animal models in addition to samples from human subjects demonstrated that these cells are involved in the production of pathogenic autoantibodies. A recent study showed increased Tfh-like cells ($CXCR5^+ICOS^+PD\text{-}1^+$) in SLE patient blood compared to healthy controls, which did not correlate with disease activity [20]. Thus, these cells may be considered as a marker of germinal center B-cell dysregulation. As detailed above, since Tfh cells are influenced by the gut microbiota, it is plausible to assume that the microbiota plays a role in the pathogenesis of human SLE. Over the last few years, exploratory studies on the contents of the microbiota in SLE have been published. A summary of four recent studies related to the human microbiota in SLE are listed in Table 21.1.

Various mechanisms have been ascribed to microbially triggered autoimmunity including molecular mimicry. As detailed also in Chap. 6, several studies in murine models of autoimmunity have established a role for commensal bacteria as potential chronic triggers, although the exact mechanisms remain unclear [25]. As the human gut microbiota provides an enormous source of persistent antigenic variation, it is plausible that molecular mimicry via cross-reactive antigen within the microbiome could be a chronic trigger of autoreactive lymphocytes, in particular those that are recognizing the earliest autoantigen in most lupus patients, the Ro60 protein, a conserved regulatory RNA-binding protein. Interestingly, certain human gut commensals encode Ro60 orthologs, which suggests that patients that are colonized with Ro60 ortholog-containing bacteria could develop cross-reactive responses to human Ro60 protein that eventually lead to pathogenic responses based on their HLA class II-related genetic predisposition. Indeed, experimental support for such a scenario is accumPulating [26].

In summary, many facets of the microbiota could influence the pathogenesis of SLE. Besides various innate immune interactions with the microbiota, adaptive immune responses described here—Treg/Th17 balances, Tfh, and IgA levels—are influenced by the microbiota and potentially dysregulated in lupus. It is important to note that there are likely even more host-microbiota interactions impinging on innate immunity that are

Table 21.1 Studies on the human microbiome in SLE patients

Source	Key findings	Comments
Intestinal dysbiosis associated with SLE [21]	16S rDNA sequencing of fecal samples from 20 SLE patients vs healthy donors revealed: (a) Comparable diversity between groups based on Shannon diversity index; significantly lower Firmicutes/Bacteroidetes ratio in SLE vs healthy as characterized in other autoimmune diseases (b) Decrease of some families within the Firmicutes, increase of Bacteroidetes opposite to obesity microbiota studies (c) In silico overrepresentation of oxidative phosphorylation and glycan utilization in SLE patient microbiota (d) Most abundant family in both subject groups was *Lachnospiraceae*	(a) Study examined only SLE patients in remission (1) Patients with more active disease are missing (2) Drug therapy prior to the study could have altered the microbiota (b) All patients were Caucasian
Ranking the impact of human health disorders on gut metabolism: Systemic lupus erythematosus and obesity as study cases [22]	(a) Statistically significant differences between patients and controls in composition of fecal metabolome (b) Mass spectroscopy (MS) signals were highly similar in all SLE patients regardless of age, BMI, disease duration, dietary intake, lifestyle, or medical history, while the MS signals of healthy subjects differed according to BMI status. SLE samples: decreased levels of components necessary for peptidoglycan cell wall synthesis; decreased molecules needed for heme synthesis (c) Conclusion: immune status of SLE is a dominant factor in the fecal metabolome, while in healthy subject BMI becomes driving factor determining microbial metabolism	– Healthy subjects but not SLE patients were selected based on BMI ranges, thereby possibly affecting the conclusions of this study
Th17 responses and natural IgM antibodies are related to gut microbiota composition in systemic lupus erythematosus patients [23]	(a) SLE fecal samples promoted lymphocyte activation and Th17 differentiation to a greater extent than healthy control microbiota (b) Enrichment of SLE microbiota with Treg-inducing bacteria reduced the Th17/Th1 balance; *Bifidobacterium bifidum* supplementation prevented $CD4^+$ lymphocyte overactivation (probiotics) (c) Ex vivo: increased Th17 and $Foxp3^+$ $IL\text{-}17^+$ populations (d) Negative correlation between $IL\text{-}17^+$ populations and Firmicutes in healthy controls (e) In SLE: proportion of Firmicutes correlated directly with serum levels of IFN-γ (f) Firmicutes/Bacteroidetes ratio reduced in SLE patients if anti-dsDNA titers increased; strong negative correlation with IL-6 serum levels; positive correlation with protective natural IgM antibodies against phosphorylcholine	– Significance of correlative findings unclear without in vitro or vivo studies to corroborate these findings
Association between *Staphylococcus aureus* nasal carriage and disease phenotype in patients affected by systemic lupus erythematosus [24]	(a) *S. aureus* colonization is frequent in patients with SLE and healthy subjects (21.4% vs 28.6%) (b) Presence of colonization associated with certain SLE phenotypes (renal involvement, autoantibody positivity) suggests that changes in the skin microbiota might be linked with SLE severity	(a) Study mainly based on questionnaires (b) No microbiome analyses performed

equally important in SLE pathogenesis, including activation of the inflammasome in lupus nephritis (LN) [27] or overstimulation of TLR signaling leading to an increased production of inflammatory cytokines and type I interferon (IFN) [28]. More research is needed to understand the multifaceted roles the microbiota may play in the pathogenesis of SLE.

The Pathogenic Microorganisms

Several studies on experimental animal models demonstrated that infectious agents are capable of breaking immunological tolerance to self-antigen inducing autoimmunity [29]. The list of microorganisms associated with human SLE includes parvovirus B19 [30], CMV [31, 32], retroviruses [31, 33], dengue virus [34], HPV vaccination or infection [35], *Toxocara canis* [36], and *Mycobacterium tuberculosis* [31], but the most compelling evidence supports a role for Epstein-Barr virus (EBV). Many SLE patients negative for anti-dsDNA antibodies showed abnormal antibody responses to EBV: they produced IgG antibodies to EBV antigens to which healthy controls did not respond and failed to make antibodies to EBV antigens seen in healthy controls [37].

It was reported that the positive rate of EBV-encoded latent membrane protein 1 (LMP1) in the renal tissues was significantly higher in young patients with LN compared to controls [38]. The positive rate was similar between patients of initial onset and relapse, and there was no detectable difference between the patients with and without infection. The findings support the hypothesis that EBV reactivation is associated with SLE induction with a potential role of EBV-encoded LMP1 in this process.

Rasmussen et al. [39] studied 57 SLE patients and 29 healthy controls using plasma galectin-3-binding protein as a surrogate marker of type I IFN activity. They showed that the marker's concentrations were significantly higher in SLE patients and associated positively with EBV early antigen diffuse (EBV EA/D)-directed antibodies and the presence of antibodies against extractable nuclear antigens [39].

In addition, Draborg et al. [40] demonstrated that there was an impaired regulation of the immune response against latent and lytic cycle EBV infection in SLE, even in the absence of lymphopenia, which further supported the proposed general dysfunction of leukocytes and their cytokine regulation in SLE patients. Reviewing the numerous experimental studies on EBV establishing an association with SLE, Draborg et al. [40] theorized that the interplay between an impaired immune system and the cumulative effects of EBV and other viruses results in frequent reactivation of EBV and enhanced cell death, leading to autoreactivity and development of SLE.

Type I INF family comprises 12 IFN-α subtypes and IFN-β, IFN-ε, IFN-κ, and IFN-ω. Normally, IFN-α and IFN-β production is strictly controlled but starts rapidly when viral or bacterial nucleic acids are sensed by pattern recognition receptors (PRRs) [41]. Two cell types capable of secreting large amounts of IFN-α and IFN-β are plasmacytoid dendritic cells (PDC) and monocytes. Monocytes respond mainly to dsRNA, certain RNA viruses such as Sendai and influenza virus, whereas PDCs can be triggered to secrete type I IFN by almost all viruses and some bacteria [42].

As microbial RNA and DNA can be recognized by multiple nucleic acid sensors and thereby induce production of type I IFNs, this may be the mechanism by which several microorganisms can contribute to the development and relapse of SLE [43]. An increase in the expression of long interspersed nuclear element 1 (LINE-1) was reported in kidney biopsies from patients with LN and transcript expression correlated with the tissue expression of type I IFN [44]. This connection may suggest that endogenous retroviruses may play a role in the initiation or amplification of the autoimmune process [43].

A recent study implicated one additional specific organism, *Enterococcus gallinarum*, as an etiologic agent of lupus. Manfredo Vieira et al. [45] studied the (NZW × BXSB)F[1] lupus model, demonstrating a role for the microbiota as evidenced by diminished disease following antibiotic therapy. Antibiotics also strengthened the gut wall barrier, preventing translocation of bacteria into the mesenteric lymph nodes, mesenteric veins, and liver. *E. gallinarum* specifically was able to weaken the barrier defense and induce pro-inflammatory intestinal changes in mice, and its translocation specifically upregulated lupus-associated autoantibody production, and vaccination against *E. gallinarum* was protective against the diseaes in mice. Finally, in humans, this organism was present in the livers of 3/3 lupus patients who underwent biopsy, compared to 0/6 healthy liver transplant donors.

The Protective Role of Infectious Agents and Parasites

Contrary to this, there are other studies that support the notion of a protective role of other organisms. Experimental animal studies showed that hepatitis B virus plays a protective role against SLE [46]. Gamma-irradiated *Plasmodium chabaudi* infection of lupus-prone BWF1 mice ameliorated the histopathological changes attributed to renal involvement in lupus [47]. Another study showed that infection of female BWF1 lupus mice with malaria parasites attenuated B-cell autoreactivity [48]. Chen et al. demonstrated that *Toxoplasma gondii* infection may prevent the progression of SLE-related nephritis in New Zealand Black/New Zealand White F1 mice and was associated with downregulated intracellular expression of IFN-γ and IL-10 [49]. Fischer et al. evaluated the seroprevalence of anti-*T. gondii* antibodies in European patients with rheumatoid arthritis (RA) and SLE. They found a higher prevalence of anti-*T. gondii* antibodies in those with RA than in SLE patients (63% vs 36%, respectively) and that the rates of seropositivity of IgG against other infectious agents were comparable between the two groups [50].

Sowalha and his group investigated the prevalence of *Helicobacter pylori* seropositivity in a cohort of 466 patients with SLE, finding a low rate of specific *H. pylori* antibodies suggesting that *H. pylori* might exert a protective role on the risk of developing SLE [51]. Furthermore, it has been reported that in filarial endemic areas in India, patients with SLE do not suffer from concomitant filariasis. Filarial infestation was found to be associated with a low plasma level of IL-17A, which may contribute to protection from the development of autoimmune disorders like SLE [52].

Many pathogens have developed efficient methods to overcome adaptive immune mechanisms, and there is growing evidence that they are capable of insinuating their own anti-immune strategies into a susceptible host. They can block antigen presentation interference with Toll-like receptor signaling and alter the cytokine milieu, which is crucial for an effective immune response. They may also cause antigenic competition, the tendency of strong antigens, particularly from infectious agents, to impair antibody responses to weaker ones, which would dampen immune responses against self-antigens [53, 54].

Risk Factors for Infection in SLE

SLE patients have an increased frequency of severe bacterial and viral infections, possibly due to inherited genetic and immunological defects as well as due to chronic immunosuppressive therapies [55].

Doaty et al. [31] in their review of literature cited innate immunity disturbance in SLE patients that included:

(a) Breakdown of epithelial barriers in SLE patients caused by rashes, ulcers, and wounds allowing entry of infectious agents in the body.
(b) Accumulation of gamma delta T cells in skin of SLE patients as compared to healthy subjects [56]. These cells are implicated in epithelial breakdown, further increasing the risk of infection [57].
(c) Impaired production of IL-8 and IL-12 by PMNs with disruption of the links between the innate and adaptive systems mediated by IL-12 [58].
(d) Deficiencies of the early components of the classical pathway of the complement system (C1q, C4, and C2). A higher prevalence of these genetic defects has been established in SLE, but acquired complement deficiency because of consumption due to immune complex disease may also play a role in predisposing SLE patients to infection by encapsulated organisms [59–61]. Furthermore, single nucleotide polymorphisms have been reported associated with mannose-binding lectin deficiency in SLE patients, further increasing their susceptibility to infection [62, 63].

(e) Decreased levels of complement receptors CR1 and CR2 on B cells, PMNs, and RBCs in SLE patents [64].
(f) Suppressed natural killer (NK)-cell cytotoxicity with fewer NK cells [65] and weaker NK response to IL-2 stimulation [66].

Inappropriate or dysfunctional antigen presentation by DCs might promote the breakdown of T-cell and B-cell tolerance in SLE and other autoimmune diseases. Patients with SLE show multiple DC abnormalities, including a reduced number of circulating conventional DCs but increased numbers of PDCs [67].

Neutrophils show several facets of dysregulation in SLE. Impaired phagocytosis by neutrophils in SLE has been described in multiple reports and might contribute to the increased susceptibility to infection associated with this disease [68]. In one study, neutrophils from patients with SLE showed reduced production of reactive oxygen species (ROS), which correlated with disease severity and end-organ damage [69]. Patients with chronic granulomatous disease, in which ROS production is defective, have a high incidence of SLE [70, 71]. Patients with SLE have an abnormal subset of neutrophils (termed low-density granulocytes) with an increased propensity for NETosis [72]. NETosis is a mechanism of cell death that occurs in response to various stimuli, including infectious organisms and oxidative stress. NETosis involves the extrusion of chromatin and other nuclear, cytoplasmic, and granular material from the cell. This extruded material, called neutrophil extracellular traps (NETs), contains proinflammatory cytokines, antimicrobial peptides, enzymes such as myeloperoxidase, and potentially antigenic citrullinated histones and dsDNA [73].

Other workers reported that leukopenia, in particular lymphopenia, was a common finding in SLE. In their work, however, it was not persistent [74]. SLE patients can also develop granulocytopenia due to anti-granulocyte antibodies or complications from chronic immunosuppression. If neutropenia is severe enough, the impaired function of PMNs in SLE predisposes to severe bacterial infections. It was reported [68] that regardless of infection status, medication, or disease activity, pediatric-onset SLE patients have impaired phagocytic ability against *Salmonella*-specific lipopolysaccharides (LPS) which is not influenced by the use of immunosuppressants. The same study [68] did not find deficiency of peroxidase production and chemotaxis activity in SLE patients; however, serum complement levels were not reported.

In the earlier review by Doaty et al. [31], they also reported adaptive immunity disturbances such as:

(a) Impaired production of IFN-γ, IL-1, IL-2, and TNF-α contributing to T-cell dysfunction [75]
(b) Reduced numbers and dysfunction of all B-cell lines: naïve, memory, and plasma cells

Hypogammaglobulinemia has been attributed to immunosuppressive therapy in SLE patients even in the absence of therapy with B-cell-depleting agents. Isolated IgM [76] and IgA [77] were reported in SLE patients; however their contribution to an increased risk of infection was not shown. Therefore, it has been recommended in one report to measure immunoglobulin levels during the course of SLE treatment [78].

More than 80 genetic loci are reported to show robust genetic associations with SLE [79–82]. More than half of these loci are connected to the type I IFN system [83]. Genome-wide association studies have revealed single nucleotide polymorphisms in the STAT4 gene, which codes for a protein involved in type I interferon receptor signal transduction, that are associated with enhanced protein production [84]. The NCF1 gene encodes the p47phox/Ncf1 protein of the NADPH oxidase (NOX2) complex, which is critical for the induction of ROS. The NCF1 gene is highly complex and has excluded SNPs in NCF1 in genome-wide association studies. It has been recently reported that an amino acid replacement in NCF1, leading to a lower capacity of inducing oxidative burst, is strongly associated with SLE [85, 86]. This observation aligns with the previously reported association of an ROS-reducing SNP in the NCF2 gene with SLE [87]. Also, some rare monogenic SLE diseases are now categorized as type I interferonopathies because of the prominent type I IFN signature [43].

In a study by Danza and Ruiz-Irastorza [88], risk factors for infection in SLE included disease activity, prednisone doses over 7.5–10 mg/day, high doses of methylprednisolone, as well as use of chemotherapeutic agents such as cyclophosphamide and multiple courses of rituximab treatment. It is difficult, however, to tease apart the therapeutics from the underlying disease severity that prompted use of these medications. Indeed, lupus patients present with multiple features that pose an increased infection risk, including hypocomplementemia, lymphopenia, and hyposplenism, and data from the 1970s prior to the introduction and widespread use of newer therapies indicated a high risk of mortality from infections early in the disease course, attesting again to the infectious risk associated with active SLE [89].

Lupus Nephritis

Renal involvement occurs in up to 60% of SLE patients [90] and remains a major determinant for morbidity and mortality among these patients [90, 91]. We will focus on this particular organ as a notorious example of the interplay between the disease and infection.

Feldman et al. [92] studied serious infections among adult Medicaid beneficiaries with SLE and LN over the years 2000–2010. They identified 33,565 patients with SLE, of whom 7113 had LN. There were 9078 serious infections reported in 7078 SLE patients, whereas in 1825 LN patients, there were 3494 reports. Infection incidence rate per 100 person-year was 10.8 in the SLE cohort and 23.9 in the LN sub-cohort.

Therapeutic modalities used in LN management, either as induction therapy or for maintenance treatment, influence the prognosis of LN. An Egyptian study retrospectively analyzed records of 928 SLE patients with biopsy-confirmed LN seen between 2006 and 2012 at Cairo University hospitals [93]. The reported complications included pneumonia requiring hospitalization in 93/575 (16.1%) patients who received intravenous cyclophosphamide as induction therapy, compared to 22 of 321 (6.9%) patients in the group that received mycophenolate. However, the difference between these two groups was not statistically significant ($p = 0.270$). Herpes zoster infection (HZI) was reported in 12 (1.3%) patients. The 5-year mortality was 7.4%. Sepsis was responsible for death in 68.1%, which was higher than the percentages reported in Europe (25%) [94] and China (60%) [95].

In India, Srivastava et al. [96] studied the outcome of LN in childhood-onset SLE (cSLE) retrospectively from 1989 to 2013. Among 205 children with cSLE, 134 had evidence of LN. During the follow-up period, 11 (8.2%) children died, and infections were the leading cause of death.

Lin et al. [97] conducted a nationwide cohort study of 7326 patients with newly diagnosed SLE and no history of end-stage renal disease (ESRD). They derived their data from Taiwan's National Health Insurance claims database from 2000 to 2011. Among all SLE patients, 316 (43%) developed ESRD. Multivariate Cox regression analysis indicated that the risk of ESRD increased with the number of infection-related hospitalizations. For patients with three or more infection-related admissions, the hazard ratio (HR) for ESRD was 5.08 (99% CI: 3.74–6.90) relative to those with no infection-related admissions. Analysis by type of infection indicated that bacteremia patients had the greatest risk for ESRD with a HR of 4.82 (95% CI: 3.40–6.85) highlighting the impact of infection on LN outcome.

In South China [98], a group of investigators studied hospital-acquired infections (HAI) in SLE patients. In a multivariate analysis, they found that a history of LN or a higher SLE disease activity index SLEDAI score correlated with HAI [OR: 3.7 ($p < 0.001$) and 1.1 ($p < 0.001$), respectively]. Moreover, treatment with high doses of glucocorticoids or cyclophosphamide was the main risk factor for HAI [OR: 2.7 ($p < 0.001$) and 2.9 ($p < 0.001$), respectively].

Murray et al. [99] studied hospitalization trends for SLE from 2000 to 2011. They identified 361,337 hospitalizations for SLE that were derived from the United States (US) Healthcare Cost and Utilization Project National Inpatient Sample (NIS). A diagnosis of SLE was associated with increased severe and opportunistic infections, including bacteremia, pneumonia, opportunistic fungal infections, herpes zoster (HZ), CMV, and *Pneumocystis jirovecii* pneumonia (PJP). They also found that among SLE hospitalization, rates of all these infections significantly rose between 2000 and 2011, with the exception of PJP which significantly declined. HZ was the only infection that disproportionally increased over time among SLE hospitalizations when compared with non-SLE hospitalizations. They attributed this to the increasingly widespread use of mycophenolate mofetil for induction and maintenance of LN and for severe non-renal lupus. It has been demonstrated that medications used to treat SLE, including prednisone, azathioprine, and cyclophosphamide, increase the risk of HZ [100–104]. In a prospective cohort study of 1485 patients with SLE, the hazard ratio for an incident diagnosis of HZ was greatest in SLE patients treated with mycophenolate mofetil (HR 5.00, 95% CI 1.40–17.60) followed by prednisone [100].

Murray et al. [99] attributed the reduction of PJP in their study to the declining use of cyclophosphamide and increasing use of mycophenolate. Even among patients receiving cyclophosphamide as induction therapy, cumulative doses may be declining over time. The Euro-Lupus Nephritis trial demonstrated equivalent efficacy and a favorable side effect profile for low-dose intravenous cyclophosphamide compared with a previously standard high-dose regime [105, 106]. Also, the American College of Rheumatology recommended mycophenolate or cyclophosphamide for induction of LN with lower cumulative doses of cyclophosphamide ("Euro-Lupus" dosing schedule), followed by mycophenolate or azathioprine for maintenance therapy [107]. Interestingly, animal studies and data from renal transplant trials suggest that mycophenolate may have antimicrobial properties against *P. jirovecii*, although data specific to lupus patients are lacking [108, 109].

Based on the Medicaid Analytic Extract database (2000–2010); Feldman et al. [92] found no difference in the rates of serious infection and mortality among new users of mycophenolate, azathioprine, or cyclophosphamide when examining the 29 most populated US states. Strikingly, antimalarial treatment of SLE patients was associated with an additional benefit in protection against serious infection [110]. In summary, patients with severe lupus, as evidenced by LN, have a high risk of serious infections, including death. It remains unclear the extent to which this higher risk is mediated by the underlying disease severity, versus its therapy. One favorable trend in recent years has been a lower incidence of PJP, potentially attributable to lower cumulative doses of cyclophosphamide and/or more widespread usage of mycophenolate.

The Heavy Burden of Infection on Morbidity and Mortality in SLE

It is well established that infection contributes significantly to the morbidity and mortality of SLE patients. In a South African study [111], the authors reviewed the records of hospitalized SLE patients admitted over a 79-month period. They found that infections accounted for 35.2% of admissions. Among those, pneumonia, cutaneous sepsis, urinary tract infections, and septicemia were the most common types of infection. Organisms commonly isolated were *Staphylococcus aureus*, *Escherichia coli*, and *Klebsiella* species, as well as *Mycobacterium tuberculosis*. The incidence rate ratio for infection in SLE was 1.49 compared to matched controls emphasizing its burden as a comorbidity in the disease [112]. It was found that infection-related hospitalizations are associated with an increased risk of end-stage renal disease in SLE, especially the juvenile-onset type [97]. Souza et al. reported that renal failure and infectious diseases were the most frequent causes of death in Brazilian SLE patients [113]. A Chinese study reported that over time (1986–2012) infections have increased gradually and have become the most frequent cause of death in SLE

[114]. Richie et al. extensively reviewed the literature and reported a total of 17 maternal deaths in women with LN within 6 weeks postpartum. In all cases where mortality was attributed to SLE and nephritis, the patients had active disease, and infection was responsible for 41.2% of deaths [115]. In a meta-analysis that included 26,101 SLE patients with 4640 deaths, the cause-specific standardized mortality ratios (SMRs) were assessed in SLE patients. The SMR for infection was reported as 4980 with a highly significant *p*-value [116]. In a multicenter Southern Chinese study that included 3815 hospitalized patients, infection was the leading cause of death. Features of infection in this group included early disease onset, higher percentage of respiratory tract involvement, and predominance of Gram-negative bacteria with emergence of multidrug-resistant strains and a variety of pathogens [117].

The Clinical Presentations of Infections in SLE

Serious infections are defined as those that lead to hospitalization or death or require intravenous antibiotic treatment [118].

Shen et al. [119] studied the temporal trends among SLE patients in the intensive care unit (ICU) as part of a national population-based study in Taiwan between 1999 and 2008. The incidence of infection rose from 39.1% to 47.2%. The study reported three poor prognostic factors (i.e., older age, infection, and organ dysfunction) that were thought to potentially lessen the temporal improvement of short-term survival in ICU patients with SLE. The authors suggested that improved treatment of SLE reduces and postpones the occurrence of acute critical illness. Their study showed that the median time for SLE diagnosis to ICU admission had increased by 4 years during the 10-year study period. However, the improved survival was achieved at the costs of immune-suppression and accrual of organ damage.

Han et al. [120] studied the clinical presentations and outcomes of SLE patients with infection admitted to the ICU. They demonstrated that SLE patients with infections in the ICU have a higher mortality rate, and a higher APACHE II score compared to SLE patients without infections. SLE with infections also had a higher maximum temperature, higher minimum and maximum systolic blood pressure compared to SLE patients with noninfectious causes of admission.

Musculoskeletal System

Odd presentations of musculoskeletal infections at unusual anatomical sites like the sacroiliac joint [121] and uncommon organisms like *Candida albicans* involving the joints [122] are frequently reported in SLE patients. One rare and frequently misdiagnosed infection in SLE is tropical pyomyositis, primary muscle abscesses most frequently due to *Staphylococcus aureus* and frequently following trauma [123]. Also, hematogenous salmonella osteomyelitis can be encountered in immunocompromised SLE patients, a finding that can be complicated by septic arthritis if not managed promptly [124]. Infection should also be considered when dealing with cases of osteonecrosis [124, 125].

Mucocutaneous and Genital Manifestations

In a retrospective multicenter cohort study involving ten pediatric rheumatology services in São Paulo, Brazil, that included 852 childhood-onset SLE patients, the researchers reported a frequency of 14% of herpes zoster infection (HZI). Hospitalization took place in 61% of these cases, and secondary bacterial infection was reported in 13%. Postherpetic neuralgia occurred in 5%. Lymphopenia and immunosuppressive therapy seemed to be the major factors underlying this complication [126].

There is a special interest concerning human papillomavirus (HPV) in SLE patients. In a meta-analysis, the authors found that cutaneous warts (CW) were present in a higher frequency in SLE patients compared to healthy controls. It is of interest that most of the articles they cited showed that the presence of CW did not correlate with the use of immunosuppressive drugs [127].

SLE female patients have also been shown to have a higher prevalence of genital HPV infection (80.7%) compared to healthy women (35%). The odds ratio (OR) for genital HPV infection in women with SLE was 7.2 [128]. There was no evidence that the use of immunosuppressive drugs was associated with a higher prevalence of HPV infection. This finding together with the study of Silva et al. [127] suggests that the high prevalence of HPV may be due to defects in immune mechanisms that are independent of immunosuppressive drugs. Another study found that in a subset of women diagnosed with SLE in the eastern Brazilian Amazon, 75% of them were HPV positive in the 1–5 years preceding the study [129].

The Urinary Tract

Lupus patients are likely to have urinary tract infections (UTI), with a prevalence of 36%. They usually manifest in the lower tract. They are community acquired, and the most frequently isolated uropathogen is *E.coli* [130].

In an Egyptian cohort of 200 SLE patients who were followed up for one year, the urinary tract was the most common site of infection (31.8%) with 74/230 infectious episodes. *E.coli* was the most common isolated bacterial organism (26/230), followed by *Klebsiella* species (11/230) and *Proteus mirabilis* (8/230), whereas nine cases had mixed infections [131].

Hematological Involvement

Lupus patients with episodes of bacteremia suffer from poor long-term outcome. *E. coli* and *S. aureus* are the leading pathogens reported in this setting. Community-acquired bacteremia and C-reactive protein levels lower than 8 mg/dl during bacteremic episodes are associated with lower long-term mortality [132]. A Danish study involving 5102 patient-years of follow-up [133] reported an increased incidence of arterial and venous thrombosis within 1 year after infection (2.18% and 2.56%, respectively) compared to patients who never had either a hospitalized infection or herpes simplex virus. Infections can also trigger catastrophic antiphospholipid syndrome [134] (see Chap. 22).

The Respiratory System

Respiratory tract infection is a common problem in SLE. Luijten et al. [135] reported the incidence of invasive pneumococcal infections to be 13 times higher in SLE patients than in the general Dutch population. The prevalence of latent tuberculosis infection was reported to be 26.5% in SLE patients [136]. The authors of the study cautioned that higher SLE disease activity index (SLEDAI) and increased glucocorticoid dose were associated with indeterminate results in interferon-gamma release assays. Fungal infections including aspergillosis can occur and may be associated with cavitary lesions that can lead to pneumothorax [137] (Fig. 21.1).

Studying the incidence of diffuse alveolar hemorrhage (DAH) in SLE patients [138], researchers reported 57 episodes of DAH of 50 patients including seven recurrences. They detected infection in 22 episodes (38.6%): 8 invasive fungal infections and 16 bacterial infections, including two patients with both types. These infections were associated with treatment for SLE, requirement for mechanical ventilation, hypocomplementemia, and high CRP levels.

The Gastrointestinal System

In a large prospective cohort study of 2258 SLE patients from the Hopkins Lupus Cohort, Fangtham et al. [139] reported 53,548 cohort visits. Oral candidiasis was diagnosed at 675 visits

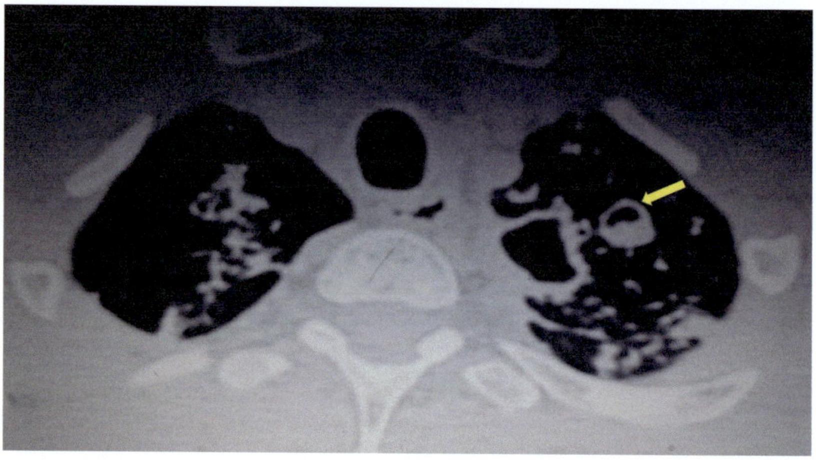

Fig. 21.1 High-resolution chest CT scan with contrast showing a case of SLE with multiple pulmonary fungal cavitary lesions. Arrow: intracavitary mycosis. Microbiological studies diagnosed the case as aspergillosis. *SLE* systemic lupus erythematosus. Courtesy of Dr. Hala El-Guendy, Professor of Internal Medicine, Cairo University

(1.25%), in 325/2258 (14%) of SLE patients. The authors recommended inspection of the oral cavity for signs of oral candidiasis, especially in patients with active disease, proteinuria, high white blood cell count, and intake of prednisone, immunosuppressive drugs, or antibiotics.

Fawzy et al. [140] reported an increase of *Giardia lamblia* infection in SLE patients: 30% in SLE patients compared to 3.3% in healthy, age- and sex-matched controls from the same geographic area. This number was even higher in those who had GI symptoms (52.9%). In acute pancreatitis, the presence of concomitant infections was associated with a poor prognosis in SLE patients [141].

Opportunistic CMV colitis can lead to colonic perforation with life-threatening consequences [142, 143]. In case of significant gastrointestinal symptoms, CMV infection should be considered in SLE patients who are immunosuppressed. SLE was also found to be significantly associated with chronic hepatitis C infection [144].

The Nervous System

Infectious brain lesions (IBLs) are rare presentations in SLE patients. They can, however, be life-threatening in this context. Xu et al. [145] described 15 patients with IBLs. They reported the following characteristics: fever in 80% of cases, headache and focal neurological signs (73.3%), associated pulmonary infection (66.7%), and associated meningitis (40%). There were ring-enhancing lesions in enhanced magnetic resonance imaging in all patients (100%) (Fig. 21.2).

Progressive multifocal leukoencephalopathy (PML) has been reported in SLE patients treated with various immunosuppressive therapies including biological drugs (e.g., rituximab or belimumab). It was suggested that severe lymphopenia may be responsible for John Cunningham virus (JCV) reactivation, the causative agent of PML. Early infection screening, antiviral therapy, and effective management of lymphopenia are important in this setting [146]. Diagnosis of PML is generally made by identification of the virus in CSF by PCR along with consistent imaging and clinical features [147]. CSF lactate is a good single indicator and a better marker, compared to other conventional markers, to distinguish bacterial meningitis from aseptic meningitis [148, 149].

Cryptococcal meningitis [150] and meningoencephalitis [151] can be fatal in SLE patients. Epidural infection, an uncommon condition, can be caused by *Salmonella enteritidis*, which was also reported in SLE [152]. An early diagnosis and prompt treatment is essential to prevent mortality.

Invasive and Disseminated Infections

Miliary TB with fatal consequences has been reported in juvenile SLE patients in Brazil. The authors stressed the importance of routine

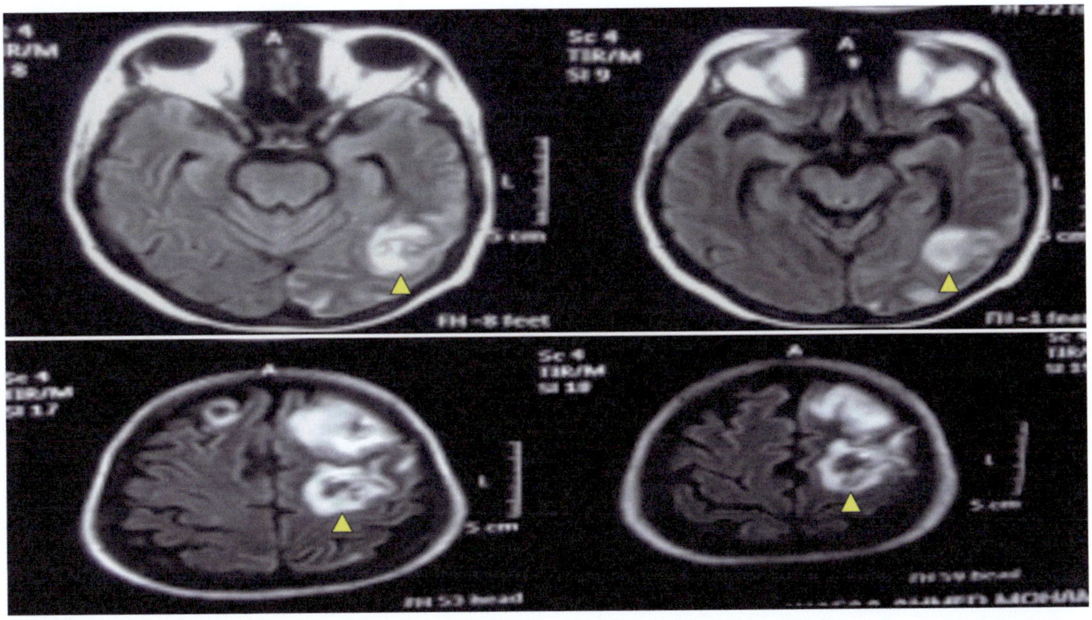

Fig. 21.2 Cranial MRI with IV contrast, T2 weighted, showing an SLE patient whose condition was complicated with subacute bacterial endocarditis (SBE) and multiple infected emboli of the brain. Arrow heads: ring-enhancing lesions. Courtesy of Dr. Hala El-Guendy, Professor of Internal Medicine, Cairo University

screening for TB in this patient population [153]. Also, the prevalence of disseminated CMV infection is rising as a complication of active treatment of SLE [154].

Invasive fungal infections (IFI) describe a group of diseases caused by cryptococcus, histoplasma, aspergillus, and candida [155]. Their frequency was 4.8% in hospitalized SLE patients in Argentina [155] and 3.9% in juvenile SLE in Brazil [156]. A Mexican study [157] found the risk of IFI in SLE to be associated with high CRP levels, high disease activity, mechanical ventilation, antibiotic treatment, hemodialysis, high dose of glucocorticoids, and treatment with mycophenolate mofetil. The mortality was four times higher in patients with IFI than in those without. *Cryptococcus neoformans* is the most frequent agent in Argentina and East Asia [155, 158], while *Candida* spp. are more common in North America [155].

IFI should be suspected in hospitalized SLE patients undergoing immunosuppressive therapy. We suggest that clinicians have a high index of suspicion for IFI in hospitalized SLE patients who have unexplained organ-specific symptoms and imaging abnormalities (e.g., neurologic, pulmonary, dermatologic, musculoskeletal, and elevated CRP with or without elevated WBC or fever). Additionally, hospitalized SLE patients who do not improve rapidly with antibiotics should undergo thorough diagnostic procedures (e.g., CSF sampling, bone marrow/tissue biopsies and/or bronchoalveolar lavage with culture, histopathology, serum antigen and antibody levels, and PCR testing) and consideration for prompt empiric antifungal treatment.

Differentiating Flare from Infection in SLE Patients

SLE follows a chronic course with intermitting flares [159]. Symptoms such as fever, fatigue, and rash may be seen in an SLE flare or as a result of infection [160]. The differentiation of SLE activity and infection in febrile or otherwise acutely ill SLE patients is extremely difficult, and several biomarkers have been recognized as potential tools to differentiate between these two conditions [161].

Serum procalcitonin (PCT) and CRP are markers with strong supportive evidence. Song et al. [162] performed a meta-analysis of published studies and found that procalcitonin is more specific and has better diagnostic accuracy than PCR for bacterial infection in systemic rheumatic diseases. Bador et al. [163] conducted a study to determine predictive values of PCT and CRP for bacterial infections in SLE patients. Bacterial infection was defined as positive culture results. PCT and CRP were measured by automated immunoassays. The areas under the receiver operating characteristic curves for PCT and CRP were not significantly different (0.797 (CCI 0.614–0.979) vs 0.755 (CI 0.600–0.910)). They found that PCT but not CRP was higher in flaring lupus patients with infection ($p = 0.019$ vs 0.195), as compared to flaring SLE patients without infection. A PCT of <0.17 ng/ml ruled out infection with a negative predictive value (NPV) of 94%. In patients in remission, CRP but not PCT was elevated during infection ($p = 0.036$ vs 0.103); a CRP <0.57 ng/dl had a NPV of 96%. They concluded that PCT may be a better marker to rule out bacterial infection in lupus flares but not in remission or general screening. Serio et al. [164] conducted a systematic review on this topic and concluded that PCT levels detected during disease flares were lower than those observed during bacterial infection and that elevated PCT levels ≥0.5 μg/l strongly suggest bacterial infection. SLE patients, including patients in remission, tend to have higher CRP baseline levels when compared with controls. CRP response during flares seems to be incomplete and did not always correlate with disease activity. Values greater than 1.0 mg/dl can indicate severe flare if neither serositis nor arthritis is associated, while higher CRP levels above 5–6 mg/dl may be associated with infection [165].

Other potential biomarkers have been identified but have limited usage to date. One is the delta neutrophil index, an index which reflects the fraction of circulating immature granulocytes associated with infection [166]. The activity of adenosine triphosphate produced by $CD4^+$ T cells was also found to be lower in patients with LN with infection compared to non-infected LN patients [167]. The ratio of erythrocyte-bound C4d to complement receptor 1 (C4d/CR1) was also studied. Febrile patients with disease flares had higher ratios and lower CRP levels than those with infection [168]. Ospina et al. [161] suggested that new scores, which include different biomarkers, might represent a better solution for differentiating infections from flares.

Prevention of Infections in SLE

Various strategies can be applied to reduce the risk of infections in SLE patients. These include vaccinations, antibacterial or antiviral prophylaxis, and intravenous immunoglobulins [169] (see also Chaps. 32 and 33).

Most non-live vaccines are immunogenic and safe in SLE patients, although antibody titers are frequently lower than those of healthy controls [170]. HPV vaccines can be given safely to SLE patients to avoid the increased incidence of anogenital warts and cervical epithelial dysplasia or carcinoma associated with high-risk viral genotypes [170]. Several experts [171] have recommended annual examinations of the cervical cytology in immunosuppressed patients.

Influenza vaccination is well tolerated and conveys a moderate protection against influenza infection in SLE. Considering that influenza runs a more severe course in SLE patients with a higher risk of disease exacerbation, influenza vaccination is recommended in patients with a low-to-moderate SLEDAI score or in those with stable disease. However, there were limited data and concern of the vaccine triggering a flare in severe disease [172]. Pneumococcal vaccination, however, is recommended for patients at any stage of their disease [171].

Live attenuated vaccines should generally be avoided in immunosuppressed patients. Recent studies, however, suggest that they can be considered in mildly immunosuppressed patients [171]. Serological screening for hepatitis B virus infection before starting immunosuppressive therapy is recommended for SLE patients to avoid viral reactivation [173].

Conclusion In summary, microbial agents are involved in various aspects of lupus including the pathogenesis, treatment complications, and long-term sequelae. Further studies are needed to fully delineate the role of commensal microbiota in the pathogenesis of SLE and the entire spectrum of acute and chronic infections (bacterial, viral, parasitic) during the lifespan of lupus patients, particularly those on chronic immunosuppressive therapies.

References

1. Mackay IR. Science, medicine, and the future: tolerance and autoimmunity. BMJ. 2000;321(7253):93–6.
2. Brown MA, Kenna T, Wordsworth BP. Genetics of ankylosing spondylitis—insights into pathogenesis. Nat Rev Rheumatol. 2016;12(2):81–91.
3. van Drongelen V, Holoshitz J. Human leukocyte antigen-disease associations in rheumatoid arthritis. Rheum Dis Clin N Am. 2017;43(3):363–76.
4. Gollwitzer ES, Marsland BJ. Impact of early-life exposures on immune maturation and susceptibility to disease. Trends Immunol. 2015;36(11):684–96.
5. Arrieta MC, Stiemsma LT, Amenyogbe N, et al. The intestinal microbiome in early life: health and disease. Front Immunol. 2014;5:427.
6. Vieira SM, Pagovich OE, Kriegel MA. Diet, microbiota and autoimmune diseases. Lupus. 2014;23(6):518–26.
7. Stadhouders R, Lubberts E, Hendriks RW. A cellular and molecular view of T helper 17 cell plasticity in autoimmunity. J Autoimmun. 2017;87:1–15.
8. Veldhoen M, Hocking RJ, Flavell RA, et al. Signals mediated by transforming growth factor-beta initiate autoimmune encephalomyelitis, but chronic inflammation is needed to sustain disease. Nat Immunol. 2006;7(11):1151–6.
9. Acosta-Rodriguez EV, Napolitani G, Lanzavecchia A, et al. Interleukins 1beta and 6 but not transforming growth factor-beta are essential for the differentiation of interleukin 17-producing human T helper cells. Nat Immunol. 2007;8(9):942–9.
10. Voo KS, Wang YH, Santori FR, et al. Identification of IL-17-producing FOXP3+ regulatory T cells in humans. Proc Natl Acad Sci U S A. 2009;106(12):4793–8.
11. Lee YK, Mukasa R, Hatton RD, et al. Developmental plasticity of Th17 and Treg cells. Curr Opin Immunol. 2009;21(3):274–80.
12. Koenen HJ, Smeets RL, Vink PM, et al. Human CD25highFoxp3pos regulatory T cells differentiate into IL-17-producing cells. Blood. 2008;112(6):2340–52.
13. Ivanov II, Atarashi K, Manel N, et al. Induction of intestinal Th17 cells by segmented filamentous bacteria. Cell. 2009;139(3):485–98.
14. Johnson BM, Gaudreau MC, Al-Gadban MM, et al. Impact of dietary deviation on disease progression and gut microbiome composition in lupus-prone SNF1 mice. Clin Exp Immunol. 2015;181(2):323–37.
15. Palm NW, de Zoete MR, Cullen TW, et al. Immunoglobulin A coating identifies colitogenic bacteria in inflammatory bowel disease. Cell. 2014;158(5):1000–10.
16. Scher JU, Ubeda C, Artacho A, et al. Decreased bacterial diversity characterizes the altered gut microbiota in patients with psoriatic arthritis, resembling dysbiosis in inflammatory bowel disease. Arthritis Rheumatol. 2015;67(1):128–39.
17. Wang NS, McHeyzer-Williams LJ, Okitsu SL, et al. Divergent transcriptional programming of class-specific B cell memory by T-bet and RORalpha. Nat Immunol. 2012;13(6):604–11.
18. Hirota K, Turner JE, Villa M, et al. Plasticity of Th17 cells in Peyer's patches is responsible for the induction of T cell-dependent IgA responses. Nat Immunol. 2013;14(4):372–9.
19. Kubinak JL, Petersen C, Stephens WZ, et al. MyD88 signaling in T cells directs IgA-mediated control of the microbiota to promote health. Cell Host Microbe. 2015;17(2):153–63.
20. Choi JY, Ho JH, Pasoto SG, et al. Circulating follicular helper-like T cells in systemic lupus erythematosus: association with disease activity. Arthritis Rheumatol. 2015;67(4):988–99.
21. Hevia A, Milani C, Lopez P, et al. Intestinal dysbiosis associated with systemic lupus erythematosus. MBio. 2014;5(5):e01548–14.
22. Rojo D, Hevia A, Bargiela R, et al. Ranking the impact of human health disorders on gut metabolism: systemic lupus erythematosus and obesity as study cases. Sci Rep. 2015;5:8310.
23. Lopez P, de Paz B, Rodriguez-Carrio J, et al. Th17 responses and natural IgM antibodies are related to gut microbiota composition in systemic lupus erythematosus patients. Sci Rep. 2016;6:24072.
24. Conti F, Ceccarelli F, Iaiani G, et al. Association between *Staphylococcus aureus* nasal carriage and disease phenotype in patients affected by systemic lupus erythematosus. Arthritis Res Ther. 2016;18:177.
25. Ruff WE, Kriegel MA. Autoimmune host-microbiota interactions at barrier sites and beyond. Trends Mol Med. 2015;21(4):233–44.
26. Greiling TM, Dehner C, Chen X, et al. Commensal orthologs of the human autoantigen Ro60 as triggers of autoimmunity in lupus. Science Translational Medicine. 2018;10(434):eaan2306.
27. Kahlenberg JM, Kaplan MJ. The inflammasome and lupus: another innate immune mechanism contributing to disease pathogenesis? Curr Opin Rheumatol. 2014;26(5):475–81.
28. Horton CG, Farris AD. Toll-like receptors in systemic lupus erythematosus: potential targets for therapeutic intervention. Curr Allergy Asthma Rep. 2012;12(1):1–7.

29. Hsieh AH, Jhou YJ, Liang CT, et al. Fragment of tegument protein pp65 of human cytomegalovirus induces autoantibodies in BALB/c mice. Arthritis Res Ther. 2011;13(5):R162.
30. Hod T, Zandman-Goddard G, Langevitz P, et al. Does parvovirus infection have a role in systemic lupus erythematosus? Immunol Res. 2017;65(2):447–53.
31. Doaty S, Agrawal H, Bauer E, et al. Infection and lupus: which causes which? Curr Rheumatol Rep. 2016;18(3):13.
32. Rigante D, Esposito S. Infections and systemic lupus Erythematosus: binding or sparring partners? Int J Mol Sci. 2015;16(8):17331–43.
33. Nelson P, Rylance P, Roden D, et al. Viruses as potential pathogenic agents in systemic lupus erythematosus. Lupus. 2014;23(6):596–605.
34. Sane P, Amritkar V, Pooja G. Dengue viral infection triggering abnormal immune response in a case of Kikuchi disease which later evolved into SLE. J Assoc Physicians India. 2016;64(1):147.
35. Soldevilla HF, Briones SF, Navarra SV. Systemic lupus erythematosus following HPV immunization or infection? Lupus. 2012;21(2):158–61.
36. Levy M, Bourrat E, Baudouin V, et al. Toxocara canis infection: unusual trigger of systemic lupus erythematosus. Pediatr Int. 2015;57(4):785–8.
37. Fattal I, Shental N, Molad Y, et al. Epstein-Barr virus antibodies mark systemic lupus erythematosus and scleroderma patients negative for anti-DNA. Immunology. 2014;141(2):276–85.
38. Ding Y, He X, Liao W, et al. The expression of EBV-encoded LMP1 in young patients with lupus nephritis. Int J Clin Exp Med. 2015;8(4):6073–8.
39. Rasmussen NS, Nielsen CT, Houen G, et al. Humoral markers of active Epstein-Barr virus infection associate with anti-extractable nuclear antigen autoantibodies and plasma galectin-3 binding protein in systemic lupus erythematosus. Lupus. 2016;25(14):1567–76.
40. Draborg AH, Sandhu N, Larsen N, et al. Impaired cytokine responses to Epstein-Barr virus antigens in systemic lupus Erythematosus patients. J Immunol Res. 2016;2016:6473204.
41. Gürtler C, Bowie AG. Innate immune detection of microbial nucleic acids. Trends Microbiol. 2013;21(8):413–20.
42. Fitzgerald-Bocarsly P, Feng D. The role of type I interferon production by dendritic cells in host defense. Biochimie. 2007;89(6–7):843–55.
43. Bengtsson AA, Ronnblom L. Role of interferons in SLE. Best Pract Res Clin Rheumatol. 2017;31(3):415–28.
44. Mavragani CP, Sagalovskiy I, Guo Q, et al. Expression of long interspersed nuclear element 1 Retroelements and induction of type I interferon in patients with systemic autoimmune disease. Arthritis Rheumatol. 2016;68(11):2686–96.
45. Manfredo Vieira S, Hiltensperger M, Kumar V, Zegarra-Ruiz D, Dehner C, Khan N, Costa FRC, Tiniakou E, Greiling T, Ruff W, Barbieri A, Kriegel C, Mehta SS, Knight JR, Jain D, Goodman AL, Kriegel MA. Translocation of a gut pathobiont drives autoimmunity in mice and humans. Science. 2018;359:1156–61.
46. Liu X, Jiao Y, Cui B, et al. The potential protective role of hepatitis B virus infection in pristane-induced lupus in mice. Lupus. 2016;25(11):1180–9.
47. Abdel-Maksoud MA, Abdel-Ghaffar FA, El-Amir A, et al. Infection with Plasmodium chabaudi diminishes plasma immune complexes and ameliorates the histopathological alterations in different organs of female BWF1 lupus mice. Eur Rev Med Pharmacol Sci. 2016;20(4):733–44.
48. Badr G, Sayed A, Abdel-Maksoud MA, et al. Infection of female BWF1 lupus mice with malaria parasite attenuates B cell Autoreactivity by modulating the CXCL12/CXCR4 Axis and its downstream signals PI3K/AKT, NFkappaB and ERK. PLoS One. 2015;10(4):e0125340.
49. Chen M, Aosai F, Norose K, et al. Toxoplasma gondii infection inhibits the development of lupus-like syndrome in autoimmune (New Zealand black × New Zealand white) F1 mice. Int Immunol. 2004;16(7):937–46.
50. Fischer S, Agmon-Levin N, Shapira Y, et al. Toxoplasma gondii: bystander or cofactor in rheumatoid arthritis. Immunol Res. 2013;56(2–3):287–92.
51. Sawalha AH, Schmid WR, Binder SR, et al. Association between systemic lupus erythematosus and helicobacter pylori seronegativity. J Rheumatol. 2004;31(8):1546.
52. Panda AK, Das BK. Diminished IL-17A levels may protect filarial-infected individuals from development of rheumatoid arthritis and systemic lupus erythematosus. Lupus. 2017;26(4):348–54.
53. Finlay BB, McFadden G. Anti-immunology: evasion of the host immune system by bacterial and viral pathogens. Cell. 2006;124(4):767–82.
54. Bach JF. Infections and autoimmune diseases. J Autoimmun. 2005;25:74–80.
55. Murdaca G, Orsi A, Spano F, et al. Vaccine-preventable infections in systemic lupus Erythematosus. Hum Vaccin Immunother. 2016;12(3):632–43.
56. Robak E, Niewiadomska H, Robak T, et al. Lymphocytes Tgammadelta in clinically normal skin and peripheral blood of patients with systemic lupus erythematosus and their correlation with disease activity. Mediat Inflamm. 2001;10(4):179–89.
57. Volc-Platzer B, Anegg B, Milota S, et al. Accumulation of gamma delta T cells in chronic cutaneous lupus erythematosus. J Investig Dermatol. 1993;100(1):84s–91s.
58. Tsai CY, Wu TH, Yu CL, et al. Decreased IL-12 production by polymorphonuclear leukocytes in patients with active systemic lupus erythematosus. Immunol Investig. 2002;31(3–4):177–89.
59. Truedsson L. Classical pathway deficiencies – a short analytical review. Mol Immunol. 2015;68(1):14–9.

60. Rupert KL, Moulds JM, Yang Y, et al. The molecular basis of complete complement C4A and C4B deficiencies in a systemic lupus Erythematosus patient with homozygous C4A and C4B mutant genes. J Immunol. 2002;169(3):1570.
61. Pickering MC, Botto M, Taylor PR, et al. Systemic lupus erythematosus, complement deficiency, and apoptosis. Adv Immunol. 2000;76:227–324.
62. Garred P, Voss A, Madsen HO, et al. Association of mannose-binding lectin gene variation with disease severity and infections in a population-based cohort of systemic lupus erythematosus patients. Genes Immun. 2001;2(8):442–50.
63. Sebastiani GD, Galeazzi M. Infection—genetics relationship in systemic lupus erythematosus. Lupus. 2009;18(13):1169–75.
64. Marquart HV, Svendsen A, Rasmussen JM, et al. Complement receptor expression and activation of the complement cascade on B lymphocytes from patients with systemic lupus erythematosus (SLE). Clin Exp Immunol. 1995;101(1):60–5.
65. Park YW, Kee SJ, Cho YN, et al. Impaired differentiation and cytotoxicity of natural killer cells in systemic lupus erythematosus. Arthritis Rheum. 2009;60(6):1753–63.
66. Tanaka T, Saiki O, Negoro S, et al. Decreased expression of interleukin-2 binding molecules (p70/75) in T cells from patients with systemic lupus erythematosus. Arthritis Rheum. 1989;32(5):552–9.
67. Jin O, Kavikondala S, Sun L, et al. Systemic lupus erythematosus patients have increased number of circulating plasmacytoid dendritic cells, but decreased myeloid dendritic cells with deficient CD83 expression. Lupus. 2008;17(7):654–62.
68. Wu SA, Yeh KW, Lee WI, et al. Impaired phagocytosis and susceptibility to infection in pediatric-onset systemic lupus erythematosus. Lupus. 2013;22(3):279–88.
69. Bengtsson AA, Pettersson A, Wichert S, et al. Low production of reactive oxygen species in granulocytes is associated with organ damage in systemic lupus erythematosus. Arthritis Res Ther. 2014;16(3):R120.
70. Magnani A, Brosselin P, Beaute J, et al. Inflammatory manifestations in a single-center cohort of patients with chronic granulomatous disease. J Allergy Clin Immunol. 2014;134(3):655–662.e8.
71. De Ravin SS, Naumann N, Cowen EW, et al. Chronic granulomatous disease as a risk factor for autoimmune disease. J Allergy Clin Immunol. 2008;122(6):1097–103.
72. Villanueva E, Yalavarthi S, Berthier CC, et al. Netting neutrophils induce endothelial damage, infiltrate tissues, and expose immunostimulatory molecules in systemic lupus erythematosus. J Immunol. 2011;187(1):538–52.
73. Smith CK, Kaplan MJ. The role of neutrophils in the pathogenesis of systemic lupus erythematosus. Curr Opin Rheumatol. 2015;27(5):448–53.
74. Lertchaisataporn K, Kasitanon N, Wangkaew S, et al. An evaluation of the association of leukopenia and severe infection in patients with systemic lupus erythematosus. J Clin Rheumatol. 2013;19(3):115–20.
75. Alarcon GS. Infections in systemic connective tissue diseases: systemic lupus erythematosus, scleroderma, and polymyositis/dermatomyositis. Infect Dis Clin N Am. 2006;20(4):849–75.
76. Goldstein MF, Goldstein AL, Dunsky EH, et al. Selective IgM immunodeficiency: retrospective analysis of 36 adult patients with review of the literature. Ann Allergy Asthma Immunol. 2006;97(6):717–30.
77. Cassidy JT, Kitson RK, Selby CL. Selective IgA deficiency in children and adults with systemic lupus erythematosus. Lupus. 2007;16(8):647–50.
78. Lim E, Tao Y, White AJ, et al. Hypogammaglobulinemia in pediatric systemic lupus erythematosus. Lupus. 2013;22(13):1382–7.
79. Chen L, Morris DL, Vyse TJ. Genetic advances in systemic lupus erythematosus: an update. Curr Opin Rheumatol. 2017;29(5):423–33.
80. Deng Y, Tsao BP. Advances in lupus genetics and epigenetics. Curr Opin Rheumatol. 2014;26(5):482–92.
81. Cui Y, Sheng Y, Zhang X. Genetic susceptibility to SLE: recent progress from GWAS. J Autoimmun. 2013;41:25–33.
82. Bentham J, Morris DL, Cunninghame Graham DS, et al. Genetic association analyses implicate aberrant regulation of innate and adaptive immunity genes in the pathogenesis of systemic lupus erythematosus. Nat Genet. 2015;47:1457.
83. Bronson PG, Chaivorapol C, Ortmann W, et al. The genetics of type I interferon in systemic lupus erythematosus. Curr Opin Immunol. 2012;24(5):530–7.
84. Abelson AK, Delgado-Vega AM, Kozyrev SV, et al. STAT4 associates with systemic lupus erythematosus through two independent effects that correlate with gene expression and act additively with IRF5 to increase risk. Ann Rheum Dis. 2009;68(11):1746–53.
85. Zhao J, Ma J, Deng Y, et al. A missense variant in NCF1 is associated with susceptibility to multiple autoimmune diseases. Nat Genet. 2017;49:433.
86. Olsson LM, Johansson ÅC, Gullstrand B, et al. A single nucleotide polymorphism in the NCF1 gene leading to reduced oxidative burst is associated with systemic lupus erythematosus. Ann Rheum Dis. 2017;76(9):1607–13.
87. Jacob CO, Eisenstein M, Dinauer MC, et al. Lupus-associated causal mutation in neutrophil cytosolic factor 2 (NCF2) brings unique insights to the structure and function of NADPH oxidase. Proc Natl Acad Sci U S A. 2012;109(2):E59–67.
88. Danza A, Ruiz-Irastorza G. Infection risk in systemic lupus erythematosus patients: susceptibility factors and preventive strategies. Lupus. 2013;22(12):1286–94.
89. Urowitz MB, Bookman AA, Koehler BE, et al. The bimodal mortality pattern of systemic lupus erythematosus. Am J Med. 1976;60(2):221–5.
90. Mok CC. Con: cyclophosphamide for the treatment of lupus nephritis. Nephrol Dial Transplant. 2016;31(7):1053–7.

91. Mills JA. Systemic lupus erythematosus. N Engl J Med. 1994;330(26):1871–9.
92. Feldman CH, Hiraki LT, Winkelmayer WC, et al. Serious infections among adult Medicaid beneficiaries with systemic lupus erythematosus and lupus nephritis. Arthritis Rheumatol. 2015;67(6):1577–85.
93. Momtaz M, Fayed A, Wadie M, et al. Retrospective analysis of nephritis response and renal outcome in a cohort of 928 Egyptian lupus nephritis patients: a university hospital experience. Lupus. 2017;26(14):1564–70.
94. Cervera R, Khamashta MA, Font J, et al. Morbidity and mortality in systemic lupus erythematosus during a 10-year period: a comparison of early and late manifestations in a cohort of 1,000 patients. Medicine (Baltimore). 2003;82(5):299–308.
95. Mok CC, Lau CS, Chan TM, et al. Clinical characteristics and outcome of southern Chinese males with systemic lupus erythematosus. Lupus. 1999;8(3):188–96.
96. Srivastava P, Abujam B, Misra R, et al. Outcome of lupus nephritis in childhood onset SLE in north and Central India: single-centre experience over 25 years. Lupus. 2016;25(5):547–57.
97. Lin CH, Hung PH, Hu HY, et al. Infection-related hospitalization and risk of end-stage renal disease in patients with systemic lupus erythematosus: a nationwide population-based study. Nephrol Dial Transplant. 2017;32(10):1683–90.
98. Zhan Z, Lao M, Su F, et al. Hospital-acquired infection in patients with systemic lupus erythematosus: a case-control study in a southern Chinese population. Clin Rheumatol. 2017;37(3):709–17.
99. Murray SG, Schmajuk G, Trupin L, et al. National lupus hospitalization trends reveal rising rates of herpes zoster and declines in pneumocystis pneumonia. PLoS One. 2016;11(1):e0144918.
100. Chakravarty EF, Michaud K, Katz R, et al. Increased incidence of herpes zoster among patients with systemic lupus erythematosus. Lupus. 2013;22(3):238–44.
101. Borba EF, Ribeiro AC, Martin P, et al. Incidence, risk factors, and outcome of herpes zoster in systemic lupus erythematosus. J Clin Rheumatol. 2010;16(3):119–22.
102. Pope JE, Krizova A, Ouimet JM, et al. Close association of herpes zoster reactivation and systemic lupus erythematosus (SLE) diagnosis: case-control study of patients with SLE or noninflammatory nusculoskeletal disorders. J Rheumatol. 2004;31(2):274–9.
103. Manzi S, Kuller LH, Kutzer J, et al. Herpes zoster in systemic lupus erythematosus. J Rheumatol. 1995;22(7):1254–8.
104. Rondaan C, de Haan A, Horst G, et al. Altered cellular and humoral immunity to varicella-zoster virus in patients with autoimmune diseases. Arthritis Rheumatol. 2014;66(11):3122–8.
105. Houssiau FA, Vasconcelos C, D'Cruz D, et al. Immunosuppressive therapy in lupus nephritis: the euro-lupus nephritis trial, a randomized trial of low-dose versus high-dose intravenous cyclophosphamide. Arthritis Rheum. 2002;46(8):2121–31.
106. Rhee C, Gohil S, Klompas M. Regulatory mandates for sepsis care--reasons for caution. N Engl J Med. 2014;370(18):1673–6.
107. Hahn BH, McMahon MA, Wilkinson A, et al. American College of Rheumatology guidelines for screening, treatment, and management of lupus nephritis. Arthritis Care Res (Hoboken). 2012;64(6):797–808.
108. Husain S, Singh N. The impact of novel immunosuppressive agents on infections in organ transplant recipients and the interactions of these agents with antimicrobials. Clin Infect Dis. 2002;35(1):53–61.
109. Oz HS, Hughes WT. Novel anti-pneumocystis carinii effects of the immunosuppressant mycophenolate mofetil in contrast to provocative effects of tacrolimus, sirolimus, and dexamethasone. J Infect Dis. 1997;175(4):901–4.
110. Herrinton LJ, Liu L, Goldfien R, et al. Risk of serious infection for patients with systemic lupus Erythematosus starting glucocorticoids with or without Antimalarials. J Rheumatol. 2016;43(8): 1503–9.
111. Dubula T, Mody GM. Spectrum of infections and outcome among hospitalized South Africans with systemic lupus erythematosus. Clin Rheumatol. 2015;34(3):479–88.
112. Rees F, Doherty M, Grainge M, et al. Burden of comorbidity in systemic lupus Erythematosus in the UK, 1999–2012. Arthritis Care Res (Hoboken). 2016;68(6):819–27.
113. Souza DC, Santo AH, Sato EI. Mortality profile related to systemic lupus erythematosus: a multiple cause-of-death analysis. J Rheumatol. 2012;39(3):496–503.
114. Fei Y, Shi X, Gan F, et al. Death causes and pathogens analysis of systemic lupus erythematosus during the past 26 years. Clin Rheumatol. 2014;33(1):57–63.
115. Ritchie J, Smyth A, Tower C, et al. Maternal deaths in women with lupus nephritis: a review of published evidence. Lupus. 2012;21(5):534–41.
116. Lee YH, Choi SJ, Ji JD, et al. Overall and cause-specific mortality in systemic lupus erythematosus: an updated meta-analysis. Lupus. 2016;25(7):727–34.
117. Chen D, Xie J, Chen H, et al. Infection in southern Chinese patients with systemic lupus erythematosus: spectrum, drug resistance, outcomes, and risk factors. J Rheumatol. 2016;43(9):1650–6.
118. Dixon WG, Watson K, Lunt M, et al. Rates of serious infection, including site-specific and bacterial intracellular infection, in rheumatoid arthritis patients receiving anti-tumor necrosis factor therapy: results from the British Society for Rheumatology biologics register. Arthritis Rheum. 2006;54(8):2368–76.
119. Shen HN, Yang HH, Lu CL. Temporal trends in characteristics and outcome of intensive care unit patients with systemic lupus erythematosus in Taiwan: a national population-based study. Lupus. 2013;22(6):644–52.

120. Han BK, Bhatia R, Traisak P, et al. Clinical presentations and outcomes of systemic lupus erythematosus patients with infection admitted to the intensive care unit. Lupus. 2013;22(7):690–6.
121. Pronk SM, van Ommen CH, Prince FH, et al. Venous thrombosis as a first sign of SLE. Ned Tijdschr Geneeskd. 2014;158:A7179.
122. Imamura H, Iwamoto T, Momohara S. Unusual case of an elbow mass caused by Candida arthritis in a patient with systemic lupus erythematosus. Hand Surg. 2014;19(3):409–11.
123. Meesiri S. Pyomyositis in a patient with systemic lupus erythematosus and a review of the literature. BMJ Case Rep. 2016. https://doi.org/10.1136/bcr-2016-214809.
124. Kim SS, Perino G, Boettner F, et al. Salmonella septic arthritis of the knees in a patient with systemic lupus erythematosus. Lupus. 2013;22(7):740–3.
125. Khammassi N, Kort Y. Osteonecrosis of the femoral condyles revealed by septic arthritis in systemic lupus erythematosus. Pan Afr Med J. 2015; 22:94.
126. Ferreira JC, Marques HH, Ferriani MP, et al. Herpes zoster infection in childhood-onset systemic lupus erythematosus patients: a large multicenter study. Lupus. 2016;25(7):754–9.
127. Silva LM, Santos WG, Santiago MB. Prevalence of cutaneous warts in patients with systemic lupus erythematosus: a systematic review. J Infect Dev Ctries. 2016;10(9):902–6.
128. Lyrio LD, Grassi MF, Santana IU, et al. Prevalence of cervical human papillomavirus infection in women with systemic lupus erythematosus. Rheumatol Int. 2013;33(2):335–40.
129. Amaral JL, Araujo MV, Dias GA, et al. Clinical and epidemiological study of human papillomavirus infection in women with systemic lupus erythematosus in eastern Brazilian amazon. Acta Reumatol Port. 2017;42(1):47–54.
130. Hidalgo-Tenorio C, Jiménez-Alonso J, de Dios Luna J, et al. Urinary tract infections and lupus erythematosus. Ann Rheum Dis. 2004;63(4):431–7.
131. Mohamed DF, Habeeb RA, Hosny SM, et al. Incidence and risk of infection in Egyptian patients with systemic lupus erythematosus. Clin Med Insights Arthritis Musculoskelet Disord. 2014;7:41–8.
132. Marcos M, Fernandez C, Soriano A, et al. Epidemiology and clinical outcomes of bloodstream infections among lupus patients. Lupus. 2011;20(9):965–71.
133. Baronaite Hansen R, Jacobsen S. Infections increase risk of arterial and venous thromboses in Danish patients with systemic lupus erythematosus: 5102 patient-years of followup. J Rheumatol. 2014;41(9):1817–22.
134. Catoggio C, Alvarez-Uria A, Fernandez PL, et al. Catastrophic antiphospholipid syndrome triggered by fulminant disseminated herpes simplex infection in a patient with systemic lupus erythematosus. Lupus. 2012;21(12):1359–61.
135. Luijten RK, Cuppen BV, Bijlsma JW, et al. Serious infections in systemic lupus erythematosus with a focus on pneumococcal infections. Lupus. 2014;23(14):1512–6.
136. Xiao P, Dong C, Yue Y, et al. Dynamic expression of microRNAs in M2b polarized macrophages associated with systemic lupus erythematosus. Gene. 2014;547(2):300–9.
137. Pamuk ON, Pamuk GE, Barutcu E, et al. The development of pulmonary aspergillosis and pneumothorax in a patient with neutropenic systemic lupus erythematosus and successful treatment of the first case. BMJ Case Rep. 2014;2014:bcr2013200818. https://doi.org/10.1136/bcr-2013-200818.
138. Martinez-Martinez MU, Sturbaum AK, Alcocer-Varela J, et al. Factors associated with mortality and infections in patients with systemic lupus erythematosus with diffuse alveolar hemorrhage. J Rheumatol. 2014;41(8):1656–61.
139. Fangtham M, Magder LS, Petri MA. Oral candidiasis in systemic lupus erythematosus. Lupus. 2014;23(7):684–90.
140. Fawzy M, Edrees A, Okasha H, et al. Gastrointestinal manifestations in systemic lupus erythematosus. Lupus. 2016;25(13):1456–62.
141. Wang Q, Shen M, Leng X, et al. Prevalence, severity, and clinical features of acute and chronic pancreatitis in patients with systemic lupus erythematosus. Rheumatol Int. 2016;36(10):1413–9.
142. Strasser C, Wolf EM, Kornprat P, et al. Opportunistic cytomegalovirus infection causing colonic perforation in a patient with systemic lupus erythematosus. Lupus. 2012;21(4):449–51.
143. Tachikawa Y, Nozawa H, Tanaka J, et al. Colonic perforation in a patient with systemic lupus erythematosus accompanied by cytomegalovirus infection: a case report. Int J Surg Case Rep. 2016;23: 70–3.
144. Mahroum N, Hejly A, Tiosano S, et al. Chronic hepatitis C viral infection among SLE patients: the significance of coexistence. Immunol Res. 2017;65(2):477–81.
145. Xu Y, Xu D, Zhang T, et al. The prevalence and clinical characteristics of systemic lupus erythematosus with infectious brain lesions in China. Scand J Rheumatol. 2012;41(6):466–71.
146. Berntsson SG, Katsarogiannis E, Lourenco F, et al. Progressive multifocal leukoencephalopathy and systemic lupus erythematosus: focus on etiology. Case Rep Neurol. 2016;8(1):59–65.
147. Williamson EML, Berger JR. Diagnosis and treatment of progressive multifocal Leukoencephalopathy associated with multiple sclerosis therapies. Neurotherapeutics. 2017;14(4):961–73.
148. Mekitarian Filho E, Horita SM, Gilio AE, et al. Cerebrospinal fluid lactate level as a diagnostic biomarker for bacterial meningitis in children. Int J Emerg Med. 2014;7(1):14.
149. Huy NT, Thao NT, Diep DT, et al. Cerebrospinal fluid lactate concentration to distinguish bacterial

from aseptic meningitis: a systemic review and meta-analysis. Crit Care. 2010;14(6):R240.
150. Zhong Y, Li M, Liu J, et al. Cryptococcal meningitis in Chinese patients with systemic lupus erythematosus. Clin Neurol Neurosurg. 2015;131:59–63.
151. Zheng H, Li M, Wang D, et al. Gender-specific contributing risk factors and outcome of female cryptococcal meningoencephalitis patients. BMC Infect Dis. 2016;16:22.
152. de Araujo DB, Daolio L, Szajubok JC, et al. Epidural abscess due to Salmonella enteritidis in a patient with systemic lupus erythematosus. Lupus. 2012;21(12):1356–8.
153. Freire PS, Montoni JD, Ribeiro AS, et al. Miliary tuberculosis: a severe opportunistic infection in juvenile systemic lupus erythematosus patients. Rev Bras Reumatol Engl Ed. 2016;56(3):274–9.
154. Berman N, Belmont HM. Disseminated cytomegalovirus infection complicating active treatment of systemic lupus erythematosus: an emerging problem. Lupus. 2017;26(4):431–4.
155. Vinicki JP, Catalan Pellet S, Pappalardo C, et al. Invasive fungal infections in argentine patients with systemic lupus erythematosus. Lupus. 2013;22(9):892–8.
156. Silva MF, Ferriani MP, Terreri MT, et al. A multicenter study of invasive fungal infections in patients with childhood-onset systemic lupus erythematosus. J Rheumatol. 2015;42(12):2296–303.
157. Martinez-Martinez MU, Herrera-Van Oostdam D, Roman-Acosta S, et al. Invasive fungal infections in patients with systemic lupus erythematosus. J Rheumatol. 2012;39(9):1814–8.
158. Chen GL, Chen Y, Zhu CQ, et al. Invasive fungal infection in Chinese patients with systemic lupus erythematosus. Clin Rheumatol. 2012;31(7):1087–91.
159. Chung SA, Brown EE, Williams AH, et al. Lupus nephritis susceptibility loci in women with systemic lupus erythematosus. J Am Soc Nephrol. 2014;25(12):2859–70.
160. Firooz N, Albert DA, Wallace DJ, et al. High-sensitivity C-reactive protein and erythrocyte sedimentation rate in systemic lupus erythematosus. Lupus. 2011;20(6):588–97.
161. Ospina FE, Echeverri A, Zambrano D, et al. Distinguishing infections vs flares in patients with systemic lupus erythematosus. Rheumatology (Oxford). 2017;56(suppl_1):i46–54.
162. Song GG, Bae SC, Lee YH. Diagnostic accuracies of procalcitonin and C-reactive protein for bacterial infection in patients with systemic rheumatic diseases: a meta-analysis. Clin Exp Rheumatol. 2015;33(2):166–73.
163. Bador KM, Intan S, Hussin S, et al. Serum procalcitonin has negative predictive value for bacterial infection in active systemic lupus erythematosus. Lupus. 2012;21(11):1172–7.
164. Serio I, Arnaud L, Mathian A, et al. Can procalcitonin be used to distinguish between disease flare and infection in patients with systemic lupus erythematosus: a systematic literature review. Clin Rheumatol. 2014;33(9):1209–15.
165. Dima A, Opris D, Jurcut C, et al. Is there still a place for erythrocyte sedimentation rate and C-reactive protein in systemic lupus erythematosus? Lupus. 2016;25(11):1173–9.
166. Pyo JY, Park JS, Park YB, et al. Delta neutrophil index as a marker for differential diagnosis between flare and infection in febrile systemic lupus erythematosus patients. Lupus. 2013;22(11):1102–9.
167. Liu J, Pan Y, Tang LJ, et al. Low adenosine triphosphate activity in CD4+ cells predicts infection in patients with lupus nephritis. Clin Exp Rheumatol. 2014;32(3):383–9.
168. Chen CH, Tai SB, Chen HC, et al. Analysis of erythrocyte C4d to complement receptor 1 ratio: use in distinguishing between infection and flare-up in febrile patients with systemic lupus Erythematosus. Biomed Res Int. 2015;2015:939783.
169. Sciascia S, Cuadrado MJ, Karim MY. Management of infection in systemic lupus erythematosus. Best Pract Res Clin Rheumatol. 2013;27(3):377–89.
170. Grein IH, Groot N, Lacerda MI, et al. HPV infection and vaccination in systemic lupus Erythematosus patients: what we really should know. Pediatr Rheumatol Online J. 2016;14(1):12.
171. Mathian A, Arnaud L, Adoue D, et al. Prevention of infections in adults and adolescents with systemic lupus erythematosus: guidelines for the clinical practice based on the literature and expert opinion. Rev Med Interne. 2016;37(5):307–20.
172. Liao Z, Tang H, Xu X, et al. Immunogenicity and safety of influenza vaccination in systemic lupus Erythematosus patients compared with healthy controls: a meta-analysis. PLoS One. 2016;11(2):e0147856.
173. Watanabe R, Ishii T, Harigae H. Pretreatment screening for hepatitis B virus infection in patients with systemic lupus erythematosus. Tohoku J Exp Med. 2015;237(1):9–15.

Antiphospholipid Syndrome 22

Gaafar Ragab, William Ruff, Derek Pearson,
Hadi Goubran, and Martin Kriegel

Abbreviations

aCL	Anticardiolipin
Anti-β2 GP1	Anti-beta 2-glycoprotein-1
APCs	Antigen-presenting cells
APS	Antiphospholipid syndrome
aPTT	Activated partial thromboplastin time
CAPS	Catastrophic antiphospholipid syndrome
CRP	C-reactive protein
CYP	Cytochrome P
dRVVT	Dilute Russell viper venom time
DVT	Deep vein thrombosis
ELISA	Enzyme-linked immunosorbent assay
EpC	Epithelial cells
HELLP syndrome	Hemolysis, elevated liver enzymes, and low platelet count
HIT	Heparin-induced thrombocytopenia
IFN	Interferon
Ig G	Immunoglobulin G
Ig M	Immunoglobulin M
LA	lupus anticoagulant
LAK	lymphokine-activated killer
LMWH	Low molecular weight heparin
MAMPs	Microbe-associated molecular patterns
MI	Myocardial infarction
NOD	Nonobese diabetic
PRRs	Pattern recognition receptors
PSA	Polysaccharide
SCFAs	Short-chain fatty acids
SFB	Segmented filamentous bacteria
SLE	Systemic lupus erythematosus
Tfh	T follicular helper cells
Th17	T helper 17 cells
TLR	Toll-like receptors
TMAO	Trimethylamine *N*-oxide
TMP/SMX	Trimethoprim/sulfamethoxazole
VTE	Venous thromboembolism

G. Ragab (✉)
Rheumatology and Clinical Immunology Unit, Department of Internal Medicine, Cairo University, Giza, Cairo, Egypt
e-mail: gragab@kasralainy.edu.eg

W. Ruff · M. Kriegel
Department of Immunobiology, Yale School of Medicine, New Haven, CT, USA
e-mail: martin.kriegel@yale.edu

D. Pearson · H. Goubran
College of Medicine, University of Saskatchewan, Saskatoon, SK, Canada

Saskatoon Cancer Centre, Saskatoon, SK, Canada

Introduction

Antiphospholipid syndrome (APS) is an autoimmune multisystem disorder characterized by arterial, venous, or small vessel thromboembolism and/

G. Ragab et al. (eds.), *The Microbiome in Rheumatic Diseases and Infection*,
https://doi.org/10.1007/978-3-319-79026-8_22

or pregnancy morbidity in the presence of persistent antiphospholipid antibodies (aPLs) [1]. aPLs are a heterogeneous group of autoantibodies which are directed against phospholipid-binding proteins.

APS occurs as a primary condition or in the setting of an underlying systemic autoimmune disease, particularly systemic lupus erythematosus (SLE). Several reports suggest the possible evolution of APS into SLE with variable rates ranging between 0 to 23% in 5–9 years [2–5].

Background

Three major aPL tests recognized by international classification criteria for APS are as follows:

- Anticardiolipin antibodies (aCL) immunoglobulin G (IgG) and/or M (IgM)
- Anti-beta2-glycoprotein I (anti-β2GPI) antibodies IgG and/or IgM
- Lupus anticoagulant (LA) test

The diagnosis of APS is made in the presence of one or more of the above aPL detected in the setting of thrombosis, recurrent fetal loss, or intrauterine growth retardation. The mere presence of such antibodies is associated with an increased thrombotic risk [1].

Epidemiology

In a large retrospective analysis including patients without known autoimmune diseases, aPLs were present in approximately 9% of patients with pregnancy losses, 14% with stroke, 11% with myocardial infarction (MI), and 10% with deep vein thrombosis (DVT) [2]. Estimates in the United States suggest that aPLs are associated with approximately 50,000 pregnancy losses, 110,000 strokes, 100,000 MIs, and 30,000 DVTs annually [3–9].

Pathogenesis

aPLs affect coagulation through procoagulant action on protein C, platelets, proteases, toll-like receptors, and alteration of fibrinolysis [10–15]. They also increase vascular tone, thereby increasing the susceptibility to atherosclerosis, fetal loss, and neurological damage [16]. Further, aPLs can interact with other antibodies through complex interactions as patients with aPLs often co-express antibodies against platelet receptors, coagulation factors, or fibrinolytic elements [17–26]. Genetic risk related to APS predisposition is also emerging, but most studies are relatively underpowered compared to studies in other autoimmune diseases [27–36].

In addition to APS-specific genetic risks, patients with increased inherited risks of thrombosis are also more likely to present with thrombotic events in the context of aPLs. In different studies, factor V Leiden, the prothrombin G20210A gene mutation, and activated protein C resistance were associated with an increased risk of venous thromboembolism (VTE) [37, 38]. Additionally, overexpression of tissue factor, the trigger for the initiation of activation of coagulation, is noted on the surface of monocytes of APS patients [39]. The most commonly accepted explanation for the development of aPLs is that they occur in genetically susceptible individuals following incidental exposure to infectious agents or in the background of rheumatic diseases such as SLE. It is widely accepted that aPLs alone are insufficient for the complete manifestation of APS and that a "second hit" is required for the syndrome to develop completely [40]. Potential candidates for the delivery of such a "second hit" are multiple; they include a long list of exposing factors to thrombosis often described in risk assessment models, e.g., smoking, prolonged immobilization, pregnancy and puerperium, hormone therapy, and malignancy [41]. In addition, infectious agents, commensal microbiota, and microparticles are implicated as additional pathogenic factors and are discussed in detail below.

aPLs interact with platelets, resulting in their activation and binding to the endothelium. Microparticles are fragments of cell membranes of apoptotic, activated, or damaged cells. They play important roles in regulating health and disease and can act as a nidus for the activation of coagulation [42, 43]. The plasma concentration of platelet and endothelial-derived microparticles is increased among patients with APS when compared to people with aPL without thrombotic events and to healthy controls [44–46].

The complement pathway is also involved in the pathogenesis of APS. Depending on the isotype, antigen-antibody interactions can lead to complement consumption. APS patients can have lower levels of CH50, C3, and C4 with increased levels of complement activation by-products [47]. The presence of increased complement deposition in the placentae of patients with APS and pregnancy-related diseases highlights its importance [48, 49]. Complement contributes also to the progression of APS into catastrophic APS (CAPS) that is characterized by micro- and macrothrombotic events in multiple organs within a short period of time [42, 43].

Besides microbial triggers, aPLs can occur in the setting of certain medications and in malignancy. A large number of medications known to alter immune system function including phenytoin, hydralazine, procainamide, and quinine, as well as oral contraceptive pills and hormonal replacement therapy that are known to increase the risk for thrombosis, have been associated with transient aPLs, often of the IgM isotype; these are rarely associated with thrombosis without additional predisposition for thrombophilia [50, 51]. aPLs have also been reported in patients with a variety of malignancies including cancers of the lung, colon, cervix, prostate, kidney, ovary, and breast as well as premalignant and malignant hematologic diseases including lymphoproliferative, myeloproliferative, and myeloid disorders [50–52].

In summary, the pathogenesis of APS is complex and multifactorial. After generation of aPLs, patients develop thrombotic events after various "second hits" that promote thrombogenesis. We next review in more depth the role of viral, bacterial, and commensal microbial agents in the initiating and propagating steps in the pathogenesis of APS.

Innate and Viral Sensors

The "interferon-α (IFN-α) signature" in patients with several systemic rheumatic diseases, in particular lupus, is well described and correlates with disease flares [53]. Since the IFN pathway is central to antiviral immune responses, this signature in autoimmune patients suggests that the virome could theoretically be involved in the pathogenesis of these diseases. In addition to infecting human host cells, viruses, specifically bacteriophages, live also within microbial cells such as the gut commensal bacteria that colonize the gut of human hosts. Thus, viruses both within the host and commensal bacteria could be a potential source for the production of interferon-α via nucleic acid sensors such as TLR7, a receptor implicated in systemic autoimmunity [54].

Type I interferons, e.g., IFN-α or INF-β, bind to a shared receptor formed by two transmembrane proteins IFNAR-1 and IFNAR-2. These form a ternary complex that initiates signaling leading to the production of secondary IFN-γ (mediating antiviral activity) and the production of IL-2, IL-6, IL-4, and IL-10 with a paradoxical proliferative response [55, 56]. Thus, the immunomodulatory effect of interferon-α depends on its ability to stimulate the production of endogenous IFN-γ and IL-2 leading to the initiation of a Th1 response with enhanced MHC class II expression by antigen-presenting cells. In the presence of interferon-γ, CD8+ T and NK cells will be activated and transformed into "lymphokine-activated killer" (LAK) cells disrupting the integrity of their virally infected target. Interferon-inducible proteins inhibit viral protein synthesis but contribute also to the antiproliferative response of interferons and lead to the often observed cytopenias, particularly thrombocytopenia observed in the context of lupus [56]. Activation of the IFN pathway has also been observed in APS patients. Interestingly, in 68 patients with primary APS, elevated type I interferon activity was detected in the circulation of patients and correlated with impaired endothelial progenitor function [57]. The possibility of a link between the virome and APS is only speculative at present but plausible given its shared pathogenesis with lupus with increased IFN activity.

aPLs, APS, and Infections

The first report of aPLs cross-reacting with infectious agents was made in 1985, with cross-reactivity identified in patients with syphilis [58]. These findings were confirmed in a larger cohort at that time [59]. Follow-up studies interestingly found that aPLs occur transiently in subjects with a variety of infections [60–62]. These aPLs are usually IgM aCL, are not long-lasting, and do not target the major autoantigen β2GPI [60]. Further, these aPLs rarely result in thrombotic events and are absent upon follow-up [60–62]. Specific examples are discussed below.

Pathogenic bacteria including *Mycobacterium tuberculosis* are implicated in aPL generation [63, 64]. Of note, a significant decrease in IgM titers against all phospholipids was observed upon anti-TB treatment [65]. This study highlighted the measurement of IgM antiphospholipid antibodies as a useful biomarker to monitor treatment response in tuberculous patients [65]. Furthermore, sporadic reports point to tuberculosis as a triggering "second hit" for clinically evident APS [66].

An association between Lyme disease and aPL has recently been described [67]. Furthermore, infection-associated aPL levels in patients with infective endocarditis were found to be related to endothelial cell activation, thrombin generation, and impairment of fibrinolysis [68]. This may contribute to the increased risk for major embolic events in these patients [68]. Patients with infective endocarditis may develop also rheumatic manifestations concurrent with autoantibodies such as rheumatoid factor, aCL, and anti-β2 GP1, with low specificity, which leads to potential misdiagnosis [69] (see Chap. 30).

The range of bacterial infections that have been reported to induce aPLs includes leptospirosis, leprosy, post-streptococcal rheumatic fever, mycoplasma, and *Klebsiella*. A large number of viral infections including hepatitis A, B, and C, mumps, human immunodeficiency virus (HIV), cytomegalovirus (CMV), Epstein-Barr virus (EBV), parvovirus B19, and rubella, as well as a number of parasites, including malaria, and fungi, e.g., *Pneumocystis jirovecii*, have been associated with aPLs or occasionally APS in predisposed patients [70–78].

Besides infectious triggers that are transient, emerging research suggests that another initial and perhaps chronic trigger for aPLs could be the microbiota, commensal bacteria that are not usually pathogenic but live on the mucosal and epithelial surfaces of the host.

Microbiota/Microbiome and Autoimmunity

The microbiome, introduced in Chap. 1, is a potential contributor to a wide variety of chronic disease states given its intimate interactions with the host and long coevolutionary history. While there are several differences between a pathogen and a commensal, the innate and adaptive immune responses can be similar. At least three, not mutually exclusive mechanisms by which infectious agents induce autoimmunity are bystander activation, epitope spreading, and molecular mimicry [79]. Growing evidence supports that the microbiota also influences autoimmunity by similar mechanisms [80]. The connection between the gut microbiota and gut diseases such as inflammatory bowel disease is long-standing. Several studies using animal models have lately also connected the gut microbiota with non-intestinal autoimmune disease. A classic example of commensal gut bacteria influencing non-gut autoimmune disease comes from the common mouse small intestine-resident bacteria referred to as segmented filamentous bacteria (SFB).

Gram-positive, spore-forming SFB are influenced by nutrient availability, such as vitamin A, and have been shown to instigate the pathogenesis of autoimmune arthritis and experimental autoimmune encephalomyelitis in animal models [81, 82]. Conversely, SFB exert a sex-specific protective effect in a mouse model of type I diabetes, the nonobese diabetic (NOD) mouse, that depends on the concomitant effects of other microbiota [83, 84]. To date, the colonization of SFB in humans remains a topic of debate, as most studies have failed to identify SFB in the intestinal tract of humans with the exception of infants [85]. Nevertheless, studies utilizing SFB offer proof of concept that gut bacteria influence the pathogenesis of non-gut autoimmunity. The dichotomy of

SFB's exacerbative or protective effects in different experimental autoimmune models is likely due to the different molecular drivers of autoimmune disease, such as CD4+ T helper cells, that are influenced by the microbiota [80].

CD4+ T helper cells, in particular T helper 17 cells (Th17) and T follicular helper cells (Tfh), are at the interface of the microbiota and autoimmunity [86]. T helper cells play a critical role in the development of autoimmune disease and autoantibodies by secreting cytokines such as IL-17A (Th17), IL-21, and IL-4 (Tfh) [87, 88]. While the full cellular and molecular mechanisms of these complex interactions remain not yet completely understood, it is well defined that the cytokine milieu in which CD4+ cells are activated by antigen-presenting cells (APCs) will dictate the differentiation of T helper cells, which in turn will influence the adaptive immune response and antibody production [87, 88]. Individual microbes or communities of microbes are known to modify the cytokine profile of both APCs and T helper cells through direct interactions, such as activation of innate pattern recognition receptors (PRRs) by microbe-associated molecular patterns (MAMPs), and indirect interactions, such as the production of metabolites like short-chain fatty acids (SCFAs) [80]. The following examples highlight our current understanding of the interaction of the adaptive immune system and the microbiome in autoimmunity.

Direct Interaction with Barrier Sites and Ag Specificity at Local and Distant Sites

Th17 cells have been associated with APS [89]. As noted above, SFB is capable of inducing the formation of Th17 cells, which in autoimmune models of arthritis and multiple sclerosis have pathogenic effects but paradoxically protective effects in NOD mice. SFB is able to induce antigen-specific and antigen-independent Th17 cells through direct interaction with the epithelial cells (EpC) of the small intestine [86, 90]. SFB, upon interaction with intestinal epithelium, causes the induction of serum amyloid A proteins, which promote the expansion of Th17 cells via the production of IL-17A and IL-22 [91]. Using adhesion molecule deficient strains of SFB, *Citrobacter*, and *E. coli* 0157 in conjugation with host-specific strains of SFB, Atarashi et al. further demonstrated that adhesion was necessary to induce Th17 cells [92]. Further, this group showed that a mix of 20 bacterial strains isolated from human samples and having EpC adhesion characteristics were able to induce Th17 cells in gnotobiotic mice, thus highlighting a role for EpC adherent human microbiota in inducing Th17 cells [92]. While these studies demonstrate one potential mechanism of Th17 induction by adherent commensals, the role of EpC adherent bacteria and Th17 cells on peripheral autoimmunity in humans, in particular APS, remains to be demonstrated. The role of the microbiota in activating antigen-specific T cells in autoimmunity was further highlighted by Caspi et al., who showed that the gut microbiota as a whole is necessary to activate autoantigen-specific T cells in the autoimmune uveitis model R161H [93]. However, due to technical limitations, the causative element(s) of the gut microbiota remains elusive. This work highlights the difficulties in identifying pathogenic members of the microbiota even when there are clear associations in a reduced experimental setting [94].

Indirect Effects Via Soluble MAMPs (PSA) and Metabolites (SCFAs)

In addition to direct interactions leading to inflammatory settings, the microbiome is the source of numerous soluble factors that lead to a pro- or anti-inflammatory state locally or systemically. Most are anti-inflammatory, which relates to the coevolutionary history of host colonization without immunologic rejection. Certain microbe-associated molecular pattern (MAMPs), such as polysaccharide A (PSA) derived from *Bacteroides fragilis*, are protective against experimental autoimmune encephalomyelitis [95]. PSA mediates the conversion of CD4+ T cells into CD39+, IL-10 secreting Tregs through the PRR TLR2 [95,

96]. It is important to note that not all *B. fragilis* strains are anti-inflammatory as it is known that enterotoxigenic strains producing the *B. fragilis* toxin are capable of driving colitis [97].

Additional tolerance-promoting microbial metabolites are SCFAs, which are produced by the microbiota by metabolizing fiber in the host's diet. SCFAs are the most abundant microbial metabolite in the gut, reaching concentrations of up to 130 nM in the proximal colon [98]. SCFAs are thought to be beneficial in autoimmune models by increasing the number and function of local and peripheral CD4+ Tregs through various mechanisms, which will decrease inflammation and limit autoimmunity [80, 99]. One mechanism by which SCFAs exert their effect on CD4+ Tregs is the direct coupling of SCFAs with chemotactic G-protein-coupled receptors 43 and 109a. Binding to these receptors on either Tregs or innate cells, such as macrophages, leads to protection in models of autoimmune gut inflammation, arthritis, and asthma due to the increase of anti-inflammatory cells and cytokines [54, 100–103]. While a direct link to SCFAs and APS has yet to be proven, altered Treg frequencies have been described in APS [104]. Whether these are related to gut microbial dysbiosis remains to be elucidated, but an ongoing microbiome study in APS that could address this question will be discussed further below. Figure 22.1 illustrates the mechanisms by which the microbiota affects the immune system and could contribute to APS pathogenesis.

Microbiota/Microbiome Paving the Way to APS Development

The host-microbiota interactions summarized in the previous section involve immune cells and pathways that are also implicated in APS. In addition, the infectious factors contributing to the

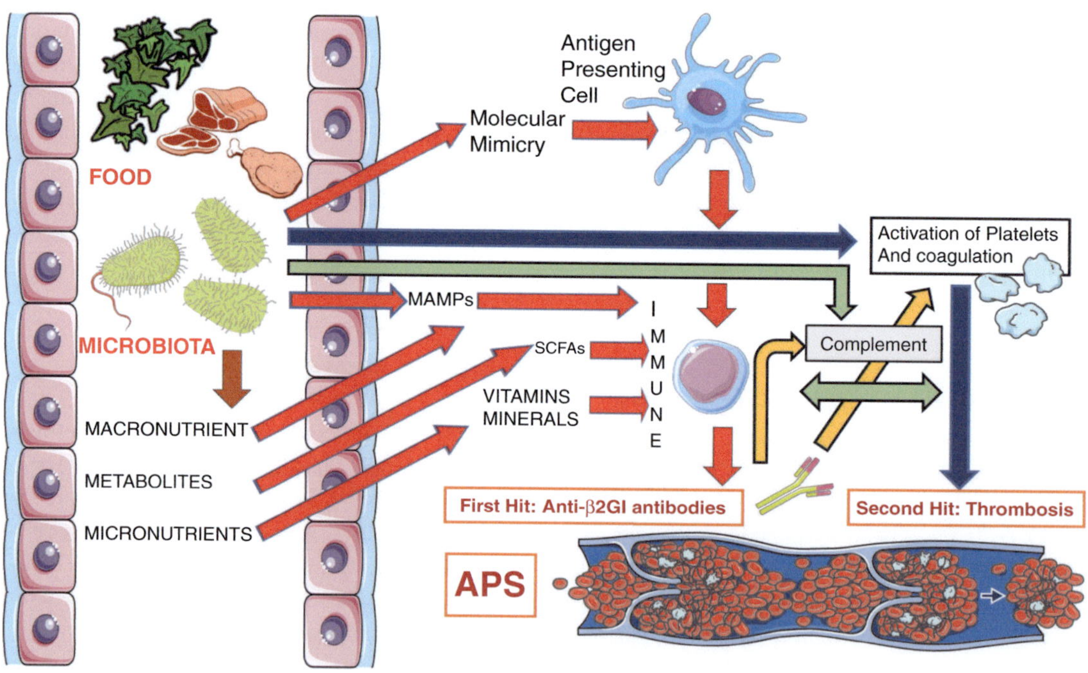

Fig. 22.1 The microbiota acts via two mechanisms: A first immune-mediated hit occurs as a result of molecular mimicry and through direct and indirect interaction with the immune system results in anti-β2GPI-antibody production. The second hit occurs when microbiota lipoprotein activates platelets and coagulation with the complement activation often acting as an intermediary. Then the combination of aPLs and activated primary and secondary hemostasis results in the full-blown picture of APS. *MAMPs* microbe-associated molecular patterns, *SCFAs* short-chain fatty acids

first and second "hits" in APS could equally be derived from commensal, instead of pathogenic, bacteria. Studies of the murine and human microbiome in APS are currently ongoing and will be summarized here to support the hypothesis that commensal bacteria are involved in the etiopathogenesis of APS. The various roles the microbiota could play in APS were recently reviewed by Manfredo Vieira et al. [105]. This work focused on potential antigenic triggers of beta-2 glycoprotein I autoreactivity via molecular mimicry, also known as cross-reactivity. Previous studies in mice have shown that pathogenic microbes including *H. influenzae*, *N. gonorrhoeae*, and a human CMV-derived peptide were capable of inducing beta-2 glycoprotein I antibodies via cross-reactivity. The cross-reactivity is thought to be mediated through recognition by B and T cells of pathogenic epitopes that share either sequence or structural homology to immunodominant epitopes of beta-2 glycoprotein I [106–108].

With current estimates of non-redundant genes present in the commensal population of the human intestinal tract at over 9.8 million, it is not surprising that commensal bacteria would also share significant homology with autoantigens in APS [105, 109–111]. It was hypothesized that cross-reactivity with gut commensal antigens might also play a role in the development of APS in the absence of overt inflammation and tissue destruction. Since transient aPLs can be induced by cross-reactive pathogens, it is plausible that APS is mediated by stably colonizing, cross-reactive gut commensals. A systematic search in silico revealed a number of possibilities including a common colonic bacterium, *Roseburia intestinalis*, as a potential cross-reactive candidate that contains B and T cell mimic epitopes [105]. In vitro and vivo studies with this organism support that commensal-mediated molecular mimicry plays a role in the activation of non-gut autoreactive T and B cells [80, 112]. However, it should be noted that bystander activation, epitope spreading, and molecular mimicry are likely to work in tandem to fully break tolerance before autoimmunity develops, and thus molecular mimicry is only one possible mechanism by which the microbiome may influence the pathogenesis of APS [80].

Further support for the role of the microbiome and the development of APS comes from the observation that a spontaneous mouse model of APS, the (NZWxBXSB) F1 hybrid, is protected by depletion of the microbiota by orally administered broad-spectrum antibiotics [105]. The NZWxBXSB F1 model is characterized by production of high titers of anti-β2GPI antibodies and clinical features of APS including thrombotic events, in particular microthrombi in the coronaries leading to myocardial infarctions, and thrombocytopenia. Broad-spectrum antibiotic depletion of the gut microbiota markedly prevented infarctions and thrombotic events in this model [105]. Interestingly, treatment with ampicillin or vancomycin alone was sufficient to protect from autoimmune mortality, suggesting that gram-positive gut bacteria are driving APS pathogenesis [105]. How gram-positive bacteria are influencing the development of APS in these mice is currently under investigation and might help clarify also how pathogenic aPLs are induced in human APS.

At the epithelial border that separates the microbiota from host tissues, resident antigen-presenting cells, epithelial TLRs, and nucleotide-binding oligomerization domain-like receptors sense MAMPs and by-products of the microbiota [113]. As summarized above, diet also influences the microbiota which in turn affects the host; for instance, fibers are metabolized by the colonic microbiota to SCFAs that are known to induce Tregs [113]. A deficiency in SCFA producing colonic microbiota could thus lead to reduced Treg numbers or function in APS. Further, lipopolysaccharide from gram-negative gut bacteria can trigger TLR4. Of note, TLR4 was shown to be required for the activation of B cells and the production of autoantibody in mice treated with β2GPI [114]. Activation of the TLR4/MyD88 pathway mediates also trophoblast damage, a process that could be implicated in obstetric APS [115]. Many more innate and adaptive immune pathways could theoretically be triggered by components of the microbiota, which represents a large area of research to explore. In the next section, we focus on a theoretical role of the microbiota in influencing the complement and coagulation systems, two ancient and related proteolytic systems that are fundamental in the pathogenesis of APS.

Microbiota-Mediated Autoimmunity Affecting the Complement and Coagulation Systems

The coagulation and complement systems are ancestrally related enzymatic cascades of the blood. Although their primary purposes have diverged over the past few 100 million years, they remain inextricably connected. Both complement and coagulation systems limit infection by pathogens through innate immune mechanisms. Recently, it has been shown that hyperactive complement (in particular, elevated C5a/C5b-9) is involved in the pathogenesis of thrombosis in diseases such as paroxysmal nocturnal hemoglobinuria, atypical hemolytic uremic syndrome, and APS [116].

In mouse models of APS, activation of the complement system is required, and interaction of complement C5a with its receptor C5aR leads to aPL-induced inflammation, placental insufficiency, and thrombosis [117]. Anti-C5 antibody and C5aR antagonist peptides prevent aPL-mediated pregnancy loss and thrombosis in these experimental models [42, 117]. Clinical studies of anti-C5 monoclonal antibody in aPL-positive patients are limited to a small number of case reports but support efficacy [42].

The mechanisms through which complement activation occurs are not fully understood. Hypothetically, activation through the lectin pathway by the microbiota is one of many possibilities [118]. Once the complement pathway is interfered with, it is likely that the microbial community composition on barrier surfaces is altered, which in turn can affect immune function. Indeed, antagonism of the C5aR leads to skin commensal dysbiosis and altered inflammatory state [117]. Autoantibodies produced against C1q, a component of complement 1, were reported to correlate with complement activation in systemic lupus erythematosus [118]. These antibodies target neoepitopes of deformed C1q bound to various molecules (i.e., anionic phospholipids) and induce accelerated complement activation. Anti-C1q antibodies are more frequently detected in primary APS patients than in control patients and in refractory APS patients with repeated thrombotic events. The titer of anti-C1q antibodies was significantly higher in refractory APS patients than in APS patients without flare. The binding of C1q to anionic phospholipids may be associated with the surge in complement activation in patients with anti-C1q antibodies when triggered by "second-hit" biological stressors such as infection or, theoretically, commensal dysbiosis. Such stressors will induce overexpression of anionic phospholipids, with subsequent increases in deformed C1q that is targeted by anti-C1q antibodies [118].

Signaling crosstalk between complement and TLRs normally serves to coordinate host immunity. However, among oral microbes, the periodontal bacterium *Porphyromonas gingivalis*, for example, expresses C5 convertase-like enzymatic activity and adeptly exploits complement-TLR crosstalk to subvert host defenses and escape elimination. Intriguingly, this defect in immune surveillance leads to the remodeling of the periodontal microbiota to a dysbiotic state that causes inflammatory periodontitis [119]. It is not known if other gut microbes share the same properties or if this bacterium plays a role in APS pathogenesis.

It is well established that aPLs predispose to thrombosis by generating a thrombogenic state mediated by endothelial damage, monocyte activation with overexpression of tissue factor, and platelet hyper-reactivity. The generation of trimethylamine *N*-oxide (TMAO) by the gut microbiota contributes directly to platelet hyper-reactivity and enhanced thrombosis potential [120]. It is therefore possible that TMAO production in APS patients contributes to the thrombogenic state besides the role in aPL induction discussed above. Gut microbial dysbiosis is also firmly linked to obesity and chronic inflammation that are disease states associated with hypercoagulability, which may be a result of both increased production of coagulant vitamin K-dependent factors and reduced fibrinolytic activity [121, 122]. The composition of the gut microbiota might also promote or inhibit coagulation if disturbed by probiotics. In a recent study of 24 participants receiving probiotics, there was a significant reduction in D-dimer levels (median change 33%, $P = 0.03$) and a trend toward reduced levels of C-reactive protein (CRP) ($P = 0.05$). Thus, probiotic interventions appear to influence markers of coagulation and inflammation that warrant further exploration in APS [123]. Overall, there are multiple ways in which the microbiota may interact with the host in APS by affecting the complement and coagulation systems. Figure 22.1 illustrates the mechanisms through which the microbiota is proposed to influence APS development.

Clinical Manifestations

APS presents usually with thrombosis either affecting veins, arteries, or small vessels, with specific pregnancy-related complications or with livedo reticularis, reduction in platelet count, or transient focal neurologic disorders. Rare presentations include MI, valve disease, pulmonary hypertension, avascular necrosis, or cutaneous ulcerations [82–85]. Venous thrombosis of the lower extremities is the most common presentation in 20–30% of cases, whereas thrombosis at unusual sites occurs less frequently [124]. Figure 22.2 illustrates the frequency of the different presenting clinical manifestations of the disease [124].

Mild thrombocytopenia ranging from 100,000 to 140,000/μl is not infrequent in APS patients, with an incidence ranging from 22 to 42% [125]. Other hematologic manifestations are also well described in APS, in particular Coombs' positive hemolytic anemia, which can be a harbinger of transition to SLE [125]. Pregnancy complications are another hallmark of APS. Such complications result partly from placental ischemia and complement-mediated damage and range from intrauterine fetal growth retardation, preeclampsia, HELLP syndrome (hemolysis, elevated liver enzymes, and low platelet count), and premature birth to fetal death. Patients with SLE and lupus anticoagulant have an increased risk of pregnancy loss as well as a poorer prognosis than aPL-negative patients [126].

Moreover, in a longitudinal analysis of outcomes of lupus nephritis in an international inception cohort using a multistate model approach, the study group found that the presence of lupus anticoagulant in lupus patients predicted less improvement in renal outcomes [127]. A small subset of patients with APS (0.8%) develop widespread thrombosis of the small vessels resulting in multiorgan failure referred to as "catastrophic APS" (CAPS) [124, 128] and is associated with significant mortality risks despite prompt treatment [129].

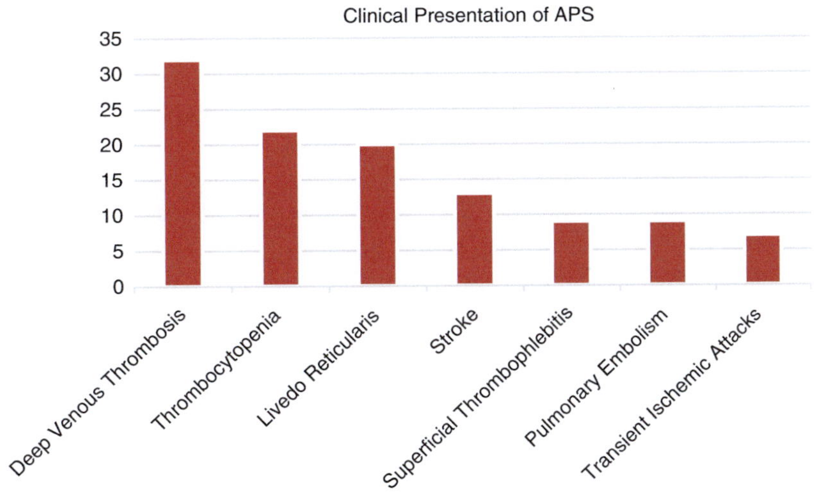

Fig. 22.2 Illustration of the presenting symptoms and signs (percent) of patients with APS [124]

The criteria to diagnose CAPS include:

- History of APS and/or presence of aPL
- Three or more new organ thromboses within a week
- Biopsy confirmation of a microthrombus
- Exclusion of other causes of multiple organ thromboses or micro-thromboses

The differential diagnoses of CAPS include heparin-induced thrombocytopenia (HIT) with or without thrombosis, disseminated intravascular coagulation, and thrombotic microangiopathy.

Diagnostic Evaluation

Patients with suspected APS should be thoroughly evaluated including a full clinical assessment with history of thromboembolic disease, pregnancy complications or associated immune disorders, and skin changes and a complete physical examination to detect findings consistent with livedo reticularis or digital ischemia and venous thrombosis [130]. Clinical assessment is often complemented by a battery of investigations usually done shortly after a clinical event, followed by confirmatory testing at least 12 weeks later and includes:

- aCL; immunoglobulin G (IgG) and/or IgM by enzyme-linked immunosorbent assay (ELISA).
- Anti-beta2-GP I antibodies; IgG and/or IgM by ELISA.
- LA testing in a three-step procedure: The first step aims at demonstrating a prolonged phospholipid-dependent screening test of hemostasis. Commonly used screening tests include the dilute Russell viper venom time (dRVVT) and an activated partial thromboplastin time (aPTT) that has been optimized for this purpose (aPTT or lupus aPTT), followed by mixing studies. In those, patient plasma is mixed with normal plasma resulting in a failure to correct the prolonged screening test(s) due to the presence of inhibitors and eliminating the possibility of a coagulation factor deficiency. The next step requires the addition of excess phospholipid shortening or correcting the prolonged coagulation test (phospholipid dependence).

Additional testing often includes a thrombophilia screen, routine laboratory evaluations for SLE as well as tests needed to exclude HIT if suspected.

According to the revised Sapporo APS classification criteria (also called the Sydney criteria), APS is present in patients who meet at least one of the clinical criteria and at least one of the laboratory criteria [131, 132]:

Clinical Criteria

1. Vascular thrombosis—One or more episodes of venous, arterial, or small vessel thrombosis with unequivocal imaging and excluding superficial venous thrombosis.
2. Pregnancy morbidity—One or more unexplained deaths of a morphologically normal fetus at ≥10 weeks of gestation, or one or more premature births of a morphologically normal neonate before 34 weeks of gestation because of eclampsia, preeclampsia, or placental insufficiency, or three or more consecutive spontaneous pregnancy losses at <10 weeks of gestation.

Laboratory Criteria

The presence of one or more aPLs on two or more occasions at least 12 weeks apart.

Approach to Therapy

The cornerstone therapy for the non-obstetric manifestations of APS uncomplicated by CAPS or other comorbidities involves outpatient treatment using antithrombotic medications which include aspirin, heparins, and warfarin [133]. Recently the new oral anticoagulant rivaroxaban has been used with some success [134–136].

In addition, any patient with concomitant lupus who is typically treated with hydroxychloroquine would also benefit from the proposed effects of this drug in primary APS [137]. Patients with comorbidities or with life-threatening VTE often require admission and inpatient hospital treatment [9].

Aspirin alone has been of minimal benefit for the prevention of thrombotic APS manifestations in patients who have experienced previous events [138, 139]. Although thrombotic events are unlikely in the absence of additional risk factors for thrombosis, some studies suggested that aspirin (81 mg/day) reduces the thrombotic risk in (aPL)-positive individuals. It should be noted that among patients with aCL antibodies, the higher the titer, the greater is possibly the risk of thrombosis [140]. It is therefore reasonable to consider primary prophylaxis using low-dose aspirin in patients with concomitant connective tissue diseases or other risk factors such as cardiovascular or genetic risks. Every attempt should be made to address modifiable risk factors for thrombosis such as thrombogenic medications, cigarette smoking, or venous stasis [141]. Other antiplatelet agents or dual antiplatelet therapy are not currently recommended [142]. The special task force of the 13th International Congress on Antiphospholipid Antibodies recommended that asymptomatic aPL carriers follow a strict control of cardiovascular risk factors and thromboprophylaxis using a low molecular weight heparin (LMWH) in the context of any added risk for thrombosis [143].

The usual approach to treat a venous thrombotic episode in a patient with APS is to initiate treatment with heparin or LMWH that is bridged to a lifelong warfarin therapy maintaining an INR between 2.0 and 3.0. High-intensity therapy (aiming at an INR 3.0–4.0) is associated with no demonstrable additional benefit and may be harmful [144, 145]. In occasional patients with a first venous event, a known transient precipitating factor, and a low aPL titer, treating for a more defined period, such as 6 months, may be acceptable [143]. Treatment failure with recurrence is observed in 7% of cases and major bleeding reported in around 2–3% of cases per year. If thrombotic events recur during warfarin therapy despite therapeutic INR levels, a high-intensity approach or the addition of low-dose aspirin may be considered.

In the context of active infections when systemic antibiotics are used in conjunction to warfarin, close monitoring of the INR is needed as many antibiotics can disturb the vitamin K-producing bacteria within the gut microbiome resulting in an enhanced warfarin action. Furthermore, antimicrobials may also inhibit cytochrome p450 (CYP450) enzymes (primarily CYP2C9 and 3A4), which are responsible for the metabolism of warfarin [145]. The antibiotics most likely to interfere with warfarin are trimethoprim/sulfamethoxazole [TMP/SMX], ciprofloxacin, levofloxacin, metronidazole, fluconazole, azithromycin, and clarithromycin, whereas low-risk agents include clindamycin, cephalexin, and penicillin G [31, 146]. Presumptive warfarin dose reductions in an attempt to avoid supra-therapeutic INRs in patients being prescribed antibiotics should be considered only in the presence of the antibiotics TMP/SMX and metronidazole [145, 146].

The treatment of arterial thrombosis is more controversial as some investigators have advocated the use of a combination of warfarin targeting an INR of 2.0–3.0 in combination with aspirin, whereas others have suggested a high-intensity warfarin therapeutic regimen [146–149]. It is reasonable to consider aspirin prophylaxis for patients with transient ischemic attacks associated with aPLs, whereas patients meeting the criteria for APS should be treated with warfarin targeting an INR of 2.0–3.0. For those with recurrent strokes despite “adequate” anticoagulation, a higher INR strategy or adding ASA 81 mg or switching to heparin can be considered [150].

With cardiac involvement, low-dose aspirin (81 mg/day) is suggested in patients with echocardiographic evidence of valvular thickening without clinical features of systemic embolization, whereas heparin followed by warfarin anticoagulation (target INR 2.0–3.0) is suggested for patients with echocardiographic evidence of vegetations, clinical evidence of systemic embolization, or aPL-associated MI [151].

Thrombocytopenia in APS is believed to result from binding of aPLs to platelet-associated phospholipids and requires no treatment if mild, although some data suggest a beneficial effect of anticoagulation [152]. Marked thrombocytopenia, on the other hand, should be managed as immune thrombocytopenia [153], whereas thrombocytopenia occurring in the context of a thrombotic microangiopathy is best addressed by plasma exchange.

Pregnancy-associated disorders are best treated with LMWH with or without aspirin. Warfarin is a teratogen and should be avoided long before the decision to conceive is made.

The management of CAPS necessitates the integration of our entire therapeutic arsenal, and the prognosis is guarded with a high mortality in the range of 30% [154]. Any identifiable infection, whether bacterial, fungal, or viral, that may have precipitated CAPS [155] should be treated promptly with the appropriate antimicrobial therapy, if possible. The treatment is generally directed at addressing thrombotic events and suppressing the cytokine cascade. This typically involves a combination of anticoagulants, systemic glucocorticoids, plasma exchange, and/or intravenous immune globulin [156]. Several case reports described the use of rituximab in resistant cases [157] or eculizumab in recurrent cases [158]. Barratt and his group applied eculizumab to treat a case of CAPS with remarkable improvement. When the drug was decreased abruptly, the patient experienced a serious relapse that was rapidly reversed following eculizumab rechallenge [42].

Summary and Conclusions

In summary, patients who survive the initial episode that leads to the diagnosis of APS remain at risk for recurrent events. Currently available treatments (oral anticoagulation or aspirin) may reduce, but do not eliminate, the risk of recurrent thrombotic, thromboembolic, or obstetrical adverse outcomes, and sometimes these events are fatal. Prompt treatment of infections in patients with aPLs in the absence of a full-blown APS may prevent the second hit needed for APS to develop.

The complex ecosystem which coevolved with humans comprises trillions of microbes with thousands of species which sustain a state of tolerance, promoting anti-inflammation. Any break in tolerance with microbial mimicry, PAMPs/MAMPs over-activating TLRs, diet-related metabolites from the microbiota, and the generation of cytokines can lead to activation of the immune system and initiation of autoimmune processes. Given the relation between aPLs and microbes, it is likely that the microbiota might play a role in the development and evolution of APS. The importance of complement activation and the activation of coagulation in APS and its progression to CAPS may also be partly influenced by our microbiota. A deeper understanding of host-microbiota interactions and the impact of infections on autoimmune-prone hosts may help in better understanding the pathophysiology of autoimmune diseases including APS. Targeting the microbiota or some of the mediators that interact with the immune system may offer future potential therapeutic targets in the management of APS.

References

1. Pengo V, Ruffatti A, Legnani C, et al. Incidence of a first thromboembolic event in asymptomatic carriers of high-risk antiphospholipid antibody profile: a multicenter prospective study. Blood. 2011;118(17):4714–8.
2. Merrill JT, Zhang HW, Shen C, et al. Enhancement of protein S anticoagulant function by beta2-glycoprotein I, a major target antigen of antiphospholipid antibodies: beta2-glycoprotein I interferes with binding of protein S to its plasma inhibitor, C4b-binding protein. Thromb Haemost. 1999;81(5):748–57.
3. Andreoli L, Chighizola CB, Banzato A, et al. Estimated frequency of antiphospholipid antibodies in patients with pregnancy morbidity, stroke, myocardial infarction, and deep vein thrombosis: a critical review of the literature. Arthritis Care Res (Hoboken). 2013;65(11):1869–73.
4. Macklon NS, Geraedts JP, Fauser BC. Conception to ongoing pregnancy: the 'black box' of early pregnancy loss. Hum Reprod Update. 2002;8(4): 333–43.

5. Stephenson MD. Frequency of factors associated with habitual abortion in 197 couples. Fertil Steril. 1996;66(1):24–9.
6. Martin JA, Hamilton BE, Ventura SJ, et al. Births: final data for 2009. Natl Vital Stat Rep. 2011;60(1):1–70.
7. Roger VL, Go AS, Lloyd-Jones DM, et al. Executive summary: heart disease and stroke statistics—2012 update: a report from the American Heart Association. Circulation. 2012;125(1):188–97.
8. White RH. The epidemiology of venous thromboembolism. Circulation. 2003;107(23 Suppl 1): I4–8.
9. www.census.gov/population/www/cen2010/glance/index.html. Accessed 19 Oct 2015.
10. Urbanus RT, Derksen RH, de Groot PG. Platelets and the antiphospholipid syndrome. Lupus. 2008;17(10):888–94.
11. Chen PP, Giles I. Antibodies to serine proteases in the antiphospholipid syndrome. Curr Rheumatol Rep. 2010;12(1):45–52.
12. Raschi E, Borghi MO, Grossi C, et al. Toll-like receptors: another player in the pathogenesis of the anti-phospholipid syndrome. Lupus. 2008;17(10):937–42.
13. Kinev AV, Roubey RA. Tissue factor in the antiphospholipid syndrome. Lupus. 2008;17(10):952–8.
14. Bu C, Gao L, Xie W, et al. beta2-glycoprotein i is a cofactor for tissue plasminogen activator-mediated plasminogen activation. Arthritis Rheum. 2009;60(2):559–68.
15. Forastiero R, Martinuzzo M. Prothrombotic mechanisms based on the impairment of fibrinolysis in the antiphospholipid syndrome. Lupus. 2008;17(10):872–7.
16. Mackworth-Young CG. Antiphospholipid syndrome: multiple mechanisms. Clin Exp Immunol. 2004;136(3):393–401.
17. Shibata S, Harpel PC, Gharavi A, et al. Autoantibodies to heparin from patients with antiphospholipid antibody syndrome inhibit formation of antithrombin III-thrombin complexes. Blood. 1994;83(9):2532–40.
18. Galli M. Non beta 2-glycoprotein I cofactors for antiphospholipid antibodies. Lupus. 1996;5(5):388–92.
19. Bidot CJ, Jy W, Horstman LL, et al. Factor VII/VIIa: a new antigen in the anti-phospholipid antibody syndrome. Br J Haematol. 2003;120(4):618–26.
20. Jones DW, MacKie IJ, Gallimore MJ, et al. Antibodies to factor XII and recurrent fetal loss in patients with the anti-phospholipid syndrome. Br J Haematol. 2001;113(2):550–2.
21. Rand JH, Wu XX, Lapinski R, et al. Detection of antibody-mediated reduction of annexin A5 anticoagulant activity in plasmas of patients with the antiphospholipid syndrome. Blood. 2004;104(9):2783–90.
22. Cesarman-Maus G, Rios-Luna NP, Deora AB, et al. Autoantibodies against the fibrinolytic receptor, annexin 2, in antiphospholipid syndrome. Blood. 2006;107(11):4375–82.
23. Munoz-Rodriguez FJ, Reverter JC, Font J, et al. Prevalence and clinical significance of antiprothrombin antibodies in patients with systemic lupus erythematosus or with primary antiphospholipid syndrome. Haematologica. 2000;85(6):632.
24. Satoh A, Suzuki K, Takayama E, et al. Detection of anti-annexin IV and V antibodies in patients with antiphospholipid syndrome and systemic lupus erythematosus. J Rheumatol. 1999;26(8):1715–20.
25. Bertolaccini ML, Sanna G, Ralhan S, et al. Antibodies directed to protein S in patients with systemic lupus erythematosus: prevalence and clinical significance. Thromb Haemost. 2003;90(4):636–41.
26. Cugno M, Cabibbe M, Galli M, et al. Antibodies to tissue-type plasminogen activator (tPA) in patients with antiphospholipid syndrome: evidence of interaction between the antibodies and the catalytic domain of tPA in 2 patients. Blood. 2004;103(6):2121–6.
27. Sebastiani GD, Iuliano A, Cantarini L, et al. Genetic aspects of the antiphospholipid syndrome: an update. Autoimmun Rev. 2016;15(5):433–9.
28. Chen X, Liang PY, Li GG, et al. Association of HLA-DQ alleles with the presence of an anti-beta2-glycoprotein I antibody in patients with recurrent miscarriage. HLA. 2016;87(1):19–24.
29. Yin H, Borghi MO, Delgado-Vega AM, et al. Association of STAT4 and BLK, but not BANK1 or IRF5, with primary antiphospholipid syndrome. Arthritis Rheum. 2009;60(8):2468–71.
30. Sanchez ML, Katsumata K, Atsumi T, et al. Association of HLA-DM polymorphism with the production of antiphospholipid antibodies. Ann Rheum Dis. 2004;63(12):1645–8.
31. Ochoa E, Iriondo M, Bielsa A, et al. Thrombotic antiphospholipid syndrome shows strong haplotypic association with SH2B3-ATXN2 locus. PLoS One. 2013;8(7):e67897.
32. Goldberg SN, Conti-Kelly AM, Greco TP. A family study of anticardiolipin antibodies and associated clinical conditions. Am J Med. 1995;99(5):473–9.
33. Lundstrom E, Gustafsson JT, Jonsen A, et al. HLA-DRB1*04/*13 alleles are associated with vascular disease and antiphospholipid antibodies in systemic lupus erythematosus. Ann Rheum Dis. 2013;72(6):1018–25.
34. Jimenez S, Tassies D, Espinosa G, et al. Double heterozygosity polymorphisms for platelet glycoproteins Ia/IIa and IIb/IIIa increases arterial thrombosis and arteriosclerosis in patients with the antiphospholipid syndrome or with systemic lupus erythematosus. Ann Rheum Dis. 2008;67(6):835–40.
35. Karassa FB, Bijl M, Davies KA, et al. Role of the Fcgamma receptor IIA polymorphism in the antiphospholipid syndrome: an international meta-analysis. Arthritis Rheum. 2003;48(7):1930–8.
36. Hirose N, Williams R, Alberts AR, et al. A role for the polymorphism at position 247 of the beta2-glycoprotein I gene in the generation of anti-beta2-

glycoprotein I antibodies in the antiphospholipid syndrome. Arthritis Rheum. 1999;42(8):1655–61.
37. Brouwer JL, Bijl M, Veeger NJ, et al. The contribution of inherited and acquired thrombophilic defects, alone or combined with antiphospholipid antibodies, to venous and arterial thromboembolism in patients with systemic lupus erythematosus. Blood. 2004;104(1):143–8.
38. Nojima J, Kuratsune H, Suehisa E, et al. Acquired activated protein C resistance is associated with the co-existence of anti-prothrombin antibodies and lupus anticoagulant activity in patients with systemic lupus erythematosus. Br J Haematol. 2002;118(2):577–83.
39. Cuadrado MJ, Lopez-Pedrera C, Khamashta MA, et al. Thrombosis in primary antiphospholipid syndrome: a pivotal role for monocyte tissue factor expression. Arthritis Rheum. 1997;40(5):834–41.
40. Erkan D, Lockshin MD. What is antiphospholipid syndrome? Curr Rheumatol Rep. 2004;6(6):451–7.
41. Motykie GD, Caprini JA, Arcelus JI, et al. Risk factor assessment in the management of patients with suspected deep venous thrombosis. Int Angiol. 2000;19(1):47–51.
42. Barratt-Due A, Floisand Y, Orrem HL, et al. Complement activation is a crucial pathogenic factor in catastrophic antiphospholipid syndrome. Rheumatology (Oxford). 2016;55(7):1337–9.
43. Cervera R, Font J, Gomez-Puerta JA, et al. Validation of the preliminary criteria for the classification of catastrophic antiphospholipid syndrome. Ann Rheum Dis. 2005;64(8):1205–9.
44. Dignat-George F, Camoin-Jau L, Sabatier F, et al. Endothelial microparticles: a potential contribution to the thrombotic complications of the antiphospholipid syndrome. Thromb Haemost. 2004;91(4):667–73.
45. Ambrozic A, Bozic B, Kveder T, et al. Budding, vesiculation and permeabilization of phospholipid membranes-evidence for a feasible physiologic role of beta2-glycoprotein I and pathogenic actions of anti-beta2-glycoprotein I antibodies. Biochim Biophys Acta. 2005;1740(1):38–44.
46. Morel O, Jesel L, Freyssinet JM, et al. Elevated levels of procoagulant microparticles in a patient with myocardial infarction, antiphospholipid antibodies and multifocal cardiac thrombosis. Thromb J. 2005;3:15.
47. Oku K, Atsumi T, Bohgaki M, et al. Complement activation in patients with primary antiphospholipid syndrome. Ann Rheum Dis. 2009;68(6):1030–5.
48. Salmon JE, Girardi G, Holers VM. Activation of complement mediates antiphospholipid antibody-induced pregnancy loss. Lupus. 2003;12(7):535–8.
49. Girardi G, Berman J, Redecha P, et al. Complement C5a receptors and neutrophils mediate fetal injury in the antiphospholipid syndrome. J Clin Invest. 2003;112(11):1644–54.
50. Triplett DA. Many faces of lupus anticoagulants. Lupus. 1998;7(Suppl 2):S18–22.
51. Dlott JS, Roubey RA. Drug-induced lupus anticoagulants and antiphospholipid antibodies. Curr Rheumatol Rep. 2012;14(1):71–8.
52. Vassalo J, Spector N, de Meis E, et al. Antiphospholipid antibodies in critically ill patients with cancer: a prospective cohort study. J Crit Care. 2014;29(4):533–8.
53. Pascual V, Chaussabel D, Banchereau J. A genomic approach to human autoimmune diseases. Annu Rev Immunol. 2010;28:535–71.
54. Vieira SM, Pagovich OE, Kriegel MA. Diet, microbiota and autoimmune diseases. Lupus. 2014;23(6):518–26.
55. Ochoa-Reparaz J, Mielcarz DW, Wang Y, et al. A polysaccharide from the human commensal Bacteroides fragilis protects against CNS demyelinating disease. Mucosal Immunol. 2010;3(5):487–95.
56. Goubran HA. Interferon therapy: from cell signaling to haematological side effects. Dig Liver Dis Suppl. 2009;3(1):13–6.
57. Grenn RC, Yalavarthi S, Gandhi AA, et al. Endothelial progenitor dysfunction associates with a type I interferon signature in primary antiphospholipid syndrome. Ann Rheum Dis. 2017;76(2):450–7.
58. Harris EN, Gharavi AE, Loizou S, et al. Crossreactivity of antiphospholipid antibodies. J Clin Lab Immunol. 1985;16(1):1–6.
59. Costello PB, Green FA. Reactivity patterns of human anticardiolipin and other antiphospholipid antibodies in syphilitic sera. Infect Immun. 1986;51(3):771–5.
60. McNeil HP, Chesterman CN, Krilis SA. Immunology and clinical importance of antiphospholipid antibodies. Adv Immunol. 1991;49:193–280.
61. Erkan D, Derksen WJ, Kaplan V, et al. Real world experience with antiphospholipid antibody tests: how stable are results over time? Ann Rheum Dis. 2005;64(9):1321–5.
62. Vila P, Hernandez MC, Lopez-Fernandez MF, et al. Prevalence, follow-up and clinical significance of the anticardiolipin antibodies in normal subjects. Thromb Haemost. 1994;72(2):209–13.
63. Adebajo AO, Charles P, Maini RN, et al. Autoantibodies in malaria, tuberculosis and hepatitis B in a west African population. Clin Exp Immunol. 1993;92(1):73–6.
64. Elkayam O, Caspi D, Lidgi M, et al. Auto-antibody profiles in patients with active pulmonary tuberculosis. Int J Tuberc Lung Dis. 2007;11(3):306–10.
65. Elkayam O, Bendayan D, Segal R, et al. The effect of anti-tuberculosis treatment on levels of anti-phospholipid and anti-neutrophil cytoplasmatic antibodies in patients with active tuberculosis. Rheumatol Int. 2013;33(4):949–53.
66. Ghosh K, Shetty S. Deep venous thrombosis associated with antiphospholipid antibodies following tuberculosis lymphadenitis in a predisposed patient. Blood Coagul Fibrinolysis. 2008;19(5):464–5.
67. Stricker RB, Johnson L. Antiphospholipid antibodies in patients with persistent Lyme disease symptoms. Lupus. 2012;21(3):346–7.

68. Kupferwasser LI, Hafner G, Mohr-Kahaly S, et al. The presence of infection-related antiphospholipid antibodies in infective endocarditis determines a major risk factor for embolic events. J Am Coll Cardiol. 1999;33(5):1365–71.
69. Bojalil R, Mazon-Gonzalez B, Carrillo-Cordova JR, et al. Frequency and clinical significance of a variety of autoantibodies in patients with definite infective endocarditis. J Clin Rheumatol. 2012;18(2): 67–70.
70. McNally T, Purdy G, Mackie IJ, et al. The use of an anti-beta 2-glycoprotein-I assay for discrimination between anticardiolipin antibodies associated with infection and increased risk of thrombosis. Br J Haematol. 1995;91(2):471–3.
71. Santiago M, Martinelli R, Ko A, et al. Anti-beta2 glycoprotein I and anticardiolipin antibodies in leptospirosis, syphilis and Kala-azar. Clin Exp Rheumatol. 2001;19(4):425–30.
72. Galli L, Gerdes VE, Guasti L, et al. Thrombosis associated with viral hepatitis. J Clin Transl Hepatol. 2014;2(4):234–9.
73. Prieto J, Yuste JR, Beloqui O, et al. Anticardiolipin antibodies in chronic hepatitis C: implication of hepatitis C virus as the cause of the antiphospholipid syndrome. Hepatology. 1996;23(2):199–204.
74. Leroy V, Arvieux J, Jacob MC, et al. Prevalence and significance of anticardiolipin, anti-beta2 glycoprotein I and anti-prothrombin antibodies in chronic hepatitis C. Br J Haematol. 1998;101(3):468–74.
75. Munoz-Rodriguez FJ, Tassies D, Font J, et al. Prevalence of hepatitis C virus infection in patients with antiphospholipid syndrome. J Hepatol. 1999;30(5):770–3.
76. Von Landenberg P, Lehmann HW, Knoll A, et al. Antiphospholipid antibodies in pediatric and adult patients with rheumatic disease are associated with parvovirus B19 infection. Arthritis Rheum. 2003;48(7):1939–47.
77. Roszkiewicz J, Smolewska E. Kaleidoscope of autoimmune diseases in HIV infection. Rheumatol Int. 2016;36(11):1481–91.
78. Gomes LR, Martins YC, Ferreira-da-Cruz MF, et al. Autoimmunity, phospholipid-reacting antibodies and malaria immunity. Lupus. 2014;23(12):1295–8.
79. Munz C, Lunemann JD, Getts MT, et al. Antiviral immune responses: triggers of or triggered by autoimmunity? Nat Rev Immunol. 2009;9(4):246–58.
80. Ruff WE, Kriegel MA. Autoimmune host-microbiota interactions at barrier sites and beyond. Trends Mol Med. 2015;21(4):233–44.
81. Wu HJ, Ivanov II, Darce J, et al. Gut-residing segmented filamentous bacteria drive autoimmune arthritis via T helper 17 cells. Immunity. 2010;32(6):815–27.
82. Lee YK, Menezes JS, Umesaki Y, et al. Proinflammatory T-cell responses to gut microbiota promote experimental autoimmune encephalomyelitis. Proc Natl Acad Sci U S A. 2011;108(Suppl 1):4615–22.
83. Kriegel MA, Sefik E, Hill JA, et al. Naturally transmitted segmented filamentous bacteria segregate with diabetes protection in nonobese diabetic mice. Proc Natl Acad Sci U S A. 2011;108(28):11548–53.
84. Yurkovetskiy L, Burrows M, Khan AA, et al. Gender bias in autoimmunity is influenced by microbiota. Immunity. 2013;39(2):400–12.
85. Ericsson AC, Hagan CE, Davis DJ, et al. Segmented filamentous bacteria: commensal microbes with potential effects on research. Comp Med. 2014;64(2):90–8.
86. Ivanov K II, Atarashi NM, et al. Induction of intestinal Th17 cells by segmented filamentous bacteria. Cell. 2009;139(3):485–98.
87. Burkett PR, Meyer zu Horste G, Kuchroo VK. Pouring fuel on the fire: Th17 cells, the environment, and autoimmunity. J Clin Invest. 2015;125(6):2211–9.
88. Craft JE. Follicular helper T cells in immunity and systemic autoimmunity. Nat Rev Rheumatol. 2012;8(6):337–47.
89. Popovic-Kuzmanovic D, Novakovic I, Stojanovich L, et al. Increased activity of interleukin-23/interleukin-17 cytokine axis in primary antiphospholipid syndrome. Immunobiology. 2013;218(2):186–91.
90. Yang Y, Torchinsky MB, Gobert M, et al. Focused specificity of intestinal TH17 cells towards commensal bacterial antigens. Nature. 2014;510(7503):152–6.
91. Sano T, Huang W, Hall JA, et al. An IL-23R/IL-22 circuit regulates epithelial serum amyloid a to promote local effector Th17 responses. Cell. 2015;163(2):381–93.
92. Atarashi K, Tanoue T, Ando M, et al. Th17 cell induction by adhesion of microbes to intestinal epithelial cells. Cell. 2015;163(2):367–80.
93. Horai R, Zarate-Blades CR, Dillenburg-Pilla P, et al. Microbiota-dependent activation of an autoreactive T cell receptor provokes autoimmunity in an immunologically privileged site. Immunity. 2015;43(2):343–53.
94. Zarate-Blades CR, Horai R, Mattapallil MJ, et al. Gut microbiota as a source of a surrogate antigen that triggers autoimmunity in an immune privileged site. Gut Microbes. 2017;8(1):59–66.
95. Round JL, Mazmanian SK. Inducible Foxp3+ regulatory T-cell development by a commensal bacterium of the intestinal microbiota. Proc Natl Acad Sci U S A. 2010;107(27):12204–9.
96. Wang Y, Telesford KM, Ochoa-Reparaz J, et al. An intestinal commensal symbiosis factor controls neuroinflammation via TLR2-mediated CD39 signalling. Nat Commun. 2014;5:4432.
97. Sears CL, Geis AL, Housseau F. Bacteroides fragilis subverts mucosal biology: from symbiont to colon carcinogenesis. J Clin Invest. 2014;124(10): 4166–72.
98. Cummings JH, Pomare EW, Branch WJ, et al. Short chain fatty acids in human large intestine, portal, hepatic and venous blood. Gut. 1987;28(10):1221–7.

99. Rooks MG, Garrett WS. Gut microbiota, metabolites and host immunity. Nat Rev Immunol. 2016;16(6):341–52.
100. Trompette A, Gollwitzer ES, Yadava K, et al. Gut microbiota metabolism of dietary fiber influences allergic airway disease and hematopoiesis. Nat Med. 2014;20(2):159–66.
101. Smith PM, Howitt MR, Panikov N, et al. The microbial metabolites, short-chain fatty acids, regulate colonic Treg cell homeostasis. Science. 2013;341(6145):569–73.
102. Maslowski KM, Vieira AT, Ng A, et al. Regulation of inflammatory responses by gut microbiota and chemoattractant receptor GPR43. Nature. 2009;461(7268):1282–6.
103. Singh N, Gurav A, Sivaprakasam S, et al. Activation of Gpr109a, receptor for niacin and the commensal metabolite butyrate, suppresses colonic inflammation and carcinogenesis. Immunity. 2014;40(1):128–39.
104. Dal Ben ER, do Prado CH, Baptista TS, et al. Decreased levels of circulating CD4+CD25+Foxp3+ regulatory T cells in patients with primary antiphospholipid syndrome. J Clin Immunol. 2013;33(4):876–9.
105. Manfredo Vieira S, Hiltensperger M, Kumar V, et al. Translocation of a gut pathobiont drives autoimmunity in mice and humans. Science. 2018;359:1156–61.
106. Blank M, Krause I, Fridkin M, et al. Bacterial induction of autoantibodies to beta2-glycoprotein-I accounts for the infectious etiology of antiphospholipid syndrome. J Clin Invest. 2002;109(6):797–804.
107. Gharavi AE, Pierangeli SS, Espinola RG, et al. Antiphospholipid antibodies induced in mice by immunization with a cytomegalovirus-derived peptide cause thrombosis and activation of endothelial cells in vivo. Arthritis Rheum. 2002;46(2):545–52.
108. Blank M, Shoenfeld Y, Cabilly S, et al. Prevention of experimental antiphospholipid syndrome and endothelial cell activation by synthetic peptides. Proc Natl Acad Sci U S A. 1999;96(9):5164–8.
109. Ausubel LJ, Kwan CK, Sette A, et al. Complementary mutations in an antigenic peptide allow for crossreactivity of autoreactive T-cell clones. Proc Natl Acad Sci U S A. 1996;93(26):15317–22.
110. Wooldridge L, Ekeruche-Makinde J, van den Berg HA, et al. A single autoimmune T cell receptor recognizes more than a million different peptides. J Biol Chem. 2012;287(2):1168–77.
111. Li J, Jia H, Cai X, et al. An integrated catalog of reference genes in the human gut microbiome. Nat Biotechnol. 2014;32(8):834–41.
112. Dangl JL, Wensel TG, Morrison SL, et al. Segmental flexibility and complement fixation of genetically engineered chimeric human, rabbit and mouse antibodies. EMBO J. 1988;7(7):1989–94.
113. Kau AL, Ahern PP, Griffin NW, et al. Human nutrition, the gut microbiome and the immune system. Nature. 2011;474(7351):327–36.
114. Cheng S, He C, Zhou H, et al. The effect of toll-like receptor 4 on beta2-glycoprotein I-induced B cell activation in mouse model. Mol Immunol. 2016;71:78–86.
115. Mulla MJ, Brosens JJ, Chamley LW, et al. Antiphospholipid antibodies induce a pro-inflammatory response in first trimester trophoblast via the TLR4/MyD88 pathway. Am J Reprod Immunol. 2009;62(2):96–111.
116. Foley JH. Examining coagulation-complement crosstalk: complement activation and thrombosis. Thromb Res. 2016;141(Suppl 2):S50–4.
117. Chehoud C, Rafail S, Tyldsley AS, et al. Complement modulates the cutaneous microbiome and inflammatory milieu. Proc Natl Acad Sci U S A. 2013;110(37):15061–6.
118. Oku K, Nakamura H, Kono M, et al. Complement and thrombosis in the antiphospholipid syndrome. Autoimmun Rev. 2016;15(10):1001–4.
119. Hajishengallis G, Lambris JD. Complement and dysbiosis in periodontal disease. Immunobiology. 2012;217(11):1111–6.
120. Zhu W, Gregory JC, Org E, et al. Gut microbial metabolite TMAO enhances platelet hyperreactivity and thrombosis risk. Cell. 2016;165(1):111–24.
121. Nieuwdorp M, Stroes ES, Meijers JC, et al. Hypercoagulability in the metabolic syndrome. Curr Opin Pharmacol. 2005;5(2):155–9.
122. Vinje S, Stroes E, Nieuwdorp M, et al. The gut microbiome as novel cardio-metabolic target: the time has come! Eur Heart J. 2014;35(14):883–7.
123. Stiksrud B, Nowak P, Nwosu FC, et al. Reduced levels of D-dimer and changes in gut microbiota composition after probiotic intervention in HIV-infected individuals on stable ART. J Acquir Immune Defic Syndr. 2015;70(4):329–37.
124. Cervera R, Piette JC, Font J, et al. Antiphospholipid syndrome: clinical and immunologic manifestations and patterns of disease expression in a cohort of 1,000 patients. Arthritis Rheum. 2002;46(4):1019–27.
125. Uthman I, Godeau B, Taher A, et al. The hematologic manifestations of the antiphospholipid syndrome. Blood Rev. 2008;22(4):187–94.
126. Yelnik CM, Laskin CA, Porter TF, et al. Lupus anticoagulant is the main predictor of adverse pregnancy outcomes in aPL-positive patients: validation of PROMISSE study results. Lupus Sci Med. 2016;3(1):e000131.
127. Hanly JG, Su L, Urowitz MB, et al. A longitudinal analysis of outcomes of lupus nephritis in an international inception cohort using a multistate model approach. Arthritis Rheumatol. 2016;68(8):1932–44.
128. Erkan D, Espinosa G, Cervera R. Catastrophic antiphospholipid syndrome: updated diagnostic algorithms. Autoimmun Rev. 2010;10(2):74–9.
129. Cervera R, Khamashta MA, Shoenfeld Y, et al. Morbidity and mortality in the antiphospholipid syndrome during a 5-year period: a multicentre prospective study of 1000 patients. Ann Rheum Dis. 2009;68(9):1428–32.

130. Ruiz-Irastorza G, Crowther M, Branch W, et al. Antiphospholipid syndrome. Lancet. 2010;376(9751): 1498–509.
131. Miyakis S, Lockshin MD, Atsumi T, et al. International consensus statement on an update of the classification criteria for definite antiphospholipid syndrome (APS). J Thromb Haemost. 2006;4(2):295–306.
132. Wilson WA, Gharavi AE, Koike T, et al. International consensus statement on preliminary classification criteria for definite antiphospholipid syndrome: report of an international workshop. Arthritis Rheum. 1999;42(7):1309–11.
133. Segal JB, Streiff MB, Hofmann LV, et al. Management of venous thromboembolism: a systematic review for a practice guideline. Ann Intern Med. 2007;146(3):211–22.
134. Arachchillage DJ, Cohen H. Use of new oral anticoagulants in antiphospholipid syndrome. Curr Rheumatol Rep. 2013;15(6):331.
135. Signorelli F, Nogueira F, Domingues V, et al. Thrombotic events in patients with antiphospholipid syndrome treated with rivaroxaban: a series of eight cases. Clin Rheumatol. 2016;35(3):801–5.
136. Haladyj E, Olesinska M. Rivaroxaban – a safe therapeutic option in patients with antiphospholipid syndrome? Our experience in 23 cases. Reumatologia. 2016;54(3):146–9.
137. Wang TF, Lim W. What is the role of hydroxychloroquine in reducing thrombotic risk in patients with antiphospholipid antibodies? Hematology Am Soc Hematol Educ Program. 2016;2016(1):714–6.
138. Khamashta MA, Cuadrado MJ, Mujic F, et al. The management of thrombosis in the antiphospholipid-antibody syndrome. N Engl J Med. 1995;332(15):993–7.
139. Barbhaiya M, Erkan D. Primary thrombosis prophylaxis in antiphospholipid antibody-positive patients: where do we stand? Curr Rheumatol Rep. 2011;13(1):59–69.
140. Ruffatti A, Del Ross T, Ciprian M, et al. Risk factors for a first thrombotic event in antiphospholipid antibody carriers. A multicentre, retrospective follow-up study. Ann Rheum Dis. 2009;68(3):397–9.
141. Ruiz-Irastorza G, Khamashta MA. The treatment of antiphospholipid syndrome: a harmonic contrast. Best Pract Res Clin Rheumatol. 2007;21(6): 1079–92.
142. Bick RL. Antiphospholipid thrombosis syndromes. Hematol Oncol Clin North Am. 2003;17(1):115–47.
143. Ruiz-Irastorza G, Cuadrado MJ, Ruiz-Arruza I, et al. Evidence-based recommendations for the prevention and long-term management of thrombosis in antiphospholipid antibody-positive patients: report of a task force at the 13th international congress on antiphospholipid antibodies. Lupus. 2011;20(2):206–18.
144. Onysko M, Holcomb N, Hornecker J. Antibiotic interactions: answers to 4 common questions. J Fam Pract. 2016;65(7):442–8.
145. PL Detail-Document #280806. Antimicrobial drug interactions with warfarin. Pharmacist's Letter/ Prescriber's Letter. 2012.
146. Lane MA, Zeringue A, McDonald JR. Serious bleeding events due to warfarin and antibiotic co-prescription in a cohort of veterans. Am J Med. 2014;127(7):657–663.e2.
147. Crowther MA, Ginsberg JS, Julian J, et al. A comparison of two intensities of warfarin for the prevention of recurrent thrombosis in patients with the antiphospholipid antibody syndrome. N Engl J Med. 2003;349(12):1133–8.
148. Finazzi G, Marchioli R, Brancaccio V, et al. A randomized clinical trial of high-intensity warfarin vs. conventional antithrombotic therapy for the prevention of recurrent thrombosis in patients with the antiphospholipid syndrome (WAPS). J Thromb Haemost. 2005;3(5):848–53.
149. Ruiz-Irastorza G, Hunt BJ, Khamashta MA. A systematic review of secondary thromboprophylaxis in patients with antiphospholipid antibodies. Arthritis Rheum. 2007;57(8):1487–95.
150. Petri M. Pathogenesis and treatment of the antiphospholipid antibody syndrome. Med Clin North Am. 1997;81(1):151–77.
151. Whitlock RP, Sun JC, Fremes SE, et al. Antithrombotic and thrombolytic therapy for valvular disease: antithrombotic therapy and prevention of thrombosis, 9th ed: American College of Chest Physicians Evidence-Based Clinical Practice Guidelines. Chest. 2012;141(2 Suppl):e576S–600S.
152. Atsumi T, Furukawa S, Amengual O, et al. Antiphospholipid antibody associated thrombocytopenia and the paradoxical risk of thrombosis. Lupus. 2005;14(7):499–504.
153. Leuzzi RA, Davis GH, Cowchock FS, et al. Management of immune thrombocytopenic purpura associated with the antiphospholipid antibody syndrome. Clin Exp Rheumatol. 1997;15(2):197–200.
154. Bucciarelli S, Espinosa G, Cervera R, et al. Mortality in the catastrophic antiphospholipid syndrome: causes of death and prognostic factors in a series of 250 patients. Arthritis Rheum. 2006;54(8):2568–76.
155. Garcia-Carrasco M, Mendoza-Pinto C, Macias-Diaz S, et al. The role of infectious diseases in the catastrophic antiphospholipid syndrome. Autoimmun Rev. 2015;14(11):1066–71.
156. Cervera R, Rodriguez-Pinto I, Colafrancesco S, et al. 14th international congress on antiphospholipid antibodies task force report on catastrophic antiphospholipid syndrome. Autoimmun Rev. 2014;13(7):699–707.
157. Rubenstein E, Arkfeld DG, Metyas S, et al. Rituximab treatment for resistant antiphospholipid syndrome. J Rheumatol. 2006;33(2):355–7.
158. Shapira I, Andrade D, Allen SL, et al. Brief report: induction of sustained remission in recurrent catastrophic antiphospholipid syndrome via inhibition of terminal complement with eculizumab. Arthritis Rheum. 2012;64(8):2719–23.

Sjögren's Syndrome

23

Luca Quartuccio, Saviana Gandolfo,
Sara Zandonella Callegher, and Salvatore De Vita

Abbreviations

AhR	Aryl hydrocarbon receptor
ATL	Adult T-cell leukaemia-lymphoma
BAFF	B-cell activating factor
CMV	Cytomegalovirus
Cp	*Chlamydia psittaci*
CV	Coxsackievirus
EBV	Epstein-Barr virus
GC	Germinal centre
GPCR	G-protein-coupled receptor
HAM/TSP	HTLV-1 associated myelopathy/ tropical spastic paraparesis
HBV	Hepatitis B virus
HCV	Hepatitis C virus
HIV	Human immunodeficiency virus
HP	*Helicobacter pylori*
HTLV-1	Human T-lymphotropic virus type 1
MALT	Mucosa-associated lymphoid tissue
MCMV	Murine CMV
MESA	Myoepithelial sialadenitis
NHL	Non-Hodgkin lymphoma
SG	Salivary gland
SLE	Systemic lupus erythematosus
SS	Sjögren's syndrome

L. Quartuccio (✉) · S. Gandolfo · S. Z. Callegher
S. De Vita
Rheumatology Clinic, Academic Hospital Santa Maria della Misericordia, Udine, Department of Medical and Biological Sciences, Udine, Italy
e-mail: luca.quartuccio@asuiud.sanita.fvg.it

Introduction: The Link Between Infections and Sjögren's Syndrome Pathogenesis

Sjögren's syndrome (SS) is a chronic autoimmune disease, more prevalent in women, affecting exocrine glands, mostly salivary and lacrimal glands, but also extraglandular tissues and organs. SS is characterized by quite specific autoantibodies, namely anti-Ro (SSA), anti-La (SSB), and by chronic lymphocytic infiltrates in exocrine glands. Ro/SSA and La/SSB represent heterogeneous ribonucleoprotein complexes consisting of antigenic proteins (two main proteins of 52 kDa [Ro52] and 60 kDa [Ro60] for Ro/SSA and one protein of 48 kDa for La/SSB) associated with small cytoplasmic RNAs (hYRNAs) [1]. The function of Ro/SSA hYRNA complexes is largely unknown, while the La/SSB protein has been suggested to participate in the transcription termination of RNA polymerase III and in the initiation of the translation of at least the poliovirus mRNA [2]. Several mechanisms, including molecular mimicry with viral antigens or antigen-driven responses, have been proposed to explain the genesis of these autoantibodies in SS. Furthermore, these autoantibodies seem to represent a link between SS and systemic lupus erythematosus, another autoimmune disease where sicca symptoms can be recognized often in association with anti-Ro/SSA and/or anti-La/SSB autoantibodies (secondary SS). These findings strongly suggest a

G. Ragab et al. (eds.), *The Microbiome in Rheumatic Diseases and Infection*,
https://doi.org/10.1007/978-3-319-79026-8_23

relationship between the biologic processes that generate these specific immunologic responses and the autoimmune sicca disorder itself. Importantly, viral infections or the induction of cellular stress by heat, UV light, and chemicals on cultured epithelial cells and keratinocytes have been shown to induce the translocation of Ro/SSA and La/SSB ribonucleoproteins to the cellular surface [3]. Similarly, in the conjunctival and salivary epithelial cells of SS patients, abnormal translocation and localization to the outer membranes of the nuclear autoantigens La/SSB have also been demonstrated [4]. Additionally, apoptosis is another cellular mechanism that possibly results in the release of autoantigens that are captured by antigen-presenting cells and presented to the immune cells, thus perpetuating and expanding the immune responses. Interestingly, in mouse models of genetic abnormalities in the programmed cell-death processes (Fas or Fas-ligand mutated mice), persistence of autoreactive T-cell clones has been shown. Notably, the infection of exocrine glands of such mutant mice by epitheliotropic viruses may result in chronic inflammatory gland lesions [5]. Furthermore, using cultured nonneoplastic cell lines, salivary gland epithelial cells have been shown to be susceptible to Fas-mediated and Fas-unrelated apoptotic death after stimulation by interferon-gamma [6]. This finding is very interesting since it suggests that epithelial cell apoptosis contributes to the glandular lesions in SS, either by the action of local infiltrating cytotoxic T-cells or via intrinsic mechanisms, possibly occurring before lymphocytic infiltration. On the other hand, recent advances have revealed a major role for activation of the type I interferon pathway in the pathogenesis of SS, as evidenced by the increased circulating type I interferon activity and an interferon "signature" in peripheral blood mononuclear cells and minor salivary gland biopsies from these patients. Polymorphisms in genes involved in the interferon-alpha pathway, such as IRF5 and STAT4, have been found to be associated with disease susceptibility. While the initial triggers of the innate immune response in SS remain elusive, preliminary evidence supports the role of inappropriately expressed endogenous LINE-1 (L1) retroelements (endogenous virus-like genomic repeat elements, normally silent), as potential triggers of type I interferon activation in SS, as well as in other systemic autoimmune diseases, possibly through Toll-like receptor (TLR)-dependent or TLR-independent pathways [7]. These observations possibly have uncovered a link between infections and autoimmune processes since the interferon pathway is also active in the innate immune defence against infections. From a clinical point of view, there is a clear relationship between infections and SS when considering the development of cryoglobulinaemia in the course of SS. In fact, cryoglobulinaemic vasculitis is the most frequent form of vasculitis in SS, and it has been well recognized as one of the most important extrahepatic manifestations during HCV infection. Moreover, both SS and HCV patients are at high risk of developing lymphoma, and cryoglobulinaemic vasculitis represents one of the most relevant red flags for lymphoma in SS. Importantly, SS and HCV infection share a number of features: the association with cryoglobulinaemia and with serum rheumatoid factor positivity, chronic salivary gland (SG) inflammation, and deep similarities in immunoglobulin gene usage, plus homology with rheumatoid factor sequences, by the related B-cell lymphoproliferation [8]. Research on the role of antigenic stimulation for the acquisition of lymphoid tissue and the development of specific subtypes of MALT lymphoma has identified in bacterial- or viral-triggered activity the first possible event [9]. The expanded B-cell clone, which often uses a combination of immunoglobulin genes encoding autoantibodies, may in turn become infectious trigger-independent, and the eradication of infection may no longer be sufficient to abolish clonal persistence and potential malignant evolution. Infectious triggers linked to B-cell lymphomagenesis have been identified in *Helicobacter pylori (HP)*, *Borrelia burgdorferi* and *B. afzelii*, *Chlamydia psittaci* (*Cp*), and *Campylobacter jejuni* for gastric, cutaneous, ocular adnexal, and small intestinal MALT lymphomas, respectively [10–13].

A role for viruses in the activation of B-cells in ectopic lymphoid structures of SS glands and in lymphomagenesis has been hypothesized.

Croia et al. [14] recently demonstrated a latent Epstein-Barr virus (EBV) infection in B-cells and lytic EBV infection in plasma cells exclusively within inflammatory infiltrates of SS salivary gland tissue, suggesting a potential EBV contribution to local growth and differentiation of self-reacting B-cells. Furthermore, a high prevalence of *Cp* subclinical infection has been recently shown in Italian patients with SS with a higher frequency of Cp detection in MALT lymphoma, as compared to myoepithelial sialadenitis (MESA) or to SS patients without a lymphoproliferative disease [15].

However, the best example of chronic antigen-driven overstimulation of B-cells, as stated before, is represented by HCV-related lymphoproliferation. In a meta-analysis, SS has been associated with HCV [16], even if the presence of HCV is an exclusion criterion for primary SS (pSS). Epidemiology studies showed a higher risk of NHL in patients with chronic HCV infection compared to healthy subjects [17]. Importantly, HCV is sialotropic, and HCV infection is linked to SG chronic inflammation and to sicca syndrome. Hence, HCV-related sicca syndrome, especially when positive for anti-SSA/SSB antibodies, could be considered as a particular subset of SS associated with a well-recognized infectious trigger [8, 18–21].

Active EBV infection appears to cause expansion and differentiation of autoreactive B-cells in SS. Latent EBV and lytic EBV infection were detected in SS salivary glands containing ectopic lymphoid follicle-like structures, and plasma cells with Ro52 immunoreactivity within the glands were frequently EBV positive. Furthermore, when transplanted into SCID mice, SS salivary glands containing ectopic lymphoid follicle-like structures produced anti-Ro52 antibodies and anti-EBV antibodies [22]. Commensal microbiota may initiate autoimmunity in SS and lupus. For instance, peptides homologous to portions of the von Willebrand factor type A from the oral microbe *Capnocytophaga ochracea* activated HLA-DR3-positive, Ro60-reactive T-cells [23]. Environmental pollutants, such as dioxin, through aryl hydrocarbon receptor (AhR), reactivate (i.e. induce a switch from latent to lytic infection) EBV in B-cells and salivary epithelial cells [24]. Finally, human T-lymphotropic virus type 1 (HTLV-1) is associated with SS in endemic areas, such as Nagasaki in Japan [25, 26]. It should be mentioned that HTLV-1 preferentially infects CD4-positive T-cells but can also infect human primary SG epithelial cells [23]. Taken together, these observations highlight the possible interaction between infections and the immune system in the very early phase of the autoimmune process that finally leads to the occurrence of an overt autoimmune disease. In this context of multifactorial diseases, other factors are certainly relevant, including host genetic background, environmental factors, and hormones.

The possible role of the following infections in the pathogenesis of SS will be described in detail: coxsackievirus (CV), EBV, HTLV-1, HP, HCV, hepatitis B virus (HBV), Cytomegalovirus (CMV), and parvovirus B19 (B19V).

Coxsackievirus

CV are cytolytic viruses, belonging to enterovirus genus of the *Picornaviridae* family, able to replicate in the submucosal lymph tissue and then disseminate to the reticuloendothelial system. For their intrinsic epithelial and lymphoid tropism, they have been hypothesized as potential environmental triggers for SS.

Interestingly, Triantafyllopoulou et al. [27] found the presence of RNA from two CV strains, CVB4 and CVA13, in minor salivary gland (MSG) samples from SS patients and also demonstrated by immunohistochemistry a positive staining for the enteroviral capsid protein VP1 in epithelial cells and lymphocytic infiltrates in MSG SS specimens, providing evidence of a possible active involvement of CV in the pathogenesis of the disease. However, a French study [28], trying to replicate the above-mentioned molecular findings by using seminested RT-PCR with specific primers for the 5′-NCR of the enteroviral genome on high-quality RNA suitable for gene expression study of SGs, was unable to find CV in any salivary gland specimens studied. The discrepant conclusions reached from these two studies could be the result of differences in geographic and/or genetic factors. It could be in fact hypothesized that the incidence of enteroviral infection might be different in Greece and in France, and this could explain for the apparently different association of CV with SS SG tissue. Moreover, genetic polymorphisms predisposing to SS are known to clearly differ between Greeks and French [29, 30]; thus, the potential viral contribution to the induction of autoimmunity could be restricted only to some genetically predisposed patients.

Stathopoulou et al. [31] have subsequently found that a synthetic peptide derived from the CV A21 protein 2B, functionally characterized as a viroporin which interacts with cellular membranes modifying permeability, presented 87% sequence homology with a region of a major linear B-cell epitope of Ro60 kD protein spanning the sequence 216–232 amino acids (pep216–232). Sera obtained from SS patients, SLE patients, healthy individuals as normal controls, and patients with rheumatoid arthritis as disease controls were tested against both peptides. The authors found that sera reacting with pep216–232 were apparently the same as those reacting with viral 2B peptide and that both peptides reacted more prominently with anti-Ro-/La-positive sera from SS patients. Purified antibodies against pep216–232 readily reacted with both peptides, while inhibition experiments revealed the specificity of this reaction. These results suggested a possible role of CV, through a molecular mimicry mechanism, in autoantibody formation and perpetuation of an autoimmune response against Ro/SSA and La/SSB in SS patients.

Human T-Lymphotropic Virus Type 1

HTLV-1 is an oncogenic retrovirus, which causes HTLV-1-associated myelopathy/tropical spastic paraparesis (HAM/TSP) and adult T-cell leukaemia-lymphoma (ATL) in individuals with dysfunctional immune responses [32, 33].

Several studies from both endemic and non-endemic areas have associated HTLV-1 with SS [34–37]. In the city of Nagasaki, Japan, which is a HTLV-1 endemic area, an epidemiologic study [36] found that 23% of SS patients were HLTV-1 seropositive compared to 3% among healthy blood donors. In another study, the prevalence of anti-HLTV-1 antibodies in SS patients was found to be higher than in the general population coming from the same area (36% vs. 10–15%) [37]. Moreover, IgA class antibodies against HTLV-1 were detected in the saliva of HTLV-1 seropositive SS patients and proposed as local biomarkers of viral replication [26].

Green et al. [38] reported that tax transgenic mice showed SS-like sialadenitis. Tax, a viral oncoprotein, is a transcription factor that is essential for HLTV-1 replication. Many authors [39–41] have reported the presence of the HTLV-I tax-like DNA in SGs of HTLV-1-seronegative SS patients suggesting that HTLV-1 might potentially be able to localize inside SGs of SS patients and stimulate autoimmunity also in noncarrier patients. Moreover, a French study showed anti-Tax antibodies in approximately half of the SS patients evaluated [17].

Nakamura et al. [42] observed a high prevalence (60%) of SS among patients with HAM. Studies conducted on HAM SS patients found a lack of the usual SG damage as assessed by magnetic resonance [43] and histopathology [44]. Interestingly, SG specimens of HTLV-1-positive, asymptomatic SS patients showed significantly less ectopic germinal centre (GC) formation than HTLV-1 seronegative SS, and a total absence of GCs was observed in HAM SS patients together with significantly lower expression of CXCL13, a crucial chemokine for B-cell GC homing, in this subset of patients [45, 46]. On the basis of these data, a preliminary hypothesis of a possible HTLV-1 role in preserving glandular function in SS patients has been formulated, but this interesting observation needs further confirmatory studies.

In seropositive SS patients, histopathological analyses have revealed the clear presence of HTLV-1proviral DNA in CD4$^+$T lymphocytes infiltrating SGs [47]. CD4$^+$T lymphocytes represent the preferential target of HTLV-1 infection, but in vitro studies [48] have demonstrated that HTLV-1 is also able to directly infect salivary gland epithelial cells. In vivo confirmation and functional consequences of this finding are still lacking.

Taken together, current evidence supports a potential role of HTLV-1 in the pathogenesis of SS, but more studies are needed to elucidate its exact etiopathogenetic importance in genetically and geographically different subsets of SS patients.

Epstein-Barr Virus

Not under Coxackie virus EBV is a ubiquitous DNA virus of the *Herpesviridae* family, transmitted in saliva and initially infecting epithelial cells in the oro- and nasopharynx. Subsequently, EBV infects B-cells and, after the primary lytic phase, persists in immortalized resting memory B-cells. EBV can also occasionally reactivate in a dynamic interaction with the immune response of the host [49].

A pathogenetic association between EBV infection and SS has been deeply studied. In SS patients an increase in EBV viral load in saliva and salivary and lacrimal gland tissues [50–54], elevated levels of circulating anti-EBV antibodies [54–56], and an increased number of circulating B-cells harbouring EBV [57, 58] have been demonstrated.

EBV antigens and DNA were found in salivary infiltrating lymphocytes and epithelial cells [54], with a selective distribution inside ectopic lymphoid structures [14]. In addition, EBV-infected plasma cells within SGs showed immunoreactivity against SS-associated autoantigen Ro52. Interestingly, following transplantation of SS SGs containing ectopic lymphoid structures into SCID mice, production of both anti-Ro52 and anti-EBV antibodies by the recipient mice was found [14]. Overall, these data suggest the potential existence of a strict link between EBV infection and expansion of differentiation of autoreactive B-cells in SS, raising the intriguing possibility that a persistent latent EBV infection could provide chronic survival signals to B-cell clones within affected tissues.

The reactivation of EBV infection, and consequently its pathogenic effects, could be dynamically influenced by activating local factors within saliva. Nagata et al. [59] have shown that saliva from SS patients is able to activate EBV, by acting on the promoter of the gene BZLF1, the first gene to be transcribed during viral replication, suggesting a more frequent reactivation of EBV in SS patients triggered by the local SG milieu.

EBV reactivation in SS patients has also been found to be linked to exogenous environmental factors, such as dioxin, via binding to the aryl hydrocarbon receptor (AhR) [24]. The binding of ligands to the AhR triggers its translocation into the nucleus and the regulation of transcription target genes. In activated B-cells and salivary epithelial cells of SS patients, the EBV BZLF1 gene has been demonstrated to be a novel target of the dioxin-activated AhR. Dioxin-enhanced BZLF1 transcription produces ZEBRA factor, which mediates the switch from latent to the lytic phase of EBV infection, suggesting a novel role for dioxin as pathogenic environmental factor for autoimmune diseases via EBV reactivation.

Novel potential mechanisms of EBV triggering of SS have also been proposed. With regard to this, it has been demonstrated that EBV-infected cells are able to release EBV-encoded small RNA forming complexes with SSB/La that would be able to bind Toll-like receptor (TLR)-3 with consequent activation of type I interferon production [60] (see Chap. 11).

Helicobacter pylori

HP is a gram-negative spiral-shaped bacterium which colonizes the human gastric mucosa and is transmitted by the faecal-oral route. It affects approximately 50% of the world's population, more frequently those living in poor sanitary conditions; however it produces disease in only a minority of patients [61, 62].

HP's most important virulence factors are urease and flagella, obligatory for the colonization of the gastric mucosa, the cytotoxins, VacA and CagA, and the neutrophil-activating protein (NapA) gene [63].

The main pathophysiological event in HP infection is the persistent presence of the bacteria in the gastric mucosa, which has the effect of chronic immune system activation with ongoing cytokine signalling, infiltration by neutrophils, macrophages, lymphocytes, as well as production of effector T-cells and antibodies [64]. Various mechanisms have been suggested in an attempt to explain the extraintestinal manifestations of HP infections: atrophic gastritis, enhancement in vascular permeability, release of inflammatory mediators, systemic immune response, molecular mimicry, microchimerism, and superantigens. All this leads to an overall downregulation of the host immune response [65, 66].

To evaluate a possible link between HP infection and SS, several groups investigated the presence of the bacterium and its related antibodies in SS-affected patients [67]. Some studies revealed that SS patients are more likely to have HP infection in comparison to patients with other connective tissue diseases [68]. In SS patients serum antibody titres to HP correlated with their disease activity index, age, disease duration, and C-reactive protein levels. Evaluation of HP infection status in older SS patients with active disease for a relatively long duration is therefore recommended, especially those who have been suffering from primary SS for more than 3 years [69]. One of the studies suggested a possible connection between antibodies produced against heat shock protein (HSP 60) of HP and SS development [70]. Contrary to previous studies, a much larger study of 164 primary SS patients from Sweden did not prove a higher seroprevalence rate of HP as compared with control group [71]. Moreover there was no association between HP status and abnormal autoantibody levels or abnormal lip biopsy in these patients. In a separate cohort of 54 SS patients, seroprevalence of HP was 57% compared to 62% in the control group ($p = 0.6$) [72]. Another study compared 36 primary SS patients to 31 patients with secondary SS and determined the HP infection prevalence was 80.6% and 71%, respectively ($p = 0.4$). Furthermore, no significant association was found between HP positivity and the presence of autoantibodies in primary or secondary SS patients [73].

The results of these studies are contradictory. Some data suggests that SS patients have a higher prevalence of HP infection. However, in a larger cohort of a homogenous population (with an overall low HP incidence), no such association was found.

Globally, there is no real evidence for a definitive association of HP infection and SS (see (Chap. 8).

Hepatitis C Virus

HCV is a small, enveloped, single-stranded, positive-sense RNA virus, a member of the family *Flaviviridae*. Chronic HCV infection has been implicated as a cause of multiple autoimmune diseases; the most commonly associated are SS (nearly half the cases), RA, and systemic lupus erythematosus [74]. HCV infection may lead to inflammatory injury of the SGs causing clinical features similar to those of SS, and this infection is currently considered an exclusion criterion for the diagnosis of SS. In some very specific cases, however, it is postulated that HCV might trigger SS [75].

A possible relationship between SS and HCV was first postulated in 1992 by Haddad et al., who reported lymphocytic sialadenitis in 57% of HCV-infected patients versus 5% of controls [76]. In a meta-analysis Wang et al. showed that HCV infection is significantly associated with SS, there being an overall 3.3-fold increase in risk compared with controls [77]. There is a higher prevalence of SS in patients with HCV infection (25.9%) compared to patients with HBV (3.4%) and higher in those with chronic HCV infection [78, 79]. A few more recent prospective studies have also reported a wide range (9–67%) for the prevalence of SS in HCV-infected patients [80, 81]. Factors possibly contributing to the wide variation include (1) differences in diagnostic criteria for SS, (2) sensitivity of the HCV test used, and (3) geographic differences in HCV seroprevalence [82, 83]. Thus, further research is required to establish an unequivocal causative link between HCV and SS [77].

HCV "sicca-like" symptoms tend to be milder compared to SS, and HCV-related SS has mild lymphocytic infiltrates that tend to locate in the pericapillary area rather than around the glandular ducts. Only mild damage of the glandular tissue is reported in HCV-related SS [80, 84]. Further, patients with HCV-related SS/sicca syndrome are distinctly different from patients with pSS in their clinical (older age at diagnosis, male sex, peripheral neuropathy, cutaneous vasculitis, hepatocarcinoma, or neoplasia-lymphoma, in particular monoclonal gammopathy (IgMκ)) and immunological (cryoglobulinaemia and hypocomplementaemia) characteristics. The latter two features are markers or predictors for the development of extrahepatic manifestations including lymphoproliferative disorders, seronegativity for SSA/SSB, and RF autoantibodies and a higher prevalence of anti-gastric parietal cell antibodies and anti-mitochondrial antibodies [84–88]. Potthoff et al. demonstrated that patients with chronic HCV infection show high titre of alpha-fodrin IgA antibodies but neither symptom severity or frequency correlated with these antibodies [89]. A clear genetic association with HLA DQB1*02 has been documented in chronic HCV infection with sicca syndrome [90].

Different mechanisms could explain the pathogenesis of the HCV-SS/sicca syndrome combination, including molecular mimicry between HCV and salivary glands, direct infection and proliferation of HCV in salivary glands, and the role of immune complexes that include HCV antigens [91]. HCV expresses tropism for lacrimal and salivary epithelial cells, and HCV RNA has been found both in saliva and salivary gland tissue of SS patients [92]. However it has not necessarily been confirmed that the presence of HCV RNAs has an immune effect, either direct or indirect, in any SG disorder [93]. Also linking HCV to SS are transgenic mice that carry HCV envelope proteins E1 and E2. These mice develop SS-like symptoms manifesting as sialadenitis. Rosa et al. have hypothesized that the E2 glycoprotein binds to CD81 and stimulates B-cell proliferation [94, 95]. HCV may provide a chronic antigen stimulus that drives clonal expansion of somatically mutated IgM memory B-cells, and some of these B-cells may be autoreactive and predispose to SS [96, 97]. However, the exact pathogenic mechanism underlying SS-like disease in HCV-infected subjects is still unclear [91].

By integrated clinical, pathologic, and molecular studies, we recently highlighted the observation that cryoglobulinaemic vasculitis has a different biologic background in SS if compared to chronic HCV infection [88]. Cryoglobulinaemic vasculitis is associated with a polyclonal B-cell lymphoproliferation in the bone marrow and is associated with salivary MALT lymphoma in SS, consistent with the primary role of salivary MALT chronic inflammation and lymphoproliferation as predisposing factors to lymphoma in this disease, which is rarely associated with HCV infection. By contrast, cryoglobulinaemic vasculitis in the course of HCV infection is primarily a liver and bone marrow autoimmune and lymphoproliferative disorder, and malignant lymphoproliferation of salivary MALT is rare in this setting. Overlapping features of SS and cryoglobulinaemic vasculitis may however occur in HCV-positive patients. Interestingly, abnormal acquisition of gastric MALT may occur both in SS and in cryoglobulinaemic syndrome. Thus, the study of the gastric microenvironment, in conjunction with that of the bone marrow, liver, and salivary glands, may be relevant for future research aimed to clarify the mechanisms leading to preferential rheumatoid factor-positive B-cell expansion in these diseases and, in general, to better explain the various components of gastric lymphomagenesis. Besides local antigenic stimulation, the mechanisms by which HCV infection and other local triggers may favour gastric acquisition of MALT and, more generally, chronic inflammation and B-cell expansion remain elusive. With regard to this issue, local cytokine networks are likely implicated. Recent results pointed out the role of HCV infection in upregulating the expression of BAFF [98], a relevant growth factor implicated in autoimmunity and B-cell lymphoproliferation. Recently, MALT lymphoma of salivary glands associated with cryoglobulinaemic vasculitis in the course of SS has been successfully treated with belimumab, a human monoclonal antibody, which targets soluble BAFF, and rituximab sequential therapy [99]. Thus, the therapeutic value of targeting the local trigger of chronic inflammation, autoimmunity, and lymphoproliferation versus other biologic targets are promising opportunities for exploration in the future (see (Chap. 12).

Hepatitis B Virus

HBV is a small DNA virus member of the family *Hepadnaviridae* that replicates through an RNA intermediate and can integrate into host genome [100]. Different studies have linked this virus with various types of autoimmune phenomena from the generation of autoantibodies, most commonly ANA and SMA, up to the development of autoimmune diseases. The principal mechanism by which HBV is supposed to induce autoimmunity is molecular mimicry and the formation of immune complexes [91, 101].

An association between SS and chronic HBV infection has rarely been investigated and remains controversial. Both HBV and HCV replicate extrahepatically and produce SS-like disease. However, only 3% of HBV patients have sicca syndrome, significantly fewer than HCV patients [102]. Chen et al. reported that in Taiwan HBV is highly endemic with 17.3% of the adult population HbsAg-positive, but the rate of HBV infection was significantly less frequent in primary SS patients when compared to the general population [103]. A Spanish study recorded a prevalence of chronic HBV infection in SS that is very similar to the prevalence in general population: only 0.83% primary SS patients were positive for HbsAg [104].

The low risk of SS-like disease in patients with HBV infection may be attributable to the following three factors: (1) in most developed countries, there are active HBV vaccination programmes; (2) because the disease progresses rapidly in patients with HBV infection, very few of them develop cirrhosis [102]; and (3) based on a study with healthy controls, Rama et al. have recently suggested that HBV infection protects against autoimmune disorders, including SS/sicca syndrome [100]. Indeed Rama et al., in spite of previous studies, found an extremely low prevalence of HBcAb in diverse autoimmune diseases when compared to healthy donors. Two theories may explain these results [100]. The former is the hygiene hypothesis, in which a previous exposure to HBV may protect the subject from eventual development of autoimmune disease via mechanisms such as antigen competition (in which the immune response to an antigen is decreased by a concomitant immune response against an unrelated antigen) or downregulation of allergic and autoimmune responses (regulatory cells stimulated by infectious agents will produce IL-10 and TGF-β whose suppressor effect will extend to other immune responses) [105, 106]. The latter theory is that patients with different autoimmune diseases are probably protected from HBV due to high levels of INF-α which acts as immunomodulator and enhances the natural immune response to HBV [107] (see (Chap. 11).

Cytomegalovirus

CMV is a DNA virus member of the family *Herpesviridae*; although it may be found throughout the body, CMV infections are frequently associated with the salivary glands in humans and other mammals [108]. The immune response to CMV appears to be associated with autoimmune disease, but there are no clear connections to SS [109]. Barzilai et al. found elevated titres of CMV IgM antibodies in a cohort of SS patients [109].

Mouse models may offer guidance in regard to a role for CMV in SS. Features of human SS were demonstrated in female NZM2328 mice upon infection of sialotropic murine CMV (MCMV). MCMV DNA levels were detectable in the SGs and lacrimal glands 14–28 days after intraperitoneal infection and interestingly correlated with acute inflammation in the submandibular gland. After latency, PCR was unable to detect the virus in the glands; however, a progressive loss in SG function and focal dacryoadenitis was observed in the females during that latent infection [110].

M33 is the MCMV homologue of HCMV UL33 G-protein-coupled receptor (GPCR), which is important for salivary gland tropism and establishment of reactivation from latency. When mice that are deficient for M33 or have an M33 mutation are infected with recombinant viruses, the mice have significantly diminished MCMV infection of the salivary glands, indicating that M33 contributes to the efficient establishment or maintenance of long-term latent MCMV infection [111, 112] (see (Chap. 11).

Human Parvovirus B19

Human parvovirus B19 is a single-stranded DNA virus member of the family *Parvoviridae*; it has a unique tropism for human erythroid progenitor cells. While B19Vconstituents may persist in salivary gland tissue without lymphocytic infiltration, there is no evidence associating this virus with SS [113]. Interestingly Ramos-Casals et al. reported that cytopenia, particularly leukopenia and thrombocytopenia, in primary SS correlated with serological evidence of past human parvovirus B19 infection [114].

Conclusion

To date, efforts in clearly identifying infectious triggers implicated in SS pathogenesis and in SS-related lymphoproliferation have failed. However, the research on the interaction between infections, epithelial cells, and immune system continuously enrich the knowledge of the role of the complex biological relationship between the humans and a variety of infectious agents in the origin of autoimmune disorders such as SS. Moreover, these studies pave the way to possible novel treatments for this "orphan" disease. Finally, new technologies, now available and applied in genetic and biological studies, may solve old questions and provide new insights into the pathogenesis and treatment of SS [115, 116].

References

1. Slobbe RL, Pruijn GJ, Van Venrooij WJ. Ro (SS-A) and La (SS-B) ribonucleoprotein complexes: structure, function and antigenicity. Ann Med Interne (Paris). 1991;142:592–600.
2. Bachmann M, Falke D, Müller WE. Is La protein involved in autoimmunization and inflammatory events during disease? Characterization of La protein as an unwinding enzyme. Mol Biol Rep. 1990;14:49–50.
3. Rosen CF, Poon R, Drucker DJ. UVB radiation-activated genes induced by transcriptional and post-transcriptional mechanisms in rat keratinocytes. Am J Phys. 1995;268:C846–55.
4. Yannopoulos DI, Roncin S, Lamour A, Pennec YL, Moutsopoulos HM, Youinou P. Conjunctival epithelial cells from patients with Sjögren's syndrome inappropriately express major histocompatibility complex molecules, La(SSB) antigen, and heat-shock proteins. J Clin Immunol. 1992;12:259–65.
5. Fleck M, Zhang HG, Kern ER, et al. Treatment of chronic sialadenitis in a murine model of Sjögren's syndrome by local fasL gene transfer. Arthritis Rheumatol. 2001;44:964–73.
6. Abu-Helu RF, Dimitriou ID, Kapsogeorgou EK, et al. Induction of salivary gland epithelial cell injury in Sjogren's syndrome: in vitro assessment of T cell-derived cytokines and Fas protein expression. J Autoimmun. 2001;17:141–53.
7. Mavragani C, Crow MK. Activation of the type I interferon pathway in primary Sjogren's syndrome. J Autoimmun. 2010;35:225–31.
8. De Re V, De Vita S, Gasparotto D, et al. Salivary gland B cell lymphoproliferative disorders in Sjögren's syndrome present a restricted use of antigen receptor gene segments similar to those used by hepatitis C virus-associated non-Hodgkin's lymphomas. Eur J Immunol. 2002;32:903–10.
9. Zucca E, Bertoni F, Vannata B, et al. Emerging role of infectious etiologies in the pathogenesis of marginal zone B-cell lymphomas. Clin Cancer Res. 2014;20:5207–16.
10. Ponzoni M, Ferreri AJ, Guidoboni M, et al. Chlamydia infection and lymphomas: association beyond ocular adnexal lymphomas highlighted by multiple detection methods. Clin Cancer Res. 2008;14:5794–800.
11. Lecuit M, Abachin E, Martin A, et al. Immunoproliferative small intestinal disease associated with *Campylobacter jejuni*. N Engl J Med. 2004;350:239–48.
12. Schollkopf C, Melbye M, Munksgaard L, et al. Borrelia infection and risk of non-Hodgkin lymphoma. Blood. 2008;111:5524–9.
13. Wotherspoon AC, Ortiz-Hidalgo C, Falzon MR, et al. *Helicobacter pylori*-associated gastritis and primary B-cell gastric lymphoma. Lancet. 1991;338:1175–6.
14. Croia C, Astorri E, Murray-Brown W, et al. Implication of Epstein-Barr virus infection in disease-specific autoreactive B cell activation in ectopic lymphoid structures of Sjogren's syndrome. Arthritis Rheumatol. 2014;66:2545–57.
15. Fabris M, Dolcetti R, Pasini E, et al. High prevalence of Chlamydophila psittaci subclinical infection in Italian patients with Sjogren's syndrome and parotid gland marginal zone B-cell lymphoma of MALT-type. Clin Exp Rheumatol. 2014;32:61–5.

16. Blank M, Shoenfeld Y, Perl A. Cross-talk of the environment with the host genome and the immune system through endogenous retroviruses in systemic lupus erythematosus. Lupus. 2009;18:1136–43.
17. Mizokami A, Eguchi K, Moriuchi R, et al. Low copy numbers of human T-cell lymphotropic virus type I (HTLV-I) tax-like DNA detected in the salivary gland of seronegative patients with Sjögren's syndrome in an HTLV-I endemic area. Scand J Rheumatol. 1998;27:435–40.
18. Mariette X. Lymphomas complicating Sjogren's syndrome and hepatitis C virus infection may share a common pathogenesis: chronic stimulation of rheumatoid factor B cells. Ann Rheum Dis. 2001;60:1007–10.
19. De Vita S, Damato R, De Marchi G, et al. True primary Sjogren's syndrome in a subset of patients with hepatitis C infection: a model linking chronic infection to chronic sialadenitis. Isr Med Assoc J. 2002;4:1101–5.
20. De Re V, De Vita S, Marzotto A, et al. Sequence analysis of the immunoglobulin antigen receptor of hepatitis C virus-associated non-Hodgkin lymphomas suggests that the malignant cells are derived from the rheumatoid factor-producing cells that occur mainly in type II cryoglobulinemia. Blood. 2000;96:3578–84.
21. De Re V, Sansonno D, Simula MP, et al. HCV-NS3 and IgG-Fc crossreactive IgM in patients with type II mixed cryoglobulinemia and B-cell clonal proliferations. Leukemia. 2006;20:1145–54.
22. Croia C, Serafini B, Bombardieri M, et al. Epstein-Barr virus persistence and infection of autoreactive plasma cells in synovial lymphoid structures in rheumatoid arthritis. Ann Rheum Dis. 2013;72:1559–68.
23. Szymula A, Rosenthal J, Szczerba BM, et al. T cell epitope mimicry between Sjogren's syndrome antigen A (SSA)/Ro60 and oral, gut, skin and vaginal bacteria. Clin Immunol. 2014;152:1–9.
24. Inoue H, Mishima K, Yamamoto-Yoshida S, et al. Aryl hydrocarbon receptor-mediated induction of EBV reactivation as a risk factor for Sjogren's syndrome. J Immunol. 2012;188:4654–62.
25. Nakamura H, Kawakami A, Eguchi K. Mechanisms of autoantibody production and the relationship between autoantibodies and the clinical manifestations in Sjogren's syndrome. Transl Res. 2006;148:281–8.
26. Hida A, Imaizumi M, Sera N, et al. Association of human T lymphotropic virus type I with Sjogren syndrome. Ann Rheum Dis. 2010;69:2056–7.
27. Triantafyllopoulou A, Tapinos N, Moutsopoulos HM. Evidence for coxsackievirus infection in primary Sjögren's syndrome. Arthritis Rheum. 2004;50:2897–902.
28. Gottenberg JE, Pallier C, Ittah M, et al. Failure to confirm coxsackievirus infection in primary Sjögren's syndrome. Arthritis Rheum. 2006;54:2026–8.
29. Papasteriades CA, Skopouli FN, Drosos AA, et al. HLA-alloantigen associations in Greek patients with Sjögren's syndrome. J Autoimmun. 1988;1:85–90.
30. Gottenberg JE, Busson M, Loiseau P, et al. In primary Sjögren's syndrome, HLA class II is associated exclusively with autoantibody production and spreading of the autoimmune response. Arthritis Rheum. 2003;48:2240–5.
31. Stathopoulou EA, Routsias JG, Stea EA, et al. Cross-reaction between antibodies to the major epitope of Ro60 kD autoantigen and a homologous peptide of Coxsackie virus 2B protein. Clin Exp Immunol. 2005;141:148–54.
32. Popovic M, Reitz MS Jr, Sarngadharan MG, et al. The virus of Japanese adult T-cell leukaemia is a member of the human T-cell leukaemia virus group. Nature. 1982;300(5887):63–6.
33. Gessain A, Barin F, Vernant JC, et al. Antibodies to human T-lymphotropic virus type-I in patients with tropical spastic paraparesis. Lancet. 1985;2:407–10.
34. Osame M, Usuku K, Izumo S, Ijichi N, Amitani H, Igata A, Matsumoto M, Tara M. HTLV-I associated myelopathy, a new clinical entity. Lancet. 1986;1:1031–2.
35. Nakamura H, Kawakami A. What is the evidence for Sjögren's syndrome being triggered by viral infection? Subplot: infections that cause clinical features of Sjögren's syndrome. Curr Opin Rheumatol. 2016;28:390–7.
36. Terada K, Katamine S, Eguchi K, et al. Prevalence of serum and salivary antibodies to HTLV-1 in Sjögren's syndrome. Lancet. 1994;344:1116–9.
37. Eguchi K, Matsuoka N, Ida H, et al. Primary Sjögren's syndrome with antibodies to HTLV-I: clinical and laboratory features. Ann Rheum Dis. 1992;51:769–76.
38. Bélec L, Georges MC, Pillot J, et al. Antibodies to HTLV-I in Sjögren's syndrome. Lancet. 1995;345:71–2.
39. Green JE, Hinrichs SH, Vogel J, et al. Exocrinopathy resembling Sjögren's syndrome in HTLV-1 tax transgenic mice. Nature. 1989;341:72–4.
40. Sumida T, Yonaha F, Maeda T, et al. Expression of sequences homologous to HTLV-I tax gene in the labial salivary glands of Japanese patients with Sjögren's syndrome. Arthritis Rheumatol. 1994;37:545–50.
41. Mariette X, Agbalika F, Daniel MT, et al. Detection of human T lymphotropic virus type I tax gene in salivary gland epithelium from two patients with Sjögren's syndrome. Arthritis Rheumatol. 1993;36:1423–8.
42. Mariette X, Cherot P, Cazals D, et al. Antibodies to HTLV-I in Sjögren's syndrome. Lancet. 1995;345:71.
43. Nakamura H, Eguchi K, Nakamura T, et al. High prevalence of Sjögren's syndrome in patients with HTLV-I associated myelopathy. Ann Rheum Dis. 1997;56:167–72.
44. Izumi M, Nakamura H, Nakamura T, et al. Sjögren's syndrome (SS) in patients with human T cell leukemia virus I associated myelopathy: paradoxical features of the major salivary glands compared to classical SS. J Rheumatol. 1999;26:2609–14.
45. Nakamura H, Kawakami A, Hayashi T, et al. Low prevalence of ectopic germinal Centre formation in patients with HTLV-I-associated Sjogren's syndrome. Rheumatology (Oxford). 2009;48:854–5.

46. Ansel KM, Ngo VN, Hyman PL, et al. A chemokine-driven positive feedback loop organizes lymphoid follicles. Nature. 2000;406:309–14.
47. Ohyama Y, Nakamura S, Hara H, et al. Accumulation of human T lymphotropic virus type I-infected T cells in the salivary glands of patients with human T lymphotropic virus type I-associated Sjögren's syndrome. Arthritis Rheumatol. 1998;41:1972–8.
48. Nakamura H, Takahashi Y, Yamamoto-Fukuda T, et al. Direct infection of primary salivary gland epithelial cells by human T lymphotropic virus type I in patients with Sjögren's syndrome. Arthritis Rheumatol. 2015;67:1096–106.
49. Thorley-Lawson DA. Epstein-Barr virus: exploiting the immune system. Nat Rev Immunol. 2001;1:75–82.
50. Fox RI, Pearson G, Vaughan JH. Detection of Epstein-Barr virus-associated antigens and DNA in salivary gland biopsies from patients with Sjogren's syndrome. J Immunol. 1986;137:3162–8.
51. Mariette X, Gozlan J, Clerc D, et al. Detection of Epstein-Barr virus DNA by in situ hybridization and polymerase chain reaction in salivary gland biopsy specimens from patients with Sjögren's syndrome. Am J Med. 1991;90:286–94.
52. Wen S, Shimizu N, Yoshiyama H, et al. Association of Epstein-Barr virus (EBV) with Sjögren's syndrome: differential EBV expression between epithelial cells and lymphocytes in salivary glands. Am J Pathol. 1996;149:1511–7.
53. Pflugfelder SC, Crouse CA, Monroy D, et al. Epstein-Barr virus and the lacrimal gland pathology of Sjögren's syndrome. Am J Pathol. 1993;143:49–64.
54. Saito I, Servenius B, Compton T, et al. Detection of Epstein-Barr virus DNA by polymerase chain reaction in blood and tissue biopsies from patients with Sjogren's syndrome. J Exp Med. 1989;169:2191–8.
55. Inoue N, Harada S, Miyasaka N, et al. Analysis of antibody titers to Epstein-Barr virus nuclear antigens in sera of patients with Sjögren's syndrome and with rheumatoid arthritis. J Infect Dis. 1991;164:22–8.
56. Yamaoka K, Miyasaka N, Yamamoto K. Possible involvement of Epstein-Barr virus in polyclonal B cell activation in Sjögren's syndrome. Arthritis Rheumatol. 1988;31:1014–21.
57. Tateishi M, Saito I, Yamamoto K, et al. Spontaneous production of Epstein-Barr virus by B lymphoblastoid cell lines obtained from patients with Sjögren's syndrome. Possible involvement of a novel strain of Epstein-Barr virus in disease pathogenesis. Arthritis Rheum. 1993;36:827–35.
58. Vaughan JH, Valbracht JR, Nguyen MD, et al. Epstein-Barr virus-induced autoimmune responses. I. Immunoglobulin M autoantibodies to proteins mimicking and not mimicking Epstein-Barr virus nuclear antigen-1. J Clin Invest. 1995;95:1306–15.
59. Nagata Y, Inoue H, Yamada K, et al. Activation of Epstein-Barr virus by saliva from Sjogren's syndrome patients. Immunology. 2004;111:223–9.
60. Iwakiri D, Zhou L, Samanta M, et al. Epstein-Barr virus (EBV)-encoded small RNA is released from EBV-infected cells and activates signaling from toll-like receptor 3. J Exp Med. 2009;206:2091–9.
61. Lehours P, Yilmaz O. Epidemiology of *Helicobacter pylori* infection. Helicobacter. 2007;12(Suppl 1):1–3.
62. Cover TL, Blaser MJ. *Helicobacter pylori* in health and disease. Gastroenterology. 2009;136:1863–73.
63. Sheu BS, Yang HB, Yeh YC, et al. *Helicobacter pylori* colonization of the human gastric epithelium: a bug's first step is a novel target for us. J Gastroenterol Hepatol. 2010;25:26–32.
64. Blaser MJ, Atherton JC. *Helicobacter pylori* persistence: biology and disease. J Clin Invest. 2004;113:321–33.
65. Raghwan R. Host cell contact induces fur-dependent expression of virulence factors CagA and VacA in *Helicobacter pylori*. Helicobacter. 2014;19:17–25.
66. Chan AO, Chu KM, Huang C, et al. Association between *Helicobacter pylori* infection and interleukin 1beta polymorphism predispose to CpG island methylation in gastric cancer. Gut. 2007;56:595–7.
67. Radić M. Role of *Helicobacter pylori* infection in autoimmune systemic rheumatic diseases. World J Gastroenterol. 2014;20:12839–46.
68. Radić M, Martinović Kaliterna D, Bonacin D, et al. Correlation between *Helicobacter pylori* infection and systemic sclerosis activity. Rheumatology (Oxford). 2010;49:1784–5.
69. Radić M, Kaliterna DM, Bonacin D, et al. Is *Helicobacter pylori* infection a risk factor for disease severity in systemic sclerosis? Rheumatol Int. 2013;33:2943–8.
70. Gasbarrini A, Massari I, Serricchio M, et al. *Helicobacter pylori* eradication ameliorates primary Raynaud's phenomenon. Dig Dis Sci. 1998;43:1641–5.
71. Showji Y, Nozawa R, Sato K, et al. Seroprevalence of *Helicobacter pylori* infection in patients with connective tissue diseases. Microbiol Immunol. 1996;40:499–503.
72. Sorrentino D, Faller G, De Vita S, et al. *Helicobacter pylori* associated antigastric autoantibodies: role in Sjögren's syndrome gastritis. Helicobacter. 2004;9:46–53.
73. El Miedany YM, Baddour M, Ahmed I, et al. Sjogren' s syndrome: concomitant H. pylori infection and possible correlation with clinical parameters. Joint Bone Spine. 2005;72:135–41.
74. Ramos-Casals M, Loustaud-Ratti V, De Vita S, et al. Sjögren syndrome associated with hepatitis C virus: a multicenter analysis of 137 cases. Medicine. 2005;84:81–9.
75. Pasoto SG, Ribeiro CA, Bonfa E. Update on infections and vaccinations in systemic lupus erythematosus and Sjögren's syndrome. Curr Opin Rheumatol. 2014;26:528–37.
76. Haddad J, Deny P, Munz-Gotheil C, et al. Lymphocytic sialadenitis of Sjogren's syndrome associated with chronic hepatitis C virus liver disease. Lancet. 1992;339:321–3.

77. Wang Y, Dou H, Liu G, et al. Hepatitis C virus infection and the risk of Sjögren or sicca syndrome: a meta-analysis. Microbiol Immunol. 2014;58:675–87.
78. Nagao Y, Hanada S, Shishido S, et al. Incidence of Sjögren's syndrome in Japanese patients with hepatitis C virus infection. J Gatroenterol Hepatol. 2003;18:258–66.
79. Ramos-Casals M, Garcia-Carrasco M, Cervera R, et al. Sjogren's syndrome and hepatitis C virus. Clin Rheumatol. 1999;18:93–100.
80. Loustaud-Ratti V, Riche A, Liozon E, et al. Prevalence and characteristics of Sjogren's syndrome or Sicca syndrome in chronic hepatitis C virus infection: a prospective study. J Rheumatol. 2001;28:2245–51.
81. Cacoub P, Renou C, Rosenthal E, et al. Extrahepatic manifestations associated with hepatitis C virus infection. A prospective multicenter study of 321 patients. Infectieuses sur le Virus de l'Hepatite C. Medicine (Baltimore). 2000;79:47–56.
82. Porter SR, Scully C, Lodi G, et al. Lack of association between hepatitis C virus and Sjogren's syndrome. Oral Dis. 1996;2:183–4.
83. Marson P, Ostuni PA, Vicarioto M, et al. Anti-hepatitis C virus serology in primary Sjogren's syndrome: no evidence of cross-reactivity between rheumatoid factor and specific viral proteins. Clin Exp Rheumatol. 1991;9:661–2.
84. Scott CA, Avellini C, Desinan L, et al. Chronic lymphocytic sialoadenitis in HCV-related chronic liver disease: comparison of Sjögren's syndrome. Histopathology. 1997;30:4–8.
85. Garcia-Carrasco M, Ramos-Casals M, Rosas J, et al. Primary Sjogren syndrome: clinical and immunologic disease patterns in a cohort of 400 patients. Medicine (Baltimore). 2002;81:270–80.
86. Himoto T, Masaki T. Extrahepatic manifestations and autoantibodies in patients with hepatitis C virus infection. Clin Dev Immunol. 2012;2012:871401.
87. Ramos-Casals M, Font J. Extrahepatic manifestations in patients with chronic hepatitis C virus infection. Curr Opin Rheumatol. 2005;17:447–55.
88. De Vita S, Quartuccio L, Salvin S, et al. Cryoglobulinaemia related to Sjogren's syndrome or HCV infection: differences based on the pattern of bone marrow involvement, lymphoma evolution and laboratory tests after parotidectomy. Rheumatology (Oxford). 2012;51:627–33.
89. Potthoff A, Witte T, Rifai K, et al. Prevalence of alpha-fodrin antibodies in patients with chronic hepatitis C infection and Sjögren syndrome. Scand J Gastroenterol. 2009;44:994–1003.
90. Smyth CM, McKiernan SM, Hagan R, et al. Chronic hepatitis C infection and sicca syndrome: a clear association with HLA DQB1*02. Eur J Gastroenterol Hepatol. 2007;19:493–8.
91. Igoe A, Scofield HR. Autoimmunity and infection in Sjögren's syndrome. Curr Opin Rheumatol. 2013;25:480–7.
92. Toussirot E, Le Huédé G, Mougin C, et al. Presence of hepatitis C virus RNA in the salivary glands of patients with Sjögren's syndrome and hepatitis C virus infection. J Rheumatol. 2002;29:2382–5.
93. Grossmann Sde MC, Teixeira R, de Oliveira GC, et al. Xerostomia, hyposalivation and sialadenitis in patients with chronic hepatitis C are not associated with the detection of HCV RNA in saliva or salivary glands. J Clin Pathol. 2010;63:1002–7.
94. Koike K, Moriya K, Ishibashi K, et al. Sialadenitis histologically resembling Sjogren syndrome in mice transgenic for hepatitis C virus envelope genes. Proc Natl Acad Sci U S A. 1997;94:233–6.
95. Rosa D, Saletti G, De Gregorio E, et al. Activation of naïve B lymphocytes via CD81, a pathogenetic mechanism for hepatitis C virus-associated B lymphocyte disorders. Proc Natl Acad Sci U S A. 2005;102:18544–9.
96. Machida K, Cheng KT-H, Pavio N, et al. Hepatitis C virus E2-CD81 interaction induces hypermutation of the immunoglobulin gene in B cells. J Virol. 2005;79:8079–89.
97. Roughan JE, Reardon KM, Cogburn KE, et al. Chronic hepatitis C virus infection breaks tolerance and drives polyclonal expansion of autoreactive B cells. Clin Vaccine Immunol. 2012;19:1027–37.
98. Fabris M, Quartuccio L, Sacco S, et al. B-Lymphocyte stimulator (BLyS) up-regulation in mixed cryoglobulinaemia syndrome and hepatitis-C virus infection. Rheumatology. 2007;46:37–43.
99. De Vita S, Quartuccio L, Salvin S, et al. Sequential therapy with belimumab followed by rituximab in Sjögren's syndrome associated with B-cell lymphoproliferation and overexpression of BAFF: evidence for long-term efficacy. Clin Exp Rheumatol. 2014;32:490–4.
100. Rama M, Anaya J-M, Barzilai O, et al. The putative protective role of hepatitis B virus (HBV) infection from autoimmune disorders. Autoimmun Rev. 2008;7:621–5.
101. Ichiki Y, He XS, Shimoda S, et al. T cell immunity in hepatitis B and hepatitis C virus infection: implications for autoimmunity. Autoimmun Rev. 2005;4:82–95.
102. Cacoub P, Saadoun D, Bourliere M, et al. Hepatitis B virus genotypes and extrahepatic manifestations. J Hepatol. 2005;43:764–70.
103. Chen M-H, Hsiao L-T, Chen M-H, et al. Clinical significance of chronic hepatitis B virus infection in patients with primary Sjögren's syndrome. Clin Rheumatol. 2012;31:309–15.
104. Marcos M, Alvarez F, Brito-Zerón P, et al. Chronic hepatitis B virus infection in Sjögren's syndrome. Prevalence and clinical significance in 603 patients. Autoimmun Rev. 2009;8:616–20.
105. Bach JF. Protective role of infections and vaccinations on autoimmune diseases. J Autoimmun. 2001;16:347–53.
106. Bach JF. The effect of infections on susceptibility to autoimmune and allergic diseases. N Engl J Med. 2002;347(12):911–20.

107. Osborn MK, Lok AS. Antiviral options for the treatment of chronic hepatitis B. J Antimicrob Chemother. 2006;57:1030–4.
108. Koichi Y, Arvin AM, Campadelli-Fiume G, et al. Human herpesviruses: biology, therapy and immunoprophylaxis. Cambridge: Cambridge University Press; 2007.
109. Barzilai O, Sherer Y, Ram M, et al. Epstein-Barr virus and cytomegalovirus in autoimmune diseases: are they truly notorious? A preliminary report. Ann N Y Acad Sci. 2007;1108:567–77.
110. Ohyama Y, Carroll VA, Deshmukh U, et al. Severe focal sialadenitis and dacryoadenitis in NZM2328 mice induced by MCMV: a novel model for human Sjogren's syndrome. J Immunol. 2006;177:7391–7.
111. Cardin RD, Schaefer GC, Allen JR, et al. The M33 chemokine receptor homolog of murine cytomegalovirus exhibits a differential tissue-specific role during in vivo replication and latency. J Virol. 2009;83:7590–601.
112. Davis-Poynter NJ, Lynch DM, Vally H, et al. Identification and characterization of a G protein-coupled receptor homolog encoded by murine cytomegalovirus. J Virol. 1997;71:1521–9.
113. De Re V, De Vita S, Battistella V, et al. Absence of human parvovirus B19 DNA in myoepithelial sialadenitis of primary Sjögren's syndrome. Ann Rheum Dis. 2002;61:855–6.
114. Ramos-Casals M, Cervera R, García-Carrasco M, et al. Cytopenia and past human parvovirus B19 infection in patients with primary Sjögren's syndrome. Semin Arthritis Rheumatol. 2000;29:373–8.
115. Gallo A, Tandon M, Illei G, Alevizos I. Discovery and validation of novel microRNAs in Sjögren's syndrome salivary glands. Clin Exp Rheumatol. 2014;32:761–2.
116. Giannopoulou EG, Elemento O, Ivashkiv LB. Use of RNA sequencing to evaluate rheumatic disease patients. Arthritis Res Ther. 2015;17:167.

24 Systemic Sclerosis

Julia Spierings, Femke C. van Rhijn-Brouwer, and Jacob M. van Laar

Abbreviations

B. burgdorferi	*Borrelia burgdorferi*
CMV	Cytomegalovirus
DcSSc	Diffuse cutaneous systemic sclerosis
EC	Endothelial cells
F. prausnitzii	*Faecalibacterium prausnitzii*
GvHD	Graft versus host disease
HBV	Hepatitis B virus
LcSSc	Limited cutaneous systemic sclerosis
SIBO	Small intestinal bacterial overgrowth
SSc	Systemic sclerosis

J. Spierings · J. M. van Laar (✉)
Department of Rheumatology and Clinical Immunology, University Medical Centre Utrecht, Utrecht, The Netherlands
e-mail: j.m.vanlaar@umcutrecht.nl

F. C. van Rhijn-Brouwer
Department of Rheumatology and Clinical Immunology, University Medical Centre Utrecht, Utrecht, The Netherlands

Department of Nephrology and Hypertension, University Medical Centre Utrecht, Utrecht, The Netherlands

Clinical Presentation and Pathogenesis of Systemic Sclerosis

Systemic sclerosis (SSc) is a rare systemic autoimmune connective tissue disease characterized by inflammation, vasculopathy, and fibrosis of the skin and visceral organs.

The clinical presentation of SSc is heterogeneous. Manifestations vary from limited skin involvement (tightening of the skin) and Raynaud's phenomenon (limited cutaneous systemic sclerosis (lcSSc)) to generalized skin involvement with severe internal organ damage (diffuse cutaneous systemic sclerosis (dcSSc) [1, 2]. LcSSc and dcSSc can partly be differentiated by their autoantibody profile. In patients with dcSSc, major organ involvement is more common.

Systemic manifestations of SSc are diverse because almost every organ system can be involved. Cardiac, pulmonary, musculoskeletal, and gastrointestinal symptoms are commonly reported [3, 4]. Pulmonary fibrosis and pulmonary arterial hypertension are the leading causes of mortality. The 10-year mortality for dcSSc with rapid increase in skin involvement and development of organ fibrosis is ~27%. The disease course of lcSSc is more indolent though life-threatening organ complications can also occur later on in the disease course in case of cardiopulmonary organ involvement, leading to a 10-year mortality of ~19% [5–7].

G. Ragab et al. (eds.), *The Microbiome in Rheumatic Diseases and Infection*,
https://doi.org/10.1007/978-3-319-79026-8_24

The pathogenesis of SSc is not entirely understood and is considered to be a complex, multifactorial process. Endothelial injury occurs early, leading to fibroproliferative vasculopathy and hypoxia. Subsequent dysfunction of fibroblasts and myofibroblasts then causes excessive production of collagen and other matrix components which accumulate in the skin, vessels, and internal organs [8, 9]. Both innate and adaptive immune systems contribute to initiation and maintenance of inflammation and formation of autoantibodies [10]. Several genetic associations with SSc have been reported, though concordance in monozygotic twins is very low, which suggests a limited role for genetic factors in the pathogenesis of SSc [11]. Several environmental factors have been identified in SSc patient population studies, such as occupational exposure to silica and solvents [12, 13].

Infections in SSc

Infections may play a role in the development and progression of SSc. Links between SSc and prior infection have been suggested but none has been firmly established. Serological reactivity and increased antibody titers against cytomegalovirus (CMV), retroviruses, parvovirus B19, hepatitis B virus (HBV), and toxoplasmosis were detected more often in patients with SSc compared with healthy controls in several studies [14–16]. Also, there are studies suggesting that CMV triggers autoimmunity through a mechanism based on molecular mimicry in SSc patients [17]. CMV can infect endothelial cells (EC) and monocytes and cause inflammation and upregulation of fibrogenic cytokines in animal models [18]. Furthermore, there is a homology between a certain epitope of the virus and proteins expressed on the surface of ECs [19]. The development of vasculopathy in animal models of CMV infection indirectly supports a role for CMV infection in SSc pathogenesis. Although these findings link infections with SSc, there is no strong evidence for a direct causal role of one specific infectious agent.

Patients with systemic sclerosis are more susceptible to infectious disease. Immune abnormalities, organ manifestations, and immunosuppressive treatments could explain this increased risk [20, 21]. In a cohort of 117 SSc patients with 310 person-years under observation, 63 infections were reported [22]. Thirty-seven events required antibiotic therapy or hospitalization. Urinary tract, skin and soft tissue, and gastrointestinal infections were most frequently found. Opportunistic infections occurred in only one patient; this low number might be explained by the limited use of immunosuppressant therapy including high-dose steroids in this cohort.

Infection has been reported as an important cause of death in SSc patients. In a prospective cohort of 5860 SSc patients, infections were responsible for a third of the non-SSc-related causes of death. Among the infections with considerable SSc-related risk factors, pneumonia predominated with esophageal reflux, aspiration, and significant immobility. Septicemia was reported in patients with significant immobility and patients with skin ulcers [23].

As mentioned earlier, skin ulcers are very common in SSc [24]. Ischemia due to vasculopathy together with repetitive microtrauma, skin alterations, and calcinosis is assumed to contribute to the development of digital ulcers in SSc [24, 25]. This avascular and atrophic tissue has a reduced wound healing capacity and is highly susceptible for infection. Consequently, superinfection of skin ulcers is a frequently reported complication, and its management can be challenging. These ulcers can become complicated by osteomyelitis [26]. In a retrospective study of 248 SSc patients with a mean follow-up time of 60.8 months, skin ulcers were observed in 119 patients; in 45 patients these ulcers were infected. Nineteen of these patients showed underlying bone involvement. The most frequently isolated pathogens were *Staphylococcus aureus and Escherichia coli.*

Successful treatment of skin infections in SSc patients requires timely and accurate diagnostic assessment, including tissue and fluid cultures and a combination of targeted antimicrobial therapy and local treatment. In addition to the treatment of pneumonia, treatment of SSc-related factors like esophageal dysmotility needs to be optimized.

Awareness of the SSc-related and treatment-related risk factors for infection is important in the prevention and timely recognition of infection.

The Microbiome in SSc

The role of microbiota is an area that is largely unexplored in SSc. Currently, there are five published studies that investigate the composition of the microbiome in the gastrointestinal tract or the skin. Though exploratory in nature, these studies suggest that microbial communities potentially contribute to both the pathogenesis of SSc and clinical symptoms of patients with early or late SSc.

The Gut Microbiome in SSc In a cross-sectional study, Andreasson et al. reported dysbiosis in 74 (76%) of 98 consecutive in-hospital SSc patients. These patients were admitted for planned, SSc-related, in-hospital care. Seventy-seven patients (78%) of this group were classified as having lcSSc and 21 (22%) as dcSSc; the median duration of disease was 6 years. Sixty-five patients (65%) reported gastrointestinal complaints; 82 patients (84%) exhibited esophageal dysfunction, which was assessed by cineradiography. Sixty patients (61%) did not use any immunosuppressive therapy and no patients were on prednisolone. Unfortunately, use of antibiotics was not reported in detail. Dysbiosis was established by analyzing stool samples with the GA-Map Dysbiosis Test (Genetic Analysis, Oslo, Norway), a ribosomal RNA probe set representing 54 bacterial species or clades; results were expressed with a Dysbiosis Index Score. In 66 (67.3%) of all patients, fewer *Faecalibacterium prausnitzii* transcripts were present compared to the GA-Map Dysbiosis Test results in a standard reference cohort from the manufacturer [27].

F. prausnitzii is a common member of the human intestinal microbiome [28]. In patients with intestinal disorders, in particular with Crohn's disease, depletion of *F. prausnitzii* is reported [29]. Interestingly, *F. prausnitzii* was shown to exhibit anti-inflammatory effects in in vitro studies and in studies using animal colitis models. In vitro peripheral blood mononuclear cell stimulation by *F. prausnitzii* led to higher production of IL-10 and lower IL-12 and IFN-gamma excretion. In mice with induced colitis, oral administration of *F. prausnitzii* improved severity of disease [30, 31].

Lower concentrations of *F. prausnitzii* reported in SSc patients could reflect a pro-inflammatory state of the SSc intestinal microbiome; however, further research is required to establish its role in this disease. Another observation reported in the study of Andreasson was a decrease in *Clostridiaceae* transcripts in 25 (26%) and an increase of *Lactobacillus* in 31 (32%) SSc patients. Additionally, Andreasson et al. found that dysbiosis was more prevalent and severe in patients with esophageal dysmotility and was associated with micronutrient deficiency and risk for malnutrition. Interestingly, the degree of dysbiosis also correlated with the presence of skin teleangiectasias, pitting scars, and pulmonary fibrosis [27]. This finding suggests a link between dysbiosis and extraintestinal manifestations of SSc, or reflects the consequences of late disease, so a causal relationship cannot be inferred. Unfortunately, this study was limited by the fact that the investigators only examined a predefined set of bacteria, as opposed to more commonly used amplicon-based or whole genome sequencing methods. Secondly, stool samples from SSc patients were compared with a standard reference cohort from the manufacturer of the predefined genome test, while comparison with healthy controls from the same background population would be preferred here. Furthermore, the study only included in-hospital patients, which may not be representative of the overall population of SSc patients.

Volkmann et al. investigated the intestinal microbiome of 17 patients with systemic sclerosis in comparison with 17 healthy age- and sex-matched controls. In contrast with the study discussed above, this study utilized a broader approach to determine the composition of the microbiome in SSc patients, namely, sequencing of the 16S ribosomal DNA. The median age of SSc patients included in the study group was 52.1 years, and the median disease duration was 7.1 years. From the 17 SSc patients, six (36%) had dcSSc, six patients had taken antibiotics in the last 3 months, three patients were on immunosuppressive agents, and three patients used probiotic oral supplements. The mean total score on the questionnaire on gastrointestinal complaints indicated moderate symptom severity (distention, constipation, social functioning, and emotional well-being) or mild severity (diarrhea). Microbiome profiles were compiled by multiplex sequencing of bacterial ribosomal RNA in colonic lavage samples. Microbial communities in the cecum and sigmoid significantly differed in SSc patients as compared with healthy controls. In samples of SSc patients, a decreased concentration of protective commensal bacteria (i.e., *Faecalibacterium* and *Clostridium*) and increased concentration of inflammatory pathologic bacteria (i.e., *Fusobacterium* and *gamma-Proteobacterium*) were found. These findings were confirmed in two independent SSc cohorts in Oslo ($n = 17$) and California ($n = 17$) compared with healthy controls ($n = 17$) [32]. The cohorts were similar in disease duration, gender distribution, age and gastrointestinal symptoms. Less severe gastrointestinal symptoms were reported in patients with higher abundance of *Clostridium*. The association of the microbial signatures of dysbiosis in the gut with gastrointestinal disease in SSc was also reported by Patrone and colleagues [33]. Fecal bacterial composition of patients with ($n = 9$) and without ($n = 9$) gastrointestinal symptoms and healthy controls ($n = 9$) were compared. Again, higher levels of *Lactobacillus, Eubacterium*, and *Acinetobacter* and lower levels of *Roseburia, Clostridium*, and *Ruminococcus* were found in SSc patient with gastrointestinal symptoms compared with healthy controls while SSc patients without gastrointestinal symptoms were more similar to the healthy controls than their symptomatic counterparts. Streptococcus salivarius was, however, over-represented in the fecal samples of SSc patients without gastrointestinal symptoms compared to SSc patients with symptoms and healthy controls.

The microbiome thus seems to reflect the inflammatory state present in SSc and differences in composition of the microbiome are associated with gastrointestinal symptoms. In agreement with the findings by Andreasson et al., both Volkmann et al. and Patrone et al. also reported an increased amount of *Lactobacillus* in SSc patients compared to healthy controls.

Interestingly, studies in patients with active Crohn's disease and ulcerative colitis also report increased levels of *Lactobacillus* in fecal and biopsy samples [34, 35]. The effects of *Lactobacillus* in the gut lumen in these patients should be further determined, as it seems to conflict with the anti-inflammatory effects reported in in vitro studies and animal models of inflammatory conditions [36]. Furthermore, several clinical trials investigating the effect of administration of *Lactobacillus* organisms have shown promising results in certain conditions, including inflammatory bowel disease, but due to inconsistency among studies, these results should be interpreted with caution [37, 38].

Further analysis of the bacterial genomic data in the study of Volkmann revealed a decreased number of genes involved in amino sugar and nucleotide sugar metabolism pathways in SSc patients. The clinical relevance of this is unknown, though impaired fructose absorption has been reported in SSc [39].

The results of the microbiome profiling were also correlated with gastrointestinal symptom severity as measured with validated questionnaires. *Bacteroides fragilis* was decreased, and *Fusobacterium* was increased in patients with gastrointestinal symptoms, compared with patients who were asymptomatic.

Although the strengths of this study are the broader investigation of the composition of the gut microbiome and the inclusion of a healthy control group, there are some limitations. The cross-sectional design does not give any information about the relationship between specific genera and clinical signs in time. Secondly, relatively long disease duration might influence the microbiome, so it would be more interesting to investigate patients early in the disease. Furthermore, confounding factors, including antibiotics, probi-

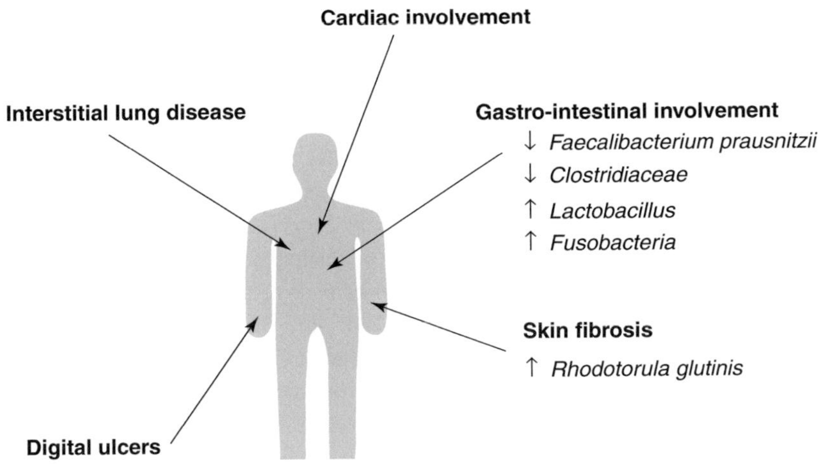

Fig. 24.1 SSc affects the skin, lungs, and gastrointestinal tract, which are prominent locations of the microbiome [3, 4]. Four studies investigating the microbiome of the gastrointestinal tract in SSc reported decreased levels of *F. prausnitzii* and *Clostridiaceae* species and an increase in *Lactobacillus* and *Fusobacteria* [27, 32, 33, 40]. One study investigated the composition of the skin microbiome in SSc and reported an increase in *R. glutinis* compared to healthy controls [43]

otics, as well as differences in diet, were present, which might alter compositions of the microbiome. Finally, although significant differences were found between the groups, this study was very small. Volkmann et al. provided valuable insights into the microbiota composition of SSc patients, but these findings have to be confirmed in other cohorts [40].

The Skin Microbiome in SSc Composition and alterations in composition of the skin microbiome are also of interest in SSc as the most obvious and early signs of this disease are its cutaneous manifestations. In other inflammatory skin diseases, such as psoriasis, studies have shown some differences in microbiota between psoriasis and normal skin [41, 42].

One study specifically investigated the composition of the skin microbiome in SSc patients (Fig. 24.1).

Arron et al. analyzed the skin transcriptome of four patients with early diffuse SSc to gain further insight in the skin microbiome in SSc. Multiplex sequencing was performed on RNA extracted from 4 mm skin biopsies of patients with early disease and four healthy controls, and results were compared after subtraction of human sequences. Interestingly, there were no differences between SSc patients and healthy controls with regard to viral or bacterial transcripts, but there were significant differences in the fungus sequences. Compared with healthy controls, patients with SSc showed higher concentrations of *Rhodotorula glutinis* species, a yeast that is a common environmental inhabitant [43]. Given the heterogeneity and limited size of the sample, further studies are needed to confirm and explore the meaning of this finding.

Plausibility of a Causative Role of the Microbiome in SSc

The aforementioned studies on the composition of the microbiome in SSc patients suggest that the microbiome is altered in SSc. However, an important question that remains is whether this reflects a cause or a consequence. In addition to this small number of studies into the microbiome of SSc patients, there are other indications that the microbiome plays a role in SSc disease pathogenesis and progression.

Firstly, gastrointestinal dysfunction affects 90% of patients with SSc and is a major cause of morbidity [44]. Clinical manifestations include esophageal dysmotility, constipation, and small intestinal bacterial overgrowth (SIBO) [45]. Whether SIBO is only a result of the disease or a contributing factor in disease progression has still to be established. However, treatment of SIBO with medications such as antibiotics and even probiotics in small pilot studies that alter the microbiota seems to reduce the severity of gastrointestinal symptoms in non-SSc patients with SIBO [46].

In SSc patients, antibiotic treatment (norfloxacin and metronidazole) aimed to eradicate SIBO led to a significant improvement of intestinal symptoms too [47, 48]. This supports the hypothesis that the composition of the microbiome influences intestinal symptoms in SSc. Unfortunately, no effects on extraintestinal symptoms were reported.

The use of erythromycin, a macrolide antibiotic, has also been proven to be effective in SSc patients with gastroesophageal reflux and SIBO. Besides antimicrobial effects, erythromycin functions as a motilin agonist, which could influence the microbial colonization of the gut in two ways, firstly by treating gastrointestinal motor abnormalities, which predisposes to bacterial overgrowth, and secondly by physically displacing microorganisms [49, 50]. A relationship between intestinal motility on the colonic mucosal microbiota was also shown in studies performed in non-SSc patients with constipation; faster transit times correlated with the presence of fewer pathogenic bacteria [51–53].

On the other hand, the use of antimicrobial therapies to prevent infections and other inflammatory conditions, such as acute graft versus host disease (GVHD), is a matter of debate because antibiotics can disrupt gut ecology and aggravate gastrointestinal symptoms and contribute to the development of resistant strains [54–56].

Interestingly, the few studies investigating the role of antimicrobial therapy in SSc aiming to decrease overall disease progression reported negative results, even though in vitro studies suggested a strong anti-fibrotic effect [57, 58]. Therefore, caution is warranted in interpreting the results of these two interventional studies in SSc patients with gastrointestinal symptoms.

As probiotics can also potentially modify the intestinal microbial colonization, improvement of symptoms after probiotic administration might signify a causal relationship between composition of the microbiome and disease symptoms. The administration of probiotics was reported to be effective in terms of resolving gastrointestinal complaints in SSc in one small open-label study. Ten SSc patients with stable organ disease and gastrointestinal complaints received *Bifidobacterium infantis* or *Lactobacillus GG* daily during 2 months. Gastrointestinal complaints were measure with the validated GIT 2.0 questionnaire. After administration of probiotics, GIT scores on reflux and distention and bloating significantly improved [59]. Unfortunately, no control group was included, so firm conclusions cannot be drawn.

Secondly, some animal studies in Crohn's disease suggest that certain microbes could have a profibrotic effect on the gut [60]. As SSc is characterized by progressive fibrosis of multiple organs, this new reported mechanism is of interest because it provides a putative explanation for the link between symptoms and microbiota. Data in SSc are lacking however.

Thirdly, another approach of investigating the influence of the microbiome on SSc disease activity is to look into the host side. Activation of subsets of immune cells associated with pathogen defense can strengthen the suggestion that infection or colonization with pathogenic microbiota is related to clinical signs of disease. In SSc, there are indications that several innate immune system effector cells are activated [61, 62].

One reported infection related to signs of disease is the association between *Borrelia burgdorferi* and morphea (local skin thickening without systemic signs). Several studies have reported the presence of *B. burgdorferi* RNA in skin biopsies. However, the interpretation of these findings is complex. Firstly, there might be a difference in subspecies of *B. burgdorferi* as in morphea patients from Venezuela, from the United States, and from Scotland; no *B. burgdorferi* could be detected [63–65]. Secondly, various types of biopsy material (unfixed, fixed) were used, which also might affect detection sensitivity. Furthermore, it is unsure whether antibiotic treatment affects morphea symptoms; results of studies are conflicting and no RCT has been conducted yet [66].

Another possible link between disease activity and pathogenic microbiota is the colonization of skin ulcers. There is a high prevalence of chronic ulcers in SSc patients [24]. In general, direct toxic effects of bacteria as well as deleterious host-pathogen interactions have been implicated in poor wound healing [67]. One retrospective study evaluated the results of bacterial cultures taken from 42 SSc patients with digital ulcers displaying clinical signs of infection. After cleaning and debridement, the ulcers were sampled with a sterile swab. Bacterial species were identified using antigen agglutination or protein/DNA sequencing. *S. aureus* was the most common pathogen, but in 26% of the patients, colonization with intestinal bacteria (i.e., *E. coli* and *Enterococcus feacalis*) was found. This highlights the importance of hygienic precautions in SSc patients with digital ulcers and suggests a link between colonization with intestinal bacteria and poor healing ulcers. However, given the retrospective nature of this study, the risk of inclusion bias due to only including patients with already infected ulcers, as well as the lack of broad genomic sequence methods, the clinical relevance of this study may be limited [26].

Periodontal disease has been linked to inflammation in a wide variety of conditions, including cardiovascular disease and rheumatoid arthritis. Periodontal disease is common in SSc [68, 69]. A link between periodontal ligament widening—a radiographic hallmark of periodontitis—and disease severity has been shown in a large Canadian cohort [70]. Though it seems very reasonable that periodontal changes are a consequence of microstomia and xerostomia, periodontal inflammation can have a profound effect on the vascular endothelium and therefore might also affect SSc progression through affecting the microcirculation [71]. As of yet, no such studies have been done to corroborate this.

Conclusion and Implications for Further Research

Very few studies have been performed in the field of the microbiome in SSc. The studies conducted so far provide tentative evidence that alterations in the microbiome can be associated with SSc, but the implications of these findings are not clear, due to the heterogeneity of the methods used, the small numbers studied, lack of controls, and confounding factors such as the use of immunosuppressive drugs, diet, antibiotics, and hospitalization. This underscores the importance of further well-designed studies of the microbiome in SSc patients with appropriate controls.

Above, we addressed various lines of hypothesis that may strengthen the rationale for further investigation of the microbiome in SSc. The fact that SSc affects the skin, lungs, and gastrointestinal tract, which are prominent locations of the microbiome, makes it more challenging to explore the role of microorganisms in the disease process. Inclusion of locally recruited healthy controls is essential to minimize potential confounders. Furthermore, it would be very interesting to determine if symptoms could be improved by influencing the microbiome of these patients. Most importantly, it has to be established if these altered populations are the cause or the result of the disease or the immunosuppressive treatment.

References

1. LeRoy EC, Medsger TA Jr. Criteria for the classification of early systemic sclerosis. J Rheumatol. 2001;28(7):1573–6.
2. van den Hoogen F, Khanna D, Fransen J, et al. 2013 classification criteria for systemic sclerosis: an American college of rheumatology/European league against rheumatism collaborative initiative. Ann Rheum Dis. 2013;72(11):1747–55. https://doi.org/10.1136/annrheumdis-2013-204424.
3. Black CM. Scleroderma–clinical aspects. J Intern Med. 1993;234(2):115–8.
4. Steen VD. Clinical manifestations of systemic sclerosis. Semin Cutan Med Surg. 1998;17(1):48–54.
5. Ferri C, Sebastiani M, Lo Monaco A, et al. Systemic sclerosis evolution of disease pathomorphosis and survival. Our experience on Italian patients' population and review of the literature. Autoimmun Rev. 2014;13(10):1026–34. https://doi.org/10.1016/j.autrev.2014.08.029.
6. Gabrielli A, Avvedimento EV, Krieg T. Scleroderma. N Engl J Med. 2009;360(19):1989–2003. https://doi.org/10.1056/NEJMra0806188.
7. Ioannidis JP, Vlachoyiannopoulos PG, Haidich AB, et al. Mortality in systemic sclerosis: an international meta-analysis of individual patient data. Am

J Med. 2005;118(1):2–10. https://doi.org/10.1016/j.amjmed.2004.04.031.
8. Allanore Y, Simms R, Distler O, et al. Systemic sclerosis. Nat Rev Dis Primers. 2015;1:15002. https://doi.org/10.1038/nrdp.2015.2.
9. Jimenez SA. Role of endothelial to mesenchymal transition in the pathogenesis of the vascular alterations in systemic sclerosis. ISRN Rheumatol. 2013;2013:835948. https://doi.org/10.1155/2013/835948.
10. Pattanaik D, Brown M, Postlethwaite BC, et al. Pathogenesis of systemic sclerosis. Front Immunol. 2015;6:272. https://doi.org/10.3389/fimmu.2015.00272.
11. Feghali-Bostwick C, Medsger TA Jr, Wright TM. Analysis of systemic sclerosis in twins reveals low concordance for disease and high concordance for the presence of antinuclear antibodies. Arthritis Rheum. 2003;48(7):1956–63. https://doi.org/10.1002/art.11173.
12. Nietert PJ, Silver RM. Systemic sclerosis: environmental and occupational risk factors. Curr Opin Rheumatol. 2000;12(6):520–6.
13. Rubio-Rivas M, Moreno R, Corbella X. Occupational and environmental scleroderma. Systematic review and meta-analysis. Clin Rheumatol. 2017;36(3):569–82. https://doi.org/10.1007/s10067-016-3533-1.
14. Arnson Y, Amital H, Guiducci S, et al. The role of infections in the immunopathogenesis of systemic sclerosis–evidence from serological studies. Ann N Y Acad Sci. 2009;1173:627–32. https://doi.org/10.1111/j.1749-6632.2009.04808.x.
15. Grossman C, Dovrish Z, Shoenfeld Y, et al. Do infections facilitate the emergence of systemic sclerosis? Autoimmun Rev. 2011;10(5):244–7. https://doi.org/10.1016/j.autrev.2010.09.010.
16. Radic M, Martinovic Kaliterna D, Radic J. Infectious disease as aetiological factor in the pathogenesis of systemic sclerosis. Neth J Med. 2010;68(11):348–53.
17. Dolcino M, Puccetti A, Barbieri A, et al. Infections and autoimmunity: role of human cytomegalovirus in autoimmune endothelial cell damage. Lupus. 2015;24(4–5):419–32. https://doi.org/10.1177/0961203314558677.
18. Muryoi T, Kasturi KN, Kafina MJ, et al. Antitopoisomerase I monoclonal autoantibodies from scleroderma patients and tight skin mouse interact with similar epitopes. J Exp Med. 1992;175(4):1103–9.
19. Randone SB, Guiducci S, Cerinic MM. Systemic sclerosis and infections. Autoimmun Rev. 2008;8(1):36–40. https://doi.org/10.1016/j.autrev.2008.07.022.
20. Heijnen T, Wilmer A, Blockmans D. Outcome of patients with systemic diseases admitted to the medical intensive care unit of a tertiary referral hospital: a single-centre retrospective study. Scand J Rheumatol. 2016;45(2):146–50. https://doi.org/10.3109/03009742.2015.1067329.
21. Woytala PJ, Morgiel E, Łuczak A, et al. The safety of intravenous cyclophosphamide in the treatment of rheumatic diseases. Adv Clin Exp Med. 2016;25(3):479–84. https://doi.org/10.17219/acem/28736.
22. Foocharoen C, Siriphannon Y, Mahakkanukrauh A, et al. A incidence rate and causes of infection in Thai systemic sclerosis patient. Int J Rheum Dis. 2012;15(3):277–83. https://doi.org/10.1111/j.1756-185X.2012.01728.x.
23. Tyndall AJ, Bannert B, Vonk M, et al. Causes and risk factors for death in systemic sclerosis: a study from the EULAR scleroderma trials and research (EUSTAR) database. Ann Rheum Dis. 2010;69(10):1809–15. https://doi.org/10.1136/ard.2009.114264.
24. Steen V, Denton CP, Pope JE, et al. Digital ulcers: overt vascular disease in systemic sclerosis. Rheumatology (Oxford). 2009;48(Suppl 3):iii19–24. https://doi.org/10.1093/rheumatology/kep105.
25. Korn JH, Mayes M, Matcci Cerinic M, et al. Digital ulcers in systemic sclerosis: prevention by treatment with bosentan, an oral endothelin receptor antagonist. Arthritis Rheum. 2004;50(12):3985–93. https://doi.org/10.1002/art.20676.
26. Giuggioli D, Manfredi A, Colaci M, et al. Scleroderma digital ulcers complicated by infection with fecal pathogens. Arthritis Care Res. 2012;64(2):295–7. https://doi.org/10.1002/acr.20673.
27. Andreasson K, Alrawi Z, Persson A, et al. Intestinal dysbiosis is common in systemic sclerosis and associated with gastrointestinal and extraintestinal features of disease. Arthritis Res Ther. 2016;18(1):278. https://doi.org/10.1186/s13075-016-1182-z.
28. Suau A, Bonnet R, Sutren M, et al. Direct analysis of genes encoding 16S rRNA from complex communities reveals many novel molecular species within the human gut. Appl Environ Microbiol. 1999;65(11):4799–807.
29. Swidsinski A, Loening-Baucke V, Vaneechoutte M, et al. Active Crohn's disease and ulcerative colitis can be specifically diagnosed and monitored based on the biostructure of the fecal flora. Inflamm Bowel Dis. 2008;14(2):147–61. https://doi.org/10.1002/ibd.20330.
30. Miquel S, Martin R, Rossi O, et al. *Faecalibacterium prausnitzii* and human intestinal health. Curr Opin Microbiol. 2013;16(3):255–61. https://doi.org/10.1016/j.mib.2013.06.003.
31. Sokol H, Pigneur B, Watterlot L, et al. *Faecalibacterium prausnitzii* is an anti-inflammatory commensal bacterium identified by gut microbiota analysis of Crohn disease patients. Proc Natl Acad Sci U S A. 2008;105(43):16731–6. https://doi.org/10.1073/pnas.0804812105.
32. Volkmann ER, Hoffman-Vold A, Chang Y, et al. Systemic sclerosis is associated with specific alterations in gastrointestinal microbiota in two independent cohorts. BMJ Open Gastroenterol. 2017;4(1):e000134.
33. Patrone V, Puglisi E, Cardinali M, et al. Gut microbiota profile in systemic sclerosis patients with and without clinical evidence of gastrointestinal involvement. Sci Rep. 2017;7(1):14874.
34. Wang W, Chen L, Zhou R, et al. Increased proportions of Bifidobacterium and the Lactobacillus group and loss of butyrate-producing bacteria in inflammatory

bowel disease. J Clin Microbiol. 2014;52(2):398–406. https://doi.org/10.1128/jcm.01500-13.
35. Willing BP, Dicksved J, Halfvarson J, et al. A pyrosequencing study in twins shows that gastrointestinal microbial profiles vary with inflammatory bowel disease phenotypes. Gastroenterology. 2010;139(6):1844–1854.e1841. https://doi.org/10.1053/j.gastro.2010.08.049.
36. Sartor RB. Therapeutic manipulation of the enteric microflora in inflammatory bowel diseases: antibiotics, probiotics, and prebiotics. Gastroenterology. 2004;126(6):1620–33.
37. Di Cerbo A, Palmieri B, Aponte M, et al. Mechanisms and therapeutic effectiveness of lactobacilli. J Clin Pathol. 2015;69(3):187–203. https://doi.org/10.1136/jclinpath-2015-202976.
38. Martinez RC, Bedani R, Saad SM. Scientific evidence for health effects attributed to the consumption of probiotics and prebiotics: an update for current perspectives and future challenges. Br J Nutr. 2015;114(12):1993–2015. https://doi.org/10.1017/s0007114515003864.
39. Marie I, Leroi AM, Gourcerol G, et al. Fructose malabsorption in systemic sclerosis. Medicine (Baltimore). 2015;94(39):e1601.
40. Volkmann ER, Chang YL, Barroso N, et al. Association of systemic sclerosis with a unique colonic microbial consortium. Arthritis Rheumatol. 2016;68(6):1483–92. https://doi.org/10.1002/art.39572.
41. Alekseyenko AV, Perez-Perez GI, De Souza A, et al. Community differentiation of the cutaneous microbiota in psoriasis. Microbiome. 2013;1(1):31. https://doi.org/10.1186/2049-2618-1-31.
42. Fahlen A, Engstrand L, Baker BS, et al. Comparison of bacterial microbiota in skin biopsies from normal and psoriatic skin. Arch Dermatol Res. 2012;304(1):15–22. https://doi.org/10.1007/s00403-011-1189-x.
43. Arron ST, Dimon MT, Li Z, et al. High Rhodotorula sequences in skin transcriptome of patients with diffuse systemic sclerosis. J Invest Dermatol. 2014;134(8):2138–45. https://doi.org/10.1038/jid.2014.127.
44. Gyger G, Baron M. Systemic sclerosis: gastrointestinal disease and its management. Rheum Dis Clin North Am. 2015;41(3):459–73. https://doi.org/10.1016/j.rdc.2015.04.007.
45. Tauber M, Avouac J, Benahmed A, et al. Prevalence and predictors of small intestinal bacterial overgrowth in systemic sclerosis patients with gastrointestinal symptoms. Clin Exp Rheumatol. 2014;32(6 Suppl 86):S-82–7.
46. Grace E, Shaw C, Whelan K, et al. Review article: small intestinal bacterial overgrowth–prevalence, clinical features, current and developing diagnostic tests, and treatment. Aliment Pharmacol Ther. 2013;38(7):674–88. https://doi.org/10.1111/apt.12456.
47. Marie I, Ducrotte P, Denis P, et al. Small intestinal bacterial overgrowth in systemic sclerosis. Rheumatology (Oxford). 2009;48(10):1314–9. https://doi.org/10.1093/rheumatology/kep226.
48. Parodi A, Sessarego M, Greco A, et al. Small intestinal bacterial overgrowth in patients suffering from scleroderma: clinical effectiveness of its eradication. Am J Gastroenterol. 2008;103(5):1257–62. https://doi.org/10.1111/j.1572-0241.2007.01758.x.
49. Ebert EC. Gastric and enteric involvement in progressive systemic sclerosis. J Clin Gastroenterol. 2008;42(1):5–12. https://doi.org/10.1097/MCG.0b013e318042d625.
50. Fiorucci S, Distrutti E, Bassotti G, et al. Effect of erythromycin administration on upper gastrointestinal motility in scleroderma patients. Scand J Gastroenterol. 1994;29(9):807–13.
51. Asama T, Kimura Y, Kono T, et al. Effects of heat-killed Lactobacillus kunkeei YB38 on human intestinal environment and bowel movement: a pilot study. Benef Microbes. 2016;7(3):337–44. https://doi.org/10.3920/bm2015.0132.
52. Attaluri A, Jackson M, Valestin J, et al. Methanogenic flora is associated with altered colonic transit but not stool characteristics in constipation without IBS. Am J Gastroenterol. 2010;105(6):1407–11. https://doi.org/10.1038/ajg.2009.655.
53. Parthasarathy G, Chen J, Chen X, et al. Relationship between microbiota of the colonic mucosa vs feces and symptoms, colonic transit, and methane production in female patients with chronic constipation. Gastroenterology. 2016;150(2):367–379.e361. https://doi.org/10.1053/j.gastro.2015.10.005.
54. Taur Y, Jenq RR, Perales MA, et al. The effects of intestinal tract bacterial diversity on mortality following allogeneic hematopoietic stem cell transplantation. Blood. 2014;124(7):1174–82. https://doi.org/10.1182/blood-2014-02-554725.
55. Wang W, Xu S, Ren Z, et al. Gut microbiota and allogeneic transplantation. J Transl Med. 2015;13:275. https://doi.org/10.1186/s12967-015-0640-8.
56. Whangbo J, Ritz J, Bhatt A. Antibiotic-mediated modification of the intestinal microbiome in allogeneic hematopoietic stem cell transplantation. Bone Marrow Transplant. 2017;52(2):183–90. https://doi.org/10.1038/bmt.2016.206.
57. Bujor AM, Haines P, Padilla C, et al. Ciprofloxacin has antifibrotic effects in scleroderma fibroblasts via downregulation of Dnmt1 and upregulation of Fli1. Int J Mol Med. 2012;30(6):1473–80. https://doi.org/10.3892/ijmm.2012.1150.
58. Mayes MD, O'Donnell D, Rothfield NF, et al. Minocycline is not effective in systemic sclerosis: results of an open-label multicenter trial. Arthritis Rheum. 2004;50(2):553–7. https://doi.org/10.1002/art.20036.
59. Frech TM, Khanna D, Maranian P, et al. Probiotics for the treatment of systemic sclerosis-associated gastrointestinal bloating/distention. Clin Exp Rheumatol. 2011;29(2 Suppl 65):S22–5.
60. Rieder F. The gut microbiome in intestinal fibrosis: environmental protector or provocateur? Sci Transl Med. 2013;5(190):190ps110. https://doi.org/10.1126/scitranslmed.3004731.
61. Sakamoto N, Kakugawa T, Hara A, et al. Association of elevated alpha-defensin levels with intersti-

tial pneumonia in patients with systemic sclerosis. Respir Res. 2015;16:148. https://doi.org/10.1186/s12931-015-0308-1.

62. van Bon L, Affandi AJ, Broen J, et al. Proteome-wide analysis and CXCL4 as a biomarker in systemic sclerosis. New Engl J Med. 2013;370(5):433–43. https://doi.org/10.1056/NEJMoa1114576.
63. Espinoza-Leon F, Hassanhi-Hassanhi M, Arocha-Sandoval F, et al. Absence of *Borrelia burgdorferi* antibodies in the sera of Venezuelan patients with localized scleroderma (morphea). Invest Clin. 2006;47(3):283–8.
64. Goodlad JR, Davidson MM, Gordon P, et al. Morphoea and *Borrelia burgdorferi*: results from the Scottish highlands in the context of the world literature. Mol Pathol. 2002;55(6):374–8.
65. Prinz JC, Kutasi Z, Weisenseel P, et al. "Borrelia-associated early-onset morphea": a particular type of scleroderma in childhood and adolescence with high titer antinuclear antibodies? Results of a cohort analysis and presentation of three cases. J Am Acad Dermatol. 2009;60(2):248–55. https://doi.org/10.1016/j.jaad.2008.09.023.
66. Weide B, Walz T, Garbe C. Is morphoea caused by *Borrelia burgdorferi*? A review. Br J Dermatol. 2000;142(4):636–44.
67. Bowler PG, Duerden BI, Armstrong DG. Wound microbiology and associated approaches to wound management. Clin Microbiol Rev. 2001;14(2):244–69. https://doi.org/10.1128/cmr.14.2.244-269.2001.
68. Dagenais M, MacDonald D, Baron M, et al. The Canadian systemic sclerosis oral health study IV: oral radiographic manifestations in systemic sclerosis compared with the general population. Oral Surg Oral Med Oral Pathol Oral Radiol. 2015;120(2):104–11. https://doi.org/10.1016/j.oooo.2015.03.002.
69. Gonzales TS, Coleman GC. Periodontal manifestations of collagen vascular disorders. Periodontol. 1999;21:94–105.
70. Baron M, Hudson M, Dagenais M, et al. Relationship between disease characteristics and oral radiologic findings in systemic sclerosis: results from a Canadian oral health study. Arthritis Care Res. 2016;68(5):673–80. https://doi.org/10.1002/acr.22739.
71. Slocum C, Kramer C, Genco CA. Immune dysregulation mediated by the oral microbiome: potential link to chronic inflammation and atherosclerosis. J Intern Med. 2016;280(1):114–28. https://doi.org/10.1111/joim.12476.

25 Systemic Vasculitides

Loïc Guillevin

Abbreviations

Ab	Antibody
Ag	Antigen
ANCA	Antineutrophil cytoplasmic antibody
HbsAg	Hepatitis B surface antigen
HBV	Hepatitis B virus
HCV	Hepatitis C virus
HIV	Human immunodeficiency virus
PAN	Polyarteritis nodosa

Viral Infections Causing Vasculitides

Virus- associated vasculitides have been described in the seventies [1, 2] and nineties [3] of the twentieth century, demontrating for the first time that viruses could be the cause of some systemic vasculitides. In the most recently revised Chapel Hill Nomenclature [4], a specific subgroup called "vasculitis associated with probable etiology" has three entries: HBV-related PAN (HBV–PAN), HCV-related cryoglobulinemic vasculitis, and syphilis-associated vasculitis. The role infectious agents play in the development of vasculitides is highlighted in that consensus document. This chapter covers only HBV-, HCV-, and HIV-related vasculitides, and we give brief overview of other microorganisms that have been associated with vasculitides.

L. Guillevin
Department of Internal Medicine, Hôpital Cochin, Assistance Publique–Hôpitaux de Paris, Université Paris Descartes, Paris Cedex 14, France
e-mail: loic.guillevin@cch.aphp.fr

HBV–PAN

Epidemiology

PAN is a rare disease that affects all racial groups. Annual incidence estimations of PAN-type systemic vasculitides per 1,000,000 inhabitants range from 4.6 in the general population in England [5] to 9.0 in Olmsted County, Minnesota, and to 77 in a hepatitis B-hyperendemic Alaskan Eskimo population [6]. An extremely low PAN incidence (0.3–0.4/1,000,000) was found in Germany and depended on the year and part of the country [7]. The northern Parisian suburb of Seine-Saint-Denis, France, had a PAN prevalence of 34/1,000,000 [8]; pertinently, a diminution of its incidence was observed in parallel with the declining HBV-infection rate [9].

In France, the last proven case of HBV dissemination via contaminated blood transfusion occurred in 1987 [9]. Unfortunately, intravenous drug abuse has replaced it as the predominant cause of HBV–PAN [9], along with sexual HBV spread to non-vaccinated individuals at risk. Anti-HBV vaccines delivered to those at risk since 1989 also help explain the subsequent drop in new cases. HBV–PAN has rarely been seen

G. Ragab et al. (eds.), *The Microbiome in Rheumatic Diseases and Infection*,
https://doi.org/10.1007/978-3-319-79026-8_25

over the past 15 years. Moreover, PAN, caused by HBV infection or not, has also declined in parallel to lifestyle changes and vaccination.

Although it is difficult to prove HBV exposure preceding PAN, an infection-transmission route could be established for 43/115 patients [9]. When identified, the mean (±SD) exposure-to-first- manifestation interval was 596 ± 628 (range, 30–1695) days. The immunological process that gives rise to PAN usually becomes evident within the first 12 months following primary HBV infection, with hepatitis remaining mostly silent prior to overt PAN.

Intriguingly, the PAN frequency seems to have been rising since 2017. All these new patients had noninfectious PAN. This increase has not yet been confirmed by prospective epidemiological studies.

Pathogenesis

Virus antigen–antibody complexes have been found in the vascular endothelium. Those deposits can activate the complement cascade, triggering the release of chemotactic factors attracting neutrophils to the site of inflammation. It has been advanced that immune complexes and local HBV replication within the endothelium serve as the pathogenic mechanism of HBV–PAN. PAN patients do not have antineutrophil cytoplasmic antibodies (ANCA); indeed, their presence in a vasculitis patient excludes the diagnosis of PAN [10].

Clinical Manifestations

The clinical symptoms of HBV–PAN are the same as those described for historically classical, non-viral PAN (Table 25.1): gastrointestinal involvement (especially perforation and bleeding), malignant hypertension, renal infarction, and/or orchiepididymitis. HBV–PAN patients' clinical findings are very similar to those for non-

Table 25.1 Relevant clinical and biological symptoms of 115 patients with HBV-associated polyarteritis nodosa [9]. With permission from © Lippincott Williams & Wilkins, Inc

Clinical symptoms	Values[a]
Age, mean ± SD (years)	51.1 ± 17
Sex ratio	74 M/41 F
General symptoms	111 (96.5)
Fever	79 (68.7)
Weight loss	100 (87)
Arthralgias	64 (55.7)
Myalgias	54 (47)

Table 25.1 (continued)

Clinical symptoms	Values[a]
Mononeuritis multiplex	96 (83.5)
Superficial peroneal	82 (71.3)
Deep peroneal	46 (40)
Cubital	25 (21.7)
Radial	12 (10.4)
Bilateral	66/91 (72.5)
GI-tract involvement	61 (53.0)
Abdominal pain	59 (51.3)
Bleeding	3 (2.6)
Appendicitis	2 (1.7)
Small intestine perforation	7 (6.1)
Cholecystitis	6 (5.2)
Pancreatitis	7 (6.1)
Renal and/or urogenital involvement	44 (38.3)
Proteinuria and/or hematuria	21 (18.3)
Glomerulonephritis[b]	1 (0.9)
Renal vasculitis	34 (29.6)
Creatininemia, mean ± SD, (mg/dl)	1.52 ± 1.39
Anuria at entry	4 (3.5)
Orchitis	18/71 (25.3)
Microaneurysms[c]	46/67 (68.6)
Renal infarcts[b, c]	19/67 (28.3)
Skin involvement	36 (31.3)
Purpura	19 (16.5)
Infiltrated purpura	13 (11.3)
Livedo	12 (10.4)
Nodules	10 (8.7)
Edema (ankles)	18 (15.7)
Vascular manifestations	21 (18.3)
Hypertension	36 (31.3)
Malignant hypertension	6 (5.2)
Cardiac insufficiency	14 (12.2)
Raynaud's phenomenon	3 (2.6)
Pericarditis	6 (5.2)
Digital ischemia	4 (3.5)
Myocardial infarction	1 (0.9)
Central nervous system involvement	11 (9.6)
Retinal vasculitis	2 (1.7)
Erythrocyte sedimentation rate > 30 mm/1st h	90 (78.3)
ANCA[d]	0

[a]Values are numbers (%), unless otherwise indicated
[b]Not related to vasculitis
[c]66 angiographies
[d]66 searches for antineutrophil cytoplasmic antibodies

viral PAN, with several notable differences: HBV–PAN occurs more often in subjects under 40 years old and is more frequently associated with malignant hypertension, renal infarction, and orchiepididymitis (25%) [9, 11]. Other frequently observed symptoms are abdominal manifestations (53%), especially surgical emergencies. Ischemia is responsible for digestive and renal involvements, with angiography-visualized infarctions and microaneurysms [12]. The latter can disappear after thrombosis and fibrotic evolution. Despite being an acute and initially severe vasculitis, HBV–PAN, when adequately treated in a timely manner, usually has an excellent outcome. Antigen (Ag)-to-antibody (Ab) seroconversion most frequently leads to recovery.

Outcomes

Without appropriate antiviral therapy, HBV–PAN outcomes are worse [9, 13–15]. Histological damage gives rise to sequelae, including vascular nephropathy, and central and/or peripheral nervous involvements. However, liver symptoms during PAN evolution remain clinically moderate, with usually modest transaminase level rises. Histological examination of liver biopsies found a chronic hepatitis pattern, indicative of the infection's progression to chronicity [16]. Most PAN cases are attributable to wild-type HBV strains, reinforcing the suspected HBeAg involvement in PAN pathophysiology. However, the few cases associated with a precore mutation preventing HBeAg formation put that etiology in doubt. Antiviral therapy successfully halted virus replication and, hence, the disease, but no potentially responsible autoimmune mechanism was identified [17]. According to a cohort study on 348 PAN patients (mean (±SD) follow-up: 68.3 ± 63.5 months), 76 (21.8%) relapsed (63 (28%) non-viral PAN versus 13 (10.6%) HBV–PAN; $P < 0.001$) and 86 (24.7%) died (44 (19.6%) non-viral PAN versus 42 (34.1%) HBV–PAN; $P = 0.002$) [11]. These results demonstrate that, when adequately treated, HBV–PAN relapses rarely. However, because of the severity of HBV–PAN, mortality is higher than in PAN without HBV infections.

Treatments

Long treated like non-viral PAN, HBV–PAN patients were prescribed corticosteroids and immunosuppressants, with or without plasma exchanges, that often achieved short-term efficacy. However, that exclusive immunosuppressive regimen allowed HBV–PAN relapses, complications attributable to virus persistence, like chronic hepatitis or liver cirrhosis, and outcomes worse than for non-viral PAN [18].

The initial rationale for prescribing a therapeutic sequence combining an antiviral and plasma exchanges and only 2 weeks of corticosteroids was as follows: first, use of corticosteroids to rapidly control the most severe life-threatening PAN manifestations; second, use of plasma exchanges to remove immune complexes and thereby control PAN and restore immune reactivity; third, use of vidarabine to block HBV replication; and, lastly, use of sudden corticosteroid withdrawal to enhance immunological clearance of HBV-infected hepatocytes and favor HBeAg-to-HBeAb seroconversion. The efficacy of that strategy was demonstrated in several prospective trials, using different antivirals as more potent ones became available over the years [14, 19].

Vidarabine [19], the first antiviral to be used in this setting, achieved full clinical recovery in 75% of the patients, HBeAg-to-HBeAb seroconversion in about half, and hepatitis B surface Ag (HBsAg)-to-HBsAb seroconversion in approximately 20%. Subsequently, small numbers of patients were given interferon-α (IFNα). Tritherapy, with plasma exchanges, corticosteroids, and IFNα, successfully treated PAN attributed to HBV with a mutant precore promoter [20]. Similar antiviral therapies achieved comparable efficacy: IFNα alone [21] or combined with famciclovir [22] or lamivudine [23–25]. First-line lamivudine also successfully treated HBV–PAN [24, 26]. Other effective, well-tolerated anti-HBV drugs (e.g., entecavir) now available should be combined with plasma exchange rather than lamivudine or IFNα.

HCV-Related Cryoglobulinemic Vasculitis

The HCV–cryoglobulinemic vasculitis link was found over 20 years ago [3]. It is well-recognized that HCV causes hepatitis, but it is also responsible for extrahepatic manifestations, e.g., cryoglobulinemia. Some rare cryoglobulinemic patients will develop small-sized vessel necrotizing vasculitis. HCV and HBV can coexist, with some PAN patients also being HCV-positive. However, HCV responsibility in medium-sized vessel vasculitis has only been reported for anecdotal cases or small series [27, 28], with 1% of 1614 HCV-positive patients developing systemic vasculitis, according to Cacoub et al. [29]. The clinical characteristics of cryoglobulinemic vasculitis [30] are given in Table 25.2.

Outcomes

Cryoglobulinemic vasculitis can cause major morbidity and mortality. Prognostic factors are age >60 years and renal involvement [31, 32], with renal failure being the main cause of death, followed by liver involvement, cardiovascular disease, infection, and lymphoma [32]. Having cryoglobulinemic vasculitis and hypogammaglobulinemia was independently associated with B-cell non-Hodgkin lymphoma [33]. The primary cause of death of cryoglobulinemic vasculitis patients is severe infections. Their deaths were frequently associated with age >60 years, renal involvement, and/or end-stage liver disease [33].

Authors of a study focusing on outcomes and comparing HCV-positive versus HCV-negative cryoglobulinemic patients reported respective 1-, 3-, 5-, and 10-year survival rates of HCV-positive patients of 96%, 86%, 75%, and 63% [34].

Treatments

A combination of antiviral drugs, e.g., pegylated-IFNα and ribavirin, used to be the standard of care for patients with mild-to-moderate vasculitis activity [35]. The responses of HCV-related vasculitis manifestations to corticosteroids alone were not improved by IFNα adjunction [36].

Table 25.2 Clinical and biological features of patients with cryoglobulinemic vasculitis according to immunochemical type and hepatitis C virus status [30]. With permission from © Lippincott Williams & Wilkins, Inc

	HCV−		HCV+
Characteristics	Monoclonal	Mixed	Mixed
Number of patients	64	242	165
Age (years)	65	63	60
Female (%)	56	69	54
Clinical features			
Skin (%)	86	83	76
Purpura (%)	69	75	71
Raynaud's phenomenon (%)	30	26	–
Necrosis (%)	28	16	1
Ulcers (%)	27	14	4
Livedo (%)	13	2	4
Joints (%)	28	40	53
Peripheral neuropathy (%)	44	52	74
Central nervous system (%)	0	2	9
Kidney (%)	30	35	34
Gastrointestinal (%)	0	5	7
Laboratory analysis[a]			
Cryoglobulin (g/l)	1.55	0.94	1.04
C4 (g/l)	0.09	0.07	0.09

[a]Normal values: cryoglobulins, <0.05 g/l; complement fraction C4, 0.14–0.40 g/l

Because immunosuppressants stimulate virus replication, they jeopardize patients' outcomes and increase mortality [37]. As for HBV–PAN, short-term corticosteroids and/or plasma exchange could be used first to control severe and life-threatening manifestations, but they do not have long-term efficacy. Antiviral use is based on direct-acting agents. Among the newer molecules, sofosbuvir (a nucleotide NS5B (nonstructural protein 5B) inhibitor) combined with ledipasvir (an NS5A (nonstructural protein 5A) inhibitor) effectively cures cryoglobulinemic vasculitis in up to 95% of patients within 3 months. That combination, like others, is more-or-less active against all genotypes. IFNα is no longer used, and ribavirin use is now limited to some genotypes and difficult-to-treat cases. Because of their efficacy, combined antivirals are the first-line treatment-of-choice for cryoglobulinemia and can cure cryoglobulinemic vasculitis, mostly non-severe forms [38].

Rituximab, an anti-CD20 monoclonal antibody, combined with antivirals, is now used extensively to treat HCV-mixed cryoglobulinemic vasculitis [39, 40].

The use of plasma exchange is now restricted to some patients, whose disease fails to respond to antivirals and rituximab.

Other Vasculitides with a Possible Infectious Etiology

Human Immunodeficiency Virus (HIV)-Associated Vasculitis

Numerous pathogens, including HIV, have been identified at vasculitis, onset and persistance. Different-sized vessels can be involved in HIV-associated vasculitis, which histologically resembles giant-cell arteritis or necrotizing vasculitis. Although HIV has been implicated in Kawasaki-like disease or PAN, most HIV-infected patients develop small-sized vessel vasculitis [41]. The pathophysiology of HIV-associated vasculitis remains unclear, with a role of immune complexes suspected but never proven. Several distinct mechanisms probably coexist: in a context of fewer than 200 CD4+ T-cells/ml, opportunistic infections can cause vasculitis, or an excess of CD8+ cells could be responsible [42].

Opportunistic infections are common in HIV/acquired immunodeficiency syndrome (AIDS) patients, like all immunocompromised individuals, and can sometimes manifest as vasculitis. Many pathogens have been directly or indirectly associated with vasculitis in HIV-infected individuals, including cytomegalovirus, *Toxoplasma gondii*, and *Pneumocystis jirovecii*. Patients with other vasculitides, who are therapeutically immunosuppressed, are also susceptible to those infections. Notably, cytomegalovirus-associated vasculitis occurs more frequently in HIV-infected patients than in the general population and, during advanced-stage AIDS, usually involves the gastrointestinal tract, lungs, central nervous system, and skin [43].

Syphilis-Associated Vasculitis

Syphilis is one of the several infectious diseases anecdotally associated with different types of vasculitides and classified in the Chapel Hill Nomenclature [4]. Notably, it was responsible for several cases of retinitis and other ocular diseases [44]. Aortitis can also be caused by syphilis [45], as can central nervous system vasculitis [46, 47].

Giant-Cell Arteritis

Giant-cell arteritis etiology is still unknown. Although infections had been considered, no microbe had been identified until 2012, when Koening et al. implicated a *Burkholderia*-like strain [48]. Should that observation be confirmed by others, it would be the first convincing documentation of a bacterium's role in this arteritis.

Miscellaneous

Despite having been implicated in the etiology of anecdotical vasculitis cases, pathogens as the causal agents have not been confirmed in larger series of patients [49–51].

References

1. Trepo C, Thivolet J. Hepatitis associated antigen and periarteritis nodosa (PAN). Vox Sang. 1970;19(3):410–1.
2. Gocke DJ, Hsu K, Morgan C, Bombardieri S, Lockshin M, Christian CL. Association between polyarteritis and Australia antigen. Lancet. 1970;2(7684):1149–53.
3. Agnello V, Chung RT, Kaplan LM. A role for hepatitis C virus infection in type II cryoglobulinemia. N Engl J Med. 1992;327(21):1490–5.
4. Jennette JC, Falk RJ, Bacon PA, Basu N, Cid MC, Ferrario F, et al. 2012 revised international Chapel Hill consensus conference nomenclature of vasculitides. Arthritis Rheum. 2013;65(1):1–11.
5. Scott DG, Bacon PA, Elliott PJ, Tribe CR, Wallington TB. Systemic vasculitis in a district general hospital 1972–1980: clinical and laboratory features, classification and prognosis of 80 cases. Q J Med. 1982;51(203):292–311.
6. McMahon BJ, Bender TR, Templin DW, Maynard JE, Barrett DH, Berquist KR, et al. Vasculitis in Eskimos living in an area hyperendemic for hepatitis B. JAMA. 1980;244(19):2180–2.
7. Reinhold-Keller E, Herlyn K, Wagner-Bastmeyer R, Gross WL. Stable incidence of primary systemic vasculitides over five years: results from the German vasculitis register. Arthritis Rheum. 2005;53(1):93–9.
8. Mahr A, Guillevin L, Poissonnet M, Aymé S. Prevalences of polyarteritis nodosa, microscopic polyangiitis, Wegener's granulomatosis, and Churg–Strauss syndrome in a French urban multiethnic population in 2000: a capture–recapture estimate. Arthritis Rheum. 2004;51(1):92–9.
9. Guillevin L, Mahr A, Callard P, Godmer P, Pagnoux C, Leray E, et al. Hepatitis B virus-associated polyarteritis nodosa: clinical characteristics, outcome, and impact of treatment in 115 patients. Medicine (Baltimore). 2005;84:313–22.
10. Henegar C, Pagnoux C, Puéchal X, Zucker JD, Bar-Hen A, Le Guern V, et al. A paradigm of diagnostic criteria for polyarteritis nodosa: analysis of a series of 949 patients with vasculitides. Arthritis Rheum. 2008;58(5):1528–38.
11. Pagnoux C, Seror R, Henegar C, Mahr A, Cohen P, Le Guern V, et al. Clinical features and outcomes in 348 patients with polyarteritis nodosa: a systematic retrospective study of patients diagnosed between 1963 and 2005 and entered into the French Vasculitis Study Group Database. Arthritis Rheum. 2010;62(2):616–26.
12. Darras-Joly C, Lortholary O, Cohen P, Brauner M, Guillevin L. Regressing microaneurysms in 5 cases of hepatitis B virus related polyarteritis nodosa. J Rheumatol. 1995;22(5):876–80.
13. Guillevin L, Lê Thi Huong D, Godeau P, Jaïs P, Wechsler B. Clinical findings and prognosis of polyarteritis nodosa and Churg–Strauss angiitis: a study in 165 patients. Br J Rheumatol. 1988;27(4):258–64.
14. Guillevin L, Lhote F, Leon A, Fauvelle F, Vivitski L, Trepo C. Treatment of polyarteritis nodosa related to hepatitis B virus with short term steroid therapy associated with antiviral agents and plasma exchanges. A prospective trial in 33 patients. J Rheumatol. 1993;20(2):289–98.
15. Trepo C, Ouzan D, Delmont J, Tremisi J. Superiorité d'un nouveau traitement étiopathogénique curateur des périarterites noueuses induites par le virus de l'hepatite B grâce a l'association corticothérapie brève, vidarabine, échanges plasmatiques. Presse Méd. 1988;17(30):1527–31.
16. Trepo C, Guillevin L. Polyarteritis nodosa and extrahepatic manifestations of HBV infection: the case against autoimmune intervention in pathogenesis. J Autoimmun. 2001;16(3):269–74.
17. Wartelle-Bladou C, Lafon J, Trepo C, Pichoud C, Picon M, Pellissier JF, et al. Successful combination therapy of polyarteritis nodosa associated with a precore promoter mutant hepatitis B virus infection. J Hepatol. 2001;34(5):774–9.
18. Guillevin L, Jarrousse B, Lok C, Lhote F, Jaïs JP, Lê Thi Huong D, et al. Longterm followup after treatment of polyarteritis nodosa and Churg–Strauss angiitis with comparison of steroids, plasma exchange and cyclophosphamide to steroids and plasma exchange. A prospective randomized trial of 71 patients. The Cooperative Study Group for Polyarteritis Nodosa. J Rheumatol. 1991;18(4):567–74.
19. Guillevin L, Merrouche Y, Gayraud M, Jarrousse B, Royer I, Leon A, et al. Périartérite noueuse du au virus de l'hépatite B. Détermination d'une nouvelle stratégie thérapeutique: 13 cas. Presse Méd. 1988;17(30):1522–6.
20. Guillevin L, Lhote F, Sauvaget F, Deblois P, Rossi F, Levallois D, et al. Treatment of polyarteritis nodosa related to hepatitis B virus with interferon-alpha and plasma exchanges. Ann Rheum Dis. 1994;53(5):334–7.
21. Simsek H, Telatar H. Successful treatment of hepatitis B virus-associated polyarteritis nodosa by interferon alpha alone. J Clin Gastroenterol. 1995;20(3):263–5.
22. Kruger M, Boker KH, Zeidler H, Manns MP. Treatment of hepatitis B-related polyarteritis nodosa with famciclovir and interferon alfa-2b. J Hepatol. 1997;26(4):935–9.
23. Auguet T, Barragan P, Ramirez R, Quer JC, Sirvent JJ, Richart C. Lamivudine in the treatment of hepatitis B virus-related polyarteritis nodosa. J Clin Rheumatol. 2007;13(5):298–9.
24. Guillevin L, Mahr A, Cohen P, Larroche C, Queyrel V, Loustaud-Ratti V, et al. Short-term corticosteroids then lamivudine and plasma exchanges to treat hepatitis B virus-related polyarteritis nodosa. Arthritis Rheum. 2004;51(3):482–7.
25. Erhardt A, Sagir A, Guillevin L, Neuen-Jacob E, Haussinger D. Successful treatment of hepatitis B virus associated polyarteritis nodosa with a combination of prednisolone, alpha-interferon and lamivudine. J Hepatol. 2000;33(4):677–83.

26. Wicki J, Olivieri J, Pizzolato G, Sarasin F, Guillevin L, Dayer JM, et al. Successful treatment of polyarteritis nodosa related to hepatitis B virus with a combination of lamivudine and interferon alpha. Rheumatology (Oxford). 1999;38(2):183–5.
27. Saadoun D, Terrier B, Semoun O, Sene D, Maisonobe T, Musset L, et al. Hepatitis C virus-associated polyarteritis nodosa. Arthritis Care Res (Hoboken). 2011;63(3):427–35.
28. Cacoub P, Lunel-Fabiani F, Du LT. Polyarteritis nodosa and hepatitis C virus infection. Ann Intern Med. 1992;116(7):605–6.
29. Cacoub P, Renou C, Rosenthal E, Cohen P, Loury I, Loustaud-Ratti V, et al. Extrahepatic manifestations associated with hepatitis C virus infection. A prospective multicenter study of 321 patients. The GERMIVIC. Groupe d'Étude et de Recherche en Médecine Interne et Maladies Infectieuses sur le Virus de l'Hépatite C. Medicine (Baltimore). 2000;79(1):47–56.
30. Terrier B, Cacoub P. Cryoglobulinemia vasculitis: an update. Curr Opin Rheumatol. 2013;25(1):10–8.
31. Tarantino A, Campise M, Banfi G, Confalonieri R, Bucci A, Montoli A, et al. Long-term predictors of survival in essential mixed cryoglobulinemic glomerulonephritis. Kidney Int. 1995;47:618–23.
32. Ferri C, Sebastiani M, Giuggioli D, Cazzato M, Longombardo G, Antonelli A, et al. Mixed cryoglobulinemia: demographic, clinical, and serologic features and survival in 231 patients. Semin Arthritis Rheum. 2004;33(6):355–74.
33. Saadoun D, Sellam J, Ghillani-Dalbin P, Crecel R, Piette JC, Cacoub P. Increased risks of lymphoma and death among patients with non-hepatitis C virus-related mixed cryoglobulinemia. Arch Intern Med. 2006;166(19):2101–8.
34. Terrier B, Krastinova E, Marie I, Launay D, Lacraz A, Belenotti P, et al. Management of noninfectious mixed cryoglobulinemia vasculitis: data from 242 cases included in the CryoVas survey. Blood. 2012;119(25):5996–6004.
35. Saadoun D, Resche-Rigon M, Thibault V, Piette JC, Cacoub P. Antiviral therapy for hepatitis C virus – associated mixed cryoglobulinemia vasculitis: a long-term followup study. Arthritis Rheum. 2006;54(11):3696–706.
36. Casato M, Agnello V, Pucillo LP, Knight GB, Leoni M, Del Vecchio S, et al. Predictors of long-term response to high-dose interferon therapy in type II cryoglobulinemia associated with hepatitis C virus infection. Blood. 1997;90(10):3865–73.
37. Terrier B, Semoun O, Saadoun D, Sene D, Resche-Rigon M, Cacoub P. Prognostic factors in patients with hepatitis C virus infection and systemic vasculitis. Arthritis Rheum. 2011;63(6):1748–57.
38. Cacoub P, Vautier M, Desbois AC, Lafuma A, Saadoun D. Effectiveness and cost of hepatitis C virus cryoglobulinaemia vasculitis treatment: from interferon-based to direct-acting antivirals era. Liver Int. 2017;37(12):1805–13. https://doi.org/10.1111/liv.13465. Epub 2017 May 29.
39. Terrier B, Saadoun D, Sene D, Sellam J, Perard L, Coppere B, et al. Efficacy and tolerability of rituximab with or without PEGylated interferon alfa-2b plus ribavirin in severe hepatitis C virus-related vasculitis: a long-term followup study of thirty-two patients. Arthritis Rheum. 2009;60(8):2531–40.
40. Zaja F, De Vita S, Mazzaro C, Sacco S, Damiani D, De Marchi G, et al. Efficacy and safety of rituximab in type II mixed cryoglobulinemia. Blood. 2003;101(10):3827–34.
41. Gisselbrecht M, Cohen P, Lortholary O, Jarrousse B, Gayraud M, Gherardi R, et al. HIV-related vasculitis: clinical presentation and therapeutic approach on six patients. AIDS. 1997;11(1):121–3.
42. Guillevin L. Vasculitides in the context of HIV infection. AIDS. 2008;22(Suppl 3):S27–33.
43. Golden MP, Hammer SM, Wanke CA, Albrecht MA. Cytomegalovirus vasculitis. Case reports and review of the literature. Medicine (Baltimore). 1994;73(5):246–55.
44. Krishnamurthy R, Cunningham ET Jr. Atypical presentation of syphilitic uveitis associated with Kyrieleis plaques. Br J Ophthalmol. 2008;92(8):1152–3.
45. Frank MW, Mehlman DJ, Tsai F, Lomasney JW, Joob AW. Syphilitic aortitis. Circulation. 1999;100(14):1582–3.
46. Gaa J, Weidauer S, Sitzer M, Lanfermann H, Zanella FE. Cerebral vasculitis due to *Treponema pallidum* infection: MRI and MRA findings. Eur Radiol. 2004;14(4):746–7.
47. Giang DW. Central nervous system vasculitis secondary to infections, toxins, and neoplasms. Semin Neurol. 1994;14(4):313–9.
48. Koening C, Katz B, Hernandez-Rodriguez J, et al. Identification of a *Burkholderia*-like strain from temporal arteries of subjects with giant cell arteritis. Arthritis Rheum. 2012;64:S373.
49. Bilge I, Sadikoglu B, Emre S, Sirin A, Aydin K, Tatli B. Central nervous system vasculitis secondary to parvovirus B19 infection in a pediatric renal transplant patient. Pediatr Nephrol. 2005;20(4):529–33.
50. Catalano-Pons C, Quartier P, Leruez-Ville M, Kaguelidou F, Gendrel D, Lenoir G, et al. Primary cytomegalovirus infection, atypical Kawasaki disease, and coronary aneurysms in 2 infants. Clin Infect Dis. 2005;41(5):e53–6.
51. Leruez-Ville M, Lauge A, Morinet F, Guillevin L, Deny P. Polyarteritis nodosa and parvovirus B19. Lancet. 1994;344(8917):263–4.

26 Cryoglobulinemic Vasculitis

Anne Claire Desbois, Cloe Comarmond,
David Saadoun, and Patrice Cacoub

Abbreviations

ANCA	Antineutrophil cytoplasmic antibodies
CMV	Cytomegalovirus
CNS	Central nervous system
CryoVas	Cryoglobulinemic vasculitis
FFS	Five-factor score
HBV	Hepatitis B virus
HCV	Hepatitis C virus
PEG-IFN	Pegylated interferon
RBV	Ribavirin
RF	Rheumatoid factor

Cryoglobulins are immune complexes that may induce systemic vasculitis, affecting small vessels and involving mainly the skin, the joints, the peripheral nerve system, and the kidneys. During the last 25 years, major progresses have been done after the discovery of the hepatitis C virus (HCV), which represents the main cause of cryoglobulins [1–3].

A. C. Desbois · C. Comarmond · D. Saadoun
P. Cacoub (✉)
Sorbonne Universités, UPMC Univ Paris 06, UMR 7211, and Inflammation-Immunopathology-Biotherapy Department (DHU i2B), Paris, France

INSERM, UMR_S 959, Paris, France

CNRS, FRE3632, Paris, France

AP-HP, Groupe Hospitalier Pitié-Salpêtrière, Department of Internal Medicine and Clinical Immunology, Referral Center for Rare Autoimmune Systemic Disorders, Paris, France
e-mail: patrice.cacoub@aphp.fr

Cryoglobulinemic Spectrum and Diagnostic Tests

Cryoglobulinemic is defined by the presence of circulating immunoglobulins that precipitate at cold temperature and dissolve with rewarming. Cryoglobulinemic is confirmed by the detection of protein precipitates in the patient's serum maintained at 4 °C during at least 7 days, which dissolved when heated at 37 °C. In most expert centers, patients are considered to have a significant cryoglobulin level when >0.05 g/L on two determinations [2]. After detection, Cryoglobulinemic is categorized by immunochemical analysis into three types [2, 4]. Type I cryoglobulins are monoclonal immunoglobulins. Type II cryoglobulins consist of a monoclonal immunoglobulin with a rheumatoid factor (RF) activity associated with polyclonal IgG, whereas type III cryoglobulins comprised polyclonal IgM and IgM with RF activity [5, 6]. Types II and III are often referred to as mixed Cryoglobulinemic. However, testing methods for Cryoglobulinemic detection have some limitations and may be influenced by artifacts arising from ex vivo cryoprecipitation after blood

G. Ragab et al. (eds.), *The Microbiome in Rheumatic Diseases and Infection*,
https://doi.org/10.1007/978-3-319-79026-8_26

drawing. Indeed, cryoglobulins are characterized by high thermal instability. For a correct evaluation of serum cryoglobulins, it is necessary to avoid false-negative results due to immunoglobulin cold precipitation which also occurs at room temperature. Blood sampling for cryoglobulin detection should be carried immediately after blood is drawn, or blood should be rapidly transported to the laboratory using a thermostable device (37 °C). In consequence, when a cryoglobulin is suspected, serum should be kept warm, tests should be carried out at 37 °C, and tests for cryoglobulin detection should be repeated if first tests are negative and clinical feature is suggestive of Cryoglobulinemic vasculitis.

Other laboratory surrogate markers, easier to detect than cryoglobulins, may provide indirect evidence of the presence of Cryoglobulinemic. Specific but inconsistent complement abnormalities are observed: decreased serum levels of early components (C1q, C2, C4) and CH50, with usually normal C3 concentration. The diagnosis of mixed cryoglobulinemic vasculitis is usually based on the association of clinical vasculitis symptoms, a Cryoglobulinemic and a decrease in C4. Rheumatoid factor activity is also often found in mixed Cryoglobulinemic, in contrast to type I cryoglobulins. Electrophoresis and immunoelectrophoresis reveal polyclonal hypergammaglobulinemia or a monoclonal component.

On pathological analysis, CryoVas is a leukocytoclastic vasculitis affecting small (arterioles, capillaries, venules) and medium vessels; it is related to an inflammatory infiltrate around the vessels predominantly composed of lymphocytes and monocytes with very few polymorphonuclears. In 20% of cases, fibrinoid necrosis around medium-size vessels may be observed and mimic features of periarteritis nodosa.

Serum cryoglobulin may also interfere with a variety of laboratory tests and have been associated with spurious quantitation of plasma proteins and erythrocyte sedimentation rate, pseudo-leukocytosis, pseudo-thrombocytosis, or pseudo-macrocytosis.

Main Features of Cryoglobulinemic Vasculitis

The disease expression is variable, ranging from mild clinical symptoms (fatigue, purpura, arthralgia) to fulminant life-threatening complications (glomerulonephritis, widespread vasculitis) [1, 7] (Table 26.1). Of note, underlying mechanisms are different, i.e., clinical symptoms are explained by intravascular precipitation of monoclonal immunoglobulin in type I Cryoglobulinemic, whereas in mixed Cryoglobulinemic, lesions are often related to small-vessel vasculitis induced by immune complex deposits.

Fatigue is the main symptom, noted in 80–90% of patients. The main cutaneous sign is a palpable purpura which is reported in 70–90% of patients. It always begins at the lower limbs and may extend to abdominal area, less frequently to the trunk and upper limbs (Fig. 26.1). It persists several days and regresses with a residual brownish pigmentation. Cutaneous ulcers may also occur in particular in type I Cryoglobulinemic. Cold associated symptoms (Raynaud's phenomenon, acrocyanosis, etc.) are seen in 25% of patients, especially in patients with type I cryoglobulin.

Arthralgia is reported in 40–60% of patients. They usually involve large joints and are

Table 26.1 Main clinical features of cryoglobulinemic vasculitis according to the type of cryoglobulin [5, 7–9]

Type of cryoglobulin	I ($n = 64$)	II–III ($n = 566$)
Skin		
Purpura	60–70%	75–90%
Raynaud phenomenon	30–40%	20–35%
Ulcers/distal skin necrosis	30%	5–15%
Cold-related symptoms	90–100%	0–10%
Livedo	10–15%	5–10%
Arthralgia/arthritis	30%	30–80%
Neurological involvement		
Peripheral neuropathy	40–50%	50–75%
Central nervous system	Rare	5–10%
Renal involvement	20–30%	20–40%
Digestive involvement	Rare	5%
Heart involvement	Rare	Rare
Pulmonary involvement	Rare	Rare

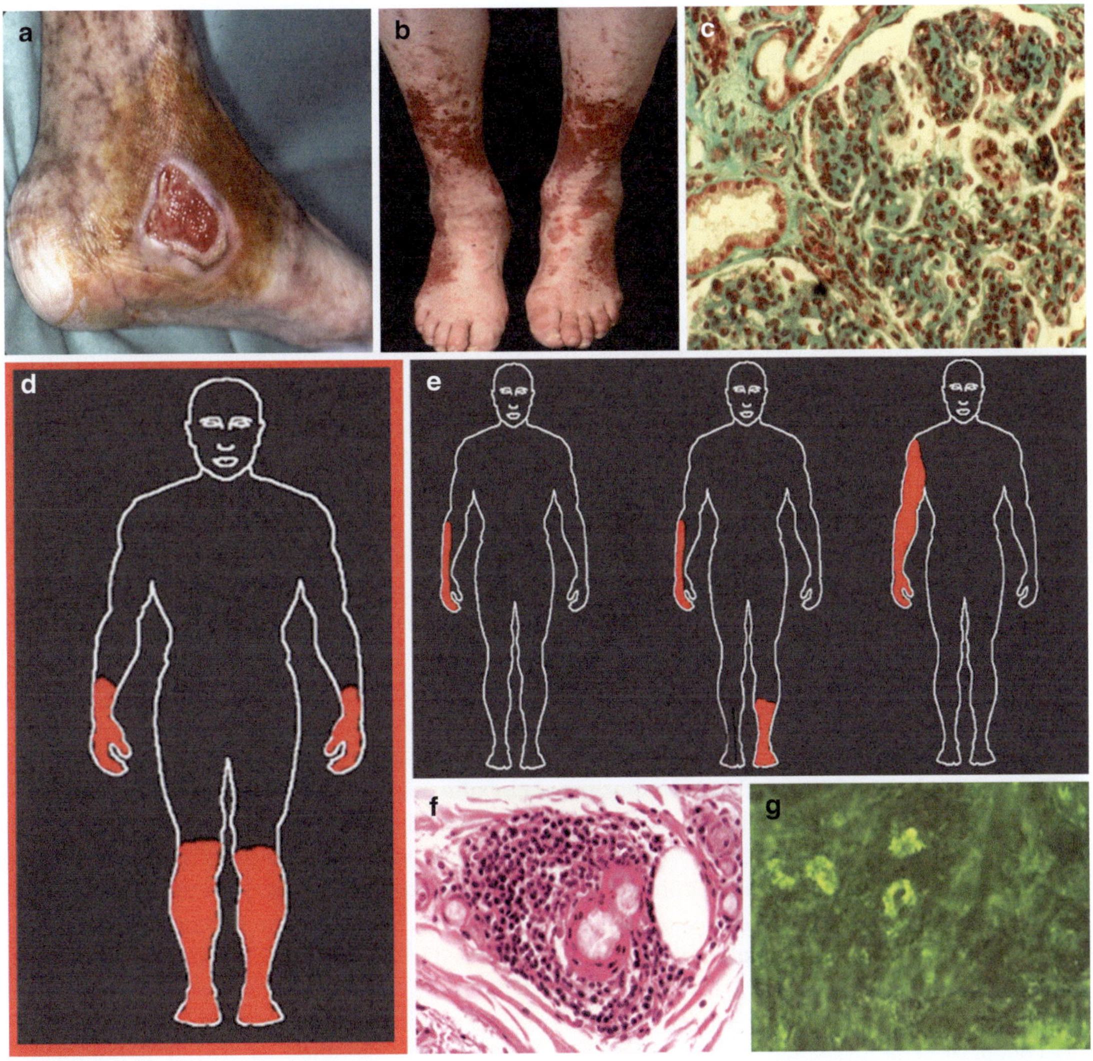

Fig. 26.1 (**a**) Skin purpura with a cutaneous ulcer in an HCV-mixed Cryoglobulinemic. (**b**) Skin purpura. (**c**) Membranoproliferative glomerulonephritis related to type II mixed Cryoglobulinemic. (**d**) Distal polyneuropathy related to mixed Cryoglobulinemic. (**e**) Mononeuropathy multiplex related to mixed Cryoglobulinemic. (**f**) Nerve biopsy showing perivascular infiltrate of T lymphocytes around small-sized vessels. (**g**) Immunofluorescence analysis of skin biopsy showing C3 deposits

bilateral and symmetric. Arthralgia involves more frequently fingers, knee, ankles, and back. Frank arthritis is reported in <10% of patients without joint deformation. A sicca syndrome has been reported in 20–40% of patients. Although sicca symptoms are very frequent in HCV-infected patients, a characterized Sjögren's syndrome defined by the presence of anti-SSA or anti-SSB antibodies and a typical salivary gland histology is uncommon.

Neurologic manifestations range from pure sensory polyneuropathy to mononeuritis multiplex (60–70%). The most frequently described form is a distal sensory or sensory-motor polyneuropathy. Polyneuropathy usually manifests as painful and asymmetric paresthesia which later becomes symmetric. Motor deficit is inconstant, mainly affects the lower limbs, and often appears from a few months to a few years after sensory symptoms. Central nervous system (CNS) involvement is infrequent (<10%) and may manifest as stroke, epilepsy, or cognitive impairment. CNS damages are the consequence of cerebral vasculitis.

Renal manifestations are reported in 20–40% of patients. The most frequent clinical presentation is proteinuria with microscopic hematuria and sometimes a variable degree of renal insufficiency. Histological analysis most often reveals an acute or chronic type I membranoproliferative glomerulonephritis with subendothelial deposits (Fig. 26.1). It represents more than 80% of cryoglobulinemic renal diseases. It is strongly associated with the presence of type II Cryoglobulinemic with IgMκ rheumatoid factor. In histological analysis, the presence of amorphous and eosinophilic intraluminal thrombi and vasculitis of small and medium-sized vessels (25%) with fibrinoid necrosis are associated with a poor outcome.

Other severe manifestations are rare (<5%). Digestive involvement may manifest as abdominal pains and gastrointestinal bleeding secondary to mesenteric vasculitis. To date, there is no data on gut microbiota in patients with Cryoglobulinemic vasculitis. Cardiac involvement is associated with significant mortality. It includes mitral valvular damages, coronary vasculitis complicated by myocardial infarction, pericarditis, or congestive heart failure. Lungs are rarely involved usually without clinical symptoms. However, some patients may present moderate exercise dyspnea, dry cough, or hemoptysis, which can be the consequence of interstitial lung fibrosis, pleural effusions, or pulmonary intra-alveolar hemorrhages.

For a patient with a vascular purpura, other causes of purpura should be excluded such as infections especially in the presence of fever (meningococcal infections, endocarditis, etc.), drugs and toxics, as well as other small-vessel vasculitis (ANCA vasculitis, IgA vasculitis, etc.).

Etiologies of Cryoglobulinemic

The production of cryoglobulins is most often the consequence of an underlying disorder that needs an etiological checkup. It is tailored, at least in part, according to the immunochemical determination of the cryoglobulin components.

In type I cryoglobulinemic vasculitis, it is mandatory to look for the presence of an underlying B-cell lymphoproliferative disorder, mainly Waldenström macroglobulinemia, multiple myeloma, or monoclonal gammopathy of unknown significance. The clinical lesions of vasculitis are explained by intravascular precipitation and "obstruction" of monoclonal immunoglobulin in small-size vessels. In this context, a cryoglobulin composed of IgM suggests a Waldenström disease, whereas Cryoglobulinemic composed of IgG is more often found in myeloma or MGUS. Type I cryoglobulins may also be observed in non-Hodgkin's lymphoma or chronic lymphocytic leukemia B, although mixed type II cryoglobulins are more common (Table 26.2).

The main etiology of mixed cryoglobulins (type II and type III) is chronic HCV infection (70–90% of mixed cryoglobulins). In large

Table 26.2 Management of cryoglobulinemic vasculitis according the type of cryoglobulin

Type I cryoglobulins		Mixed cryoglobulins (type II or III)	
MGUS	B-cell disorder (myeloma, lymphoma)	HCV+	HCV−
Treatment of MGUS: Corticosteroids *IgG* • Bortezomib • Alkylating agents • Thalidomide or lenalidomide *IgM* • Rituximab • Plasmapheresis • Ilomedine	*Treatment of myeloma* (bortezomib, alkylating agents, thalidomide, stem cell autograft) *Or lymphoma* (chemotherapy) • Plasmapheresis • Ilomedine	*Antiviral IFN-free treatment* • Rituximab • Plasmapheresis • Ilomedine	*Treatment of etiology (autoimmune disease, lymphoma)* Corticosteroids • Rituximab • Alkylating agents (cyclophosphamide) • Chemotherapy (for lymphoma) • Plasmapheresis • Ilomedine

prospective series, the presence of a mixed cryoglobulin is found in about 50% of HCV-infected patients. However, only one third of these cryoglobulin-positive HCV patients will develop a symptomatic vasculitis. In case of persistent mixed cryoglobulin despite HCV clearance, the presence of a B-cell lymphoma should be considered [10]. For mixed cryoglobulins not associated with HCV (10–30% of mixed cryoglobulins), main causes include other infectious diseases (HBV, HIV), B-cell malignancies, and autoimmune diseases (notably systemic lupus and Sjögren's syndrome). Other infectious triggers are listed in Table 26.3. Non-HCV-related infectious Cryoglobulinemic are mainly caused by virus (HBV, CMV, and HIV), bacterial pathogens (endocarditis, *Streptococcus*, *Brucella*), or parasites (leishmaniosia). In a recent study including 242 patients with noninfectious mixed Cryoglobulinemic, 30% had autoimmune disorders (Sjögren's syndrome, lupus, scleroderma), 22% had a hemopathy (marginal zone lymphoma, non-Hodgkin's B-cell lymphoma, lymphoplasmacytic lymphoma), and no cause was found in 48% of patients [11].

Table 26.3 Main infectious triggers of mixed Cryoglobulinemic

Main infectious triggers
Virus
Hepatitis C virus (HCV)
Hepatitis B virus (HBV)
Epstein-Barr virus
Cytomegalovirus
Hepatitis A virus
Human immunodeficiency virus (HIV)
Adenovirus
Parvovirus B19
Bacteria
Endocarditis
Streptococcus
Brucellosis
Coxiella
Mycobacterium leprae
Lyme disease
Syphilis
Parasites
Malaria
Leishmania
Toxoplasma
Schistosomiasis
Echinococcosis
Fungi
Candida
Coccidioidomycosis

Prognosis of Cryoglobulinemic Vasculitis

Cryoglobulinemic vasculitis is associated with increased morbidity and mortality. Some studies before the HCV era underlined the bad prognostic factor of renal involvement [10]. More recent studies defined prognostic factors of Cryoglobulinemic vasculitis according to the presence of HCV infection and the type of cryoglobulinemic [7, 12].

In a cohort of 151 HCV-associated mixed cryoglobulinemic vasculitis, the 1-year, 3-year, 5-year, and 10-year survival rates were 96%, 86%, 75%, and 63%, respectively. In HCV-associated cryoglobulinemic vasculitis, liver-related complications and severe vasculitis involvements are the main factors associated with a poor prognosis. Baseline factors associated with a poor prognosis were the presence of severe liver fibrosis (hazard ratio [HR] 5.31), central nervous system involvement (HR 2.74), kidney involvement (HR 1.91), and heart involvement (HR 4.2). The five-factor score (FFS) [13], a vasculitis scoring system based on five clinical items (proteinuria >1 gr/day, serum creatinine >140 μmol/L, cardiomyopathy, severe gastrointestinal involvement, and central nervous system involvement), was significantly associated with outcome. In multivariate analysis, severe fibrosis (HR 10.8) and the FFS (HR 2.49) were significantly associated with a poor prognosis [12]. In different studies, the most common causes of death were infection, end-stage liver disease, cardiovascular disease, vasculitis (mainly renal involvement complicated with end-stage renal and CNS involvement), and lymphoma/neoplasia [7, 12, 14]. In HCV-related cryoglobulinemic vasculitis, the overall risk of B-cell non-Hodgkin's lymphoma is about 35 times higher than in the general population. Interestingly, among patients without severe liver fibrosis, the

FFS was a good predictor of outcome, while among those with severe fibrosis, the severity of vasculitis had no prognostic value. Treatment with the combination of pegylated interferon plus ribavirin was associated with a good prognosis (HR 0.34), whereas treatment with immunosuppressive/glucocorticosteroid agents (but not rituximab and plasmapheresis) was associated with a poor outcome, even after adjustment for the severity of vasculitis (HR 4.05) [12]. Regarding response to therapy, complete clinical, immunologic, and sustained virological responses were associated with a good prognosis. In a recent study including 205 HCV-mixed cryoglobulinemic patients with renal failure, adjusted multivariate Cox regression analysis identified age (HR 1.036) and the use of antiviral therapy (HR, 0.296) as the risk factors associated with survival.

In patients with noninfectious mixed cryoglobulinemic vasculitis, baseline factors associated with prognosis have been recently reported in a large study [8, 15]. One-year, two-year, five-year, and ten-year overall survival rates were 91%, 89%, 79%, and 65%, respectively. Deaths were related to serious infections (50%), vasculitis flare, and cardiovascular disease. The cause of mixed cryoglobulinemic did not predict the outcome. Pulmonary and gastrointestinal involvements, glomerular filtration rate <60 ml/min, and age >65 years were independently associated with death. The CryoVas score (CVS), a prognostic score including these four variables, was derived for the prediction of survival at 5 years. At 5 years, the death rates were 2.6%, 13.1%, 29.6%, and 38.5% for a CVS of 0, 1, 2, and ≥3, respectively. At 1 year, the death rates were 0%, 3.2%, 18.5%, and 30.8% for a CVS of 0, 1, 2, and ≥3, respectively. The area under the curve for the CVS was higher compared with the FFS, indicating a better performance of the CVS [15]. Increased risk of lymphoma in the follow-up of such patients should also be underlined [16].

Data on the prognosis of type I cryoglobulinemic vasculitis have been reported on a series of 64 patients [5]. The 1-year, 3-year, 5-year, and 10-year survival rates were 97%, 94%, 94%, and 87%, respectively. Compared to MGUS, type I CryoVas related to hematologic malignancy tended to be associated with a poorer prognosis (p = 0.06). Deaths were mainly explained by infections (n = 2/4) and hemopathy.

Management

In type I cryoglobulinemic, the treatment of cryoglobulinemic vasculitis is that of the B-cell lymphoproliferative disorder, i.e., chemotherapy for underlying lymphoma or myeloma (including bortezomib, thalidomide, lenalidomide, or an alkylating agent) [17] (Table 26.2). A stem cell autograft may also be indicated for myeloma. In the case of MGUS linked to IgG (plasmocytes proliferation), myeloma treatments are used, whereas in the case of IgM (lymphoplasmocytic proliferation), rituximab is more readily used [9]. Specific treatment may also be indicated, including plasma exchange (in particular in severe cutaneous or renal involvement) and Ilomedine [5].

In type II and III cryoglobulinemic (mixed cryoglobulinemic), the main etiological agent is by far HCV infection. HCV-induced mixed cryoglobulinemic vasculitis manifestations respond to clearance of HCV, i.e., sustained virological response (SVR). International guidelines recommend to treat HCV-infected patients with extrahepatic manifestations such as mixed cryoglobulinemic vasculitis. During the decade 2002–2012, using a combination antiviral therapy with pegylated interferon (PegIFN) plus ribavirin for 12 months permitted to achieve a SVR in 50–60% of patients [18]. Patients who relapsed for HCV infection after responding to antiviral therapy usually relapsed for the vasculitis with the return of viremia [19]. The use of a more potent triple HCV therapy with PegIFN/ribavirin and a specifically targeted antiviral agent (NS3/4A protease inhibitor, i.e., boceprevir or telaprevir) led to improved SVR rates (65–70%) in HCV genotype 1 infection [11, 20]. However, such combination should be given for a long time (48 weeks), and serious adverse events occurred in up to 47% of patients, mostly in patients with baseline severe liver fibrosis and a low platelet count [11]. Numerous other direct-acting antivirals are now available. The NS3/4A inhibitor simeprevir and NS5B inhibitor sofosbuvir allow shortened courses of combination IFN-free therapy, which are associated with high (>95%) SVR rates and relatively few toxicities. In a prospective, open-label trial, including 24 HCV-mixed cryoglobulinemic patients (50% genotype 1, 50% with stage 4 liver fibrosis) treated with sofosbuvir and ribavirin, clinical complete remission was achieved in 87.5% at the end of treatment. A SVR was obtained in 74% of patients at week 12 after the end of treatment [17]. In a retrospective case series, including 12 HCV patients (50% cirrhosis, 67% G1, seven patients with kidney involvement) treated with sofosbuvir plus simeprevir or ribavirin, the rate of SVR was 83% at 12 weeks after the end of treatment. It is mandatory to also take into account other HCV complications, such as cirrhosis or renal insufficiency, for the choice of antiviral treatment and the initiation of specific treatment of such complications. For cryoglobulinemic vasculitis related to other pathogens (HBV, CMV, etc.), the treatment is also based on therapy targeting the infectious pathogen (i.e., antivirals against HBV) associated with plasmapheresis.

Rituximab is also an interesting therapeutic strategy in patients with mixed cryoglobulinemic, as it targets B-cells, which are responsible for cryoglobulin production and finally vasculitis lesions. In a prospective cohort study of 38 HCV-mixed cryoglobulinemic patients, rituximab plus Peg-IFN-α-/ribavirin-treated patients had a shorter time to clinical remission, better renal response rates, and higher rates of cryoglobulin clearance compared with Peg-IFN-α/ribavirin [9]. A prospective randomized trial confirmed the benefice of combination of rituximab and antivirals, showing a complete response rate of 54.5% and 33.3% in patients who received rituximab plus IFNa/RBV and Peg-IFNa/RBV alone, respectively ($p < 0.05$) [21]. More recent studies have reported that rituximab has a better efficacy than conventional immunosuppressive treatment (i.e., glucocorticosteroids, azathioprine, cyclophosphamide, and plasmapheresis) in patients refractory to antiviral treatment [22, 23]. In case of life-threatening vasculitis, plasmapheresis should have also been considered, particularly in rapidly progressing renal failure, central nervous system lesions, or cardiac/severe digestive involvement.

To summarize, the management must be individualized according to the underlying disorder and the severity of disease. In HCV-mixed cryoglobulinemic vasculitis with mild to moderate disease, an optimal antiviral treatment alone should be given. For patients with severe vasculitis (i.e., worsening of renal function, mononeuritis multiplex, extensive skin disease, intestinal ischemia, etc.), the control of disease with plasmapheresis and/or rituximab is usually required in association with the concomitant initiation of antiviral therapy.

Follow-Up

During immunosuppressive and/or antiviral treatment (for HCV-related cryoglobulinemic vasculitis), signs and symptoms gradually improve, after a follow-up of weeks (i.e., purpura, glomerulonephritis, and arthralgia) or months (peripheral neuropathy). With treatment, most patients can achieve a partial or complete clinical remission. In HCV-related cryoglobulinemic vasculitis, the clinical and immunological response is closely related to the viral response.

Long-term outcome is dependent on the occurrence of complications. Patients with non-HCV-related cryoglobulinemic vasculitis have an increased risk of death, primarily due to sepsis, and a fourfold increased risk of developing B-cell non-Hodgkin's lymphoma [8]. In HCV-related cryoglobulinemic vasculitis, the overall risk of B-cell non-Hodgkin's lymphoma is about 35 times higher than in the general population. These patients are also exposed to HCV chronic infection-induced liver disease, i.e., liver fibrosis, cirrhosis, and hepatocellular carcinoma.

Funding Sources None.

Disclosure Pr Patrice Cacoub has received consultancies, honoraria, advisory board, and speakers' fees from AbbVie, AstraZeneca, Bayer,

Boehringer Ingelheim, Gilead, GlaxoSmithKline, Janssen Pharmaceutica, Merck Sharp & Dohme, Pfizer, Roche, Servier, and Vifor Pharma.

- Pr Patrice Cacoub is an inventor of a patent application owned by his academic institution and licensed to ILTOO pharma, a biotechnology company developing low-dose IL-2 in autoimmune diseases, in which it holds shares.
- Dr Anne Claire has received speakers' fees from Gilead.
- Dr Chloe Comarmond has no conflict of interest.
- Dr David Saadoun has received consultancies, honoraria, advisory board, and speakers' fees from AbbVie, Roche, Bristol-Myers Squibb, and Gilead.

References

1. Cacoub P, Poynard T, Ghillani P, Charlotte F, Olivi M, Piette JC, Opolon P. Extrahepatic manifestations of chronic hepatitis C. MULTIVIRC group. Multidepartment virus C. Arthritis Rheum. 1999;42:2204–12. https://doi.org/10.1002/1529-0131(199910)42:10<2204::AID-ANR24>3.0.CO;2-D.
2. Brouet JC, Clauvel JP, Danon F, Klein M, Seligmann M. Biologic and clinical significance of cryoglobulins. A report of 86 cases. Am J Med. 1974;57:775–88.
3. Terrier B, Cacoub P. Cryoglobulinemic vasculitis: an update. Curr Opin Rheumatol. 2013;25:10–8. https://doi.org/10.1097/BOR.0b013e32835b15f7.
4. Musset L, Diemert MC, Taibi F, Du LTH, Cacoub P, Leger JM, Boissy G, Gaillard O, Galli J. Characterization of cryoglobulins by immunoblotting. Clin Chem. 1992;38:798–802.
5. Terrier B, Karras A, Kahn J-E, Le Guenno G, Marie I, Benarous L, Lacraz A, Diot E, Hermine O, de Saint-Martin L, Cathébras P, Leblond V, Modiano P, Léger J-M, Mariette X, Senet P, Plaisier E, Saadoun D, Cacoub P. The spectrum of type I Cryoglobulinemic vasculitis: new insights based on 64 cases. Medicine (Baltimore). 2013;92:61–8. https://doi.org/10.1097/MD.0b013e318288925c.
6. Trejo O, Ramos-Casals M, García-Carrasco M, Yagüe J, Jiménez S, de la Red G, Cervera R, Font J, Ingelmo M. Cryoglobulinemic: study of etiologic factors and clinical and immunologic features in 443 patients from a single center. Medicine (Baltimore). 2001;80:252–62.
7. Ferri C, Sebastiani M, Giuggioli D, Cazzato M, Longombardo G, Antonelli A, Puccini R, Michelassi C, Zignego AL. Mixed Cryoglobulinemic: demographic, clinical, and serologic features and survival in 231 patients. Semin Arthritis Rheum. 2004;33:355–74.
8. Terrier B, Krastinova E, Marie I, Launay D, Lacraz A, Belenotti P, de Saint-Martin L, Quemeneur T, Huart A, Bonnet F, Le Guenno G, Kahn J-E, Hinschberger O, Rullier P, Diot E, Lazaro E, Bridoux F, Zénone T, Carrat F, Hermine O, Léger J-M, Mariette X, Senet P, Plaisier E, Cacoub P. Management of noninfectious mixed Cryoglobulinemic vasculitis: data from 242 cases included in the CryoVas survey. Blood. 2012;119:5996–6004. https://doi.org/10.1182/blood-2011-12-396028.
9. Saadoun D, Resche Rigon M, Sene D, Terrier B, Karras A, Perard L, Schoindre Y, Coppere B, Blanc F, Musset L, Piette J-C, Rosenzwajg M, Cacoub P. Rituximab plus peg-interferon-alpha/ribavirin compared with peg-interferon-alpha/ribavirin in hepatitis C-related mixed Cryoglobulinemic. Blood. 2010;116:326–34. https://doi.org/10.1182/blood-2009-10-248518.
10. Landau D-A, Saadoun D, Halfon P, Martinot-Peignoux M, Marcellin P, Fois E, Cacoub P. Relapse of hepatitis C virus–associated mixed Cryoglobulinemic vasculitis in patients with sustained viral response. Arthritis Rheum. 2008;58:604–11. https://doi.org/10.1002/art.23305.
11. Saadoun D, Rigon MR, Pol S, Thibault V, Blanc F, Pialoux G, Karras A, Bazin-Kara D, Cazorla C, Vittecoq D, et al. PegIFNα/ribavirin/protease inhibitor combination in severe hepatitis C virus-associated mixed Cryoglobulinemic vasculitis. J Hepatol. 2015;62:24–30.
12. Terrier B, Semoun O, Saadoun D, Sène D, Resche-Rigon M, Cacoub P. Prognostic factors in patients with hepatitis C virus infection and systemic vasculitis. Arthritis Rheum. 2011;63:1748–57. https://doi.org/10.1002/art.30319.
13. Guillevin L, Pagnoux C, Seror R, Mahr A, Mouthon L, Toumelin PL. The five-factor score revisited: assessment of prognoses of systemic necrotizing vasculitides based on the French vasculitis study group (FVSG) cohort. Medicine (Baltimore). 2011;90:19–27. https://doi.org/10.1097/MD.0b013e318205a4c6.
14. Landau D-A, Scerra S, Sene D, Resche-Rigon M, Saadoun D, Cacoub P. Causes and predictive factors of mortality in a cohort of patients with hepatitis C virus-related cryoglobulinemic vasculitis treated with antiviral therapy. J Rheumatol. 2010;37:615–21. https://doi.org/10.3899/jrheum.090790.
15. Terrier B, Carrat F, Krastinova E, Marie I, Launay D, Lacraz A, Belenotti P, de Saint Martin L, Quemeneur T, Huart A, Bonnet F, Le Guenno G, Kahn J-E, Hinschberger O, Rullier P, Hummel A, Diot E, Pagnoux C, Lzaro E, Bridoux F, Zenone T, Hermine O, Leger J-M, Mariette X, Senet P, Plaisier E, Cacoub P. Prognostic factors of survival in patients with non-infectious mixed cryoglobulinaemia vasculitis: data from 242 cases included in the CryoVas survey. Ann

Rheum Dis. 2013;72:374–80. https://doi.org/10.1136/annrheumdis-2012-201405.
16. Saadoun D, Sellam J, Ghillani-Dalbin P, Crecel R, Piette J-C, Cacoub P. Increased risks of lymphoma and death among patients with non–hepatitis C virus–related mixed Cryoglobulinemic. Arch Intern Med. 2006;166:2101–8.
17. Saadoun D, Thibault V, Si Ahmed SN, Alric L, Mallet M, Guillaud C, Izzedine H, Plaisier A, Fontaine H, Costopoulos M, Le Garff-Tavernier M, Hezode C, Pol S, Musset L, Poynard T, Cacoub P. Sofosbuvir plus ribavirin for hepatitis C virus-associated cryoglobulinaemia vasculitis: VASCUVALDIC study. Ann Rheum Dis. 2016;75(10):1777–82. https://doi.org/10.1136/annrheumdis-2015-208339.
18. Saadoun D, Resche-Rigon M, Thibault V, Piette J-C, Cacoub P. Antiviral therapy for hepatitis C virus – associated mixed Cryoglobulinemic vasculitis: a long-term followup study. Arthritis Rheum. 2006;54:3696–706. https://doi.org/10.1002/art.22168.
19. Terrier B, Saadoun D, Sène D, Sellam J, Pérard L, Coppéré B, Karras A, Blanc F, Buchler M, Plaisier E, Ghillani P, Rosenzwajg M, Cacoub P. Efficacy and tolerability of rituximab with or without PEGylated interferon alfa-2b plus ribavirin in severe hepatitis C virus-related vasculitis: a long-term followup study of thirty-two patients. Arthritis Rheum. 2009;60:2531–40. https://doi.org/10.1002/art.24703.
20. Gragnani L, Fabbrizzi A, Triboli E, Urraro T, Boldrini B, Fognani E, Piluso A, Caini P, Ranieri J, Monti M, Laffi G, Zignego AL. Triple antiviral therapy in hepatitis C virus infection with or without mixed cryoglobulinaemia: a prospective, controlled pilot study. Dig Liver Dis. 2014;46:833–7. https://doi.org/10.1016/j.dld.2014.05.017.
21. Dammacco F, Tucci FA, Lauletta G, Gatti P, De Re V, Conteduca V, Sansonno S, Russi S, Mariggiò MA, Chironna M, Sansonno D. Pegylated interferon-alpha, ribavirin, and rituximab combined therapy of hepatitis C virus-related mixed Cryoglobulinemic: a long-term study. Blood. 2010;116:343–53. https://doi.org/10.1182/blood-2009-10-245878.
22. De Vita S, Quartuccio L, Isola M, Mazzaro C, Scaini P, Lenzi M, Campanini M, Naclerio C, Tavoni A, Pietrogrande M, Ferri C, Mascia MT, Masolini P, Zabotti A, Maset M, Roccatello D, Zignego AL, Pioltelli P, Gabrielli A, Filippini D, Perrella O, Migliaresi S, Galli M, Bombardieri S, Monti G. A randomized controlled trial of rituximab for the treatment of severe cryoglobulinemic vasculitis. Arthritis Rheum. 2012;64:843–53. https://doi.org/10.1002/art.34331.
23. Sneller MC, Hu Z, Langford CA. A randomized controlled trial of rituximab following failure of antiviral therapy for hepatitis C virus-associated cryoglobulinemic vasculitis. Arthritis Rheum. 2012;64:835–42. https://doi.org/10.1002/art.34322.

27 Behçet Disease

Ahmet Gül

Abbreviations

BD	Behçet disease
HLA	Human leukocyte antigen
HSP60	Heat shock protein 60-kDa
HSP65	Heat shock protein 65-kDa
ICR	Institute of Cancer Research

Introduction

Behçet disease (BD) is a multi-system inflammatory disorder characterized by recurrent flares affecting mucocutaneous and ocular tissues as well as joints, blood vessels, and gastrointestinal and central nervous systems. The prevalence of BD is higher in countries along the historical Silk Road from the coastal Mediterranean and Middle East to Japan, and it runs a more severe course in young males. The hyper-inflammatory nature of BD has been associated with a complex genetic tendency, and several microbial agents have been claimed as triggers of the disease manifestations starting with its first definition [1, 2].

A. Gül
Istanbul University, Istanbul Faculty of Medicine, Department of Internal Medicine, Division of Rheumatology, Istanbul, Turkey
e-mail: agul@istanbul.edu.tr

Behçet Disease and Viruses

Professor Hulusi Behçet first described his triple symptom complex consisting of recurrent oral and genital aphthous ulcers and uveitis as cardinal manifestations of an independent disease, possibly caused by a specific agent in 1937 [2]. His claims of a possible generalized infection affecting the entire body were based on his observations of simultaneous or sequential appearance of the typical manifestations during flares as well as increased duration of intervals between attacks with only systemic treatments in the first two patients, who were followed for 20 and 7 years, respectively [2, 3].

Professor Behçet tried to isolate the causative agent responsible for this unique combination of manifestations, and his collaboration with Professor Hugo Braun of the Department of Microbiology, Istanbul Faculty of Medicine, helped to document structures resembling elementary particles of a virus, which were seen in the smears prepared from the base of the aphthous ulcers and stained by Giemsa and Herzberg methods [2, 3]. He reported that the sizes of both the intra- and extracellular particles were similar to that of smallpox virus; but inoculation studies failed to culture these virus-like elementary particles.

Professor Necdet Sezer from Istanbul University later reported that he isolated a filterable neurotropic virus from the vitreous of the

G. Ragab et al. (eds.), *The Microbiome in Rheumatic Diseases and Infection*,
https://doi.org/10.1007/978-3-319-79026-8_27

enucleated eye of one patient and the subretinal serous fluids of two other patients with BD [4, 5]. He was successful in culturing the putative agent by inoculating the collected samples into the chorioallantoic membranes. Inoculation of the cultivated viral material induced encephalitis, cutaneous manifestations and thrombophlebitis in the legs of white mice, and uveitis with vitritis and hypopyon as well as encephalitis and cutaneous manifestations in rabbits [4]. He reported that electron microscopic investigations revealed viral particles with a diameter around 100 nm, and they were different from herpes simplex, lymphocytic choriomeningitis, or Theiler's viruses [4]. Professor Sezer also suggested that serologic studies with complement-fixation and neutralization tests with sera from the patients with BD and controls supported the specificity of the isolated agent for the disease [4, 5]. However, no other investigator replicated his findings, and a unique virus responsible for BD manifestations could not be demonstrated so far.

On the other hand, several investigators reported findings associated with herpes simplex virus infection in BD. Eglin and colleagues detected complementary RNA to herpes simplex virus by using ^{125}I-labeled viral DNA probes in peripheral blood mononuclear cells of patients with BD, especially in those with ocular and articular involvements, as well as of those patients with aphthous stomatitis [6]. An impaired cellular response by CD4 and CD8 T cells was observed in patients with BD, similar to those individuals with recurrent herpetic infections [7]. However, antiviral treatment with acyclovir provided no help for the aphthous ulcers or other manifestations of the disease in a randomized trial [8].

Sohn and colleagues developed an animal model for BD with mimicking mucocutaneous, ocular, and articular manifestations using herpes simplex virus in the ICR (Institute of Cancer Research) mice [9, 10]. Characteristics of the manifestations of this model were compatible with herpetic infections, and analysis of several inbred mouse strains indicated no direct effect of MHC alleles in the development of BD-like findings induced by herpes simplex virus infection [11].

BD-like manifestations were also reported in patients with other viral infections, including retroviruses, Epstein-Barr virus, and cytomegalovirus [12–15]. None of them were considered as pathogenic associations, and the development of these findings was viewed as clinical mimics.

Hypersensitivity to Streptococcal Antigens

Professor Hulusi Behçet discussed the role of focal infections in the oral cavity as possible triggers of exacerbations in his following publications; and he reported only slight improvement in the clinical course of the patients with the treatment of dental infections [16]. Later studies further supported the association of oral hygiene with the severity of BD [17].

The role of certain streptococcal strains in oral microbiota and a hypersensitivity to streptococcal antigens have long been claimed to be part of the pathogenesis of BD [18, 19]. An uncommon serotype of *Streptococcus sanguinis* KTH-1 (so-called BD113-20 strain) with its own bacterial and enzymatic properties was found to be detected at higher frequencies in patients with BD compared to healthy controls; and an increased immunoreactivity against it was suggested to play a role in the pathogenesis [20–24]. Exacerbations of systemic manifestations following dental treatments or with skin prick tests using streptococcal antigens further supported the critical role of certain *Streptococcus* strains as potential triggers of BD [25, 26]. A similar flare was also observed following 23-valent polysaccharide *Streptococcus pneumoniae* vaccine [27]. This streptococcal hypersensitivity was even suggested to be used as a diagnostic test by applying a skin prick test with self-saliva, which was considered to be the source of pathogenic streptococcal antigens [19].

Heat shock protein 65-kDa (HSP65) and Bes-1 were isolated as the immunogenic antigens of *S. sanguinis* with a potential cross-reactivity to self-proteins such as HSP60 and retinal BRN3B, respectively [18, 28]. Lehner and colleagues proposed a shared antigen hypothesis with a cross-reactivity between microbial and human HSP antigens [29]. Cross-reactive epitopes were identified between HSP65 of *Mycobacterium tuberculosis*, *S. sanguinis*, and *S. pyogenes*. Also, immunoglobulin A (IgA) and IgG antibodies against those HSP65 epitopes were detected in the serum samples from patients with BD, and antibodies against *S. sanguis* KTH-1, KTH-2, and KTH-3 were limited to BD patients compared to other disease controls including patients with recurrent aphthous stomatitis [29]. By stimulating T cells with overlapping sequences of HSP65 of *Mycobacterium tuberculosis*, four peptides (111–125, 154–172, 219–233, and 311–325) were identified as T cell epitopes inducing lymphoproliferative responses in patients with BD compared to disease and healthy controls [30]. With an exception of 154–172, these peptides stimulated only CD4 T cells; and no evidence was detected for restriction of this response by human leukocyte antigen (HLA)-B*51, which is the major genetic susceptibility factor for BD potentially affecting the immune response [30]. Also, peptides with corresponding sequences of human HSP60 induced similar or stronger lymphoproliferative responses. Subsequent studies showed that subcutaneous immunization with HSP60-derived peptide 336–351 induced CD4 T cell-mediated uveitis in Lewis rats [31, 32], and the 336–351 peptide linked to recombinant cholera toxin B subunit adjuvant was successfully used to induce oral tolerization, which resulted in the prevention of recurrences of uveitis and discontinuation of immunosuppressive drugs in a small group of patients with BD [33].

These findings also led to treatments aiming to control streptococcal infections, and some studies documented favorable effects on the disease manifestations with benzathine penicillin [34, 35], azithromycine [36], and minocycline therapies [37], mediated by either their antimicrobial or immunomodulatory mechanisms.

A recent study, which documented the immunoreactivity with neurofilament-medium filaments in the brain, retina, and scrotal skin tissues of mice by using serum samples of Behçet patients, showed a cross-reactivity with these antibodies and microbial HSP65 epitopes [38]. The mechanism associated with hypersensitivity to streptococcal and other microbial antigens has yet to be clarified; and pathogenic significance of the cross-reactivity with microbial and host proteins in the immunopathogenesis of BD needs to be explored further.

Microbiota in Behçet Disease

Limited number of microbiota studies in fecal and oral samples suggested some form of dysbiosis with possible unfavorable results in BD. A comparative study of fecal microbiota of 22 Italian BD patients with 16 healthy controls, sharing the same diet and lifestyle, showed significant depletion of *Roseburia* and *Subdoligranulum* in the patients. This study also demonstrated a significantly reduced production of butyrate in patients with BD compared to their cohabiting controls, which may play a role in the differentiation of regulatory T cells [39].

On the other hand, comparison of fecal microbiota of 12 Japanese BD patients with those of 12 healthy controls revealed a significant increase in the genera of *Bifidobacterium* and *Eggerthella* and a decrease in the genera of *Megamonas* and *Prevotella* among the patients [40].

Seoudi and colleagues investigated the microbiota of salivary and oral mucosal samples from ulcer and non-ulcer sites in 54 patients with BD, 8 patients with recurrent aphthous stomatitis, and 25 healthy controls [41]. In patients with BD, colonization of oral aphthous ulcer sites was significantly higher with *Streptococcus salivarius* compared to those of recurrent aphthous stomatitis and with *Streptococcus sanguinis* compared to healthy controls. On the other hand, an increased colonization with *Rothia dentocariosa* was detected in the non-ulcer sites of both patients with BD and those with recurrent aphthous stomatitis. Increased colonization with *Neisseria* and *Veillonella* was observed in the oral mucosa of healthy controls compared to both disease groups.

Coit and colleagues analyzed the salivary microbiota using samples from 31 Turkish BD patients and 15 healthy controls [42]. Microbial community structure was found to be less diverse in BD patients, and a repeat analysis in nine patients following treatment of periodontal disease in the short term had no effect on this structure. The most abundant species in the saliva of BD patients was *Haemophilus parainfluenzae*, and the most depleted ones included *Alloprevotella rava* and species in the genus of *Leptotrichia*.

No skin microbiota study was conducted in BD. But one study reported that microbiology of pustular skin lesions of BD was different from that of acne vulgaris with significantly increased prevalence of *Staphylococcus aureus* and *Prevotella* species [43].

It is obvious that there was no consistent pattern for fecal and oral microbiota changes despite some alterations in their distribution. Therefore, it is necessary to be cautious in the interpretation of these microbiota changes as causative or reactive, because of the possible roles of genetic, geographic, dietary, disease activity and treatment-related factors affecting the results [42].

Genetic Factors and Susceptibility to Microbial Triggers

BD shows a familial aggregation with a very high sibling recurrence risk ratio ($\lambda s = 11.4–52.5$), and it is usually thought to be associated with shared genetic factors within the family rather than a communicable pathogen spreading within the household [44]. BD has a complex genetic background, and genome-wide association studies and screenings for rare mutations revealed several variations increasing the susceptibility to BD [45–47]. Some of the variants are associated with defects in the sensing and processing of microbial and endogenous danger signals and others in the type and extent of inflammatory response [45]. Among the identified genes, a considerable similarity was noticed between the variations associated with susceptibility to BD and Crohn's disease, such as IL10, NOD2, TLR4, FUT2, LACC1, ADO-EGR2, RIPK2, IRF8, IL12A, and STAT4 [46, 47]. However, despite involvement of several overlapping variations in the tendency to both diseases, direction of the association in some genes reveals critical differences in the pathogenesis of these conditions. TLR4 variants such as D299G and T399I, associated with reduced response to lipopolysaccharide, and NOD2 variants such as R702W, G908R, and L1007 fs that are associated with reduced response to muramyl dipeptide are associated with an increased risk for Crohn's disease yet are protective for BD. These findings suggest that increased reactivity to intestinal microbiota is critical for BD, but a dampened immune reactivity with associated dysbiosis is important for Crohn's disease [46]. Dense genotyping of immune-related loci by the Immunochip of BD patients also revealed additional susceptibility factors overlapping with tendency for leprosy [47]. Associations with these variants implicate alterations in the host responses to microbial exposure including leprosy in BD. It is not clear whether BD represents a form of immunodeficiency by causing tendency for infections by certain microorganisms or associates with a shared inflammatory response such as erythema nodosum, arthritis, or uveitis induced by different microbial agents.

Conclusion and Implications

After the description of the triple symptom complex by Professor Behçet, no specific viral or other microbial agent could be demonstrated as causative. However recent studies documented the critical role of genetic susceptibility factors affecting the interactions between host and different pathogens and dangerous insults as well as the type and extent of inflammatory response. Despite the initial emphasis on viral triggers, later studies provided more information on uncommon streptococcal strains as possible triggers of the disease manifestations. Hypersensitivity to streptococcal antigens and possibility of cross-reactivity with self-proteins require further studies for elucidation of their diagnostic and therapeutic potentials. Decreasing disease prevalence with better hygiene underlines the public health potential of dealing with microbial triggers in the management of patients with BD, and identification of the genetic and immunologic basis of the disordered host—microbial interactions is expected to provide insights to reduce the impact of disease in patients as well as in high-risk populations [48, 49].

References

1. Gul A. Pathogenesis of Behcet's disease: autoinflammatory features and beyond. Semin Immunopathol. 2015;37(4):413–8.
2. Behcet H. Über rezidivierende, apthöse durch ein Virus verursachte Geschwüre am Mund, am Auge und an der Genitalen. Dermatol Wochenschr. 1937;105:1152–7.
3. Behcet H, Matteson EL. On relapsing, aphthous ulcers of the mouth, eye and genitalia caused by a virus. 1937. Clin Exp Rheumatol. 2010;28(4 Suppl 60):S2–5.
4. Sezer FN. The isolation of a virus as the cause of Behcet's diseases. Am J Ophthalmol. 1953;36(3):301–15.
5. Sezer N. Further investigations on the virus of Behcet's disease. Am J Ophthalmol. 1956;41(1):41–55.
6. Eglin RP, Lehner T, Subak-Sharpe JH. Detection of RNA complementary to herpes-simplex virus in mononuclear cells from patients with Behcet's syndrome and recurrent oral ulcers. Lancet. 1982;2(8312):1356–61.
7. Young C, Lehner T, Barnes CG. CD4 and CD8 cell responses to herpes simplex virus in Behcet's disease. Clin Exp Immunol. 1988;73(1):6–10.
8. Davies UM, Palmer RG, Denman AM. Treatment with acyclovir does not affect orogenital ulcers in Behcet's syndrome: a randomized double-blind trial. Br J Rheumatol. 1988;27(4):300–2.
9. Sohn S. Etiopathology of Behcet's disease: herpes simplex virus infection and animal model. Yonsei Med J. 1997;38(6):359–64.
10. Sohn S, Lee ES, Bang D, Lee S. Behcet's disease-like symptoms induced by the herpes simplex virus in ICR mice. Eur J Dermatol. 1998;8(1):21–3.
11. Sohn S, Lee ES, Lee S. The correlation of MHC haplotype and development of Behcet's disease-like symptoms induced by herpes simplex virus in several inbred mouse strains. J Dermatol Sci. 2001;26(3):173–81.
12. Buskila D, Gladman DD, Gilmore J, Salit IE. Behcet's disease in a patient with immunodeficiency virus infection. Ann Rheum Dis. 1991;50(2):115–6.
13. Kanazawa H, Ijichi S, Eiraku N, Igakura T, Higuchi I, Nakagawa M, et al. Behcet's disease and Sjogren syndrome in a patient with HTLV-I-associated myelopathy. J Neurol Sci. 1993;119(1):121–2.
14. Park BM, Ahn JS, Lee JB, Won YH, Yun SJ. Chronic active Epstein-Barr virus infection-associated hydroa vacciniforme-like eruption and Behcet's-like orogenital ulcers. Dermatology. 2013;226(3):212–6.
15. Annigeri RA, Rajagopalan M, Mani RM, Kaveripattu SS. Cytomegalovirus infection inducing flare of Behcet's disease with possible recurrence of glomerulonephritis after renal transplantation. Indian J Nephrol. 2016;26(1):45–8.
16. Behcet H. Some observations on the clinical picture of the so-called triple symptom complex. Dermatologica. 1940;81:73–83.
17. Mumcu G, Ergun T, Inanc N, Fresko I, Atalay T, Hayran O, et al. Oral health is impaired in Behcet's disease and is associated with disease severity. Rheumatology (Oxford). 2004;43(8):1028–33.
18. Kaneko F, Oyama N, Yanagihori H, Isogai E, Yokota K, Oguma K. The role of streptococcal hypersensitivity in the pathogenesis of Behcet's disease. Eur J Dermatol. 2008;18(5):489–98.
19. Kaneko F, Togashi A, Nomura E, Nakamura K. A new diagnostic way for Behcet's disease: skin prick with self-saliva. Genet Res Int. 2014;2014:1–10.
20. Isogai E, Ohno S, Kotake S, Isogai H, Tsurumizu T, Fujii N, et al. Chemiluminescence of neutrophils from patients with Behcet's disease and its correlation with an increased proportion of uncommon serotypes of *Streptococcus sanguis* in the oral flora. Arch Oral Biol. 1990;35(1):43–8.
21. Yokota K, Hayashi S, Araki Y, Isogai E, Kotake S, Yoshikawa K, et al. Characterization of *Streptococcus sanguis* isolated from patients with Behcet's disease. Microbiol Immunol. 1995;39(9):729–32.
22. Narikawa S, Suzuki Y, Takahashi M, Furukawa A, Sakane T, Mizushima Y. *Streptococcus oralis* previously identified as uncommon '*Streptococcus sanguis*' in Behcet's disease. Arch Oral Biol. 1995;40(8):685–90.
23. Hirohata S, Oka H, Mizushima Y. Streptococcal-related antigens stimulate production of IL6 and interferon-gamma by T cells from patients with Behcet's disease. Cell Immunol. 1992;140(2):410–9.
24. Yokota K, Hayashi S, Fujii N, Yoshikawa K, Kotake S, Isogai E, et al. Antibody response to oral streptococci in Behcet's disease. Microbiol Immunol. 1992;36(8):815–22.
25. Mizushima Y, Matsuda T, Hoshi K, Ohno S. Induction of Behcet's disease symptoms after dental treatment and streptococcal antigen skin test. J Rheumatol. 1988;15(6):1029–30.
26. Skin hypersensitivity to streptococcal antigens and the induction of systemic symptoms by the antigens in Behcet's disease--a multicenter study. The Behcet's disease research Committee of Japan. J Rheumatol. 1989;16(4):506–11.
27. Hugle T, Bircher A, Walker UA. Streptococcal hypersensitivity reloaded: severe inflammatory syndrome in Behcet's disease following 23-valent polysaccharide *Streptococcus pneumoniae* vaccine. Rheumatology (Oxford). 2012;51(4):761–2.
28. Yoshikawa K, Kotake S, Kubota T, Kimura K, Isogai E, Fujii N. Cloning and sequencing of BeS-1 gene encoding the immunogenic antigen of *Streptococcus sanguis* KTH-1 isolated from the

patients with Behcet's disease. Zentralbl Bakteriol. 1998;287(4):449–60.
29. Lehner T, Lavery E, Smith R, van der Zee R, Mizushima Y, Shinnick T. Association between the 65-kilodalton heat shock protein, *Streptococcus sanguis*, and the corresponding antibodies in Behcet's syndrome. Infect Immun. 1991;59(4):1434–41.
30. Pervin K, Childerstone A, Shinnick T, Mizushima Y, van der Zee R, Hasan A, et al. T cell epitope expression of mycobacterial and homologous human 65-kilodalton heat shock protein peptides in short term cell lines from patients with Behcet's disease. J Immunol. 1993;151(4):2273–82.
31. Stanford MR, Kasp E, Whiston R, Hasan A, Todryk S, Shinnick T, et al. Heat shock protein peptides reactive in patients with Behcet's disease are uveitogenic in Lewis rats. Clin Exp Immunol. 1994;97(2):226–31.
32. Hu W, Hasan A, Wilson A, Stanford MR, Li-Yang Y, Todryk S, et al. Experimental mucosal induction of uveitis with the 60-kDa heat shock protein-derived peptide 336-351. Eur J Immunol. 1998;28(8):2444–55.
33. Stanford M, Whittall T, Bergmeier LA, Lindblad M, Lundin S, Shinnick T, et al. Oral tolerization with peptide 336-351 linked to cholera toxin B subunit in preventing relapses of uveitis in Behcet's disease. Clin Exp Immunol. 2004;137(1):201–8.
34. Calguneri M, Kiraz S, Ertenli I, Benekli M, Karaarslan Y, Celik I. The effect of prophylactic penicillin treatment on the course of arthritis episodes in patients with Behcet's disease. A randomized clinical trial. Arthritis Rheum. 1996;39(12):2062–5.
35. Calguneri M, Ertenli I, Kiraz S, Erman M, Celik I. Effect of prophylactic benzathine penicillin on mucocutaneous symptoms of Behcet's disease. Dermatology. 1996;192(2):125–8.
36. Mumcu G, Inanc N, Ozdemir FT, Tulunay A, Eksioglu-Demiralp E, Ergun T, et al. Effects of azithromycin on intracellular cytokine responses and mucocutaneous manifestations in Behcet's disease. Int J Dermatol. 2013;52(12):1561–6.
37. Kaneko F, Oyama N, Nishibu A. Streptococcal infection in the pathogenesis of Behcet's disease and clinical effects of minocycline on the disease symptoms. Yonsei Med J. 1997;38(6):444–54.
38. Lule S, Colpak AI, Balci-Peynircioglu B, Gursoy-Ozdemir Y, Peker S, Kalyoncu U, et al. Behcet disease serum is immunoreactive to neurofilament medium which share common epitopes to bacterial HSP-65, a putative trigger. J Autoimmun. 2017;84:87–96.
39. Consolandi C, Turroni S, Emmi G, Severgnini M, Fiori J, Peano C, et al. Behcet's syndrome patients exhibit specific microbiome signature. Autoimmun Rev. 2015;14(4):269–76.
40. Shimizu J, Kubota T, Takada E, Takai K, Fujiwara N, Arimitsu N, et al. Bifidobacteria abundance-featured gut Microbiota compositional change in patients with Behcet's disease. PLoS One. 2016;11(4):e0153746.
41. Seoudi N, Bergmeier LA, Drobniewski F, Paster B, Fortune F. The oral mucosal and salivary microbial community of Behcet's syndrome and recurrent aphthous stomatitis. J Oral Microbiol. 2015;7:27150.
42. Coit P, Mumcu G, Ture-Ozdemir F, Unal AU, Alpar U, Bostanci N, et al. Sequencing of 16S rRNA reveals a distinct salivary microbiome signature in Behcet's disease. Clin Immunol. 2016;169:28–35.
43. Hatemi G, Bahar H, Uysal S, Mat C, Gogus F, Masatlioglu S, et al. The pustular skin lesions in Behcet's syndrome are not sterile. Ann Rheum Dis. 2004;63(11):1450–2.
44. Gul A, Inanc M, Ocal L, Aral O, Konice M. Familial aggregation of Behcet's disease in Turkey. Ann Rheum Dis. 2000;59(8):622–5.
45. Gul A. Genetics of Behcet's disease: lessons learned from genomewide association studies. Curr Opin Rheumatol. 2014;26(1):56–63.
46. Kirino Y, Zhou Q, Ishigatsubo Y, Mizuki N, Tugal-Tutkun I, Seyahi E, et al. Targeted resequencing implicates the familial Mediterranean fever gene MEFV and the toll-like receptor 4 gene TLR4 in Behcet disease. Proc Natl Acad Sci U S A. 2013;110(20):8134–9.
47. Takeuchi M, Mizuki N, Meguro A, Ombrello MJ, Kirino Y, Satorius C, et al. Dense genotyping of immune-related loci implicates host responses to microbial exposure in Behcet's disease susceptibility. Nat Genet. 2017;49(3):438–43.
48. Direskeneli H, Mumcu G. A possible decline in the incidence and severity of Behcet's disease: implications for an infectious etiology and oral health. Clin Exp Rheumatol. 2010;28(4 Suppl 60):S86–90.
49. Kirino Y, Ideguchi H, Takeno M, Suda A, Higashitani K, Kunishita Y, et al. Continuous evolution of clinical phenotype in 578 Japanese patients with Behcet's disease: a retrospective observational study. Arthritis Res Ther. 2016;18(1):217.

28 Autoinflammatory Diseases

Donato Rigante, Antonio Vitale, and Luca Cantarini

List of Abbreviations

AA	Amyloid A
AD	Autosomal dominant
AIDs	Autoinflammatory diseases
AR	Autosomal recessive
CAPS	Cryopyrin-associated periodic syndrome
CINCAs	Chronic infantile neurological cutaneous articular syndrome
CRMO	Chronic recurrent multifocal osteomyelitis
DAMPs	Damage-associated molecular patterns
FCAS	Familial cold autoinflammatory syndrome
FMF	Familial Mediterranean fever
IL	Interleukin
MEFV	Mediterranean fever
MKD	Mevalonate kinase deficiency
MVK	Mevalonate kinase
MWS	Muckle-Wells syndrome
NLRP3	NOD-like receptor-related protein 3
NOD	Nucleotide-binding and oligomerization domain
NOD2	Nucleotide-binding and oligomerization domain-containing protein 2
NOMID	Neonatal-onset multisystem inflammatory disease
PAMPs	Pathogen-associated molecular patterns
PFAPA	Periodic fever, aphthous stomatitis, pharyngitis, and cervical adenitis
PRR	Pattern recognition receptors
SAPHO	Synovitis, acne, pustulosis, hyperostosis, and osteitis
sJIA	Systemic juvenile idiopathic arthritis
TLR	Toll-like receptors
TNF	Tumor necrosis factor
TNFRSF1A	Tumor necrosis factor receptor superfamily member 1A
TRAPS	Tumor necrosis factor receptor-associated periodic fever syndrome

D. Rigante
Institute of Pediatrics, Università Cattolica Sacro Cuore, Fondazione Policlinico Universitario "A. Gemelli", Rome, Italy

A. Vitale · L. Cantarini (✉)
Research Center of Systemic Autoinflammatory Diseases, Behçet's Disease and Rheumatology-Ophthalmology Collaborative Uveitis Center, Department of Medical Sciences Surgery and Neurosciences, University of Siena, Siena, Italy

Introduction

Autoinflammatory diseases (AIDs) represent a relatively new group of rare disorders determined by deregulation of specific components of innate immunity. They can be subdivided into monogenic

G. Ragab et al. (eds.), *The Microbiome in Rheumatic Diseases and Infection*, https://doi.org/10.1007/978-3-319-79026-8_28

and multifactorial disorders, with the former being caused by mutations of genes involved in the regulation of innate immune system and the latter recognizing a combination of genetic background and environmental factors at the start of the pathogenic process [1, 2].

The most widely known monogenic AIDs are familial Mediterranean fever (FMF), the most frequent autosomal recessive (AR) autoinflammatory condition caused by mutations in the Mediterranean fever (MEFV) gene that encodes for pyrin, a protein associated with the inflammasome, an intracellular multiprotein complex involved in the maturation of interleukin (IL)-1β and IL-18; mevalonate kinase deficiency (MKD), the second AR disease caused by *MVK* mutations and loss of function of the mevalonate kinase enzyme, the first in the cholesterol biosynthesis enzymatic pathway; tumor necrosis factor (TNF) receptor-associated periodic fever syndrome (TRAPS), an autosomal dominant (AD) disorder related to mutations involving type 1 TNF receptor (*TNFRSF1A*); cryopyrin-associated periodic syndrome (CAPS), a group of AD disorders associated with mutations in the *NLRP3* gene that encodes for cryopyrin, a component of the NOD-like receptor-related protein 3 (NLRP3) inflammasome; and Blau syndrome/early-onset sarcoidosis, an AD disease caused by mutations in the *NOD2* gene, encoding for a key regulator of innate immunity which works as bacterial detector in the inflammatory signaling response [1, 3, 4].

The number of multifactorial AIDs is quickly increasing: indeed, during the last decade, the innate immune system has been found to participate in a wide range of systemic disorders previously recognized as metabolic disorders or degenerative conditions, including diabetes mellitus type 2, atherosclerosis, Alzheimer's disease, and fibrosing lung diseases. In a genuine rheumatologic context, Behçet's disease, systemic juvenile idiopathic arthritis, adult-onset Still's disease, gouty arthritis, and chondrocalcinosis are all recognized as polygenic and multifactorial autoinflammatory entities in which the innate immune system plays a crucial role in both pathogenesis and clinical expression. In addition, Schnitzler's disease and periodic fever, aphthous stomatitis, pharyngitis, and cervical adenitis (PFAPA) syndrome represent further disorders with an autoinflammatory basis [1, 5, 6].

Pathogenesis

From a pathogenic point of view, most AIDs are characterized by overproduction of IL-1, a master proinflammatory cytokine involved in a host of inflammatory reactions, apoptosis and pyroptosis, a specific type of cell death. For these reasons, inhibition of IL-1 with biologic agents has proved to be an effective therapeutic option in the vast majority of AIDs [7].

Monogenic AIDs

At a clinical level, monogenic AIDs share the recurrence of apparently inexplicable febrile episodes associated with increase of acute-phase reactants. High body temperature combines with a protean spectrum of inflammatory manifestations, including variable involvement of the skin, joints, gastrointestinal tract, serosal membranes, and central nervous system. More specifically, FMF is characterized by fever generally lasting 1–3 days, mono- or polyserositis presenting with chest and/or abdominal pain, arthralgia or arthritis often involving one large joint of the lower limbs, and erysipelas-like erythema [8]. Patients with MKD show recurrent febrile episodes lasting 4–7 days, different types of rashes, oral aphthosis, vomiting, diarrhea, abdominal pain, lymph node enlargement, arthralgia, and headache [8]. TRAPS) manifests with fever lasting up to 3 weeks, migratory erythematous plaques with underlying myalgia owing to monocytic fasciitis, painful periorbital edema, conjunctivitis, and diffuse joint symptoms. Serosal membrane inflammation may also occur, mainly in the form of pericarditis [8]. The clinical spectrum of CAPS ranges from familial cold autoinflammatory syndrome (FCAS), which is the mildest phenotype, to Muckle-Wells syndrome

(MWS) which is characterized by intermediate severity, and chronic infantile neurological cutaneous articular syndrome (CINCAs), the most severe phenotype, also defined neonatal-onset multisystem inflammatory disease (NOMID). In particular, FCAS presents with recurrent fevers, urticarial rash, arthralgia, and conjunctivitis typically triggered by generalized cold exposure. Ocular abnormalities and progressive sensorineural deafness add to FCAS symptoms in patients with MWS, while children with CINCAs/NOMID are also characterized by destructive arthropathy, chronic aseptic meningitis, intracranial hypertension, and different sequelae of neurological involvement [9]. Blau syndrome and early-onset sarcoidosis are, respectively, the familial and sporadic forms of pediatric granulomatous arthritis, which displays noncaseating epithelioid granulomas inducing arthritis, macular-papular-nodular dermatitis, and granulomatous uveitis [10] (Table 28.1).

Renal amyloid A (AA) amyloidosis is the most serious long-term complication of monogenic AIDs, occurring in 2–25% of patients based on the specific disease, clinical severity, and different penetrance of specific mutations. Although initially confined to the pediatric world, monogenic AIDs are a current matter for adult care physicians. In addition, adult-onset monogenic AIDs can be often related to low-penetrance mutations and manifest with incomplete and/or atypical manifestations. In this context, recurrent acute pericarditis resistant to conventional treatments may arise as unique manifestation of TRAPS, and

Table 28.1 General details and clinical clues of the most frequently recognized monogenic autoinflammatory diseases

Autoinflammatory disease		Gene, locus	Protein mutated	Specific clinical peculiarity
Familial Mediterranean fever		*MEFV*, 16p13.3	Pyrin (marenostrin)	Fever, serositis, erysipelas-like erythema, recurrent arthritis, amyloidosis in untreated or noncompliant patients
Tumor necrosis factor receptor-associated periodic syndrome		*TNFRSF1A*, 12p13.3	Tumor necrosis factor receptor 1 (p55) or CD120a	Fever, migrating erythematous skin rash, conjunctivitis, periorbital edema, arthralgia, serosal involvement, amyloidosis
Cryopyrin-associated periodic syndrome	FCAS	*NLRP3*, 1q44	Cryopyrin	Fever, urticaria-like rash, conjunctivitis, headache, joint symptoms
	MWS			Fever, urticaria-like rash, conjunctivitis, arthralgia, neurosensorial deafness, amyloidosis
	CINCAs/NOMID			Fever, urticaria-like rash, chronic arthropathy, chronic aseptic meningopathy, neurosensorial deafness, uveitis, papilledema, amyloidosis
Mevalonate kinase deficiency		*MVK*, 12q24	Mevalonate kinase	Fever, polymorphous skin rash, abdominal pain, diarrhea, lymph node enlargement, joint symptoms, oral aphthosis
Blau syndrome/early-onset sarcoidosis		*CARD15* (*NOD2*), 16q12.1–13	Caspase recruitment domain-containing protein 15 (CARD15) or nucleotide-binding oligomerization domain 2 (NOD2)	Typical triad of granulomatous arthritis, dermatitis and panuveitis

CINCAs/NOMID chronic infantile neurological cutaneous and articular syndrome/neonatal-onset multisystem inflammatory disease, *FCAS* familial cold autoinflammatory syndrome, *MWS* Muckle-Wells syndrome atypical joint involvement or unusually long-lasting inflammatory attacks may be observed even in FMF patients: this requires a careful clinical evaluation in referral centers for complex patients with ambiguous presentation [2, 3, 11].

Polygenic AIDs

Polygenic AIDs are a large group of diseases with heterogeneous clinical manifestations. Systemic juvenile idiopathic arthritis (sJIA) and adult-onset Still's disease, the adult counterpart to sJIA, are clinically characterized by high-grade fever, arthritis/arthralgia, salmon-colored rash, neutrophil leukocytosis, changes in liver function, and a significant increase in serum ferritin with reduced glycosylated ferritin (<20%). sJIA and Still's disease course may be also complicated by hemophagocytic lymphohistiocytosis, potentially lethal if not adequately treated [12, 13].

PFAPA syndrome is characterized by recurrent fever accompanied by aphthous stomatitis, pharyngitis, and cervical lymphadenitis. Erythematous or papular skin rash, abdominal pain, arthralgia, and headache have been also reported as additional manifestations. Although more commonly identified before the age of 5, PFAPA syndrome has been more recently described as a possible adult-onset febrile entity [14].

Schnitzler's syndrome manifests more frequently between 40 and 50 years with fever, urticarial rash, arthralgia, headache, increased inflammatory markers, and monoclonal gammopathy, especially of IgM type: skin biopsy in these patients usually shows a marked neutrophil infiltration. The clinical picture may progress to a lymphoproliferative disorder, and monoclonal components tend to increase over time; however, risk factors for hematologic progression have not yet been identified [15].

The Role of Infections in AIDs

Systemic inflammation characterizing AIDs is independent of adaptive immune disorders and infections. Conversely, AIDs clinical manifestations are due to hyperactivation of the innate immune system that plays a pivotal role in first-line host defense against infections and in the early healing of tissue injury in a physiologic context [16]. Innate immunity system activity depends on specific sensors defined as pattern recognition receptors (PRR), developed in the inflammatory cells to detect pathogens or stress factors. Both membrane and cytoplasm sensors are known, with toll-like receptors (TLR) being the prototype of transmembrane receptors and nucleotide-binding and oligomerization domain (NOD)-like receptors being the intracellular ones [17]. PRR may be activated by pathogen-associated molecular patterns (PAMPs), responsible for infectious agent-induced inflammation, and damage-associated molecular patterns (DAMPs), which are involved in sterile inflammation related to any tissue lesion. The former are components of pathogens such as muramyl dipeptide, flagellin/rod proteins, bacterial toxins, nucleic acids, and other structural parts of pathogens; the latter are part of damaged cells or extracellular matrix released or degraded after tissue injury. PAMPs and DAMPs do not work independently, as infections may induce cell death with consequent release of DAMPs, resulting in amplification of inflammation. PRR work by inducing the formation of inflammasome, a multimeric protein complex that activates caspase-1. In turn, this results in the activation of IL-1β and IL-18, on one hand, and the induction of highly inflammatory cell death pyroptosis, on the other. Pyroptosis is a key defense against microbial infections, as it is thought to halt the replication of intracellular pathogens by eliminating infected immune cells and amplifying the inflammatory response and presence of phagocytes [18–20].

In addition, the innate inflammatory response activated through the inflammasome may also promote protective adaptive immunity to pathogens. In this regard, it has been demonstrated that the NLRP3 inflammasome is required for protective immunity against *Streptococcus pneumoniae* respiratory infections, *Listeria monocytogenes* and chlamydial infections. On the other hand, pathogens try to contain the inflammasome activity to guarantee their own survival, as for *Legionella pneumophila* and *Yersinia enterocolitica*

Also viruses interact with the inflammasome. Indeed, NLRP3-deficient mice were shown to have increased mortality to influenza infection when compared to wild-type mice. Moreover, influenza A virus and many other viruses have been found to inhibit inflammasome-mediated cytokine production. Equally, NLRP3 inflammasome has also been reported to play an active role against fungal pathogens, such as *Candida albicans*, and helminths, such as *Schistosoma mansoni* [21].

The Role of the Microbiome in AIDs

Great interest has been directed to the role of the microbiome in the development of "sterile" inflammation. Recent studies have proved that either depletion or elimination of the microbiome or changes in diet with accompanying changes in gut microbiota lead to the improvement of inflammasome-mediated osteomyelitis and gouty arthritis. Indeed, recent studies have claimed that sterile inflammation is at least partially depending on the presence of PAMPs derived from commensal microbes, while the autoinfectome, a term used to describe the history of infectious and commensal microbes encountered over time, seems to be deeply involved in the development of systemic inflammatory diseases. In this context, the disruption of intestinal milieu and the impairment of gut homeostasis have been thought of as main contributors for susceptibility to inflammatory bowel diseases and also AIDs [22].

In the case of FMF, restructuring of the gut microbiome during febrile attacks has been described with depletion of total numbers of bacteria, loss of diversity, and shift toward *Bacteroides*, *Firmicutes*, and *Proteobacteria*. Conversely, during symptom-free periods the number of bacteria seems to be comparable to the control group, though bacterial diversity is already deviant from the norm [23]. Of note, gut bacterial diversity has been found to depend on the allele carrier status, while treatment with colchicine, the mainstay of FMF therapy, does not normalize these profiles [24]. Also, a systemic reactivity against commensal gut microbiota has been found in FMF patients as a potential consequence of hypersensitivity of the inflammasome, leading to inflammation and secondary translocation of bacteria and bacterial antigens through the gut barrier [25].

A few data are currently available on the role of the microbiome on other monogenic AIDs, as for adult-onset Still's disease and Schnitzler's disease. In this context, chronic recurrent multifocal osteomyelitis (CRMO) represents a paradigm of AIDs conditioned by the microbiome. This is a rare autoinflammatory bone disorder characterized by a wide clinical spectrum ranging from asymptomatic inflammation of single bones to CRMO. Especially among adults, CRMO is frequently associated with skin neutrophilic manifestations and might occur in the context of SAPHO, an acronym indicating CRMO associated with synovitis, acne, pustulosis, hyperostosis, and osteitis. Although the pathogenesis is unknown, recent findings have shown that disturbances in the gut microbiome may contribute to sterile bone inflammation. In detail, CRMO mice on a high-fat diet have shown a protection from the development of aseptic osteomyelitis. Accordingly, a high-fat diet exhibited a shift toward *Lactobacillus* spp. in the gut microbiome along with a reduced IL-1β expression, while mice on a low-fat diet exhibited a number of inflammation-associated microbes, including *Prevotella* spp. Interestingly, fecal transplant from high-fat diet mice to young mice resulted in protection from CRMO, while transplant from low-fat diet mice accelerated the development of osteomyelitis. Data on the effects of diet or other environmental factors on CRMO are currently lacking in humans. However, although bone cultures are typically sterile and antibiotic therapy is usually unsuccessful, an aberrant response to bacteria, especially *Propionibacterium acnes*, has been postulated in adults with SAPHO syndrome [26, 27] (see also Chap. 33).

In the case of PFAPA syndrome, the curative role of tonsillectomy has led to explore the microbiome of tonsils as an inflammatory stimulus or disease modulator. In particular, tonsils from

PFAPA patients seem to contain more likely *Candida albicans*, cyanobacteria, *Prevotella* and *Synergistetes* and less likely (or with less abundance) *Staphylococcus aureus* and *varicella-zoster virus* than controls. Conversely, to date no differences have emerged in the frequency of nasopharyngeal pathogens in PFAPA patients [28].

Conclusions

Current data on the role of the microbiome in AIDs are lacking. However, the few studies performed on this issue seem to suggest that commensal microbes may consistently influence both pathogenesis and clinical manifestations of these diseases. Although further studies are required, these clues have been glimpsed at in patients with FMF and PFAPA syndrome along with animal models of CRMO. However, they need to be investigated in all other monogenic AIDs. Therefore, how microbes may influence disease onset, clinical course, severity, and response to treatments are all topics for research in the near future. In the same way, how microbial components and metabolites in the blood may serve as surrogate markers in daily clinical practice and whether reorienting the gut microbiome may represent a therapeutic opportunity in some cases are also attractive sparks for future research.

References

1. Masters SL, et al. Horror autoinflammaticus: the molecular pathophysiology of autoinflammatory disease. Annu Rev Immunol. 2009;27:621–68.
2. Rigante D, et al. The hereditary autoinflammatory disorders uncovered. Autoimmun Rev. 2014;13(9):892–900.
3. Cantarini L, et al. Bridging the gap between the clinician and the patient with cryopyrin-associated periodic syndromes. Int J Immunopathol Pharmacol. 2011;24(4):827–36.
4. Rigante D. A systematic approach to autoinflammatory syndromes: a spelling booklet for the beginner. Expert Rev Clin Immunol. 2017;13(6):571–97.
5. Rigante D, et al. Autoinflammatory diseases and cardiovascular manifestations. Ann Med. 2011;43(5):341–6.
6. Stabile A, et al. The clinical spectrum and treatment options of macrophage activation syndrome in the pediatric age. Eur Rev Med Pharmacol Sci. 2006;10(2):53–9.
7. Lopalco G, et al. Interleukin-1 as a common denominator from autoinflammatory to autoimmune disorders: premises, perils, and perspectives. Mediat Inflamm. 2015;2015:194864.
8. Stojanov S, Kastner DL. Familial autoinflammatory diseases: genetics, pathogenesis and treatment. Curr Opin Rheumatol. 2005;17(5):586–99.
9. Kuemmerle-Deschner JB, et al. Diagnostic criteria for cryopyrin-associated periodic syndrome (CAPS). Ann Rheum Dis. 2017;76(6):942–7.
10. Rose CD, et al. Blau syndrome: cross-sectional data from a multicentre study of clinical, radiological and functional outcomes. Rheumatology (Oxford). 2015;54(6):1008–16.
11. Rigante D, et al. The pharmacologic basis of treatment with colchicine in children with familial Mediterranean fever. Eur Rev Med Pharmacol Sci. 2006;10(4):173–8.
12. Kadavath S, Efthimiou P. Adult-onset Still's disease-pathogenesis, clinical manifestations, and new treatment options. Ann Med. 2015;47(1):6–14.
13. Cimaz R. Systemic-onset juvenile idiopathic arthritis. Autoimmun Rev. 2016;15(9):931–4.
14. Vigo G, Zulian F. Periodic fevers with aphthous stomatitis, pharyngitis, and adenitis (PFAPA). Autoimmun Rev. 2012;12(1):52–5.
15. de Koning HD. Schnitzler's syndrome: lessons from 281 cases. Clin Transl Allergy. 2014;4:41.
16. Manthiram K, et al. The monogenic autoinflammatory diseases define new pathways in human innate immunity and inflammation. Nat Immunol. 2017;18(8):832–42.
17. Dolasia K, et al. TLRs/NLRs: shaping the landscape of host immunity. Int Rev Immunol. 2017;37:3–19.
18. Carta S, et al. Dysregulated IL-1beta secretion in autoinflammatory diseases: a matter of stress? Front Immunol. 2017;8:345.
19. Kim YK, Shin JS, Nahm MH. NOD-like receptors in infection, immunity, and diseases. Yonsei Med J. 2016;57(1):5–14.
20. Lamkanfi M, Dixit VM. Mechanisms and functions of inflammasomes. Cell. 2014;157(5):1013–22.
21. Dunne A. Inflammasome activation: from inflammatory disease to infection. Biochem Soc Trans. 2011;39(2):669–73.
22. Lupfer CR, Rodriguez A, Kanneganti TD. Inflammasome activation by nucleic acids and nucleosomes in sterile inflammation... or is it sterile? FEBS J. 2017;284(15):2363–74.
23. Khachatryan ZA, et al. Predominant role of host genetics in controlling the composition of gut microbiota. PLoS One. 2008;3(8):e3064.
24. Ktsoyan ZA, et al. Management of familial Mediterranean fever by colchicine does not normalize the altered profile of microbial long chain fatty acids in the human metabolome. Front Cell Infect Microbiol. 2013;3:2.

25. Manukyan GP, et al. Elevated systemic antibodies towards commensal gut microbiota in autoinflammatory condition. PLoS One. 2008;3(9):e3172.
26. Hofmann SR, et al. Chronic nonbacterial osteomyelitis: pathophysiological concepts and current treatment strategies. J Rheumatol. 2016;43(11):1956–64.
27. Ferguson PJ, Laxer RM. New discoveries in CRMO: IL-1beta, the neutrophil, and the microbiome implicated in disease pathogenesis in Pstpip2-deficient mice. Semin Immunopathol. 2015;37(4):407–12.
28. Manthiram K, Lapidus S, Edwards K. Unraveling the pathogenesis of periodic fever, aphthous stomatitis, pharyngitis, and cervical adenitis through genetic, immunologic, and microbiologic discoveries: an update. Curr Opin Rheumatol. 2017;29(5):493–9.

Histiocytoses

29

Augusto Vaglio, Rossana Rocco, Julien Haroche, and Jean-François Emile

Abbreviations

CNS	Central nervous system
CTLs	Cytotoxic T cells
ECD	Erdheim-Chester disease
HHV6	Human herpesvirus 6
HIV	Human immunodeficiency virus
HLH	Haemophagocytic lymphohistiocytosis
IFN-y	Interferon-y
IFNα	Interferon-α
IL-12	Interleukin-12
LCH	Langerhans cell histiocytosis
MRI	Magnetic resonance imaging
mTOR	Mammalian target of rapamycin
NK	Natural killer
PET	Positron emission tomography
RDD	Rosai-Dorfman disease
Th1	T-helper 1

A. Vaglio (✉) · R. Rocco
Nephrology Unit, University Hospital, Parma, Italy
e-mail: augusto.vaglio@virgilio.it

J. Haroche
Department of Internal Medicine, French Reference Center for Rare Auto-immune and Systemic Diseases, Institut E3M, AP-HP, Pitié-Salpêtrière Hospital, Paris, France

Université Pierre et Marie Curie, University Paris 6, Paris, France

J.-F. Emile
EA4340 and Pathology Department, Versailles University and Ambroise Paré Hospital, Boulogne, France

Introduction

Histiocytoses are rare, often systemic diseases hallmarked by tissue infiltration by abnormal histiocytes bearing peculiar morphological and immunohistochemical characteristics. Despite the significant advances made in the past decades in defining the clinical and molecular profile of this spectrum of diseases, the cells of origin of the different forms of histiocytosis are still incompletely understood. The abnormal histiocytes that infiltrate target organs or tissues share the phenotype of dendritic cells and monocytes/macrophages. Macrophages are usually large ovoid cells with pleiotropic functions (e.g. clearance of apoptotic cells and pathogens), whereas dendritic cells are stellate cells specialised in antigen presentation and T-cell activation. Langerhans cells are a subset of dendritic cells physiologically residing in the skin; they express characteristic antigens such as CD1a and possess Birbeck granules that can be seen on electron microscopy [1].

Until recently, the histiocytoses were classified as Langerhans cell, non-Langerhans cell and malignant. Studies performed during the past few

G. Ragab et al. (eds.), *The Microbiome in Rheumatic Diseases and Infection*,
https://doi.org/10.1007/978-3-319-79026-8_29

years have revolutionised the field: in particular, the discovery of recurrent somatic mutations of some proto-oncogenes shed light on the aetiopathogenesis of several histiocytic disorders and provided the rationale for targeted treatments that have now largely replaced previous empirical approaches. In parallel, large cohort studies have been performed; these have allowed a better understanding of the natural history of the disease, contributed to a better phenotyping of these disorders and their subsets and led to the identification of previously unrecognised overlap forms of Langerhans and non-Langerhans cell histiocytoses [2], which suggest a common ontogeny of the pathologic histiocytes. These significant advances have culminated into a new classification of histiocytoses and neoplasms of the macrophage-dendritic cell lineages (Table 29.1) that comprises five distinct groups: the "L" group, including classical Langerhans cell histiocytosis (LCH), Erdheim-Chester disease (ECD) and overlap forms; the "C" group, mainly including cutaneous and mucocutaneous forms; the "M" group, encompassing primary malignant and secondary malignant forms, the latter occurring after or sometimes simultaneously with another haematologic neoplasm; the "R" group, covering Rosai-Dorfman disease (RDD) and other non-cutaneous, non-Langerhans cell histiocytoses; and the "H" group, comprising haemophagocytic lymphohistiocytosis (HLH), either primary or secondary to infectious or immune-mediated diseases [3].

Table 29.1 Revised classification of histiocytoses according to Emile et al. (adapted from Ref. [3])

L group
Langerhans cell histiocytosis
Erdheim-Chester disease
Indeterminate cell histiocytosis
Mixed Langerhans cell and Erdheim-Chester (overlap histiocytosis)
C group
Cutaneous non-Langerhans cell histiocytosis
Xanthogranuloma family (e.g. juvenile xanthogranulomatosis, adult xanthogranuloma)
Non-xanthogranuloma family (e.g. cutaneous Rosai-Dorfman disease)
Cutaneous non-Langerhans cell histiocytosis with a major systemic component
R group
Familial Rosai-Dorfman disease
Sporadic Rosai-Dorfman disease (e.g. classical and extra-nodal, associated with neoplasia or autoimmune disease)
M Group
Primary malignant histiocytoses
Secondary malignant histiocytoses (e.g. following or associated with another haematologic malignancy)
H group
Primary haemophagocytic lymphohistiocytosis (e.g. monogenic inherited conditions)
Secondary haemophagocytic lymphohistiocytosis (non-Mendelian)
Haemophagocytic lymphohistiocytosis of unknown/uncertain origin

Since this *textbook* focuses on systemic rheumatic disorders and their relationships with infections, this *chapter* will mainly deal with systemic forms of histiocytosis of the L, R and H groups, as they may share clinical features with rheumatic diseases or recognise, in some cases, infectious triggers.

Langerhans Cell Histiocytosis

LCH is an often systemic histiocytic disorder characterised by tissue infiltration by $CD1a^+$/$CD207^+$ histiocytes (Fig. 29.1). The pathologic histiocytes in LCH are mononucleated cells with coffee bean- or kidney-shaped nuclei that diffusely infiltrate target tissues, often accompanied by abundant eosinophils and multinucleated giant cells [3]. Electron microscopy may reveal the presence of Birbeck granules, although the search for this hallmark ultrastructural feature has been replaced in clinical practice by immunohistochemical analysis on paraffin-embedded samples for typical Langerhans cell markers such as CD1a and CD207 (Figs. 29.1 and 29.2) [3]. Elegant studies have explored the origin of pathologic histiocytes in LCH: transcriptional profiling showed that LCH cells are more similar to their bone marrow-derived monocyte and dendritic cell precursors than to epidermal Langerhans cells [4]. In line with this view, studies tracking the $BRAF^{V600E}$ mutation (which is found in LCH lesions in approximately 55% of the cases) in

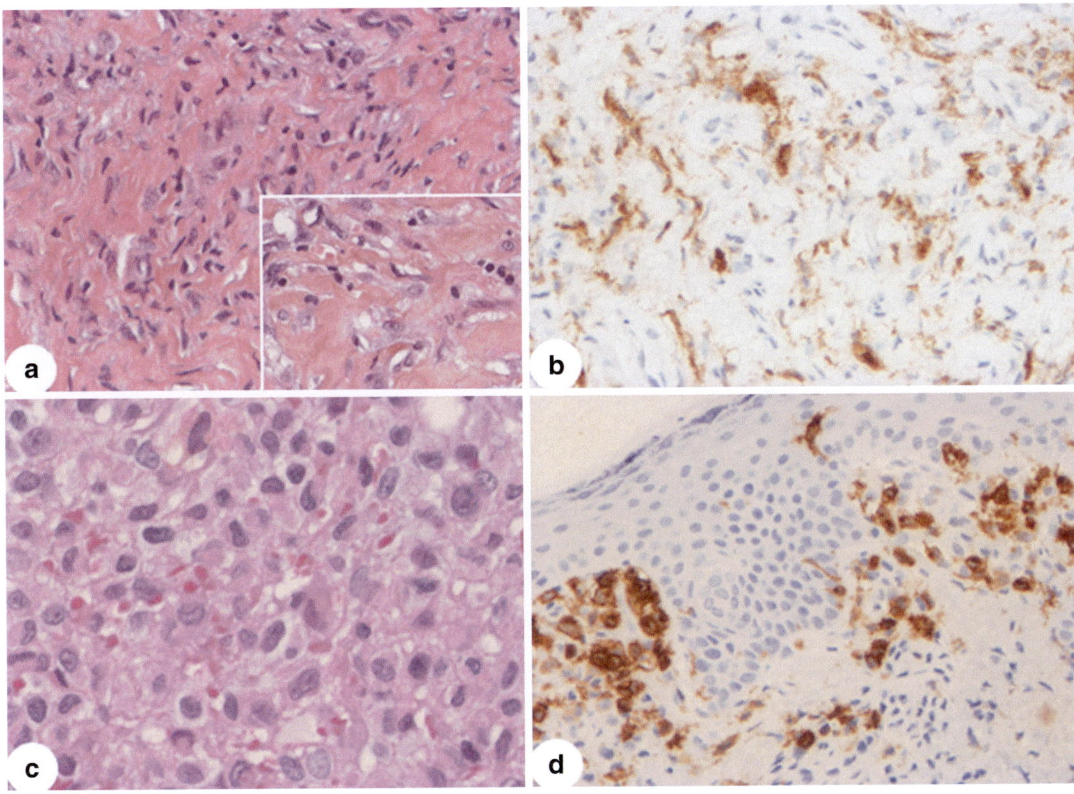

Fig. 29.1 Main histopathologic characteristics of Erdheim-Chester disease (ECD) and Langerhans cell histiocytosis (LCH). (**a**) Perirenal tissue biopsy from a patient with ECD showing fibrosis with histiocytes (some of which have a foamy cytoplasm) and small lymphocytes (inset). Haematoxylin and eosin (H&E), original magnification 200× (400× in the inset). (**b**) CD68+ immunostaining decorates the histiocytes in an ECD case. (**c**) Skin biopsy from an LCH patient shows infiltration by histiocytes with small, round or oval nuclei (H&E, 400×). In (**d**) the histiocytes shown in C are CD207+ (200×)

haematopoietic precursors were able to detect this mutation in $CD34^+$ bone marrow cells in some (although not all) cases [5]. These data suggest that LCH derives from aberrant progenitor cells that acquire somatic mutations such as *BRAF*^{V600E} and that eventually infiltrate target tissues. Mutations other than *BRAF*^{V600E} have been detected in LCH, such as those involving *MAP2K1*, which encodes MEK1; *BRAF* and *MAP2K1* mutations seem to be mutually exclusive [6]. Overall, the genetic abnormalities encountered in LCH lead to activation of the RAF-MEK-ERK pathway.

LCH is more frequent in children; its annual incidence is 5–9 cases/million in subjects younger than 15 years of age and declines to 1 case/million in patients older than 15 years of age [7]. In adults, LCH with lung involvement is strongly associated with smoking. LCH may vary from organ-limited, clinically silent forms to disseminated and life-threatening forms. Although nearly all organs or systems can be involved, the most frequently affected sites are the bone (80% of patients), the skin (30–40%), the pituitary gland (25%), the bone marrow, the liver, the spleen and the lungs (all around 10–15%) [8]. Lung involvement is more frequent in adults [1]. The main "risk organ" is the haematopoietic system, whose involvement is commonly associated with liver and spleen infiltration.

Bone lesions are very common in LCH and frequently involve the skull, the jaw, the spine (especially the cervical tract), the ribs, the pelvis and the long bones. Bone lesions in LCH are usu-

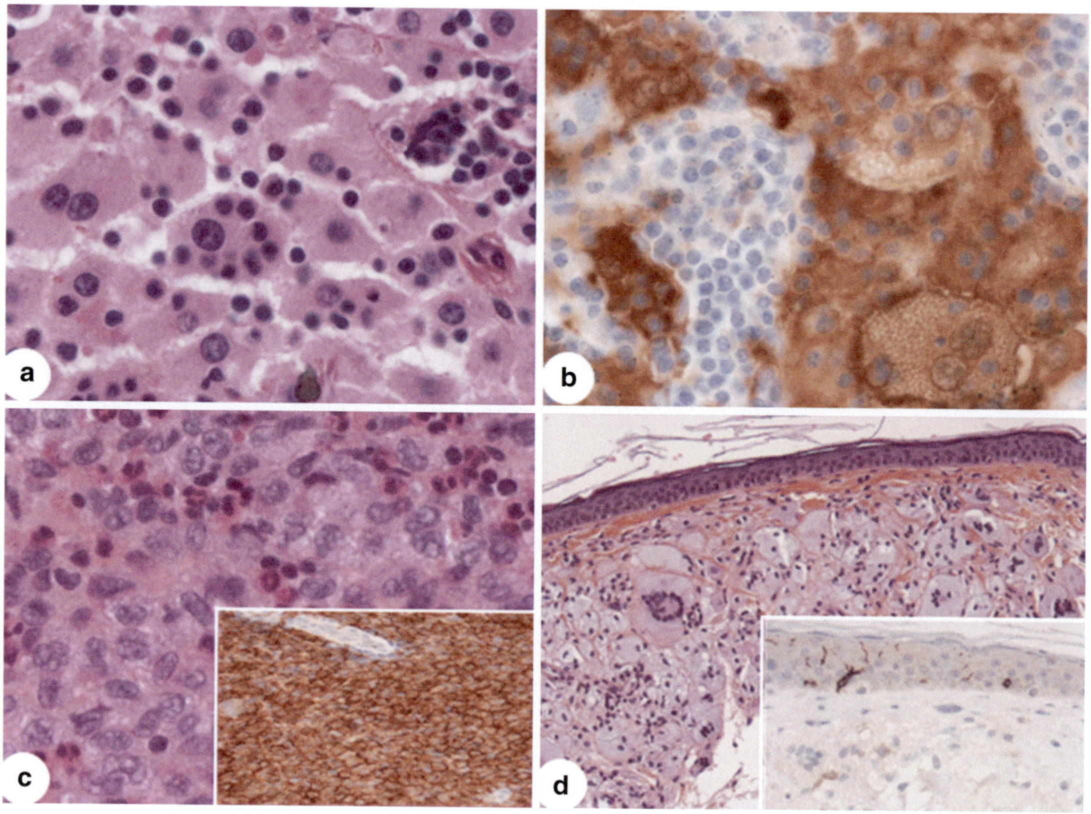

Fig. 29.2 Main histopathologic features of Rosai-Dorfman disease and of a case with overlap Langerhans cell histiocytosis (LCH) and Erdheim-Chester disease (ECD). (**a**) Lymph node biopsy in a patient with RDD showing small lymphocytes, plasma cells and histiocytes with images of emperipolesis (see text for details) (H&E, 400×). (**b**) In an RDD biopsy, the histiocytes are S-100+ and show emperipolesis (400×). (**c**, **d**) Showing images of a patient with overlap LCH-ECD. (**c**) Tissue biopsy showing LCH histiocytes which stain positive for CD1a (H&E, 400×, CD1a staining in the inset, 200×). (**d**) Skin biopsy from an ECD lesion showing diffuse infiltration by foamy histiocytes with large cytoplasm and small nuclei; multinucleated Touton giant cells are also observed (H&E, 100×); the histiocytes are CD1a negative (inset, 200×)

ally lytic (Fig. 29.3) but may be accompanied by soft tissue masses. They may cause fractures or vertebral collapse, or when localised to the maxillofacial bones or the skull base, they can cause scalp or facial swelling, otitis media, hearing loss, mastoiditis, loss of teeth and other cranial or central nervous system (CNS) manifestations [1].

CNS involvement may be severe and usually consists of either tumour-like or degenerative lesions, which may coexist. Patients with tumour-like lesions have a wide spectrum of neurological manifestations, ranging from focal neurological deficits to cranial nerve palsies, seizures and symptoms secondary to intracranial hypertension. Conversely, neurodegenerative complications of LCH lead to progressive cerebellar syndrome, cognitive impairment, tetrapyramidal syndrome and other slowly progressive manifestations. Focal CNS lesions may mimic primary or metastatic CNS neoplasms, granulomatous or infectious diseases, and can involve almost every portion of the CNS, with particular tropism for the hypothalamic-pituitary axis and the brainstem [1].

Skin lesions include brown to purplish papules, eczematous rashes resembling *Candida* infections and pustular, purpuric, vesicular or papulo-nodular lesions; oral lesions such as intra-

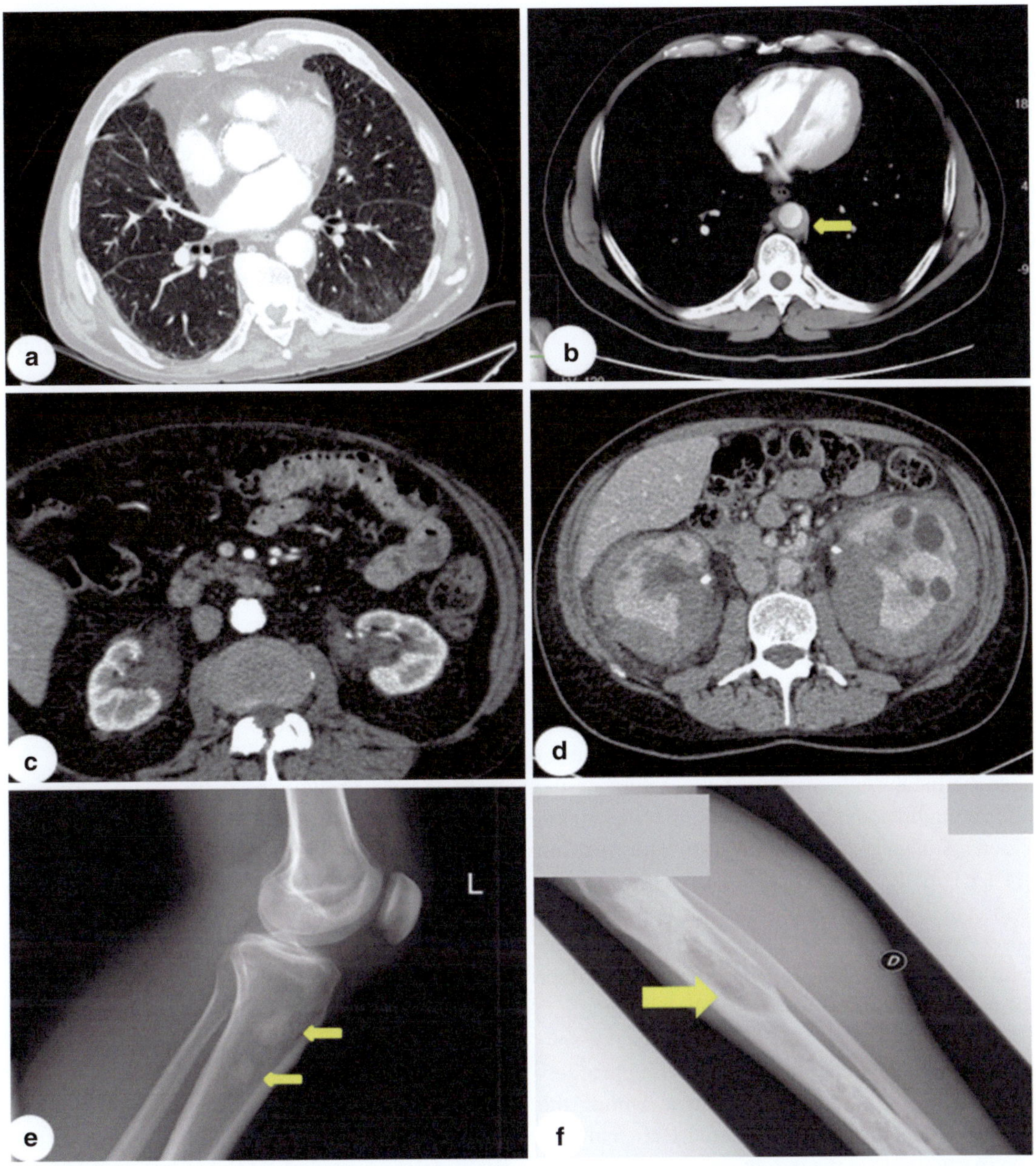

Fig. 29.3 Imaging findings in patients with Erdheim-Chester disease (ECD) and overlap Langerhans cell histiocytosis and ECD (LCH-ECD). (**a**, **b**) Showing thoracic involvement in LCH-ECD cases: (**a**) CT scan showing interstitial lung fibrosis, well represented in interlobular septa; (**b**) CT scan of thoracic aorta involvement (periaortitis) (arrow). (**c**, **d**) Showing abdominal involvement in patients with ECD: (**c**) abdominal CT scan shows infiltration of both kidneys around the renal pelvis; (**d**) CT scan showing perirenal infiltration with typical "hairy kidney" appearance. (**e**, **f**) Showing bone involvement in ECD and overlap LCH-ECD: (**e**) plain radiograph of osteosclerotic bone lesions localised in the diaphysis of the tibia in ECD (arrows); (**f**) plain radiograph of osteolytic bone lesion localised in the tibia in a LCH-ECD overlap case (arrow)

oral masses, gingivitis, ulcers and loose teeth may also occur. The involvement of the haematopoietic system represents an adverse prognostic factor in LCH. Patients with bone marrow involvement often show peripheral blood count abnormalities such as anaemia and thrombocytopenia, but some patients may have no abnormalities at all. Importantly, bone marrow involvement is usually associated with liver and spleen infiltration leading to organomegaly, tumour-like or cystic lesions and eventually organ failure.

Among the other LCH-associated manifestations, it is worth mentioning that diabetes insipidus is the most frequent endocrinopathy; it can precede or be the sole clinical manifestation of LCH in many cases. About 15% of patients with an apparently isolated diabetes insipidus were found to have LCH [9]. Lung involvement is rare and is best diagnosed using high-resolution computed tomography, which usually reveals interstitial thickening (Fig. 29.3) as well as small cysts and nodules especially in the upper and mid lung.

The diagnosis of LCH relies on histological examination of the affected tissue and immunohistochemical confirmation of the nature of the infiltrating histiocytes. Biopsy of the bone or skin lesions is usually preferred, but its interpretation must be in the context of the systemic disease manifestations and the possible differential diagnoses, which include ECD (that can also overlap with LCH), juvenile xanthogranuloma, other forms of histiocytosis and multiple myeloma.

Treatment of LCH is based on the use of several chemotherapeutic drugs along with glucocorticoids and, in some cases, surgery. Among the most used chemotherapeutic agents are vinblastine (particularly in the induction phase, in combination with glucocorticoids) and cladribine [1]. Response to treatment is better for symptomatic tumour-like lesions than for degenerative lesions, for which treatment options are mainly empirical and include all-trans retinoic acid and intravenous immunoglobulins. LCH patients bearing the $BRAF^{V600E}$ mutation have an increased frequency of risk organ involvement and show poorer response to standard therapy with glucocorticoids and vinblastine; additionally, they are more prone to relapse and more frequently experience permanent sequelae of disease and treatment [8]. To date, selective inhibition of $BRAF^{V600E}$ with vemurafenib or other agents is not yet of proven efficacy. Further studies are needed to evaluate the efficacy of targeted therapies and to tailor treatment on the basis of the underlying mutations.

Erdheim-Chester Disease

ECD is a rare histiocytosis of the L group mainly occurring in adulthood, hallmarked by the accumulation of "foamy" histiocytes staining positive for CD68, negative for CD1a and CD207 (Langerin) (Figs. 29.1 and 29.2) and usually negative for S100. In addition to tissue accumulation of foamy, lipid-laden macrophages, the pathology of ECD also shows abundant fibrosis, chronic lymphoplasmacytic infiltrates and often Touton giant cells. ECD is usually a multisystemic disease, with its hallmark feature being the symmetric involvement of the long bones that typically produces osteosclerotic lesions (Fig. 29.3) [10].

ECD was initially thought to be a primary inflammatory disease: in the affected tissues, the pathologic histiocytes express several chemokines and their receptors and also produce pro-inflammatory cytokines. In addition, serum cytokine profiling of ECD patients showed a prominent T-helper 1 (Th1) polarisation, with upregulation of interleukin (IL)-12, interferon (IFN)-g-inducible protein-10 and monocyte chemotactic protein-1 [11]. However, the recent identification of mutations or translocations in several proto-oncogenes or genes controlling cell proliferation such as *BRAF*, *MAP2K1*, *NRAS* and *KRAS* supports the hypothesis that ECD is a clonal disease [12]. The infiltrating histiocytes in ECD also show activation of the mammalian target of rapamycin (mTOR) pathway, which is involved in the control of cell metabolism and proliferation [13]. The clinical relevance of these findings is strongly supported by the evidence that targeting the mutated kinases and mTOR often leads to objective responses in ECD patients [14]. Overall, a new concept of inflammatory myeloid neoplasia is emerging for ECD as well as for LCH [1]. However, the cell of origin of the ECD histiocytes is still unclear.

ECD is an extremely rare disease, with no more than 800 cases reported up to 2016; however, its prevalence has dramatically increased in the last decade, mainly due to increased recognition of the disease. ECD usually occurs in adults with only few paediatric cases reported in the literature; it affects men more frequently than women (M:F ratio of approximately 3:1), and its incidence peaks in the fifth decade [1].

Among the clinical complications of ECD, involvement of the long bones is definitely the most common as it occurs in nearly 90% of the cases. The diaphyses and metaphyses of long bones (particularly of the lower limbs) are usually involved symmetrically (Fig. 29.3). They show increased ^{99}Tc uptake on bone scans; X-rays or other imaging studies such as computed tomography or magnetic resonance imaging (MRI) demonstrate that these lesions are generally osteosclerotic. Bone pain is common in ECD patients, as it occurs in 50% of the cases.

Another typical finding in ECD is retroperitoneal infiltration, which usually involves the adipose surrounding the kidneys, the renal pelvis and the proximal ureter, giving rise to the so-called hairy kidneys; peri-ureteral infiltration is a common cause of ureteral obstruction (Fig. 29.3) with consequent hydronephrosis and sometimes renal failure. The abdominal aortic wall and the surrounding retroperitoneum are also commonly infiltrated, and so is the adventitia of thoracic aorta (Fig. 29.3) and of the origin of the epiaortic arteries; the involvement of the whole (thoraco-abdominal) aorta is usually referred to as "coated aorta" and is found in 30% of the cases [10]. Heart involvement is also a prominent feature of ECD (40% of patients) and is also considered an adverse prognostic factor. ECD affects the pericardium (often with pericardial effusion which can lead to tamponade) and the myocardium, where the infiltration almost invariably involves the right atrium and the right atrioventricular sulcus (Fig. 29.4). Entrapment of the right coronary artery is not uncommon. Interestingly, heart involvement is usually associated with a disseminated disease [15].

The CNS is involved in 25–50% of the cases. ECD lesions are often located in the brainstem and in the dentate nuclei of the cerebellum but may develop almost anywhere in the CNS and also involve the meninges; these lesions are usually tumour-like and gadolinium enhancing on MRI (Fig. 29.4) and may mimic meningiomas, granulomatous diseases or even CNS infiltration by LCH or Rosai-Dorfman disease. Spinal cord infiltration is also reported. As in LCH, CNS infiltration in ECD can also cause degenerative lesions especially in the cerebellum. Overall, CNS lesions clinically cause a variety of neurological syndromes, the most frequent of which include cerebellar (ataxia and dysarthria) and brainstem symptoms. Interestingly, ECD patients also have diffuse grey matter reduction and may progressively develop cognitive dysfunction [16].

Other manifestations of ECD include skin lesions, particularly xanthelasmas, neuroendocrine abnormalities such as diabetes insipidus, other endocrine dysfunctions (e.g. hypogonadism, adrenal insufficiency), infiltration of serosa and effusion, interstitial lung disease and orbital infiltration with consequent exophthalmos (Fig. 29.4) [10].

The diagnosis of ECD relies on the demonstration of typical long bone lesions and compatible histology, according to the criteria proposed by Veyssier-Belot et al. [17]. Biopsies of the affected lesions are currently required not only for the diagnosis but also for molecular testing of the aforementioned mutations involving *BRAF* and other genes. Skin and perirenal tissue lesions are the easiest to biopsy and usually yield representative material. A thorough evaluation of disease extent and severity is based on a combination of imaging techniques dedicated to the study of specific organs or systems (e.g. cardiac or CNS MRI, bone scintigraphy) and laboratory tests; however, metabolic imaging studies such as positron emission tomography (PET) have become crucial in the evaluation of disease activity and response to therapy [13, 14].

The treatment of ECD has been empirical for several years, based on the use of various chemotherapeutic or immunosuppressive agents and

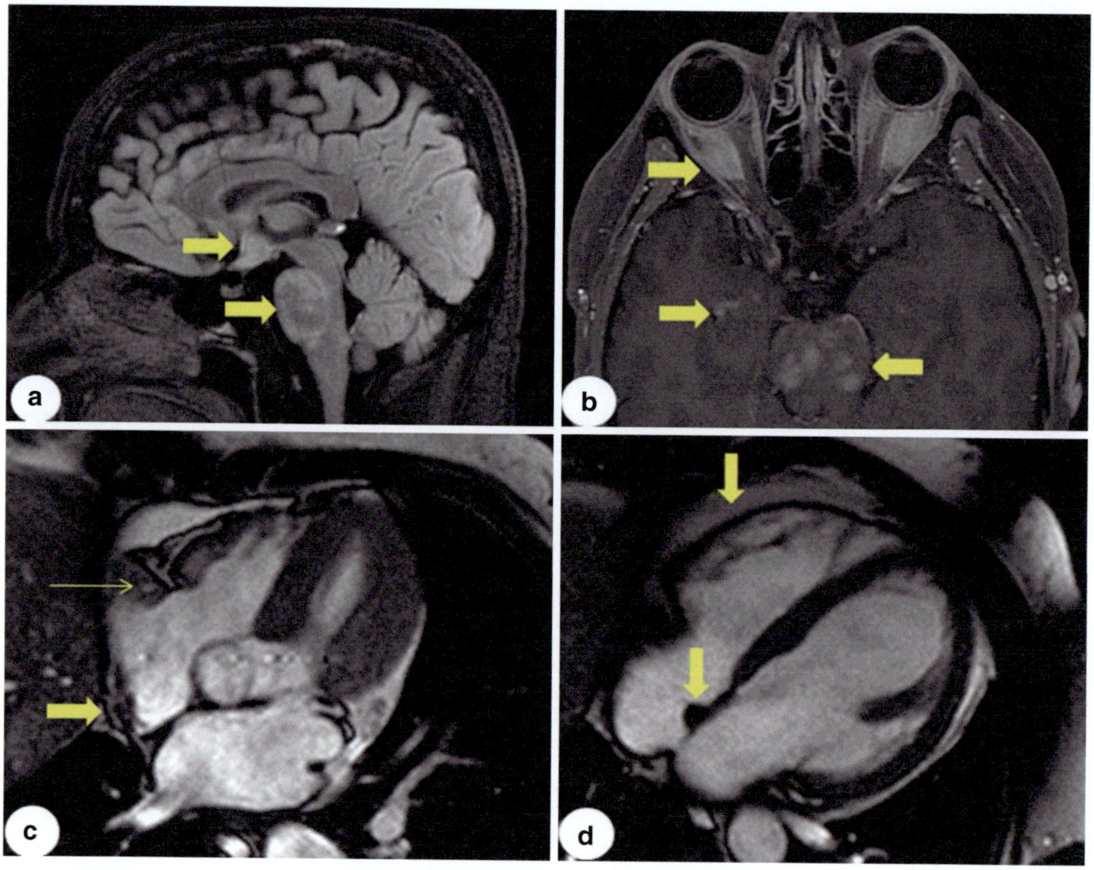

Fig. 29.4 Brain and cardiac imaging findings in patients with Erdheim-Chester disease (ECD) and overlap Langerhans cell histiocytosis and ECD (LCH-ECD). (**a**, **b**) Central nervous system involvement in an ECD patient: (**a**) brain MRI (sagittal) showing pathologic and increased gadolinium uptake in the hypothalamus (upper arrow) and pons (lower arrow). (**b**) Brain MRI (axial): irregularly increased intensity in the pons (right-hand arrow), parahippocampal region (lower left-hand arrow) and retro-orbital space (upper left-hand arrow), where the pathologic solid tissue surrounds the optical nerve. (**c**, **d**) Heart involvement in ECD and in an overlap LCH-ECD: (**c**) cardiac MRI (four-chamber view) in a case of LCH-ECD overlap form: solid tissue in the posterior wall of the right atrium (thick arrow) and in the right atrium-ventricle sulcus, surrounding the right coronary artery (thin arrow); (**d**) cardiac MRI in a ECD case: pericardial thickening with effusion (upper arrow) and a round mass within the right side of the atrial septum wall (lower arrow)

glucocorticoids. A major breakthrough was the discovery of the efficacy of interferon-α (IFNα), which is thought to induce terminal differentiation or immune-mediated killing of immature, pathologic histiocytes. IFNα (or its pegylated form, peg-IFNα) has largely been used for ECD; it is able to induce objective responses and still represents the first-line therapy for ECD in *BRAF* wild-type patients, although its use is limited by significant toxicity [18].

The discovery of the high prevalence of *BRAF*^{V600E} mutations in ECD (approximately 55–60% of the cases) led to the use of its specific inhibitor vemurafenib, which proved dramatically effective in inducing rapid and sustained objective responses [14]. Vemurafenib is therefore considered the first-line therapeutic option in *BRAF*^{V600E} patients with multisystemic or organ-threatening disease [1]. A panoply of other drugs have been proposed for ECD, including biologic agents targeting the IL-1 receptor [19], the MEK inhibitor cobimetinib [20] and the mTOR inhibitor sirolimus [15]. Overall, the advances made in the diagnosis and management of ECD have dramatically changed its prognosis: while in the late 1990s the 3-year mortality associated with the disease was reported to be up to 60% [17], it has dropped to approximately 20% in most recent years [1]. However, long-term follow-up studies are needed to ascertain the efficacy and safety of newer agents for the treatment of ECD.

Rosai-Dorfman Disease

RDD, also known as "sinus histiocytosis with massive lymphadenopathy" since Rosai's and Dorfman's seminal description, is another rare form of non-Langerhans cell histiocytosis characterised by tissue (often lymph node) infiltration by $CD68^+/CD1a^-/S100^+$ histiocytes; the infiltrating histiocytes show emperipolesis, a non-destructive form of phagocytosis of lymphocytes and erythrocytes (Fig. 29.2) [21]. In the affected lymph nodes, there is marked sinusoidal dilation containing histiocytes, plasma cells and lymphocytes. In the affected extra-nodal sites, pathologic examination discloses increased amounts of fibrosis and fewer histiocytes; as $IgG4^+$ plasma cells are not uncommon in RDD lesions, RDD- and IgG4-related disease may be in differential diagnosis.

RDD is hallmarked by heterogeneity both in its phenotype and clinical course. Patients with RDD may have concurrent haematologic (e.g. Hodgkin and non-Hodgkin's lymphoma) or autoimmune disorders (e.g. systemic lupus erythematosus, juvenile idiopathic arthritis) and overlapping histiocytic diseases such as LCH and ECD [1]. Interestingly, systemic lesions whose pathology is compatible with RDD can be found in patients with autoimmune lymphoproliferative syndromes and hereditary histiocytic conditions [22]. This broad spectrum of RDD-associated disorders suggests that RDD has an uncertain pathogenesis and that multiple mechanisms can be involved. Unlike LCH and ECD, RDD does not seem to be driven by *BRAF*^{V600E} mutations; evidence supporting the role of other somatic mutations is lacking. Only in extremely rare cases of familial RDD have germline mutations in the *SLC29A3* gene been described [23]. Therefore, it has been hypothesised that immune-mediated mechanisms leading to the accumulation of pathologic histiocytes in the tissue are involved. Infectious triggers have also been postulated; this topic will be discussed below in the paragraph on infections and histiocytoses.

RDD arises more commonly in children or young adults, although it can really occur at any age; it seems to be more frequent in African-Americans than in Caucasians and has male predominance. Most RDD patients present with symptoms of fever, sometimes night sweats, weight loss and massive, usually non-painful, cervical lymphadenopathy, which raises the suspicion of lymphoma. Actually, the diagnostic work-up of RDD is similar to that of lymphoma; in addition, autoimmune diseases and viral infections must be searched for [24].

According to the revised classification of histiocytoses by the Histiocyte Society [3] (Table 29.1), classic RDD (with isolated involvement of single or regional lymph nodes) must be distinguished from RDD involving the skin or other organs. Extra-nodal RDD accounts for up to 40% of all RDD cases, the most frequently involved sites being the skin, the head and neck region, the bone (with mostly osteosclerotic lesions) and the CNS. Intracranial RDD has an intriguing presentation as it often develops without extracranial lymphadenopathy and may present as masses involving the meninges (commonly with pleocytosis in the cerebrospinal fluid); unlike in LCH and ECD, intracranial lesions in RDD do not cause neurodegenerative complications [1].

The clinical course of RDD is extremely variable: sustained phases of remission and disease flares may alternate, and the disease is often considered to be self-limiting. However, extra-nodal RDD, involving particularly the brain or the head and neck and therefore potentially causing life-threatening manifestations, requires prompt treatment that can be surgical (debulking or complete resection) and/or medical, using a variety of chemotherapeutic or immunosuppressive drugs. Given the rarity of the disease and its extremely protean clinical manifestations, no trials have been performed. Among the drugs most frequently reported in the literature are vinca alkaloids, anthracyclines, alkylating agents and cladribine but also IFN-α, methotrexate and the anti-CD20 rituximab [24].

Haemophagocytic Lymphohistiocytosis

HLH includes a spectrum of diseases characterised by excessive immune activation and tissue infiltration by macrophages and histiocytes that clinically presents with fever, cytopenias, hepatosplenomegaly and hyperferritinemia. Other common abnormalities include hypertriglyceridemia, coagulopathy, low fibrinogen levels, high transaminase levels and neurological symptoms. Although not routinely available, testing soluble CD25 (soluble IL2-receptor) serum levels may be of diagnostic help and denotes lymphocyte activation [25].

HLH has traditionally been divided into primary and secondary forms, where the former are due to disorders with Mendelian inheritance linked to gene mutations affecting immune function, while the latter occur as a consequence of infections, solid or haematologic malignancies or autoimmune disorders (e.g. rheumatoid arthritis, systemic lupus erythematosus). HLH associated with systemic rheumatic disorders is usually referred to as macrophage-activation syndrome (MAS) (also see Chap. 14); for this HLH subset, the term MAS-HLH has been suggested [3]. Actually, infections may trigger both primary and secondary HLH, and genetic defects have also been found in patients with suspected secondary HLH. In clinical practice, the distinction between primary and secondary HLH is not essential for the diagnosis and initial management of the disease, while it becomes crucial for the subsequent follow-up.

The pathology of HLH shows a diffuse accumulation of lymphocytes and macrophages with frequent evidence of haemophagocytosis in the affected tissues, particularly the spleen, the liver (where the disease mimics chronic persistent hepatitis) and the bone marrow [26].

Although a review of the pathogenic mechanisms of the different forms of HLH is beyond the scope of this chapter, it is worthwhile mentioning that the main cell types involved in the development of the disease are natural killer (NK) cells, cytotoxic T cells (CTLs) and macrophages. In HLH, NK cells and CTLs are deficient, and activated macrophages accumulate. As a result, there is excessive macrophage activation and production of cytokines (particularly IFN-γ), which are thought to be main mediators of damage in HLH. NK- and CTL-mediated destruction of macrophages is usually a perforin-dependent mechanism; this enables NK cells and CTLs to release cytotoxic granules (containing proteases, granzyme B) into the macrophage. Genetic defects involving this cell death pathway may be involved in primary forms of HLH [26]. Infectious triggers are also usually necessary to initiate the disease and will be discussed below in the following paragraph.

The diagnostic work-up of HLH requires the exclusion of cancer using appropriate laboratory and imaging studies; MRI of the brain as well as cerebrospinal fluid evaluation is also required in almost all cases. Bone marrow aspiration or biopsy is warranted to investigate the cause(s) of cytopenia and demonstrates haemophagocytosis and macrophage infiltration and can also be sent for culture. Molecular analysis of mutations in genes involved in primary HLH forms should be performed in specialised centres, particularly in cases occurring in childhood and with no evidence of an associated rheumatological disorder.

If left untreated, HLH is a life-threatening disorder with a survival of weeks to months, but HLH-specific therapy is able to dramatically improve prognosis and overall survival [27]. Clinically stable patients should be carefully screened and receive treatment for potential underlying conditions (e.g. infection, autoimmune disorder). Conversely, acutely ill and rapidly deteriorating patients should receive cytolytic therapy with etoposide and dexamethasone, with intrathecal steroids and methotrexate for those with severe CNS involvement. The use of cyclosporine is debated. Other options include alemtuzumab (anti-CD52 antibody). Patients with HLH gene mutations or with refractory disease, haematologic malignancies that cannot be cured, or severe CNS involvement usually require allogeneic haematopoietic cell transplantation.

Infections and Histiocytoses

There is no clear evidence supporting a role for infections in the pathogenesis of LCH and ECD. The hypothesis that these two forms of histiocytosis are clonal disorders is now well accepted, especially after the discovery of recurrent somatic mutations (particularly *BRAF*^{V600E}) impacting on the activation of the RAS-RAF-MEK-ERK pathway. It must also be acknowledged that both LCH and ECD show intense inflammation and fibrosis in addition to histiocyte proliferation, which has led to the concept of inflammatory myeloid neoplasia. Whether an accompanying infectious trigger drives inflammation is still unknown.

On the other hand, the clinical presentation and the disease associations of RDD and HLH suggest, at least in some cases, a "reactive" nature of these conditions. In RDD, some evidence suggests a role of viruses in disease pathogenesis. In particular, the human herpesvirus 6 (HHV6) antigen has been demonstrated in RDD histiocytes [28], although HHV6 is so common in lymphoid tissues that its pathogenic significance in RDD remains questionable. In addition, immunohistochemistry for parvovirus B19 antigens VP1/VP2 was found to be positive in some cases of RDD [29], although this finding has not been consistently replicated. Other viral infections, caused by Epstein-Barr and polyoma viruses, have been implicated, but there is no solid evidence supporting these data. Finally, RDD-like changes in draining lymph nodes were also found during the course of bacterial infections (e.g. *Salmonella*) [30].

With regard to HLH, clear evidence supports a causal role for infections. In fact, although infections can act as triggers also in primary forms of HLH, secondary forms may recognise a purely infectious aetiology and are therefore divided into secondary to viral, bacterial, parasitic and fungal infections. Epstein-Barr virus, Cytomegalovirus, influenza virus and human immunodeficiency virus (HIV) are the most common causes of HLH associated with viral infection. It is interesting to note that HLH may develop soon after the initiation of antiretroviral therapy for HIV infection. Among the bacterial causes, mycobacteria certainly play a central role, as do *Leishmania* and different plasmodia species among parasitic infections. Finally, histoplasmosis is probably the main cause of secondary HLH associated with fungal infections [3]. Notably, infections with *Mycobacterium tuberculosis*, cytomegalovirus or *Histoplasma* can occur in patients with rheumatological conditions (which may predispose to HLH per se) after specific immunosuppressive therapies such as those with antitumour necrosis factor-α antibodies [31].

It is also important to underline that the conditions predisposing to HLH include various types of immunodeficiency, which can in turn expose patients to an increased risk of infections. These can therefore activate a vicious circle that promotes infections, and infections can act as triggers of HLH.

Conclusions

Histiocytoses encompass a broad spectrum of conditions characterised by accumulation of pathologic histiocytes in the affected tissues. These syndromes can be due to primary histiocytic neoplasia such as LCH or ECD, which can be multisystemic and recognise recurrent mutations activating the RAS-RAF-MEK-ERK pathway as main drivers; however, as is the case of HLH or RDD, these can be of inherited monogenic origin, or associated with infections or other immune-mediated disorders, and probably have a "reactive" origin. Further studies investigating the potential role of infectious triggers are warranted.

References

1. Haroche J, Cohen-Aubart F, Rollins BJ, et al. Histiocytoses: emerging neoplasia behind inflammation. Lancet Oncol. 2017;18:e113–25.
2. Hervier B, Haroche J, Arnaud L, et al. Association of both Langerhans cell histiocytosis and Erdheim-Chester disease linked to the BRAF V600E mutation. Blood. 2014;124:1119–26.

3. Emile JF, Abla O, Fraitag S, et al. Revised classification of histiocytoses and neoplasms of the macrophage-dendritic cell lineages. Blood. 2016;127:2672–81.
4. Allen CE, Li L, Peters TL, et al. Cell-specific gene expression in Langerhans cell histiocytosis reveals a distinct profile compared with epidermal Langerhans cells. J Immunol. 2010;184:4557–67.
5. Berres ML, Lim KP, Peters T, et al. BRAF V600E expression in precursor versus differentiated dendritic cells defines clinically distinct LCH risk groups. J Exp Med. 2014;211:669–83.
6. Brown NA, Furtado LV, Betz BL, et al. High prevalence of somatic MAP 2K1 mutations in BRAF V600E negative Langerhans cell histiocytosis. Blood. 2014;124:1655–8.
7. Guyot-Goubin A, Donadieu J, Barkaoui M, et al. Descriptive epidemiology of childhood Langerhans cell histiocytosis in France, 2000-2004. Pediatr Blood Cancer. 2008;51:76–81.
8. Héritier S, Emile JF, Barkaoui MA, et al. BRAF mutation correlates with high-risk Langerhans cell histiocytosis and increased resistance to first-line therapy. J Clin Oncol. 2016;34:3023–30.
9. Donadieu J, Rolon MA, Thomas C, et al. Endocrine involvement in pediatric-onset Langerhans' cell histiocytosis: a population-based study. J Pediatr. 2004;144:344–50.
10. Diamond E, Dagna L, Hyman DM, et al. Consensus guidelines for the diagnosis and clinical management of Erdheim-Chester disease. Blood. 2014;124:483–92.
11. Arnaud L, Gorochov G, Charlotte F, et al. Systemic perturbation of cytokine and chemokine network in Erdheim-Chester disease: a single center series of 37 patients. Blood. 2011;117:2783–90.
12. Diamond E, Durham BH, Haroche J, et al. Diverse and targetable kinase alterations drive histiocytic neoplasms. Cancer Discov. 2016;6:154–65.
13. Gianfreda D, Nicastro M, Galetti M, et al. Sirolimus plus prednisone for Erdheim-Chester disease: an open-label trial. Blood. 2015;126:1163–71.
14. Haroche J, Cohen-Aubart F, Emile JF, et al. Reproducible and sustained efficacy of targeted therapy with vemurafenib in patients with BRAF (V600E)-mutated Erdheim-Chester disease. J Clin Oncol. 2015;33:411–8.
15. Gianfreda D, Palumbo AA, Rossi E, et al. Cardiac involvement in Erdheim-Chester disease: an MRI study. Blood. 2016;128:2468–71.
16. Diamond EL, Hatzoglou V, Patel S, et al. Diffuse reduction of cerebral grey matter volumes in Erdheim-Chester disease. Orphanet J Rare Dis. 2016;11:109.
17. Veyssier-Belot C, Cacoub P, Caparros-Lefebvre D, et al. Erdheim-Chester disease. Clinical and radiologic characteristics of 59 cases. Medicine (Baltimore). 1996;75:157–69.
18. Hervier B, Arnaud L, Charlotte F, et al. Treatment of Erdheim-Chester disease with long-term high-dose interferon-α. Semin Arthritis Rheum. 2012;41:907–13.
19. Cohen-Aubart F, Maksud P, Saadoun D, et al. Variability in the efficacy of the interleukin-1 receptor inhibitor anakinra for treating Erdheim-Chester disease. Blood. 2016;127:1509–12.
20. Cohen-Aubart F, Emile JF, Maksud P, et al. Efficacy of the MEK inhibitor cobimetinib for wild-type BRAF Erdheim-Chester disease. Br J Haematol. 2016;180(1):150–3.
21. Rosai J, Dorfman RF. Sinus histiocytosis with massive lymphadenopathy. A newly recognized benign clinicopathological entity. Arch Pathol. 1969;87:63–70.
22. Maric I, Pittaluga S, Dale JK, et al. Histologic features of sinus histiocytosis with massive lymphadenopathy in patients with autoimmune lymphoproliferative syndrome. Am J Surg Pathol. 2005;29:903–11.
23. Morgan NV, Morris MR, Cangul H, et al. Mutations in SLC29A3, encoding an equilibrative nucleoside transporter ENT3, cause a familial histiocytosis syndrome (Faisalabad histiocytosis) and familial Rosai-Dorfman disease. PLoS Genet. 2010;6:e1000833.
24. Dalia S, Sagatys E, Sokol L, et al. Rosai-Dorfman disease: tumor biology, clinical features, pathology and treatment. Cancer Control. 2014;21:322–7.
25. Komp DM, McNamara J, Buckley P. Elevated soluble interleukin-2 receptor in childhood hemophagocytic histiocytic syndromes. Blood. 1989;73:2128–32.
26. Henter JI, Horne A, Aricò M, et al. HLH-2004: diagnostic and therapeutic guidelines for hemophagocytic lymphohistiocytosis. Pediatr Blood Cancer. 2007;48:124–31.
27. Parikh SA, Kapoor P, Letendre L, et al. Prognostic factors and outcomes of adults with hemophagocytic lymphohistiocytosis. Mayo Clin Proc. 2014;89:484–92.
28. Luppi M, Barozzi P, Garber R, et al. Expression of human herpesvirus-6 antigens in benign and malignant lymphoproliferative diseases. Am J Pathol. 1998;15:815–23.
29. Mehraein Y, Wagner M, Remberger K, et al. Parvovirus B19 detected in Rosai-Dorfman disease in nodal and extranodal manifestations. J Clin Pathol. 2006;59:1320–6.
30. Ip YT, Loo KT, Ting SH, et al. Rosai–Dorfman disease-like changes in mesenteric lymph nodes secondary to Salmonella infection. Histopathology. 2011;58:792–807.
31. Brito-Zerón P, Bosch X, Pérez-de-Lis M, et al. Infection is the major trigger of hemophagocytic syndrome in adult patients treated with biological therapies. Semin Arthritis Rheum. 2016;45:391–9.

30 Subacute Bacterial Endocarditis

Gaafar Ragab and Hussien Rizk

Abbreviations

AAV	ANCA-associated vasculitis
ACL	Anticardiolipin antibodies
ANA	Antinuclear antibodies
ANCA	Antineutrophil cytoplasmic antibodies
ARF	Acute renal failure
CAE	Community-acquired IE
cANCA/PR3	cANCA/proteinase 3
CGN	Crescentic GN
CNS	Central nervous system
CRF	Chronic renal failure
CSGN	Chronic sclerotic GN
HACEK	*Haemophilus* species, *Aggregatibacter actinomycetemcomitans*, *Cardiobacterium hominis*, *Eikenella corrodens*, and *Kingella kingae*
HAE	Healthcare-associated IE
IE	Infective endocarditis
MGN	Mesangial GN
pANCA	Perinuclear anti-neutrophil cytoplasmic antibodies
pANCA/MPO	pANCA/myeloperoxidase
PCR	Polymerase chain reaction
PVE	Prosthetic valve endocarditis
RPGN	Rapidly progressive glomerulonephritis
SBE	Subacute bacterial endocarditis
SNGN	Segmental necrotizing GN
TRF	Terminal renal failure

G. Ragab (✉)
Department of Internal Medicine,
Faculty of Medicine, Cairo University, Cairo, Egypt
e-mail: gragab@kasralainy.edu.eg

H. Rizk
Department of Cardiology, Faculty of Medicine,
Cairo University, Cairo, Egypt

Introduction

Subacute bacterial endocarditis (SBE) is causally related to infective agents. Its inclusion in this text dealing with rheumatic diseases is however predicated on two features it can present with: (1) vascular manifestations either due to direct invasion of the vessel wall by the causative microorganism or through immunological mechanisms and (2) a multitude of autoimmune phenomena. The clinical course of illness is also capable of displaying a constellation of rheumatic manifestations making it mandatory to consider SBE in many settings.

These two features of SBE were considered among the minor criteria of Duke's diagnostic criteria and again confirmed by the more recent European modifications [1].

G. Ragab et al. (eds.), *The Microbiome in Rheumatic Diseases and Infection*,
https://doi.org/10.1007/978-3-319-79026-8_30

Definition

Infective endocarditis (IE) is defined as a microbial infection of the endocardium, heart valves, or intravascular device. The disease is rare among community dwellers. Incidence ranges from 5 to 15 cases per 100,000 person/year in most western communities [2], with no reliable figures reported from third world nations. The major risk factors for the community-acquired type of this disease are older age, IV drug abuse, poor dental health, structural heart disease (essentially rheumatic valve disease in developing countries) [3], prosthetic heart valves [4], and HIV infection. Up to 30% of IE cases are healthcare associated [5]. These are often associated with intravascular devices, cardiac pacemaker/defibrillators, central or peripheral venous lines, and hemodialysis [6].

Major Pathogens

The major pathogens for community-acquired IE (CAE) are *Staphylococcus aureus*, *Streptococci*, and the HACEK group of Gram-negative bacilli (*Haemophilus* species, *Aggregatibacter actinomycetemcomitans*, *Cardiobacterium hominis*, *Eikenella corrodens*, and *Kingella kingae*) [4]. *Streptococcus bovis* is a common pathogen associated with inflammatory and neoplastic bowel disease. Zoonotic infections due to *Brucella*, *Coxiella*, and *Bartonella species* are infrequent, but they are important to identify, as they require specific antibiotic therapy [7]. Community-acquired IE in intravenous drug abusers is commonly due to staphylococci, and a sizable minority is caused by non-HACEK Gram-negative bacilli and fungi. Anaerobic bacteria are very rare causes of IE. Healthcare-associated IE (HAE) is often due to much more antibiotic-resistant organisms, mainly methicillin-resistant *Staphylococcus aureus* (MRSA), enterococci, non-HACEK Gram-negative bacilli, and fungi [6].

Clinical Presentations

Fever is the most constant feature, being the leading symptom in over 90% of patients. It varies widely in magnitude, pattern, and duration prior to diagnosis. Common patterns are persistent, hectic, and intermittent fever. Prostration and anorexia are also very common. Petechiae on the skin, nails (splinter hemorrhage), conjunctiva, or palate may be present in up to 40% of patients. Osler's nodes and Janeway lesions are given great emphasis among the clinical signs of bacterial endocarditis but are seldom seen in

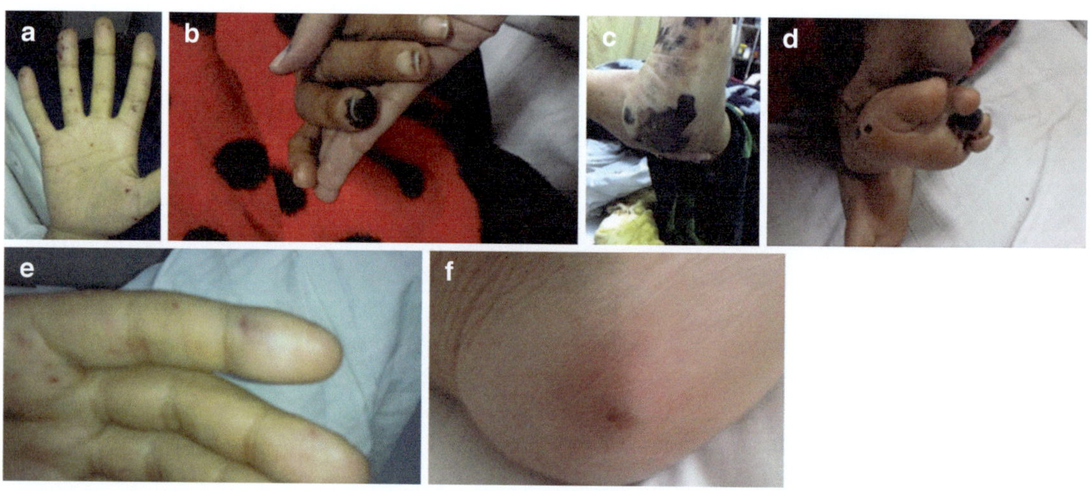

Fig. 30.1 (**a–d**) Janeway lesions. Classically start as purple-colored patches on palm and sole and may progress in severe forms to patches of superficial gangrene. (**e**, **f**) Osler's nodes. Appear as small painful nodules (Courtesy of Dr. Marwa Mashaal, Lecturer, Cardiology Department, Cairo University)

practice [8] (Fig. 30.1). They are considered among the autoimmune phenomena which will be discussed in detail. Retinal Roth spots may be observed. Skin lesions are more commonly observed in cases of late diagnosis [1].

Complications may be the presenting clinical manifestation in a sizable portion of patients. Heart failure complicates about 50% of patients. Stroke may be the presenting symptom in about one third. Septic emboli occur in about 25% of patients; renal or splenic infarctions, acute limb ischemia, and septic pulmonary emboli in patients with right-sided endocarditis are common examples. Metastatic infection, e.g., vertebral osteomyelitis, is sometimes encountered [9].

Owing to the diversity of clinical presentation, the differential diagnosis of IE includes influenza-like illness, rheumatic fever, atrial myxoma, primary neurological disease, occult cancer, pneumonia, prosthetic valve malfunction, fever of unknown origin, systemic lupus erythematosus, acute limb ischemia, and unexplained anemia [10].

Prosthetic Valve Endocarditis (PVE)

Infection involving prosthetic heart valves may occur early (within the first postoperative year) or later than this. Early PVE is often a surgical infection. It is caused by *Staphylococcus aureus*, coagulase-negative staphylococci, and rarely fungi. Late PVE is caused by organisms similar to community-acquired native valve IE. Prosthetic valve infection is commonly associated with valve ring abscess, dehiscence, and prosthesis malfunction. Vegetations are less frequently observed than in those cases involving native valve disease. Medical treatment failure and need for surgery are more frequent in PVE. Almost all patients with early PVE, particularly over metallic prostheses, as compared to bioprosthetic valves, will require early surgery [11, 12].

Diagnostic Evaluation

Microbiological Diagnosis

The mainstay of laboratory work-up is the blood culture. Culture methods may not be helpful, however, when bacterial species are difficult to isolate or following the administration of antibiotics [13]. Molecular techniques can help in these circumstances. Habib and Lancellotti et al. [1] proposed a diagnostic algorithm where in suspected blood culture-negative infective endocarditis, specific serological tests should be done. If these are negative, blood polymerase chain reaction (PCR) is the following step.

Imaging

Echocardiography: the essential imaging technique in case of suspected IE is transthoracic and commonly transesophageal echocardiography [11]. The echocardiographic findings are considered among diagnostic criteria [1, 14] (Fig. 30.2).

Other imaging techniques: neuroimaging using either CT scans or magnetic resonance imaging can help to detect subclinical central nervous system (CNS) emboli. CT scan can also help to detect other sites of embolization (Fig. 30.3). PET scanning with fluorodeoxyglucose (FDG) may show evidence of inflammation around valves or other structures [14].

Diagnosis

The diagnosis of IE requires a high index of suspicion. The presence of any two of the following findings should alert the clinician to the possibility: (a) fever lasting more than a few days, (b) heart murmur or known structural heart disease, or (c) evidence of systemic or pulmonary emboli. Clinical suspicion should lead to appropriate blood cultures and echocardiographic examination. Repeating clinical examination at close intervals is necessary since findings may change,

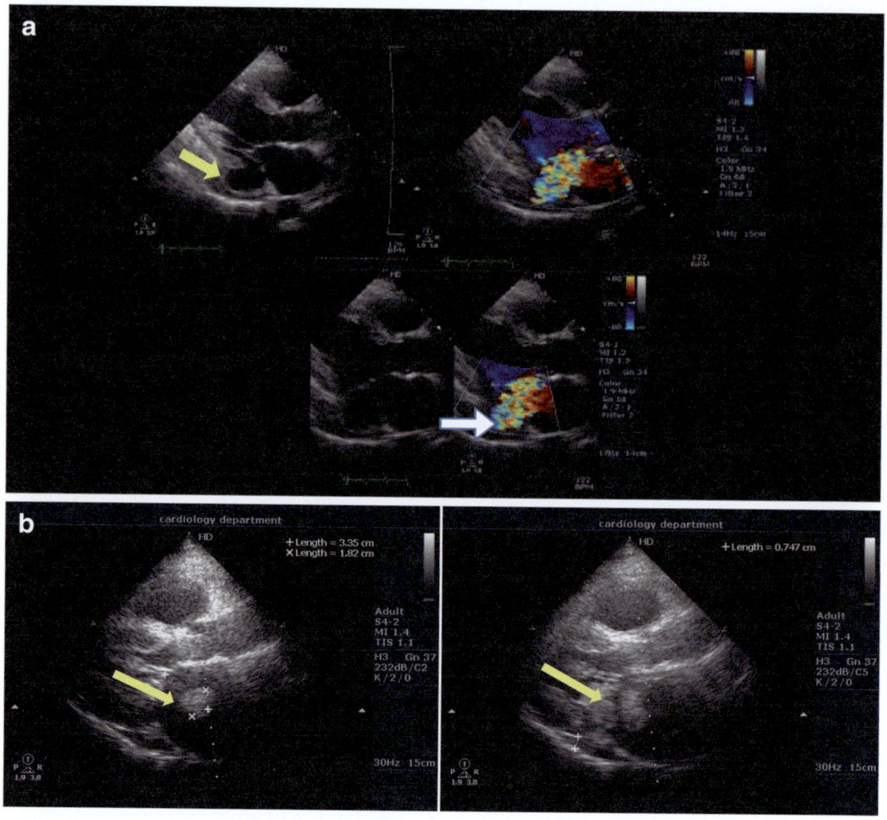

Fig. 30.2 Echocardiographic findings in SBE: (**a**) Mitral ring abscess (yellow arrow), severe mitral regurgitation (white arrow); (**b**) Vegetations of the posterior mitral leaflet (arrows). (Courtesy of Dr. Marwa Mashaal, Lecturer, Cardiology Department, Cairo University)

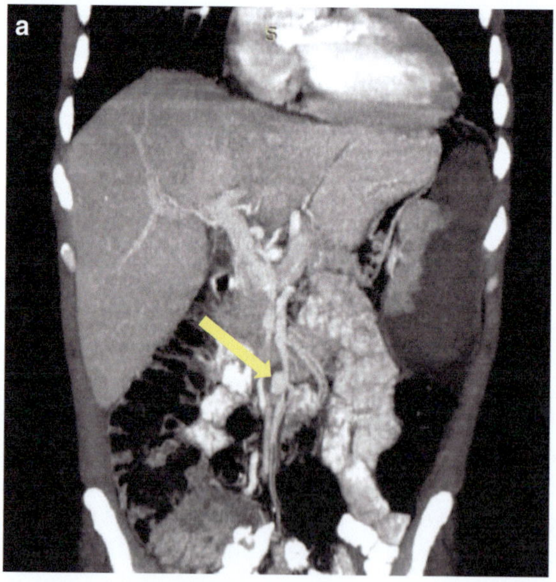

Fig. 30.3 Mycotic aneurysms : (**a**) Angeographic abdominal CT scan with contrast showing inferior mesenteric artery mycotic aneurysm (arrow); (**b**) Chest CT scan with contrast showing pulmonary artery mycotic aneurysms (arrows); (**c**) Reformatted angiography CT scan of the aorta and iliac arteries showing mycotic aneurysms of lower segment of aorta (left arrow) and left internal iliac artery (right arrow) (Courtesy of Dr. Marwa Mashaal, Lecturer, Cardiology Department, Cairo University)

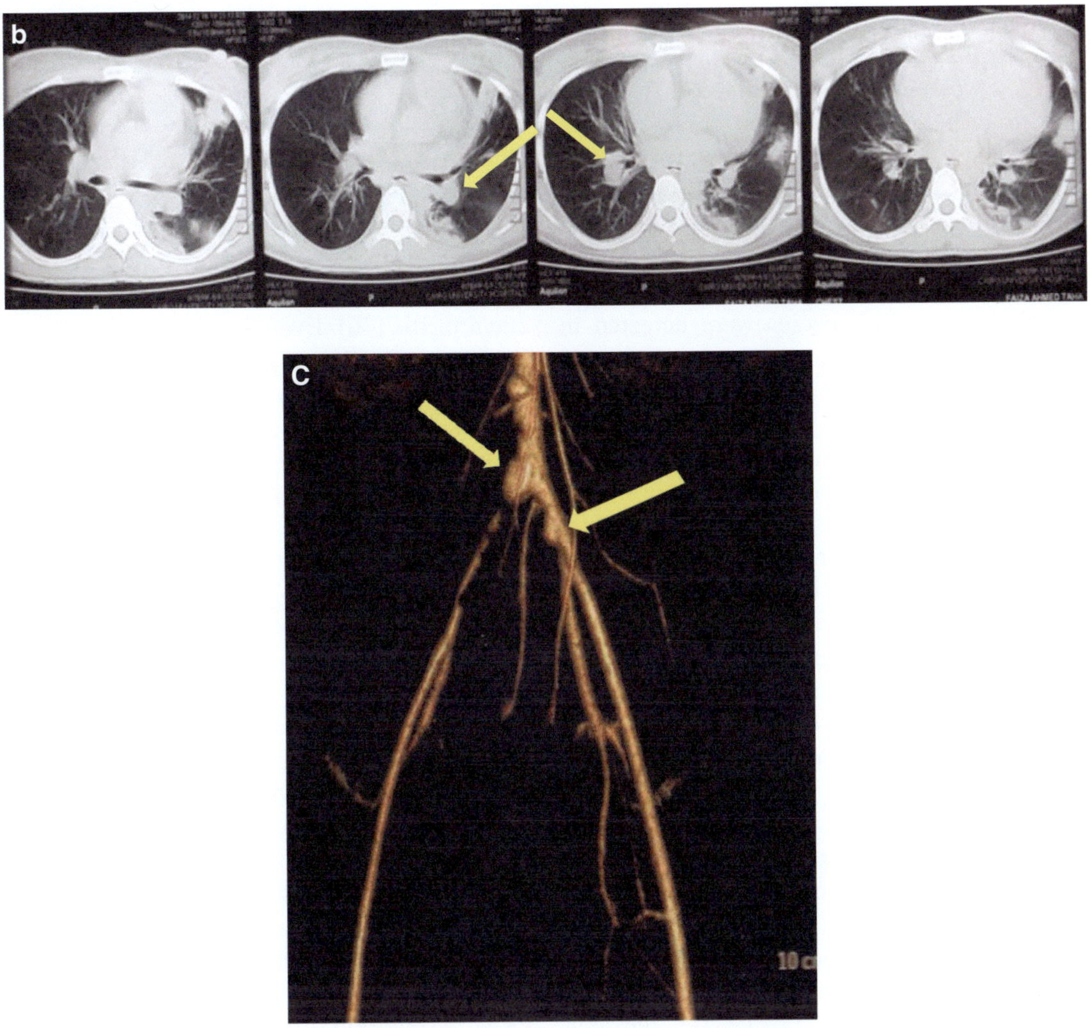

Fig. 30.3 (continued)

often due to development of complications such as valvular regurgitation, prosthesis malfunction, heart failure, atrioventricular conduction defects, renal failure, new skin or eye lesions, and systemic or pulmonary emboli [15].

The case definition of IE as currently based on the modified Duke's criteria has been previously appraised [16]. The later modification of these criteria adopted by the latest European Society of Cardiology guidelines [1] helps to increase the sensitivity of Duke's criteria.

Microbiota and SBE

Oral Sources

It has been shown that professional dental treatments as well as oral practices such as tooth brushing, flossing, and food chewing can cause bacteremia [17]. Nakano et al. studied bacterial DNA from 35 surgically obtained heart valve specimens extirpated under diagnosis of aortic, mitral, or tricuspid regurgitation from patients with treated bacterial endocarditis. *Streptococcus mutans* was detected in 77.8% of cases. They speculated that it was due to bacteremia caused by oral infection [18]. Nomura and Nakano et al. [13] studied nine heart valve specimens from infective endocarditis: six SBE and three acute cases. Bacterial species were identified by two molecular methods and compared with a culture technique. Multiple species were detected in most of the cases by both molecular techniques, although they were not the same by the two methods. Also, the species determined by blood culture were not always detected by the molecular methods. The significance of such findings needs to be investigated further. Dental plaque specimens were collected from three of their patients who were referred to the department of dentistry and oral surgery before their cardiovascular operations. Comparison of bacterial profiles between heart valve and dental plaque specimens in this small number failed to show a clear correlation. The authors related this to the fact that plaque specimens only represent the bacterial profiles of the collection site, whereas saliva specimens represent the profile of the entire oral cavity. The authors recommended focusing on bacterial profiles in saliva specimens in future studies [13].

Other sources of infective agents include the gastrointestinal tract (GIT) [19–21], the skin [22–27], mastoiditis complicating otitis media [28], upper respiratory tract [29], blood access [22], as well as ventriculoatrial shunts [30].

Immunological Phenomena

Many serological abnormalities are described. These include rheumatoid factor [31], antinuclear antibodies (ANA) [31, 32], low serum complement C3 and C4 [31, 32], anticardiolipin antibodies, and anti-β2 glycoprotein 1 of the IgM and IgG isotypes [31, 32], as well as mixed cryoglobulinemia types II and III [32–35]. Antineutrophil cytoplasmic antibody (ANCA) positivity has been repeatedly described (Table 30.1). This deserves special consideration under the vasculitic manifestations.

Rheumatological Manifestations

Musculoskeletal Manifestations

These include myalgia [30], arthralgia [32], and arthritis [36]. Even if it is caused by direct infectivity, SBE is a great mimicker, and its diagnosis can be mistaken for nonspecific back pain [37], pyomyositis which can sometimes be confused with sciatica [38], septic arthritis [29, 39], or polymyalgia rheumatica [40, 41].

Renal Manifestations

Renal involvement may be the earliest manifestation of SBE in about 20% of patients. Hematuria and mild proteinuria are common, while hypertension and nephrotic syndrome are rare [42]. The spectrum of renal involvement is broad in its presentation and diverse in its laboratory features. It includes acute nephritis [40, 43], shunt nephritis with nephrotic syndrome [30], rapidly progressive glomerulonephritis (RPGN) with cANCA/proteinase 3 (cANCA/PR3) association [44], as well as cANCA/MPO (Table 30.1). Interestingly, diffuse proliferative GN with a "full-house" deposition in immunofluorescence study (positive for C3, C4, C1q, IgG, IgA, and IgM) resembling class IV lupus nephritis has also been reported [35]. The last case reported by Lee and Lam et al. [35] improved after antibiotics. Other histopathological findings include mesangial GN (MGN), segmental necrotizing GN (SGN), crescentic GN (CGN), and chronic sclerotic GN (CSGN) [32].

The pathogenic role of circulating immune complexes in causing proliferative lesions is supported by the presence of immunoglobulins and complement components in immunofluorescence

Table 30.1 Describes case reports of SBE with positive ANCA

Reference / cases*	ANCA type	Clinical presentation and Other Investigations	Line of treatment	Causative organism
[48]	cANCA	Cutaneous small vessel vasculitis	Antibiotics (ampicillin + gentamycin), aortic valve replacement	*Enterococcus faecalis*
[36]/two cases	ANCA/PR3/MPO	Cutaneous vasculitis	ANCA titer resolved or decreased during initial steroid therapy for suspected vasculitis	*Streptococcus viridans*
[47]	cANCA	Palpable purpura, GN, RF + ve, ANA + ve, low C3, normal total complement and C4	Anti-infective therapy	*Caused by Bartonella quintana, culture negative. Diagnosis based on serology and PCR RFLP analysis*
[49]	P-ANCA/MPO	Pulmonary opacity, brain infractions, multiple cavitary parenchymal lung lesions	Antibiotics with full recovery	*Staphylococcus aureus*
[50]	P-ANCA/MPO	Diagnosed at autopsy: necrotizing arteritis of interlobular arteritis in the kidneys	Misdiagnosed and received pulse steroids, improved initially, and then deteriorated	*Missed diagnosis*
[32]/seven cases	P-ANCA/MPO	Fever, arthralgia, hematuria, *MGN*	Antibiotics	*Streptococcus viridans*
	cANCA/PR3 + MPO	Fever, arthralgia, hematuria, *SNGN*	Antibiotics	*Streptococcus viridans*
	cANCA/PR3	Fever, arthralgia, hematuria, *SNGN*	Antibiotics	*Streptococcus viridans*
	cANCA/PR3-MPO	Fever, lung infiltrate, nephrotic syndrome, ARF, splenomegaly, CGN	Antibiotics, IVIG: death	*Enterococcus*
	cANCA/PR3	Fever, hematuria, SNGN	Antibiotics: CRF	*Coagulase-negative Staphylococcus*
	cANCA/PR3-MPO	Fever, ARF, hepatosplenomegaly, CGN	Antibiotics: TRF	*Coagulase-negative Staphylococcus*
	P-ANCA/MPO	Fever, arthralgia, ARF, CGN	Antibiotics + corticosteroids: death after 2.5 months	*Staphylococcus aureus*
[43]	cANCA/PR3	GN: biopsy; immune complex-mediated acute diffuse proliferative GN	Antibiotics + valve replacement (required repeat valve replacement)	*Enterococcus faecalis*
[31]/three cases	cANCA/PR3	Acute kidney injury, cerebral embolism aortic valve destruction	Antimicrobial + diuresis	*Enterococcus faecalis*
[46]	cANCA/PR3	Lung: by CT intraparenchymal and subpleural nodules, alveolar capillaritis similar to vasculitis with polyangiitis, but no granuloma	Antibiotics: resolution of ANCA titers, GN and pulmonary nodules	Culture negative
		Renal: GN/biopsy; membranoproliferative GN with crescents; palpable purpura + hepatosplenomegaly		

(continued)

Table 30.1 (continued)

Reference / cases*	ANCA type	Clinical presentation and Other Investigations	Line of treatment	Causative organism
[51]	cANCA/ PR3 + MPO	Pauci-immune GN/renal biopsy; acute eosinophilic interstitial nephritis	Antibiotic improved fever, but CNS symptoms deteriorated. They improved when corticosteroids and cyclophosphamide were added to antibiotics	*Streptococcus mutans*
[44]	cANCA/ PR3	RPGN, had rheumatoid factor and hypocomplementemia	Antibiotics and valve surgery	*Enterococcus faecalis*
[52]/three cases	ANCA/PR3	Nephritis, proteinuria, hematuria, hypoalbuminemia, decreased kidney function, elevated CRP, anemia	1st case: aortic valve replacement (aortic resurge + vegetation)	*Enterococcus faecalis*
			2nd case: tricuspid valve replacement + closure of VSD (tricuspid regurge + vegetation)	
			Plus antibiotics	
			No steroids	

ANA antinuclear antibodies, *ANCA* antineutrophil cytoplasmic antibodies, *ANCA/MPO* ANCA/myeloperoxidase, *ARF* acute renal failure, *cANCA/PR3* cANCA/proteinase 3, *CGN* crescentic GN, *CRF* chronic renal failure, *CRP* C rective protein, *CSGN* chronic sclerotic GN, *IVIG* intravenous immunoglobulin, *MGN* mesangial GN, *PCR* polymerase chain reaction, *RF* rheumatoid factor, *RFLP* restriction fragment length polymorphism, *RPGN* rapidly progressive glomerulonephritis, *SNGN* segmental necrotizing GN, *TRF* terminal renal failure, *VSD* ventricular septal defect, (*) Each reference represents one case unless otherwise stated studies and also by the detection of deposits by electron microscopy [42].

The association of renal involvement with ANCA is discussed in more detail in Table 30.1.

Vasculitic Manifestations

These are common in SBE and are included among the diagnostic minor criteria [1]. The microorganisms can involve the vessel wall directly resulting in mycotic aneurysms (Fig. 30.3) or indirectly through immune mechanisms.

The chronic peripheral signs of SBE include Osler's nodes and Janeway lesions [45]. Clinically, Osler's nodes and Janeway lesions describe small vessel disease (Fig. 30.1). Osler's nodes are violaceous tender nodules on fingers or toes. Janeway lesions are non-tender plaque-like lesions on palms and soles. Dermatopathologically, they are both leukocytoclastic vasculitis but without microabscess formation [8]. Gunson and Oliver [8] presumed, however, that the histological picture depends on the nature of causative organisms, while the clinical appearance varies according to the anatomical site. Palpable purpura [36, 46–48], interlobular arteritis of the kidney, and also alveolar capillaritis [46] have all been reported.

The Special Case of ANCA Positivity

Although ANCA/PR3 and ANCA/myeloperoxidase (ANCA/MPO) are serological markers for ANCA-associated vasculitis (AAV), the interpretation of their positivity should consider the possibility of protracted infection [32], as these antibodies have been described with many infectious agents [31].

Autoimmune manifestations of SBE associated with ANCA positivity have been repeatedly reported. We conducted a PubMed search in December 2016 for the preceding 10 years that was updated in May 2017 entering keyword "Subacute Bacterial Endocarditis." The search yielded 182 publications. We identified 18 studies citing ANCA positivity. A meta-analysis of the 18 studies is displayed in Table 30.1. The results showed that there were 22 cases: 10 (45.5%) with PR3 and 4 (18.2%) with MPO positivity. Six cases (27.3%) had PR3 and MPO dual positivity, while two cases were not specified. Renal involvement was reported in 17 (77.3%) cases with variable clinical, serological, and histopathological presentations, making the kidneys the most frequent target. The lung was involved in three cases including one case that was due to embolization. There were four cases with cutaneous vasculitis. Apparently, the causative organism did not have an impact on the presentation.

In spite of sharing similar features, AAV patients and ANCA-positive cases with protracted infections have different serological profiles. Patients with protracted infection more frequently have concomitant PR3 and MPO-ANCA positivity, ANA, IgM anticardiolipin (ACL), IgG and IgM anti-β2 glycoprotein 1 (GP1), cryoglobulins, and low C3 and/or C4. Concomitant presence of ANCA, cryoglobulins, and complement consumption with infections was associated with a severe course of GN [32].

In summary, SBE is a great vasculitis mimicker and should always be part of the broader differential diagnosis of vasculitis [49].

Is There an Indication for Immunosuppression in SBE with Rheumatologic Features?

The immunological features and rheumatological façade that clinicians encounter when dealing with SBE raise the issue of immune suppression. There are few reports on the use of steroids in the context of SBE. Addition of steroids before the correct diagnosis of SBE was established has resulted in either deterioration [50] or serological improvement [36]. In some reports, after establishing the diagnosis, a good result could only be achieved after adding corticosteroids and cyclophosphamide to antibiotics [51]. We do not currently have sufficient data to recommend this practice. We believe that a decision regarding the use of corticosteroids or other immunosuppressive medications should be made on a case-to-case basis.

Conclusion

SBE is a great mimicker of many rheumatic diseases. Maintaining a high index of suspicion, especially in high-risk patients, will allow for timely management and avoidance of unnecessary or potentially harmful immune suppression.

References

1. Habib G, Lancellotti P, Antunes MJ, et al. ESC guidelines for the management of infective endocarditis: the task force for the management of infective endocarditis of the European Society of Cardiology (ESC) Endorsed by: European Association for Cardio-Thoracic Surgery (EACTS), the European Association of Nuclear Medicine (EANM). Eur Heart J. 2015;36(44):3075–128.
2. Mulder BJ. Endocarditis in congenital heart disease: who is at highest risk? Circulation. 2013;128(13):1396–7.
3. Sorour KA. Rheumatic heart disease in Egypt: gloomy past and promising future. Egypt Heart J. 2014;66(2):139–42.
4. Farouk H, Shaker A, El-Faramawy A, et al. Adult congenital heart disease registry at Cairo University. World J Pediatr Congenital Heart Surg. 2015;6(1):53–8.
5. Marom D, Levy I, Gutwein O, et al. Healthcare-associated versus community-associated infective endocarditis in children. Pediatr Infect Dis J. 2011;30(7):585–8.
6. Murdoch DR, Corey GR, Hoen B, et al. Clinical presentation, etiology, and outcome of infective endocarditis in the 21st century: the international collaboration on endocarditis-prospective cohort study. Arch Intern Med. 2009;169(5):463–73.
7. Hill EE, Herijgers P, Claus P, et al. Infective endocarditis: changing epidemiology and predictors of 6-month mortality: a prospective cohort study. Eur Heart J. 2007;28(2):196–203.
8. Gunson TH, Oliver GF. Osler's nodes and Janeway lesions. Australas J Dermatol. 2007;48(4):251–5.
9. Castillo FJ, Anguita M, Castillo JC, et al. Changes in clinical profile, epidemiology and prognosis of left-sided native-valve infective endocarditis without predisposing heart conditions. Rev Esp Cardiol (Engl Ed). 2015;68(05):445–8.
10. Colen TW, Gunn M, Cook E, et al. Radiologic manifestations of extra-cardiac complications of infective endocarditis. Eur Radiol. 2008;18(11):2433–45.
11. Habib G, Badano L, Tribouilloy C, et al. Recommendations for the practice of echocardiography in infective endocarditis. Eur J Echocardiogr. 2010;11(2):202–19.
12. Wang A, Athan E, Pappas PA, et al. Contemporary clinical profile and outcome of prosthetic valve endocarditis. JAMA. 2007;297(12):1354–61.
13. Nomura R, Nakano K, Nemoto H, et al. Molecular analyses of bacterial DNA in extirpated heart valves from patients with infective endocarditis. Oral Microbiol Immunol. 2009;24(1):43–9.
14. Li JS, Sexton DJ, Mick N, et al. Proposed modifications to the Duke criteria for the diagnosis of infective endocarditis. Clin Infect Dis. 2000;30(4):633–8.
15. Baddour LM, Wilson WR, Bayer AS, et al. Infective endocarditis in adults: diagnosis, antimicrobial therapy, and Management of Complications: a scientific statement for healthcare professionals from the American Heart Association. Circulation. 2015;132(15):1435–86.
16. Habib G, Derumeaux G, Avierinos JF, et al. Value and limitations of the Duke criteria for the diagnosis of infective endocarditis. J Am Coll Cardiol. 1999;33(7):2023–9.
17. Seymour RA, Lowry R, Whitworth JM, et al. Infective endocarditis, dentistry and antibiotic prophylaxis; time for a rethink? Br Dent J. 2000;189(11):610–6.
18. Nakano K, Inaba H, Nomura R, et al. Detection of cariogenic Streptococcus mutans in extirpated heart valve and atheromatous plaque specimens. J Clin Microbiol. 2006;44(9):3313–7.
19. Mello R, da Silva Santos M, Golebiosvki W, et al. Streptococcus bovis endocarditis: analysis of cases between 2005 and 2014. Braz J Infect Dis. 2015;19(2):209–12.
20. Kasmi G, Andoni R, Mano V, et al. Streptococcus bovis isolated in haemoculture a signal of malignant lesion of the colon. Clin Lab. 2011;57(11–12):1007–9.
21. Cesari W, Stewart C, Panda M. Getting to the heart of rectal bleeding: subacute bacterial endocarditis presenting as anaemia and a GI bleed. BMJ Case Rep. 2011;2011:bcr0920114814.
22. Kenzaka T, Takamura N, Kumabe A, et al. A case of subacute infective endocarditis and blood access infection caused by Enterococcus durans. BMC Infect Dis. 2013;13:594.
23. Elegino-Steffens D, Stratton A, Geimer-Flanders J. Subacute *Staphylococcus epidermidis* bacterial endocarditis complicated by mitral-aortic Intervalvular Fibrosa Pseudoaneurysm. Case Rep Cardiol. 2012;2012:467210.
24. Tsuneoka H, Yanagihara M, Otani S, et al. A first Japanese case of Bartonella henselae-induced endocarditis diagnosed by prolonged culture of a specimen from the excised valve. Diagn Microbiol Infect Dis. 2010;68(2):174–6.
25. Lejko-Zupanc T, Slemenik-Pusnik C, Kozelj M, et al. Native valve endocarditis due to Bartonella henselae in an immunocompetent man. Wien Klin Wochenschr. 2008;120(7–8):246–9.
26. Tse D, Khan S, Clarke S. Bacterial endocarditis complicating body art. Int J Cardiol. 2009;133(1):e28–9.
27. Barkan D, Abu Fanne R, Elazari-Scheiman A, et al. Navel piercing as a cause for Streptococcus viridans endocarditis: case report, review of the literature and implications for antibiotic prophylaxis. Cardiology. 2007;108(3):159–60.

28. Smith CP, Jackson C, Stewart R. Subacute bacterial endocarditis secondary to mastoiditis: a rare complication. BMJ Case Rep. 2012;2012:bcr2012007247.
29. Tsui K, Tsai CR, Lin LC, et al. Aggregatibacter aphrophilus pyogenic liver abscess in an immunocompetent young woman. J Microbiol Immunol Infect. 2012;45(5):385–9.
30. Burstrom G, Andresen M, Bartek J Jr, et al. Subacute bacterial endocarditis and subsequent shunt nephritis from ventriculoatrial shunting 14 years after shunt implantation. BMJ Case Rep. 2014;2014:bcr2014204655.
31. Satake K, Ohsawa I, Kobayashi N, et al. Three cases of PR3-ANCA positive subacute endocarditis caused by attenuated bacteria (Propionibacterium, Gemella, and Bartonella) complicated with kidney injury. Mod Rheumatol. 2011;21(5):536–41.
32. Bonaci-Nikolic B, Andrejevic S, Pavlovic M, et al. Prolonged infections associated with antineutrophil cytoplasmic antibodies specific to proteinase 3 and myeloperoxidase: diagnostic and therapeutic challenge. Clin Rheumatol. 2010;29(8):893–904.
33. Jadhav AP, Pryor JC, Nogueira RG. Onyx embolization for the endovascular treatment of infectious and traumatic aneurysms involving the cranial and cerebral vasculature. J Neurointerv Surg. 2013;5(6):562–5.
34. Sim BW, Koo RM, Hawkins C, et al. Granulicatella adiacens subacute bacterial endocarditis as the underlying cause of type II mixed cryoglobulinaemia. BMJ Case Rep. 2015;2015:bcr2014206091.
35. Lee LC, Lam KK, Lee CT, et al. "Full house" proliferative glomerulonephritis: an unreported presentation of subacute infective endocarditis. J Nephrol. 2007;20(6):745–9.
36. Tiliakos AM, Tiliakos NA. Dual ANCA positivity in subacute bacterial endocarditis. J Clin Rheumatol. 2008;14(1):38–40.
37. Starosta RT, Rivero R, de Oliveira FH, et al. Misdiagnosis of Streptococcus gallolyticus endocarditis. Autops Case Rep. 2016;6(3):29–33.
38. Hsu WC, Hsu JY, Chen MY, et al. Obturator internus pyomyositis manifested as sciatica in a patient with subacute bacterial endocarditis: a rare case report. Medicine (Baltimore). 2016;95(30):e4340.
39. Yombi J, Belkhir L, Jonckheere S, et al. Streptococcus gordonii septic arthritis: two cases and review of literature. BMC Infect Dis. 2012;12:215.
40. Bonfante HL, Bonfante HL, Azevedo CB, et al. Endocarditis with negative blood cultures and immunological alterations: a grand challenge. Acta Reumatol Port. 2011;36(3):282–6.
41. De Socio GV, Mencacci A, Bini P, et al. Fusobacterium nucleatum endocarditis mimicking polymyalgia rheumatica. South Med J. 2009;102(10):1082–4.
42. Lusco MA, Fogo AB, Najafian B, et al. AJKD atlas of renal pathology: subacute bacterial endocarditis-associated glomerulonephritis. Am J Kidney Dis. 2016;68(2):e11–2.
43. Uh M, McCormick IA, Kelsall JT. Positive cytoplasmic antineutrophil cytoplasmic antigen with PR3 specificity glomerulonephritis in a patient with subacute bacterial endocarditis. J Rheumatol. 2011;38(7):1527–8.
44. Fukasawa H, Hayashi M, Kinoshita N, et al. Rapidly progressive glomerulonephritis associated with PR3-ANCA positive subacute bacterial endocarditis. Intern Med. 2012;51(18):2587–90.
45. Chong Y, Han SJ, Rhee YJ, et al. Classic peripheral signs of subacute bacterial endocarditis. Korean J Thorac Cardiovasc Surg. 2016;49(5):408–12.
46. Peng H, Chen WF, Wu C, et al. Culture-negative subacute bacterial endocarditis masquerades as granulomatosis with polyangiitis (Wegener's granulomatosis) involving both the kidney and lung. BMC Nephrol. 2012;13:174.
47. Sugiyama H, Sahara M, Imai Y, et al. Infective endocarditis by Bartonella quintana masquerading as antineutrophil cytoplasmic antibody-associated small vessel vasculitis. Cardiology. 2009;114(3):208–11.
48. Chirinos JA, Corrales-Medina VF, Garcia S, et al. Endocarditis associated with antineutrophil cytoplasmic antibodies: a case report and review of the literature. Clin Rheumatol. 2007;26(4):590–5.
49. Riding AM, D'Cruz DP. A case of mistaken identity: subacute bacterial endocarditis associated with p-antineutrophil cytoplasmic antibody. BMJ Case Rep. 2010;2010:bcr0920103299.
50. Wang KY, Shimajiri S, Yoshida T, et al. An autopsy case of microscopic polyangiitis associated with bacterial endocarditis. J UOEH. 2010;32(3):273–9.
51. Konstantinov KN, Harris AA, Hartshorne MF, et al. Symptomatic anti-neutrophil cytoplasmic antibody-positive disease complicating subacute bacterial endocarditis: to treat or not to treat? Case Rep Nephrol Urol. 2012;2(1):25–32.
52. Hirai K, Miura N, Yoshino M, et al. Two cases of proteinase 3-anti-neutrophil cytoplasmic antibody (PR3-ANCA)-related nephritis in infectious endocarditis. Intern Med. 2016;55(23):3485–9.

31 Chronic Recurrent Multifocal Osteomyelitis (CRMO)

Polly J. Ferguson

Abbreviations

CMO	Chronic multifocal osteomyelitis
CNO	Chronic nonbacterial osteomyelitis
DIRA	Deficiency of the IL-1 receptor antagonist
HFD	High-fat diet
LFD	Low-fat diet
LPS	Lipopolysaccharide
NBO	Nonbacterial osteomyelitis
NLRP3	Nlr family pyrin domain containing 3
NSAID	Nonsteroidal anti-inflammatory drug
PSTPIP2	Proline-serine-threonine phosphatase-interacting protein 2
SAPHO	Synovitis, acne, pustulosis, hyperostosis, osteitis
WB-MRI	Whole-body magnetic resonance imaging

Background and Clinical Manifestations of Chronic Recurrent Multifocal Osteomyelitis

Nomenclature

Chronic recurrent multifocal osteomyelitis (CRMO) is a painful chronic inflammatory disease that predominantly affects children. Unlike infectious osteomyelitis, which is usually unifocal, most cases of CRMO are multifocal [1]. The disease was first described by Giedion in 1972 as a symmetric sterile multifocal form of osteomyelitis [2]. The term CRMO was later coined due to the recurrent nature of the disease [3]. More recently, the terms chronic nonbacterial osteomyelitis (CNO) and nonbacterial osteitis (NBO) have been used in the literature due to the observation that some individuals only have unifocal disease [1, 4]. Yet, if followed over time, most patients ultimately develop multifocal disease. Further complicating the nomenclature is that the term synovitis, acne, pustulosis, hyperostosis, osteitis (SAPHO) syndrome is used to describe adults with an autoinflammatory bone disease that phenotypically and histologically closely resembles CRMO [5]. In this chapter, the term CRMO will be utilized.

Distribution and Incidence

CRMO has a worldwide distribution and can affect all races and ethnicities, but the majority of

P. J. Ferguson
University of Iowa Carver College of Medicine, Iowa City, IA, USA
e-mail: polly-ferguson@uiowa.edu

G. Ragab et al. (eds.), *The Microbiome in Rheumatic Diseases and Infection*,
https://doi.org/10.1007/978-3-319-79026-8_31

cases are Caucasians with Western or Northern European ancestry. It is a rare disease. In Germany, the incidence of CRMO is estimated at 0.4/100,000 [6]. The incidence in other populations is not well delineated.

Clinical Characteristics of CRMO

CRMO is predominantly a disease of childhood although it can occur at any age. There is a slight predilection for females (2 to 4:1 female to male ratio), and the peak age of onset is around 9 years of age [1, 7–13]. Bone pain is the typical presenting symptom. The pain may be acute in onset, but more often, it is insidious. Fever is present in a minority of patients. Objective evidence of inflammation may be present on the physical examination including localized swelling, warmth, erythema, or tenderness overlying one or more bones. However, the physical examination may be completely normal, even in the presence of active bone disease. Laboratory studies are nondiagnostic. Inflammatory markers may be anywhere from normal to markedly elevated. Complete blood counts are often normal. The symptoms often wax and wane in severity or be unremitting. Nearly any bone in the body can be involved, but involvement of the long bones, vertebral bodies, clavicles, and pelvis predominates [8, 10].

CRMO is most frequently accompanied by inflammatory disease of the skin, intestine, and joints. Palmar plantar pustulosis, psoriasis vulgaris, and Crohn's disease are the most common comorbid inflammatory conditions of the skin and gut. Synovitis is common. It can be near the site of bone inflammation or less frequently at sites distant from active osteitis. When looked at rigorously in a pediatric CRMO cohort, inflammatory arthritis occurs in up to 80% of children [4] initially or during the course of the disease, and 17% satisfied the European Spondyloarthropathy Study Group criteria for spondyloarthropathy [4]. In SAPHO syndrome, up to 33% had spondylodiskitis or spondylitis [14, 15]. Maugars et al. reported that 43% of patients with SAPHO in their cohort (n = 19) met criteria of the European Spondyloarthropathy Study Group for spondyloarthropathy [16]. With long-term follow-up, CRMO and SAPHO may evolve into a classic spondyloarthropathy [9, 16–20]. Synovial biopsies show histologic synovitis in CRMO [4]. Cutaneous involvement occurs in 1/3 of cases usually as palmar-plantar pustulosis or psoriasis vulgaris [1, 8, 9]. Crohn's disease occurs in ~10% of children with CRMO [1, 9, 21], and nearly half of the 1st- and 2nd-degree relatives of children with CRMO have psoriasis, inflammatory bowel disease, or inflammatory arthritis (psoriatic arthritis or rheumatoid arthritis), demonstrating a substantial genetic component to the disease [1, 22].

Radiologic studies are a critical part of evaluating a patient with CRMO. One reason that imaging is so helpful is that asymptomatic lesions are common in CRMO. Typical imaging findings include osteolytic and sclerotic bone lesions involving the metaphyses of the long bones, clavicles, vertebrae, and pelvis seen on plain radiographs [23, 24]. However, plain films may be normal. In the past, Tc99 bone scans have been used to assess for multifocal disease which have largely been replaced by whole-body MRI (WB-MRI) which is more sensitive [25–28]. WB-MRI often provides key information to establish a diagnosis of CRMO and for guiding therapy as it can establish that the disease process is multifocal rather than unifocal. It also allows one to identify if the spine is involved which may lead to the use of more aggressive treatment.

Bone biopsy is performed to rule out infectious osteomyelitis and malignancy when the diagnosis is not clear based on other features. Histologic features mimic infectious osteomyelitis with acute, chronic, or mixed inflammatory infiltrate present depending on the timing of the biopsy. Neutrophilic infiltration tends to be dominant in early lesions, whereas a chronic lymphocytic infiltrate with sclerosis, fibrosis, new bone formation, and scattered granulomas may be seen in longer-standing disease [29]. Cultures are typically negative, and antibiotics rarely result in improvement [4, 30]. However, in adults with SAPHO syndrome, bone cultures positive for

Propionibacterium acnes, a skin commensal, has been reported by several groups [31], and there are reports of improvement with azithromycin in a few cases [32]. When assessed with molecular biology tools, there was no microbial signature in pediatric CRMO [4].

The treatment of CRMO remains largely empiric. Nonsteroidal anti-inflammatory drugs (NSAIDs) are first-line treatment, but many patients have an incomplete response [33]. Practice varies widely regarding how to treat NSAID failures [34]. Disease-modifying anti-rheumatic medications, cytokine-blocking agents, and bisphosphonates are utilized with variable success [35]. For severe disease, particularly if the spine is involved, tumor necrosis factor-blocking agents or bisphosphonates are typically utilized with reported success [35–40].

Etiology, Pathogenesis, and Genetics of Human CRMO

CRMO is an immunologically mediated disorder that can have a strong genetic basis. The syndromic forms of the disease are driven by dysregulation of the interleukin-1 (IL-1) pathway due to single gene defects and fit the classification of autoinflammatory disorders [41]. Deficiency of the IL-1 receptor antagonist (DIRA) is an autosomal recessive disorder caused by mutations in *IL1RN,* which encodes the IL-1 receptor antagonist [42, 43]. This results in the absence of functional IL-1 receptor antagonist causing unfettered signaling through the IL-1 receptor [42]. Onset is in infancy with pustular rash and multifocal osteomyelitis, typically without fever. There is marked systemic inflammation in DIRA and, if undiagnosed and untreated, results in death from systemic inflammatory response syndrome [42]. Treatment is with anakinra, the recombinant IL-1 receptor antagonist, which is given subcutaneously and replaces the very protein that these children are missing [42–46]. Majeed syndrome is due to mutation in *LPIN2* [47] which encodes LIPIN2, a phosphatidate phosphatase that plays an important role in lipid metabolism. It presents with CRMO and dyserythropoietic anemia that may be accompanied by periodic fever, neutrophilic dermatosis, and failure to thrive [48]. The CRMO in Majeed syndrome is usually of early onset, severe, and less likely to relent. Most present prior to the age of 2 years old; however, there can be phenotypic variability with later, milder presentation [49]. Labs show elevated inflammatory markers, and radiographs resemble those of non-syndromic CRMO. Translational studies demonstrate that the osteomyelitis in Majeed syndrome is IL-1β-driven disease as there is sustained clinical, laboratory, and radiologic improvement with therapeutic agents that antagonize the IL-1 receptor or block IL-1β [50]. Consistent with the clinical response to IL-1 blockade, Lorden et al. demonstrated that Lipin-2 regulates the Nlr family pyrin domain containing 3 (Nlrp3) inflammasome by affecting $P2X_7$ receptor activation [51]. The most recently identified CRMO susceptibility gene, filamin-binding LIM protein 1 (*FLBIM1*), was identified utilizing genomic information from the cmo mouse model of the disease and is discussed below [52].

There is a report of a CRMO susceptibility locus on chromosome 18 in non-syndromic CRMO, but this has not been replicated [53]. Mutations in *LPIN2*, *IL1RN*, and *FBLIM1* explain only a fraction of the genetic susceptibility in CRMO. For the majority of patients that present with typical CRMO (with age of onset late in the first decade), the genetic basis is yet to be defined. Hofmann et al. reported an association with CRMO and impaired specificity protein 1 signaling, reduced IL-10 promotor phosphorylation, and reduced IL-10 secretion by lipopolysaccharide (LPS)-stimulated myeloid cells [54]. This suggests that epigenetic differences may play a role in disease susceptibility. Decreased IL-10 production could explain the imbalance in pro- and anti-inflammatory cytokines seen in CRMO [55].

Animal Models of CRMO

There are murine models of CRMO that are due to recessive mutations in *Pstpip2*, a gene that encodes the proline-serine-threonine phosphatase-interacting protein 2 [56–58] that results in either absence of or significantly reduced protein. The chronic multifocal osteomyelitis (cmo) mouse is the best characterized model [56, 59–62]. The disease manifests itself as tail kinks and paw deformities by 3 months of age. Both sexes are affected. Disease in the cmo mouse is IL-1 mediated as cmo mice that lack a functional IL-1 receptor (cmo. IL-1R−/−) are protected from disease. The disease is IL-1β-, not IL-1α-, driven disease and can occur in the absence of a functional Nlrp3 inflammasome [61, 62]. The neutrophils, not bone marrow-derived macrophages, hyper-produce IL-1β and are critical for disease pathogenesis [61, 63]. Beyond this, little is known about the role of proline-serine-threonine phosphatase-interacting protein 2 (Pstpip2) in the process of regulating the IL-1 pathway. This data supports the role of Pstpip2 as an anti-inflammatory molecule in an Nlrp-3 inflammasome-independent pathway.

Gene expression studies performed on tissues from cmo mice and cmo.IL-1R-deficient mice identified *Fblim1* as the most differentially expressed gene in the cmo mouse [52]. *Fblim1* encodes filamin-binding LIM protein-1 that is described as an anti-inflammatory molecule that is regulated by STAT3 and involved in bone remodeling [64, 65]. Utilizing whole exome sequencing, we identified two unrelated children with CRMO and mutations in *FBLIM1*. A homozygous mutation in the filamin-binding domain was found in a child with consanguineous healthy parents and another in an unrelated child with compound heterozygous mutation in *FBLIM1* including a novel frameshift mutation and a mutation that alters enhancer activity [52].

Microbiota in CRMO

The role of the microbiota in human CRMO remains unexplored, yet Lukens et al. reported that sterile osteomyelitis in the cmo mouse can be prevented by diet-induced alterations in the microbiota [63]. They fed newly weaned cmo mice a high-fat diet (HFD) and discovered that it provided nearly complete protection from the development of osteomyelitis. By 100 days of age, mice fed standard low-fat chow (LFD) had developed disease, whereas 100% of mice fed the HFD had yet to develop disease. With further aging, a few mice did develop evidence of inflammatory bone disease, but by 125 days, >90% of the HFD-fed cmo mice remained disease-free [63]. Radiologic and histologic analysis confirmed the near-complete protection from inflammatory bone disease in mice on the HFD. At 10–12 weeks of age, the HFD-fed cmo mice had marked alterations in their microbiota compared to cmo mice fed the normal LFD. Notably, the disease-prone cmo mice on a standard LFD had relative enrichment of inflammation-associated microbes including *Prevotella* accompanied by reductions in *Lactobacillus* species, compared to those on a HFD. Pro-IL-1β levels are upregulated in cmo mice fed a LFD compared to those on a HFD [63].

Proof that this protection was mediated by alterations in the microbiota came from fecal transplant studies. Specifically, fecal transplant of stool from cmo on a LFD into young unaffected cmo mice accelerated the development of osteomyelitis, whereas stool from a cmo fed a HFD transplanted into young unaffected cmo mice was associated with relative decreases in *Prevotella* and with relative protection from disease [63]. Replication followed by determination of the specific components in the diet that alter disease susceptibility in the mouse will be important prior to taking these observations from the bench to the bedside. The diets used by Lukens et al. differed not only in fat content but also in other dietary components such as gluten (present in LFD but not HFD). Data on the effect of diet on CRMO disease in humans is lacking. It is premature to offer any advice on dietary changes for human CRMO.

References

1. Jansson A, et al. Classification of non-bacterial osteitis: retrospective study of clinical, immunological and genetic aspects in 89 patients. Rheumatology (Oxford). 2007;46(1):154–60.
2. Giedion A, et al. Subacute and chronic "symmetrical" osteomyelitis. Ann Radiol (Paris). 1972;15(3):329–42.
3. Probst FP, Bjorksten B, Gustavson KH. Radiological aspect of chronic recurrent multifocal osteomyelitis. Ann Radiol (Paris). 1978;21(2–3):115–25.

4. Girschick HJ, et al. Chronic non-bacterial osteomyelitis in children. Ann Rheum Dis. 2005;64(2):279–85.
5. Chamot AM, et al. Acne-pustulosis-hyperostosis-osteitis syndrome. Results of a national survey. 85 cases. Rev Rhum Mal Osteoartic. 1987;54(3):187–96.
6. Jansson AF, Grote V, E.S. Group. Nonbacterial osteitis in children: data of a German incidence surveillance study. Acta Paediatr. 2011;100(8):1150–7.
7. Job-Deslandre C, Krebs S, Kahan A. Chronic recurrent multifocal osteomyelitis: five-year outcomes in 14 pediatric cases. Joint Bone Spine. 2001;68(3):245–51.
8. Schultz C, et al. Chronic recurrent multifocal osteomyelitis in children. Pediatr Infect Dis J. 1999;18(11):1008–13.
9. Huber AM, et al. Chronic recurrent multifocal osteomyelitis: clinical outcomes after more than five years of follow-up. J Pediatr. 2002;141(2):198–203.
10. Wipff J, et al. A large national cohort of French patients with chronic recurrent multifocal osteitis. Arthritis Rheumatol. 2015;67(4):1128–37.
11. Hedrich CM, et al. Autoinflammatory bone disorders with special focus on chronic recurrent multifocal osteomyelitis (CRMO). Pediatr Rheumatol Online J. 2013;11(1):47.
12. El-Shanti HI, Ferguson PJ. Chronic recurrent multifocal osteomyelitis: a concise review and genetic update. Clin Orthop Relat Res. 2007;462:11–9.
13. Morbach H, et al. Autoinflammatory bone disorders. Clin Immunol. 2013;147(3):185–96.
14. Toussirot E, Dupond JL, Wendling D. Spondylodiscitis in SAPHO syndrome. A series of eight cases. Ann Rheum Dis. 1997;56(1):52–8.
15. Sonozaki H, et al. Clinical features of 53 cases with pustulotic arthro-osteitis. Ann Rheum Dis. 1981;40(6):547–53.
16. Maugars Y, et al. SAPHO syndrome: a follow-up study of 19 cases with special emphasis on enthesis involvement. J Rheumatol. 1995;22(11):2135–41.
17. Vittecoq O, et al. Evolution of chronic recurrent multifocal osteitis toward spondylarthropathy over the long term. Arthritis Rheum. 2000;43(1):109–19.
18. Boutin RD, Resnick D. The SAPHO syndrome: an evolving concept for unifying several idiopathic disorders of bone and skin. AJR Am J Roentgenol. 1998;170(3):585–91.
19. Kahn MF. Why the "SAPHO" syndrome? J Rheumatol. 1995;22:2017–9.
20. Jurik AG. Chronic recurrent multifocal osteomyelitis. Semin Musculoskelet Radiol. 2004;8(3):243–53.
21. Bousvaros A, et al. Chronic recurrent multifocal osteomyelitis associated with chronic inflammatory bowel disease in children. Dig Dis Sci. 1999;44(12):2500–7.
22. Ferguson PJ, El-Shanti HI. Autoinflammatory bone disorders. Curr Opin Rheumatol. 2007;19(5):492–8.
23. Khanna G, Sato TS, Ferguson P. Imaging of chronic recurrent multifocal osteomyelitis. Radiographics. 2009;29(4):1159–77.
24. Khanna L, El-Khoury GY. SAPHO syndrome—a pictorial assay. Iowa Orthop J. 2012;32:189–95.
25. Guerin-Pfyffer S, et al. Evaluation of chronic recurrent multifocal osteitis in children by whole-body magnetic resonance imaging. Joint Bone Spine. 2012;79(6):616–20.
26. Mandell GA, et al. Bone scintigraphy in the detection of chronic recurrent multifocal osteomyelitis. J Nucl Med. 1998;39(10):1778–83.
27. Fritz J. The contributions of whole-body magnetic resonance imaging for the diagnosis and management of chronic recurrent multifocal osteomyelitis. J Rheumatol. 2015;42(8):1359–60.
28. Kennedy MT, et al. Whole body MRI in the diagnosis of chronic recurrent multifocal osteomyelitis. Orthop Traumatol Surg Res. 2012;98(4):461–4.
29. Bjorksten B, Boquist L. Histopathological aspects of chronic recurrent multifocal osteomyelitis. J Bone Joint Surg Br. 1980;62(3):376–80.
30. Girschick HJ, et al. Chronic recurrent multifocal osteomyelitis in children: diagnostic value of histopathology and microbial testing. Hum Pathol. 1999;30(1):59–65.
31. Sharma M, Ferguson PJ. Autoinflammatory bone disorders: update on immunologic abnormalities and clues about possible triggers. Curr Opin Rheumatol. 2013;25(5):658–64.
32. Schilling F, Wagner AD. Azithromycin: an anti-inflammatory effect in chronic recurrent multifocal osteomyelitis? A preliminary report. Z Rheumatol. 2000;59(5):352–3.
33. Beck C, et al. Chronic nonbacterial osteomyelitis in childhood: prospective follow-up during the first year of anti-inflammatory treatment. Arthritis Res Ther. 2010;12(2):R74.
34. Zhao Y, et al. Physicians' perspectives on the diagnosis and treatment of chronic nonbacterial osteomyelitis. Int J Rheumatol. 2017;2017:7694942.
35. Zhao Y, Laxer RM, Ferguson PJ. Treatment advances in chronic non-bacterial osteomyelitis and other autoinflammatory bone conditions. Curr Treat Options Rheum. 2017;3(1):17–32.
36. Ferguson PJ, Sandu M. Current understanding of the pathogenesis and management of chronic recurrent multifocal osteomyelitis. Curr Rheumatol Rep. 2012;14(2):130–41.
37. Eleftheriou D, et al. Biologic therapy in refractory chronic non-bacterial osteomyelitis of childhood. Rheumatology. 2010;49(8):1505–12.
38. Roderick M, et al. Efficacy of pamidronate therapy in children with chronic non-bacterial osteitis: disease activity assessment by whole body magnetic resonance imaging. Rheumatology (Oxford). 2014;53(11):1973–6.
39. Hofmann SR, et al. Chronic nonbacterial osteomyelitis: pathophysiological concepts and current treatment strategies. J Rheumatol. 2016;43(11):1956–64.
40. Hofmann C, et al. A standardized clinical and radiological follow-up of patients with chronic nonbacterial osteomyelitis treated with pamidronate. Clin Exp Rheumatol. 2014;32(4):604–9.

41. Park H, et al. Lighting the fires within: the cell biology of autoinflammatory diseases. Nat Rev Immunol. 2012;12(8):570–80.
42. Aksentijevich I, et al. An autoinflammatory disease with deficiency of the interleukin-1-receptor antagonist. N Engl J Med. 2009;360(23):2426–37.
43. Reddy S, et al. An autoinflammatory disease due to homozygous deletion of the IL1RN locus. N Engl J Med. 2009;360(23):2438–44.
44. Jesus AA, et al. A novel mutation of IL1RN in the deficiency of interleukin-1 receptor antagonist syndrome: description of two unrelated cases from Brazil. Arthritis Rheum. 2011;63(12):4007–17.
45. Minkis K, et al. Interleukin 1 receptor antagonist deficiency presenting as infantile pustulosis mimicking infantile pustular psoriasis. Arch Dermatol. 2012;148(6):747–52.
46. Jesus AA, Goldbach-Mansky R. IL-1 blockade in autoinflammatory syndromes. Annu Rev Med. 2014;65:223–44.
47. Ferguson PJ, et al. Homozygous mutations in LPIN2 are responsible for the syndrome of chronic recurrent multifocal osteomyelitis and congenital dyserythropoietic anaemia (Majeed syndrome). J Med Genet. 2005;42(7):551–7.
48. Majeed HA, et al. The syndrome of chronic recurrent multifocal osteomyelitis and congenital dyserythropoietic anaemia. Report of a new family and a review. Eur J Pediatr. 2001;160(12):705–10.
49. Rao AP, et al. Phenotypic variability in Majeed syndrome. J Rheumatol. 2016;43(6):1258–9.
50. Herlin T, et al. Efficacy of anti-IL-1 treatment in Majeed syndrome. Ann Rheum Dis. 2013;72(3):410–3.
51. Lorden G, et al. Lipin-2 regulates NLRP3 inflammasome by affecting P2X7 receptor activation. J Exp Med. 2016;214(2):511–28.
52. Cox AJ, Darbro BW, Laxer RM, Velez G, Bing X, Finer AL, Erives A, Mahajan VB, Bassuk AG, Ferguson PJ. Recessive coding and regulatory mutations in FBLIM1 underlie the pathogenesis of chronic recurrent multifocal osteomyelitis (CRMO). PLoS One. 2017;12(3):e0169687.
53. Golla A, et al. Chronic recurrent multifocal osteomyelitis (CRMO): evidence for a susceptibility gene located on chromosome 18q21.3-18q22. Eur J Hum Genet. 2002;10(3):217–21.
54. Hofmann SR, et al. Chronic non-bacterial osteomyelitis is associated with impaired Sp1 signaling, reduced IL10 promoter phosphorylation, and reduced myeloid IL-10 expression. Clin Immunol. 2011;141(3):317–27.
55. Hofmann SR, et al. Update: cytokine dysregulation in chronic nonbacterial osteomyelitis (CNO). Int J Rheumatol. 2012;2012:310206.
56. Ferguson PJ, et al. A missense mutation in pstpip2 is associated with the murine autoinflammatory disorder chronic multifocal osteomyelitis. Bone. 2006;38(1):41–7.
57. Grosse J, et al. Mutation of mouse Mayp/Pstpip2 causes a macrophage autoinflammatory disease. Blood. 2006;107(8):3350–8.
58. Liao HJ, et al. Increased neutrophil infiltration, IL-1 production and a SAPHO syndrome-like phenotype in PSTPIP2-deficient mice. Rheumatology (Oxford). 2015;54(7):1317–26.
59. Byrd L, et al. Chronic multifocal osteomyelitis, a new recessive mutation on chromosome 18 of the mouse. Genomics. 1991;11(4):794–8.
60. Chitu V, et al. Primed innate immunity leads to autoinflammatory disease in PSTPIP2-deficient cmo mice. Blood. 2009;114(12):2497–505.
61. Cassel SL, et al. Inflammasome-independent IL-1beta mediates autoinflammatory disease in Pstpip2-deficient mice. Proc Natl Acad Sci U S A. 2014;111(3):1072–7.
62. Lukens JR, et al. Critical role for inflammasome-independent IL-1beta production in osteomyelitis. Proc Natl Acad Sci U S A. 2014;111(3):1066–71.
63. Lukens JR, et al. Dietary modulation of the microbiota affects autoinflammatory disease. Nature. 2014;516(7530):246–9.
64. Xiao G, et al. Critical role of filamin-binding LIM protein 1 (FBLP-1)/migfilin in regulation of bone remodeling. J Biol Chem. 2012;287(25):21450–60.
65. Hutchins AP, Poulain S, Miranda-Saavedra D. Genome-wide analysis of STAT3 binding in vivo predicts effectors of the anti-inflammatory response in macrophages. Blood. 2012;119(13):e110–9.

Part V

Practical Aspects

32 Vaccinations in Rheumatology

Paul A. Bryant, Anoma Nellore,
and John W. Baddley

Abbreviations

ABT	Abatacept
ACIP	Advisory Committee on Immunization Practices
HAV	Hepatitis A virus
HBV	Hepatitis B virus
HPV	Human papilloma virus
HZ	Herpes zoster
JIA	Juvenile idiopathic arthritis
LAIV	Live attenuated influenza vaccine
MMR	Measles mumps and rubella (vaccine)
MSM	Men who have sex with men
MTX	Methotrexate
PCV	Pneumococcal conjugate vaccine
PPSV	Pneumococcal polysaccharide vaccine
PsA	Psoriatic arthritis
Pso	Psoriasis
PY	Person-years
RA	Rheumatoid arthritis
RD	Rheumatic diseases
RTX	Rituximab
SLE	Systemic lupus erythematosus
TAC	Tacrolimus
TNF-I	Tumor necrosis factor inhibitors
VZV	Varicella zoster virus

P. A. Bryant · A. Nellore
Department of Medicine, Division of Infectious Diseases, University of Alabama at Birmingham, Birmingham, AL, USA

J. W. Baddley (✉)
Department of Medicine, Division of Infectious Diseases, University of Alabama at Birmingham, Birmingham, AL, USA

Medical Service, Birmingham VA Medical Center, Birmingham, AL, USA
e-mail: jbaddley@uabmc.edu

Introduction

Treatment modalities for the rheumatic diseases (RD) have vastly improved over the past decade with the increased use of biological therapies. But, as a consequence of these therapies, the risk of infection is increased. The implementation of immunization strategies for a large number of infectious agents has brought about substantial progress in disease prevention. Vaccinations targeted at high-risk populations, such as in those with aberrant immune function, have led to decreases in infection-related morbidity and mortality [1].

Recommended immunization schedules for healthy adults and children are published periodically by the US Centers for Disease Control and other organizations [2, 3]. While well studied in healthy populations, vaccine efficacy and safety in those with RD on immunosuppressive medications have been less well characterized. Few studies have evaluated clinical outcomes following immunization, and several have sought to characterize the immune response as a surrogate

G. Ragab et al. (eds.), *The Microbiome in Rheumatic Diseases and Infection*,
https://doi.org/10.1007/978-3-319-79026-8_32

marker [4] and provide data on short-term safety issues following vaccine administration. This chapter will focus on vaccination among patients with RD.

Vaccine Immune Response

The development of an enduring antibody response, mediated by the humoral immune system, is the hallmark of vaccine protection, although the exact mechanisms that underpin durable antibody production remain unclear [5]. Vaccine antigens are delivered via draining lymphatics to secondary lymphoid tissues. Within these tissues, non-cognate B cells load vaccine antigens onto follicular dendritic cells for subsequent antigen presentation and activation of cognate B cells [6]. With co-stimulatory help from follicular T helper cells, cognate B cells undergo serial rounds of maturation in the dark zone of lymphoid follicles, in order to increase affinity for vaccine antigens. This process, termed the germinal center reaction [7], produces long-lived plasma cells that home to the bone marrow and generate durable, lifelong antibodies to vaccine antigens as well as long-lived memory B cells that form a second wave of defense against infectious challenge by rapidly differentiating into new antibody-secreting cells. Direct interrogation of long-lived plasma cells or memory B cells after vaccination is not the standard of current vaccine clinical trials, precluding our ability to mechanistically understand how vaccine-induced humoral immune responses change with endogenous immunocompromised or exogenous immunomodulatory agents. However, in vitro data, serologic responses, and the characterization of short-lived, largely antigen-specific plasmablasts after vaccination can provide some mechanistic insights into the impairments of humoral immunity after vaccination of patients with rheumatologic diseases [8].

The breakdown of peripheral immune tolerance, as manifested by the development of autoantibodies from self-reactive B cells, contributes to the development of rheumatologic diseases. A recent, novel study of plasmablasts from influenza-vaccinated systemic lupus erythematosus (SLE) subjects demonstrates that self-reactive B cells may be recruited into germinal center responses against vaccine antigens and generate flu antibodies that have an increased avidity and neutralizing capacity compared to flu antibodies from vaccinated healthy controls. In this study, there was no correlation between immunosuppressive regimen and generation of high avidity flu antibodies, suggesting that the endogenous immune deficits associated with SLE pathogenesis may have solely contributed to altered humoral immune responses to flu vaccine antigens [9].

In the context of humoral immunity, cytokines promote B cell differentiation into antibody-secreting cells [10]. Prednisone and other disease-modifying rheumatologic agents (DMARDs), like TNF-alpha inhibitors (TNF-I), methotrexate (MTX), and newer biologics like tocilizumab, modify the cytokine microenvironment as part of their therapeutic mechanism of action. Therefore, it follows that these agents may abrogate the cytokine signals B cells require to become antibody-secreting cells after vaccination. For example, recent in vitro data suggest a critical role for the cytokine IL-6 in sustaining a positive feedback loop between plasmablasts and follicular T helper cells, both critical to forming vaccine-induced humoral responses. Tocilizumab acts by inhibiting IL-6, and in vitro assays of PBMCs from rheumatoid arthritis (RA) patients on tocilizumab demonstrate impaired cross talk between plasmablasts and follicular T helper cells [11].

Disruption of B cell homeostasis is another mechanism by which immunomodulatory agents compromise vaccine responses. For example, rituximab (RTX) is a monoclonal anti-CD20 antibody that depletes the B cell pool. It is FDA approved for the treatment of refractory RA and is often used off-label for the treatment of other autoimmune rheumatologic diseases, including SLE. Vaccine response after RTX likely varies by efficacy of B cell ablation and repopulation of peripheral memory B cell subsets after treatment. RTX may selectively deplete tissue-specific memory B cells poised to differentiate into antibody-secreting cells for several years after drug receipt and thus may significantly impair the development of both peripheral and mucosal humoral immunity after vaccination [12, 13]. Similarly, TNF-I, like etanercept, reduces peripheral memory B cells, germinal center B cells, and follicular dendritic cells, compromising the development of affinity-matured memory B cell responses to vaccines [14, 15].

Vaccination remains the mainstay of infection prevention. Novel adjuvants, vaccine prime-boost schedules, and delivery platforms are being developed for optimal immune responses after vaccination. Although the mechanisms that may impact humoral immune responses after vaccination of patients with rheumatologic diseases are reviewed above, certain vaccines, like live attenuated influenza vaccine (LAIV), protect an individual by inducing mucosal cytolytic T cell responses to limit infection [16, 17]. Future vaccines and particularly vaccines against complex pathogens (e.g., CMV and HIV) may utilize cytolytic T cell responses as a prime means to contain disease [5]. The effects of DMARDs and the underlying immune deficits of rheumatologic diseases on the development of cytolytic T cell responses after vaccination are not completely known. Further research into the development, maintenance, and alteration of vaccine-induced immune responses in patients with rheumatologic diseases is needed to facilitate future rational vaccine designs for this patient population.

Vaccine Timing and Indications

In general, killed or surface moiety vaccines (e.g., influenza, pneumococcus) are safe for those individuals with altered immunocompetence. In contrast, live vaccines (e.g., measles, mumps, and rubella (MMR), zoster) may be contraindicated due to risks of vaccine-related infection or underlying disease exacerbation, depending on the degree of immunosuppression [2, 3]. In general, live vaccines should be administered ≥4 weeks prior to immunosuppression and should be avoided within 2 weeks of initiation of immunosuppression [2, 3]. Recommendations for vaccination in RD patients as related to degree of immunosuppression are outlined in Table 32.1.

Inactivated Vaccines

Influenza

Several influenza vaccine formulations (trivalent or quadrivalent) are currently available in the USA. Influenza virus vaccine is well studied in terms of safety and immunogenicity and is recommended for all individuals ≥6 months of age without contraindications, according to the US Advisory Committee on Immunization Practices (ACIP). There is increased effort placed on vaccinating high-risk individuals such as the elderly, healthcare workers, and immunocompromised persons [18, 19]. Over the past decade, several studies have investigated the use, efficacy, and safety of seasonal influenza vaccination in RD patients.

Safety and Efficacy

Influenza vaccination in RD patients has been shown to be safe and immunogenic; however, there are limited data regarding clinical efficacy [2, 3]. Patients with RA have been studied more frequently with regard to vaccine safety and immune response, compared to other rheumatic diseases [3, 20–24]. A 2006 Israeli study evaluated seroconversion and disease activity in 82 RA patients and controls following administration of split-virion inactivated influenza vaccine containing three antigens [20]. Both groups saw a significant rise in mean antibody titers to all antigens tested, but the vaccine was not uniformly immunogenic. One of the three antigens provided a significantly higher rate of response (defined as at least a fourfold rise in titers by 6 weeks) in controls compared to RA patients (87% vs. 67%, $p = 0.05$). Overall, humoral response was adequate in both groups. In addition, no increase in RA disease activity was noted by 6 weeks. Response also appeared to be independent of RA therapy, including corticosteroids, MTX, infliximab, etanercept, and other DMARDs. An Italian study that same year compared SLE/RA patients vaccinated with a non-adjuvanted flu vaccine to non-vaccinated SLE/RA patients and vaccinated healthy controls [21]. There was a significant increase in antibody response in all groups, with no difference observed in either response or rate of adverse events. The study participants all had low-level or stable disease activity, and most were taking corticosteroids plus MTX or cyclosporine. The two patients that were on a TNF-I at the time of vaccination showed good tolerability, with no reported adverse events.

More recent studies have evaluated the effect of newer biological therapies. A small Israeli study demonstrated that RTX use in RA patients partially blunts the humoral response with flu vaccination compared to those patients on traditional DMARDs [22]. However, some protective benefit was achieved depending on the antigen tested, and there was no difference between groups in terms of disease activity. A similarly powered Dutch trial also showed decreased humoral response to influenza antigens in RTX-treated RA participants, but a restored response 6–10 months after RTX had been discontinued [23]. There was no laboratory or clinically measured increase in RA disease activity during the postvaccination follow-up period.

An Italian case-control study further evaluated non-adjuvanted flu vaccination in RA patients on TNF-I during 2005–2008 [24]. Patients were receiving TNF-I plus prednisone and MTX. RA patients fulfilled criteria for full protection in the 2007–2008 season, whereas they only achieved a protective response to influenza A vaccine in the first two seasons. The healthy controls only met criteria in the second season. No significant increase in RA disease activity score or antinuclear antibody titer was observed as a consequence of the vaccine [19, 20].

More promising results were obtained in a recent analysis evaluating the effects of influenza vaccine in patients with psoriatic arthritis (PsA) ($n = 63$) and psoriasis (Pso) ($n = 4$) [25]. Just over half of patients were on TNF-I, and approximately 30% were treated with a traditional DMARD. A similar immune response was achieved in healthy controls and all PsA/Pso patients regardless of their prescribed treatment modality. There was no increase in disease activity. Similarly, a prospective, Japanese pediatric study evaluated 49 children with juvenile idiopathic arthritis (JIA) ($n = 23$), SLE ($n = 12$), juvenile dermatomyositis ($n = 6$), and other RD ($n = 8$) who received a trivalent flu vaccine. No difference in immunogenicity or safety was observed among all groups, but in this study only one patient was on biological therapy [26].

The 2009–2010 influenza A/H1N1 pandemic resulted in statements by the World Health Organization encouraging the development of vaccines containing adjuvant [27, 28]. Adjuvants, such as aluminum, are frequently added to vaccines to boost immunogenicity [29, 30]. Adjuvanted influenza vaccine administered during the 2009–2010 flu pandemic showed similar results in terms of safety and efficacy [31–38] compared to the seasonal flu vaccine, with two studies recommending a booster vaccine in RD patients to produce an adequate antibody response [34, 35]. Studies with adjuvanted pandemic flu vaccine have produced variable yet still favorable results in terms of immunogenicity and safety, with one study noting a mild increase in RA-related symptoms [38].

Influenza Vaccination and Newer Biologics

Few studies have addressed influenza vaccine use in patients on newer biologic agents [39–41]. A small Japanese study showed that flu vaccination in JIA patients treated with tocilizumab was safe and effective compared to healthy controls [39]. A randomized trial with RA patients on the TNF-I certolizumab pegol or placebo showed comparable humoral responses to influenza vaccination but somewhat diminished responses with concomitant MTX use [40]. Similar results have been reported for the soluble fusion protein abatacept (ABT), in moderate-to-severe RA [41]. There are no studies to date that report a drastic difference in immunogenicity or tolerability to influenza vaccination with the newer biologics.

Clinical Outcomes and Influenza Vaccination

Incidence rates of viral infections and secondary bacterial complications are reduced in RD patients following influenza vaccination [19]. In RA and SLE patients, influenza vaccination has been shown to decrease the number of viral and secondary bacterial infections while also reducing the risk of RA/SLE exacerbations that result as a consequence of infection [42]. Milanovic et al. showed in a 2013 study that SLE patients had a significantly lower rate of total viral infections (including influenza) with 26% vs. 91% ($p < 0.01$) in the vaccinated and unvaccinated subgroups, respectively [43]. The RA and Sjögren's syndrome groups had similar results, although postvaccination antibody titers were lower in these groups. Likewise, a large cohort study of RA patients in Japan showed a decreased influenza attack rate in vaccinated patients measured over four flu seasons from 2000 to 2007 but included few patients on biologics [44].

Streptococcus pneumoniae

There are two FDA-approved vaccines available in the USA for protection against invasive pneumococcal disease: a polysaccharide vaccine (PPSV23) and a conjugate vaccine (PCV13). In the USA, PPSV23 is indicated for all adults aged > 65 years of age and in individuals >19 years of age with select chronic or immunocompromising conditions (Table 32.1, [45]). PCV13 carries the same indications but is also recommended for infants >6 weeks old, children, and adolescents to prevent otitis media and invasive pneumococcal disease and is part of the routine childhood immunization series [45]. Both vaccines should be routinely administered to patients with autoimmune RD, as these patients are at increased risk for pneumococcal disease, with especially higher rates of respiratory infections and mortality in RA and SLE patients [46–49]. In addition, these vaccines are indicated in patients on long-term corticosteroids or other immunosuppressive medications such as biologics or traditional DMARDs (Table 32.1). Of note, the PCV13 vaccine replaced the previously administered PCV7 in 2010. Many of the studies evaluating use of the conjugate pneumococcal

Table 32.1 Adult and pediatric vaccine recommendations for rheumatic disease patients based on degree of immunosuppression [2, 3]

Vaccine	Low-level immunosuppression[a]	High-level immunosuppression[b]
Influenza (inactivated)	R	R
Influenza (live attenuated)	X	X
Pneumococcal polysaccharide (PPSV23)	R	R
Pneumococcal conjugate (PCV13)	R	R
Hepatitis A	R	R
Hepatitis B	R	R
Human papillomavirus (HPV)	R	R
Diphtheria, tetanus, acellular pertussis (DTaP); tetanus, diphtheria, acellular pertussis (Tdap); or Td booster	R	R
Measles, mumps, rubella (live)	X	X
Varicella (live)	V[c]	X
Zoster (live)	R	X
Haemophilus influenzae b conjugate	R	R
Rotavirus (live)	X	X
Polio (inactivated)	R	R
Meningococcal conjugate	R	R

R routine, per usual guidelines for immunocompetent individuals, *X* contradicted, *V* variable

[a]Low-level immunosuppression includes prednisone <2 mg/kg/day (maximum 20 mg/day), methotrexate ≤0.4 mg/kg/week, azathioprine ≤3 mg/kg/day, or 6-mercaptopurine ≤1.5 mg/kg/day

[b]High-level immunosuppression includes medication dosages higher than those listed in the low-level immunosuppression category as well as biologic agents such as TNF inhibitors

[c]The Infectious Diseases Society of America (IDSA) recommends varicella vaccination to chronic inflammatory disease patients on low-dose immunosuppression. This deviates from ACIP recommendations

vaccine use this earlier formulation, as will be discussed.

Safety and Efficacy of Polysaccharide Vaccine (PPSV23)

Most studies have used humoral immune response as a marker of efficacy, with few reports on clinical outcomes following vaccination against pneumococcus in RD patients. Patients with RA and SLE have been more rigorously evaluated, with older reports using polysaccharide vaccine and confirming safety [50–52].

PPSV23 is tolerable in SLE and RA patients, but immunogenicity is variable, with a study in 2002 revealing no or poor (i.e., to only one serotype) response in 33.3% and 20.8% of RA ($n = 42$) and SLE ($n = 15$) patients, respectively. All controls responded ($p = 0.004$) [53]. Type of immunosuppressive agent did not influence response, but patients receiving biologics were not included [53, 54]. Moreover, disease activity did not increase from baseline, and no major adverse events were reported. A larger study in 2006 including 149 RA patients treated with a TNF-I plus MTX ($n = 50$), TNF-I alone or in combination with other DMARDs ($n = 62$), or MTX alone ($n = 37$) showed that PPSV23 antibody responses were present in all groups but were significantly impaired when MTX was used, regardless of TNF-I presence [55]. Similarly, an analysis of PsA patients receiving the TNF-I etanercept or placebo showed similar responses to PPSV23, but concomitant MTX use was associated with lower mean antibody titers [56].

Migita and colleagues evaluated 133 RA patients immunized with PPSV23 who were on therapy with tacrolimus (TAC) ($n = 29$), MTX ($n = 55$), or TAC/MTX ($n = 14$). Controls were classified as being treated with other DMARDs or corticosteroids ($n = 35$) [57]. Patients receiving TAC alone had comparable rates of IgG antibody response to the serotypes tested (6B, 23F), compared to RA controls. Of note, rates of response for patients on TAC monotherapy were significantly higher than for those on MTX. Mori et al. conducted a similar study with RA patients on tocilizumab that demonstrated adequate IgG response to the same serotypes of PPVS23, compared to RA controls [58]. There were no serious adverse events noted in the treatment groups. In addition, MTX use was associated with decreased vaccine efficacy, consistent with other reports [55–57]. A larger study, consisting of 130 RD patients, 51.5% of whom had RA followed in frequency by PsA, ankylosing spondylitis, or inflammatory bowel disease-associated spondyloarthritis, reported on the long-term efficacy of PPSV23 [59]. Of the 88 patients who had long-term (0–10 years) data available, there was no association between expected decreases in antibody titers and TNF-I, tocilizumab, or low-dose prednisone. However, MTX use was associated with significantly lower antibody levels.

A nested immunogenicity study was recently conducted within a randomized trial evaluating PPSV23 efficacy in RA patients, with incidence of pneumonia as the primary endpoint [60]. The focus of this 2015 Japanese study was to evaluate the effect of ABT on PPSV23 response in RA. The design was similar to other studies with three main groups: RA controls (non-ABT DMARDs; $n = 35$), MTX ($n = 55$), and ABT ($n = 24$). ABT produced no decrease in antibody functionality (measured as an opsonization index), despite leading to overall decrease in total IgG produced, and this appeared to be independent of MTX use. No safety issues were reported. Alten et al. showed that 83.9% of RA patients on ABT (with most also receiving MTX) achieved a protective level of antibodies postvaccination with PPSV23, but no control group was available for comparison [41]. RTX has also been shown to reduce humoral immune responses to polysaccharide vaccine [4, 61, 62] and conjugate vaccine [63], although tocilizumab was not shown to impair antibody response.

Conjugate Pneumococcal Vaccine (PCV7 and PCV 13)

As previously mentioned, most studies evaluating the conjugate pneumococcal vaccine in persons with RD have used the PCV7 formulation. These have primarily reported on pediatric patients. Studies involving the newer conjugate pneumococcal vaccine (PCV13) use are lacking.

Pediatric JIA patients undergoing treatment with TNF-I plus conventional DMARDs compared to DMARDs alone achieved protective antibody levels to PCV7 in a 2010 study [64]. While the mean antibody titers were lower in the TNF-I group, none of the patients developed a serious respiratory tract infection or proven invasive pneumococcal disease at 24 months of follow-up. In a recent study involving 302 adult patients with RA or spondyloarthritis on stable medication for 18 months who received PCV7, only concomitant TNF-I and MTX use were negative predictors of persistent antibody protection [65]. Long-term clinical efficacy was further evaluated in a cohort of 497 RA/PsA patients 4.5 years after a single dose of PCV7 and showed that development of serious infections was associated with older age and steroid use, rather than TNF-I or MTX [66].

There is a lack of data on use of the PCV13 vaccine in RD populations. A 2016 study included 22 RA patients on etanercept monotherapy or in combination with MTX and showed comparable immunogenicity and safety profile compared to osteoarthritis controls not on treatment [67].

Hepatitis A

Safety and Efficacy

ACIP recommends hepatitis A vaccine for all individuals >12 months of age and in select unvaccinated adult populations such as men who have sex with men (MSM) or those traveling to countries with high or intermediate levels of endemic hepatitis A (Table 32.1; [68]). A study from Turkey included 47 children with JIA who received the hepatitis A virus (HAV) vaccination series and reported that the vast majority of patients reached the study's definition of protective anti-HAV IgG levels [69]. While no increases in disease activity or serious adverse events were reported, four children who had active disease and were on TNF-I therapy did not respond. In contrast, patients on MTX and steroids mounted an appropriate immune response to a two-dose series. A more recent report included 53 nonimmune adult RA patients on active therapy with TNF-I, TNF-I plus MTX, or MTX alone [70]. While 86% of the participants reached protective antibody levels by 24 months following a two-dose series, protection was not adequate after only one dose early in the series. This is consistent with a prior study showing lack of protection after only one dose of HAV vaccine in patients on immunosuppressive medication [71]. Of note, the level of seroprotection was much higher in the TNF-I-only group compared to both groups that included MTX as part of the treatment regimen [70]. No increase in disease activity was observed.

Hepatitis B

Safety and Efficacy

ACIP recommends hepatitis B vaccine for all neonates prior to hospital discharge, unvaccinated children, and unvaccinated adults, especially those with high-risk behavior such as MSM or injection drug users, medical workers, travelers to endemic countries, and certain medical conditions such as diabetes or chronic renal disease (Table 32.1; [72, 73]). Hepatitis B virus (HBV) vaccination was shown to produce a protective immune response in an earlier study involving RA patients, with approximately 68% (15/22 patients) developing protective antibodies 1 month following the third dose in a complete series [74]. Furthermore, 80% (16/20) of JIA patients were later shown to achieve an adequate level of seroprotection following completion of the vaccine series, compared to 100% of healthy controls [75]. The response did not appear to be influenced by immunosuppressive regimen; however, no children on biologics were included in the study. Likewise, another small study showed that SLE patients could achieve a response rate of 93%, but in this particular study only patients with stable disease not on immunosuppressants (except low-dose prednisone) were included [76]. A recent study suggests a blunting of HBV vaccine response in patients on TNF-I [77].

Prior case reports have suggested that there is a risk of developing autoimmune disease following vaccination for HBV [78–80], but a larger, retrospective study [81] found no association between HBV vaccine and development of RA. In the previously discussed studies, no disease flares or adverse reactions from the vaccine itself were reported [74–76].

Human Papillomavirus (HPV)

Safety and Efficacy

ACIP currently recommends routine vaccination for HPV in females and males aged 11–12, for the prevention of cervical, anal, vulvar, and penile cancer, as well as possibly decreasing risk of male to female transmission (Table 32.1; [82–84]). Genital HPV is the most common sexually transmitted infection in the USA [85], and HPV types 16 and 18 are considered to be high risk, as they predispose to cervical cell abnormalities that can lead to cervical cancer [86–88]. SLE patients are at particular risk for infection with high-risk HPV types [89, 90], with a recent meta-analysis reporting a pooled odds ratio of 8.66 (95% CI, 3.75–20.0) for the risk of high-grade squamous intraepithelial lesions in SLE patients compared to controls [90], similar to a previous Canadian cohort analysis [91].

The bivalent HPV vaccine has been evaluated in two studies by Heijstek et al. [92, 93] and one by Esposito et al. [94]. It was initially suggested in a small pilot study that a high proportion of female SLE and juvenile dermatomyositis patients could attain seropositivity following vaccination [92]. In a larger prospective, cohort analysis, 68 female JIA participants and healthy controls all achieved seropositivity to either HPV16 or 18, or both [93]. While patients had consistently lower antibody concentrations than controls, this difference was not statistically significant. Immunosuppressive therapy did not appear to affect seropositivity, but the number of patients on TNF-I was too low to draw any definitive conclusions. Esposito et al. reached similar conclusions with a smaller number of female JIA participants [94]. No increase in underlying disease activity or flares could be attributed to vaccination.

The quadrivalent HPV4 vaccine (including types 6, 11, 16, 18) was shown to be immunogenic in SLE patients when compared to controls in an analysis by Mok et al. [95]. After 12 months, the seroconversion rate for HPV types 6, 11, 16, and 18 was 82%, 89%, 95%, and 76% for patients and 98%, 98%, 98%, and 80% for controls, respectively. There was no difference in SLE disease activity between the two groups at the end of the study. Similarly, a smaller study showed seropositivity rates >94% to all four HPV types in SLE patients [96].

Case series and epidemiological studies have shown an association between the HPV4 vaccine and increased risk of certain autoimmune adverse events such as SLE development or flares, vasculitis, and RA [97, 98] but no increased risk of Guillain-Barré syndrome [98]. The previously mentioned studies did not report an increased risk of underlying disease activity or flares following vaccination against HPV [92–96].

Live Vaccines

Measles, Mumps, and Rubella

Safety and Efficacy

ACIP recommends beginning the MMR vaccine series in all children aged 12 months and select unvaccinated adults such as healthcare workers (Table 32.1; [99]). A retrospective study on 207 JIA patients receiving MMR vaccination demonstrated no increase in disease activity or need for medication dose adjustment after 6 months [100]. This included a subset analysis of patients on MTX, where no major differences were noted relative to those that were unvaccinated. A small number of patients experienced mild joint aggravation ($n = 9$), fevers or malaise ($n = 6$), or rash ($n = 2$). No cases of measles, mumps, or rubella were reported in the follow-up period. Immunogenicity was assessed in a study by Heijstek et al., in which 400 patients with JIA who had previously received a single dose of the MMR vaccine were given an MMR booster and compared to healthy controls [101]. Vaccine-specific protective antibody concentrations were lower in JIA patients for mumps (OR 0.4; 95% CI 0.3–0.6) and rubella (OR 0.4; 0.3–0.7) but did not differ significantly for measles (OR 1.4; 0.8–2.5) compared to controls. The use of glucocorticoids or MTX did not appear to influence immune response. Importantly, this study did not assess the safety of administering the initial dose of the MMR vaccine to children on immunosuppressive medications.

Varicella

Safety and Efficacy

ACIP recommends varicella vaccination for all persons 12 months and older, especially for non-immune persons with close contact with children, as well as healthcare workers, travelers, and close contacts of immunocompromised patients (Table 32.1; [102]). While the varicella zoster virus causes both primary infection (chickenpox) and reactivation following primary infection (shingles), varicella vaccine formulation contains a much lower dose of antigen than the zoster vaccine [102].

While varicella (chickenpox) vaccine is safe and effective in patients with certain pediatric RD (e.g., SLE, vasculitis, juvenile dermatomyositis) [103], most experience has been in patients with JIA [104, 105]. A 2010 study evaluated 25 patients (predominantly with JIA) compared to controls following varicella vaccination [104]. All patients were receiving MTX (mean dosage of 16.4 mg/m^2/week, range 10–27) with 13 also on prednisone (mean total dosage of 4.2 mg/day, range 3–20), while five received other DMARDs. None were on TNF-I. Varicella zoster virus (VZV) IgG titers were similar in patients and controls during the 32-month median follow-up period, and no increase in disease activity was noted even in those on higher doses of prednisone and MTX. One patient developed severe, complicated varicella, but this patient had been started on TNF-I therapy during the follow-up period and was also exposed to an active case of varicella. A smaller prospective study with six JIA patients on biologics (TNF-I or tocilizumab) showed that five of six participants were able to seroconvert following vaccination, but one patient developed mild varicella 4 months later, even with evidence of low level of protective antibodies [105]. No increase in disease activity was observed.

Herpes Zoster Virus

In adults, the prevention of herpes zoster (HZ), or shingles, due to reactivation of latent varicella zoster virus has been shown to improve quality of life and decrease morbidity from postherpetic neuralgia [106, 107]. Several studies report an increased risk for VZV reactivation in RD patients compared to age-matched controls, especially those on immunosuppressive therapy [108–128]. A study by Zhang and colleagues demonstrated that vaccinated RD patients have lower rates of HZ compared to unvaccinated RD controls [129]. This was followed in 2012 by a larger, retrospective cohort study evaluating administrative data. In this cohort, consisting of over 460,000 patients with RA, Pso, PsA, ankylosing spondylitis, and/or inflammatory bowel disease, the risk of HZ in the immediate postvaccination period, as well as the vaccine's long-term efficacy, was evaluated [130]. Approximately 4% of the patients received HZ vaccine during the 2-year follow-up period. Of the 633 vaccinated RD patients who were exposed to TNF-I or other biologics, none developed varicella or HZ in the 42 days following receipt of the live zoster vaccine. Overall, the incidence of HZ in the vaccinated group during the 2-year median follow-up period was 6.7 cases per 1000 person-years (PY) compared to 11.6 cases per 1000 PY in the unvaccinated group (rate ratio of 0.58; $p < 0.0001$). The most common adverse event reported was injection site reactions.

A novel subunit vaccine for zoster, HZ/su, has recently been approved. It contains 50 ug of recombinant VZV glycoprotein E formulated with ASO1 adjuvant. To date, there are limited data of its use in immunosuppressed patients. However, data from early trials in HIV or autologous stem cell transplant recipients suggest that the vaccine is safe and immunogenic [131, 132].

Travel-Related Vaccinations

Travel-related vaccinations in the immunosuppressed RD patient present unique challenges depending on the travel destination (Table 32.2; [3, 133]). Vaccines such as hepatitis A, MMR, and varicella are commonly recommended for nonimmune patients prior to international travel. Certain vaccines, such as yellow fever or Japanese encephalitis virus vaccine, are recommended only for travelers to specific endemic countries (Table 32.2).

There is a lack of published data on safety, efficacy, or clinical outcomes in immunosuppressed RD patients with use of the Japanese encephalitis virus [134] or typhoid vaccines [135]. However, a single retrospective safety study has been published assessing the live virus yellow fever vaccine in these patients [136]. This study evaluated 70 patients with RD (RA, SLE, spondyloarthritis) on immunosuppression (including nine on biologics) and found that 22.5% of participants reported a mild adverse effect, such as an injection site reaction. No adverse events were reported. ACIP recommends immunocompromised persons not to travel to yellow fever-endemic countries if at all possible [137].

Conclusion

Patients with rheumatic diseases, especially those on immunosuppressive therapy, are at increased risk for a wide range of both common and opportunistic infections. In general, vaccination appears to be an appropriate strategy to reduce overall infectious risk in these patients. While large, prospective trials are limited, killed vaccines appear to be safe and pose little risk in terms of disease exacerbation or induction compared to unvaccinated controls. Among the traditional DMARDs, MTX in particular may blunt the immune response, as has been observed in studies

Table 32.2 Recommendations for travel vaccines not included in routine immunization schedules

Vaccine	Low-level immunosuppression[a]	High-level immunosuppression[b]	Comments
Japanese encephalitis virus (inactivated)	Caution, theoretically safe	Caution, theoretically safe	No safety/efficacy data available in RD patients. Indicated for travelers to endemic areas for >1 month stay, mainly Southeast Asia, Indonesia, and parts of Australia
Japanese encephalitis virus (live, attenuated, not available in the USA)	X	X	No safety/efficacy data available in RD patients
Typhoid (oral, live), from the Ty21a strain of *Salmonella typhi*	X	X	Indicated for travelers to endemic areas, close contacts of potentially exposed individuals, and laboratory workers with exposure
Typhoid (IM, inactivated), Vi capsular polysaccharide vaccine	Caution, theoretically safe	Caution, theoretically safe	No safety/efficacy data available in RD patients. May be safe for immunosuppressed RD patients
Yellow fever (live)	X	X	Limited data in RD patients. Indicated for travelers to endemic areas in South America and Africa

X = contraindicated

[a]Low-level immunosuppression includes prednisone <2 mg/kg/day (maximum 20 mg/day), methotrexate ≤0.4 mg/kg/week, azathioprine ≤3 mg/kg/day, or 6-mercaptopurine ≤1.5 mg/kg/day

[b]High-level immunosuppression includes medication dosages higher than those listed in the low-level immunosuppression category as well as biologic agents such as TNF inhibitors

[c]Recommendation to consider vaccine "Contraindicated" is based on general ACIP recommendations for live vaccines, as specific data for most travel-related vaccines in RD patients are not available

involving PPSV23 and persons with RA and SLE. TNF-I therapy appears to only affect immunogenicity to a small degree depending on the drug, while other biologics such as RTX and ABT may negatively impact the humoral response. Analyses of clinical outcomes following vaccination are more limited, but some prospective studies suggest that despite a decrease in mean antibody titers in certain immunosuppressed groups, overall incidence rates of infection are similar to vaccinated controls.

While live vaccines are generally avoided in immunosuppressed groups, the available data suggest that patients with stable rheumatic disease on low-dose immunosuppression may be candidates to receive certain vaccines, such as herpes zoster. The general approach for use of live vaccines in these individuals, if unavoidable, is to administer the vaccine ≥4 weeks prior to immunosuppression and avoid administration within 2 weeks of initiation of immunosuppression [2, 3]. A risk-benefit analysis prior to giving live vaccines to immunosuppressed patients should be made on a case-by-case basis.

While immunizations should continue to be administered according to national guidelines, additional data regarding long-term immunogenicity and clinical outcomes are needed. Vaccine adherence in patients with RD should be encouraged given the efficacy and excellent safety profile of most vaccines.

References

1. Glück T, Müller-Ladner U. Vaccination in patients with chronic rheumatic or autoimmune diseases. Clin Infect Dis. 2008;46:1459–65.
2. Centers for Disease Control and Prevention. General recommendations on immunization, recommendations of the advisory committee on immunization practices (ACIP). MMWR. 2011;60(RR-2):3–34.
3. Rubin LG, Levin MJ, Ljungman P, et al. Infectious Diseases Society of America. 2013 IDSA clinical practice guideline for vaccination of the immunocompromised host. Clin Infect Dis. 2014;58(3):44–100.
4. Papadopoulou D, Tsoulas C, Tragiannidis A, Sipsas NV. Role of vaccinations and prophylaxis in rheumatic diseases. Best Pract Res Clin Rheumatol. 2015;29(2):306–18.
5. Amanna IJ, Slifka MK. Contributions of humoral and cellular immunity to vaccine-induced protection in humans. Virology. 2011;411(2):206–15.
6. Phan TG, et al. Subcapsular encounter and complement-dependent transport of immune complexes by lymph node B cells. Nat Immunol. 2007;8(9):992–1000.
7. Mesin L, Ersching J, Victora GD. Germinal center B cell dynamics. Immunity. 2016;45(3):471–82.
8. Wrammert J, et al. Broadly cross-reactive antibodies dominate the human B cell response against 2009 pandemic H1N1 influenza virus infection. J Exp Med. 2011;208(1):181–93.
9. Kaur K, et al. High affinity antibodies against influenza characterize the Plasmablast response in SLE patients after vaccination. PLoS One. 2015;10(5):e0125618.
10. Moens L, Tangye SG. Cytokine-mediated regulation of plasma cell generation: IL-21 takes Center stage. Front Immunol. 2014;5:65.
11. Chavele KM, Merry E, Ehrenstein MR. Cutting edge: circulating plasmablasts induce the differentiation of human T follicular helper cells via IL-6 production. J Immunol. 2015;194(6):2482–5.
12. Anolik JH, et al. Insights into the heterogeneity of human B cells: diverse functions, roles in autoimmunity, and use as therapeutic targets. Immunol Res. 2009;45(2–3):144–58.
13. Sanz I, et al. Phenotypic and functional heterogeneity of human memory B cells. Semin Immunol. 2008;20(1):67–82.
14. Kobie JJ, et al. Decreased influenza-specific B cell responses in rheumatoid arthritis patients treated with anti-tumor necrosis factor. Arthritis Res Ther. 2011;13(6):R209.
15. Ravikumar R, Anolik J, Looney RJ. Vaccine responses in patients with rheumatoid arthritis. Curr Rheumatol Rep. 2007;9(5):407–15.
16. Chen GL, et al. Seasonal influenza infection and live vaccine prime for a response to the 2009 pandemic H1N1 vaccine. Proc Natl Acad Sci U S A. 2011;108(3):1140–5.
17. Peng Y, et al. Boosted influenza-specific T cell responses after H5N1 pandemic live attenuated influenza virus vaccination. Front Immunol. 2015;6:287.
18. Uyeki TM. Preventing and controlling influenza with available interventions. N Engl J Med. 2014;370(9):789–91.
19. Grohskopf LA, Sokolow LZ, Broder KR, et al. Prevention and control of seasonal influenza with vaccines. MMWR Recomm Rep. 2016;65(5):1–54.
20. Fomin I, Caspi D, Levy V, et al. Vaccination against influenza in rheumatoid arthritis: the effect of disease modifying drugs, including TNF alpha blockers. Ann Rheum Dis. 2006;65(2):191–4.

21. Del Porto F, Laganà B, Biselli R, et al. Influenza vaccine administration in patients with systemic lupus erythematosus and rheumatoid arthritis: safety and immunogenicity. Vaccine. 2006;24(16):3217–23.
22. Oren S, Mandelboim M, Braun-Moscovici Y, et al. Vaccination against influenza in patients with rheumatoid arthritis: the effect of rituximab on the humoral response. Ann Rheum Dis. 2008;67(7):937–41.
23. van Assen S, Holvast A, Benne CA, et al. Humoral responses after influenza vaccination are severely reduced in patients with rheumatoid arthritis treated with rituximab. Arthritis Rheum. 2010;62(1):75–81.
24. Salemi S, Picchianti-Diamanti A, Germano V, et al. Influenza vaccine administration in rheumatoid arthritis patients under treatment with TNF alpha blockers: safety and immunogenicity. Clin Immunol. 2010;134(2):113–20.
25. Polachek A, Korobko U, Mader-Balakirski N, et al. Immunogenicity and safety of vaccination against seasonal 2012 influenza virus among patients with psoriatic arthritis and psoriasis. Clin Exp Rheumatol. 2015;33(2):181–6.
26. Ogimi C, Tanaka R, Saitoh A, Oh-Ishi T. Immunogenicity of influenza vaccine in children with pediatric rheumatic diseases receiving immunosuppressive agents. Pediatr Infect Dis J. 2011;30(3):208–11.
27. Diez-Domingo J, Garces-Sanchez M, Baldo JM, et al. Immunogenicity and safety of H5N1A/Vietnam/1194/2004 (clade 1) AS03-adjuvanted prepandemic candidate influenza vaccines in children aged 3 to 9 years: a phase II, randomized, open, controlled study. Pediatr Infect Dis J. 2010;29:35–46.
28. Schwarz TF, Horacek T, Knuf M, et al. Single dose vaccination with AS03- adjuvanted H5N1 vaccines in a randomized trial induces strong and broad immune responsiveness to booster vaccination in adults. Vaccine. 2009;27:6284–90.
29. Reed SG, Orr MT, Fox CB. Key roles of adjuvants in modern vaccines. Nat Med. 2013;19(12):1597–608.
30. Schijns V, Tartour E, Michalek J, et al. Immune adjuvants as critical guides directing immunity triggered by therapeutic cancer vaccines. Cytotherapy. 2014;16(4):427–39.
31. Aikawa NE, Campos LMA, Silva CA, et al. Glucocorticoid: major factor for reduced immunogenicity of 2009 influenza a (H1N1) vaccine in patients with juvenile autoimmune rheumatic disease. J Rheumatol. 2012;39:167–73.
32. Lu CC, Wang YC, Lai JH, et al. A/H1N1influenza vaccination in patients with systemic lupus erythematosus: safety and immunity. Vaccine. 2011;29:444–50.
33. Urowitz MB, Anton A, Ibanez D, Gladman DD. Autoantibody response to adjuvant and nonadjuvant H1N1 vaccination in systemic lupus erythematosus. Arthritis Care Res. 2011;63:1517–20.
34. Saad CGS, Borba EF, Aikawa NE, et al. Immunogenicity and safety of the & 2009 nonadjuvanted influenza A/H1N1 vaccine in a large cohort of autoimmune rheumatic diseases. Ann Rheum Dis. 2011;70:1068–73.
35. Aikawa NE, Trudes G, Campos LM, et al. Immunogenicity and safety of two doses of a nonadjuvanted influenza A H1N1/2009 vaccine in young autoimmune rheumatic diseases patients. Lupus. 2013;22(13):1394–8.
36. Adler S, Krivine A, Weix J, et al. Protective effect of A/H1N1 vaccination in & immune-mediated disease: a prospectively controlled vaccination study. Rheumatology. 2012;51:695–700.
37. Gabay C, Bel M, Combescure C, et al. Impact of synthetic and biologic disease-modifying anti-rheumatic drugs on antibody responses to the AS03-adjuvanted pandemic influenza vaccine: a prospective, openlabel, parallel-cohort, single-center study. Arthritis Rheum. 2011;63:1486–96.
38. Milanetti F, Germano V, Nisini R, et al. Safety and immunogenicity of co-administered MF59-adjuvanted 2009 pandemic and plain 2009-10 seasonal influenza vaccines in rheumatoid arthritis patients on biologicals. Clin Exp Immunol. 2014;177(1):287–94.
39. Shinoki T, Hara R, Kaneko U, et al. Safety and response to influenza vaccine in patients with systemic-onset juvenile idiopathic arthritis receiving tocilizumab. Mod Rheumatol. 2012;22(6):871–6.
40. Kivitz AJ, Schechtman J, Texter M, Fichtner A, de Longueville M, Chartash EK. Vaccine responses in patients with rheumatoid arthritis treated with certolizumab pegol: results from a single-blind randomized phase IV trial. J Rheumatol. 2014;41(4):648–57.
41. Alten R, Bingham CO 3rd, Cohen SB, et al. Antibody response to pneumococcal and influenza vaccination in patients with rheumatoid arthritis receiving abatacept. BMC Musculoskelet Disord. 2016;17:231.
42. Stojanovich L. Influenza vaccination of patients with systemic lupus erythematosus (SLE) and rheumatoid arthritis (RA). Clin Dev Immunol. 2006;13(2–4):373–5.
43. Milanovic M, Stojanovich L, Djokovic A, Kontic M, Gvozdenovic E. Influenza vaccination in autoimmune rheumatic disease patients. Tohoku J Exp Med. 2013;229(1):29–34.
44. Kobashigawa T, Nakajima A, Taniguchi A, et al. Vaccination against seasonal influenza is effective in Japanese patients with rheumatoid arthritis enrolled in a large observational cohort. Scand J Rheumatol. 2013;42(6):445–50.
45. Tomczyk S, Bennett NM, Stoecker C, et al. Use of PCV-13 and PPSV-23 vaccine among adults aged 65 and older: recommendations of the ACIP. MMWR. 2014;63(37):822–5.
46. Salonen PH, Säilä H, Salonen JH, et al. Bloodstream infections among children with juvenile idiopathic arthritis: a prospective study from the onset of disease. Clin Exp Rheumatol. 2014;32(6):979–83.
47. Bijl M, Agmon-Levin N, Dayer JM, Israeli E, Gatto M, Shoenfeld Y. Vaccination of patients with auto-

immune inflammatory rheumatic diseases requires careful benefit-risk assessment. Autoimmun Rev. 2012;11(8):572–6.
48. Furst DE. The risk of infections with biologic therapies for rheumatoid arthritis. Semin Arthritis Rheum. 2010;39(5):327–46.
49. Greenberg SB. Infections in the immunocompromised rheumatologic patient. Crit Care Clin. 2002;18:56–931.
50. McDonald E, Jarrett MP, Schiffman G, Grayzel AI. Persistence of pneumococcal antibodies after immunization in patients with systemic lupus erythematosus. J Rheumatol. 1984;11:306–8.
51. Battafarano DF, Battafarano NJ, Larsen L, et al. Antigen-specific antibody responses in lupus patients following immunization. Arthritis Rheum. 1998;41:1828–34.
52. Tarjan P, Sipka S, Marodi L, et al. No short-term immunological effects of pneumococcus vaccination in patients with systemic lupus erythematosus. Scand J Rheumatol. 2002;31:211–5.
53. Elkayam O, Paran D, Caspi D, et al. Immunogenicity and safety of pneumococcal vaccination in patients with rheumatoid arthritis or systemic lupus erythematosus. Clin Infect Dis. 2002;34(2):147–53.
54. Elkayam O, Ablin J, Caspi D. Safety and efficacy of vaccination against streptococcus pneumonia in patients with rheumatic diseases. Autoimmun Rev. 2007;6(5):312–4.
55. Kapetanovic MC, Saxne T, Sjöholm A, Truedsson L, Jönsson G, Geborek P. Influence of methotrexate, TNF blockers and prednisolone on antibody responses to pneumococcal polysaccharide vaccine in patients with rheumatoid arthritis. Rheumatology (Oxford). 2006;45(1):106–11.
56. Mease PJ, Ritchlin CT, Martin RW, et al. Pneumococcal vaccine response in psoriatic arthritis patients during treatment with etanercept. J Rheumatol. 2004;31(7):1356–61.
57. Migita K, Akeda Y, Akazawa M, et al. Pneumococcal polysaccharide vaccination in rheumatoid arthritis patients receiving tacrolimus. Arthritis Res Ther. 2015;17:149.
58. Mori S, Ueki Y, Akeda Y, et al. Pneumococcal polysaccharide vaccination in rheumatoid arthritis patients receiving tocilizumab therapy. Ann Rheum Dis. 2013;72(8):1362–6.
59. Broyde A, Arad U, Madar-Balakirski N, et al. Long term efficacy of an antipneumococcal polysaccharide vaccine among patients with autoimmune inflammatory rheumatic diseases. J Rheumatol. 2016;43(2):267–72.
60. Migita K, Akeda Y, Akazawa M, et al. Effect of abatacept on the immunogenicity of 23-valent pneumococcal polysaccharide vaccination (PPSV23) in rheumatoid arthritis patients. Arthritis Res Ther. 2015;17:357.
61. Rehnberg M, Brisslert M, Amu S, et al. Vaccination response to protein and carbohydrate antigens in patients with rheumatoid arthritis after rituximab treatment. Arthritis Res Ther. 2010;12(3):R111.
62. Bingham IIICO, Looney RJ, Deodhar A, et al. Immunization responses in rheumatoid arthritis patients treated with rituximab: results from a controlled clinical trial. Arthritis Rheum. 2009;62(1):64–74.
63. Crnkic Kapetanovic M, Saxne T, Jönsson G, Truedsson L, Geborek P. Rituximab and abatacept but not tocilizumab impair antibody response to pneumococcal conjugate vaccine in patients with rheumatoid arthritis. Arthritis Res Ther. 2013;15(5):R171.
64. Farmaki E, Kanakoudi-Tsakalidou F, Spoulou V, et al. The effect of anti-TNF treatment on the immunogenicity and safety of the 7-valent conjugate pneumococcal vaccine in children with juvenile idiopathic arthritis. Vaccine. 2010;28(31):5109–13.
65. Crnkic Kapetanovic M, Saxne T, Truedsson L, Geborek P. Persistence of antibody response 1.5 years after vaccination using 7-valent pneumococcal conjugate vaccine in patients with arthritis treated with different antirheumatic drugs. Arthritis Res Ther. 2013;15(1):R1.
66. Nagel J, Geborek P, Saxne T, et al. The association between antibody levels before and after 7-valent pneumococcal conjugate vaccine immunization and subsequent pneumococcal infection in chronic arthritis patients. Arthritis Res Ther. 2015;17:124.
67. Rákóczi É, Perge B, Végh E, et al. Evaluation of the immunogenicity of the 13-valent conjugated pneumococcal vaccine in rheumatoid arthritis patients treated with etanercept. Joint Bone Spine. 2016;83(6):675–9.
68. Fiore AE, Wasley A, Bell BP, Advisory Committee on Immunization Practices (ACIP). Prevention of hepatitis A through active or passive immunization: recommendations of the advisory committee on immunization practices (ACIP). MMWR Recomm Rep. 2006;55:1–23.
69. Erguven M, Kaya B, Hamzah OY, Tufan F. Evaluation of immune response to hepatitis A vaccination and vaccine safety in juvenile idiopathic arthritis. J Chin Med Assoc. 2011;74(5):205–8.
70. Askling HH, Rombo L, van Vollenhoven R, et al. Hepatitis A vaccine for immunosuppressed patients with rheumatoid arthritis: a prospective, open-label, multi-Centre study. Travel Med Infect Dis. 2014;12(2):134–42.
71. van den Bijllaardt W, Siers HM, Timmerman-Kok C, et al. Seroprotection after hepatitis A vaccination in patients with drug-induced immunosuppression. J Travel Med. 2013;20:278–82.
72. Mast EE, Margolis HS, Fiore AE, et al. A comprehensive immunization strategy to eliminate transmission of hepatitis B virus infection in the United States: recommendations of the advisory committee on immunization practices (ACIP) part I: immunization of infants, children, and adolescents. MMWR Recomm Rep. 2005;54(RR-16):1–23.

73. Mast EE, Weinbaum CM, Fiore AE, et al. A comprehensive immunization strategy to eliminate transmission of hepatitis B virus infection in the United States: recommendations of the advisory committee on immunization practices (ACIP) part II: immunization of adults. MMWR Recomm Rep. 2006;55(RR-16):1–33.
74. Elkayam O, Yaron M, Caspi D. Safety and efficacy of vaccination against hepatitis B in patients with rheumatoid arthritis. Ann Rheum Dis. 2002;61(7):623–5.
75. Aytac MB, Kasapcopur O, Aslan M, Erener-Ercan T, Cullu-Cokugras F, Arisoy N. Hepatitis B vaccination in juvenile systemic lupus erythematosus. Clin Exp Rheumatol. 2011;29(5):882–6.
76. Kuruma KA, Borba EF, Lopes MH, de Carvalho JF, Bonfá E. Safety and efficacy of hepatitis B vaccine in systemic lupus erythematosus. Lupus. 2007;16(5):350–4.
77. Salinas GF, De Rycke L, Barendregt B, et al. Anti-TNF treatment blocks the induction of T cell-dependent humoral responses. Ann Rheum Dis. 2013;72(6):1037–43.
78. Stübgen JP. Immune-mediated myelitis following hepatitis B vaccination. Autoimmun Rev. 2012;12(2):144–9.
79. Zafrir Y, Agmon-Levin N, Paz Z, Shilton T, Shoenfeld Y. Autoimmunity following hepatitis B vaccine as part of the spectrum of 'Autoimmune (auto-inflammatory) syndrome induced by Adjuvants' (ASIA): analysis of 93 cases. Lupus. 2012;21(2):146–52.
80. Agmon-Levin N, Zafrir Y, Paz Z, Shilton T, Zandman-Goddard G, Shoenfeld Y. Ten cases of systemic lupus erythematosus related to hepatitis B vaccine. Lupus. 2009;18(13):1192–7.
81. Ray P, Black S, Shinefield H, et al. Risk of rheumatoid arthritis following vaccination with tetanus, influenza and hepatitis B vaccines among persons 15-59 years of age. Vaccine. 2011;29(38):6592–7.
82. Kim DK, Bridges CB, Harriman KH. Advisory committee on immunization practices. Advisory committee on immunization practices recommended immunization schedule for adults aged 19 years or older: United States, 2016. Ann Intern Med. 2016;164:184.
83. Petrosky E, Bocchini JA Jr, Hariri S, et al. Use of 9-valent human papillomavirus (HPV) vaccine: updated HPV vaccination recommendations of the advisory committee on immunization practices. MMWR Morb Mortal Wkly Rep. 2015;64:300.
84. Strikas RA, Centers for Disease Control and Prevention (CDC), Advisory Committee on Immunization Practices (ACIP), ACIP Child/Adolescent Immunization Work Group. Advisory committee on immunization practices recommended immunization schedules for persons aged 0 through 18 years--United States, 2015. MMWR Morb Mortal Wkly Rep. 2015;64:93.
85. Satterwhite CL, Torrone E, Meites E, et al. Sexually transmitted infections among US women and men: prevalence and incidence estimates, 2008. Sex Transm Dis. 2013;40:187–93.
86. Múnoz N, Bosch FX, de Sanjose S, et al. Epidemiologic classification of human papillomavirus types associated with cervical cancer. N Engl J Med. 2003;348:518–27.
87. IARC Working Group on the Evaluation of Carcinogenic Risks to Humans. Biological agents. Volume 100 B: a review of human carcinogens. IARC Monogr Eval Carcinog Risks Hum. 2012;100(Pt B):1–441.
88. Markowitz LE, Dunne EF, Saraiya M, et al. Human papillomavirus vaccination: recommendations of the advisory committee on immunization practices (ACIP). MMWR. 2014;63(RR-5):1–23.
89. Tam LS, Chan AY, Chan PK, et al. Increased prevalence of squamous intraepithelial lesions in systemic lupus erythematosus: association with human papillomavirus infection. Arthritis Rheum. 2004;50(11):3619–25.
90. Zard E, Arnaud L, Mathian A, et al. Increased risk of high-grade cervical squamous intraepithelial lesions in systemic lupus erythematosus: a meta-analysis of the literature. Autoimmun Rev. 2014;13(7):730–5.
91. Cibere J, Sibley J, Haga M. Systemic lupus erythematosus and the risk of malignancy. Lupus. 2001;10:394–400.
92. Heijstek MW, Scherpenisse M, Groot N, Wulffraat NM, Van Der Klis FR. Immunogenicity of the bivalent human papillomavirus vaccine in adolescents with juvenile systemic lupus erythematosus or juvenile dermatomyositis. J Rheumatol. 2013;40(9):1626–7.
93. Heijstek MW, Scherpenisse M, Groot N, et al. Immunogenicity and safety of the bivalent HPV vaccine in female patients with juvenile idiopathic arthritis: a prospective controlled observational cohort study. Ann Rheum Dis. 2014;73(8):1500–7.
94. Esposito S, Corona F, Barzon L, et al. Immunogenicity, safety and tolerability of a bivalent human papillomavirus vaccine in adolescents with juvenile idiopathic arthritis. Expert Rev Vaccines. 2014;13(11):1387–93.
95. Mok CC, Ho LY, Fong LS, To CH. Immunogenicity and safety of a quadrivalent human papillomavirus vaccine in patients with systemic lupus erythematosus: a case-control study. Ann Rheum Dis. 2013;72(5):659–64.
96. Soybilgic A, Onel KB, Utset T, Alexander K, Wagner-Weiner L. Safety and immunogenicity of the quadrivalent HPV vaccine in female systemic lupus erythematosus patients aged 12 to 26 years. Pediatr Rheumatol Online J. 2013;11:29.
97. Gatto M, Agmon-Levin N, Soriano A, et al. Human papillomavirus vaccine and systemic lupus erythematosus. Clin Rheumatol. 2013;32(9):1301–7.
98. Geier DA, Geier MR. Quadrivalent human papillomavirus vaccine and autoimmune adverse events: a case-control assessment of the vaccine adverse event

reporting system (VAERS) database. Immunol Res. 2016;65(1):46–54.
99. McLean HQ, Fiebelkorn AP, Temte JL, Wallace GS, Centers for Disease Control and Prevention. Prevention of measles, rubella, congenital rubella syndrome, and mumps, 2013: summary recommendations of the advisory committee on immunization practices (ACIP). MMWR Recomm Rep. 2013;62(RR-04):1–34.
100. Heijstek MW, Pileggi GC, Zonneveld-Huijssoon E, et al. Safety of measles, mumps and rubella vaccination in juvenile idiopathic arthritis. Ann Rheum Dis. 2007;66(10):1384–7.
101. Heijstek MW, van Gageldonk PG, Berbers GA, Wulffraat NM. Differences in persistence of measles, mumps, rubella, diphtheria and tetanus antibodies between children with rheumatic disease and healthy controls: a retrospective cross-sectional study. Ann Rheum Dis. 2012;71(6):948–54.
102. Marin M, Guris D, Chaves SS, Schmid S, Seward JF, Advisory Committee on Immunization Practices, Centers for Disease Control and Prevention (CDC). Prevention of varicella: recommendations of the advisory committee on immunization practices (ACIP). MMWR Recomm Rep. 2007;56(RR-4):1–40.
103. Heijstek MW, Ott de Bruin LM, Bijl M, et al. EULAR recommendations for vaccination in paediatric patients with rheumatic diseases. Ann Rheum Dis. 2011;70(10):1704–12.
104. Pileggi GS, de Souza CB, Ferriani VP. Safety and immunogenicity of varicella vaccine in patients with juvenile rheumatic diseases receiving methotrexate and corticosteroids. Arthritis Care Res. 2010;62(7):1034–9.
105. Toplak N, Avčin T. Long-term safety and efficacy of varicella vaccination in children with juvenile idiopathic arthritis treated with biologic therapy. Vaccine. 2015;33(33):4056–9.
106. Johnson RW, Rice AS. Clinical practice. Postherpetic neuralgia. N Engl J Med. 2014;371(16):1526–33.
107. Oxman MN, Levin MJ, Johnson GR, Shingles Prevention Study Group, et al. A vaccine to prevent herpes zoster and postherpetic neuralgia in older adults. N Engl J Med. 2005;352(22):2271–84.
108. Kahl LE. Herpes zoster infections in systemic lupus erythematosus: risk factors and outcome. J Rheumatol. 1994;21(1):84–6.
109. Zisman D, Bitterman H, Shalom G, et al. Psoriatic arthritis treatment and the risk of herpes zoster. Ann Rheum Dis. 2016;75(1):131–5.
110. Smitten AL, Choi HK, Hochberg MC, et al. The risk of herpes zoster in patients with rheumatoid arthritis in the United States and the United Kingdom. Arthritis Rheum. 2007;57(8):1431–8.
111. Pappas DA, Hooper MM, Kremer JM, et al. Herpes zoster reactivation in patients with rheumatoid arthritis: analysis of disease characteristics and disease-modifying antirheumatic drugs. Arthritis Care Res. 2015;67(12):1671–8.
112. McDonald JR, Zeringue AL, Caplan L, et al. Herpes zoster risk factors in a national cohort of veterans with rheumatoid arthritis. Clin Infect Dis. 2009;48(10):1364–71.
113. Curtis JR, Xie F, Yun H, Bernatsky S, Winthrop KL. Real-world comparative risks of herpes virus infections in tofacitinib and biologic-treated patients with rheumatoid arthritis. Ann Rheum Dis. 2016;75(10):1843–7.
114. Winthrop KL, Park SH, Gul A, et al. Tuberculosis and other opportunistic infections in tofacitinib-treated patients with rheumatoid arthritis. Ann Rheum Dis. 2016;75(6):1133–8.
115. Winthrop KL, Silverfield J, Racewicz A, et al. The effect of tofacitinib on pneumococcal and influenza vaccine responses in rheumatoid arthritis. Ann Rheum Dis. 2016;75(4):687–95.
116. Winthrop KL, Yamanaka H, Valdez H, et al. Herpes zoster and tofacitinib therapy in patients with rheumatoid arthritis. Arthritis Rheumatol. 2014;66(10):2675–84.
117. Ramiro S, Gaujoux-Viala C, Nam JL, et al. Safety of synthetic and biological DMARDs: a systematic literature review informing the 2013 update of the EULAR recommendations for management of rheumatoid arthritis. Ann Rheum Dis. 2014;73(3):529–35.
118. Smolen JS, Landewé R, Breedveld FC, et al. EULAR recommendations for the management of rheumatoid arthritis with synthetic and biological disease-modifying antirheumatic drugs: 2013 update. Ann Rheum Dis. 2014;73(3):492–509.
119. Youssef J, Novosad SA, Winthrop KL. Infection risk and safety of corticosteroid use. Rheum Dis Clin N Am. 2016;42(1):157–76.
120. Tafuri SS, Chironna MM, Quarto MM, Germinario CC. Risk of zoster in patients on immunosuppressant therapy: evaluation of current data. Am J Infect Control. 2015;43(4):420–1.
121. Murdaca G, Spanò F, Contatore M, et al. Infection risk associated with anti-TNF-α agents: a review. Expert Opin Drug Saf. 2015;14(4):571–82.
122. Che H, Lukas C, Morel J, Combe B. Risk of herpes/herpes zoster during anti-tumor necrosis factor therapy in patients with rheumatoid arthritis. Systematic review and meta-analysis. Joint Bone Spine. 2014;81(3):215–21.
123. Zhang N, Wilkinson S, Riaz M, Östör AJ, Nisar MK. Does methotrexate increase the risk of varicella or herpes zoster infection in patients with rheumatoid arthritis? A systematic literature review. Clin Exp Rheumatol. 2012;30(6):962–71.
124. García-Doval I, Pérez-Zafrilla B, Descalzo MA, BIOBADASER 2.0 Study Group, et al. Incidence and risk of hospitalisation due to shingles and chickenpox in patients with rheumatic diseases treated with TNF antagonists. Ann Rheum Dis. 2010;69(10):1751–5.
125. Wolfe F, Michaud K, Chakravarty EF. Rates and predictors of herpes zoster in patients with

rheumatoid arthritis and non-inflammatory musculoskeletal disorders. Rheumatology (Oxford). 2006;45(11):1370–5.

126. Kang TY, Lee HS, Kim TH, Jun JB, Yoo DH. Clinical and genetic risk factors of herpes zoster in patients with systemic lupus erythematosus. Rheumatol Int. 2005;25(2):97–102.

127. Yun H, Xie F, Delzell E, et al. Risks of herpes zoster in patients with rheumatoid arthritis according to biologic disease-modifying therapy. Arthritis Care Res. 2015;67(5):731–6.

128. Winthrop KL, Novosad S, Baddley JW, et al. Opportunistic infections and biologic therapies in immune-mediated inflammatory diseases: consensus recommendations for infection reporting during clinical trials and postmarketing surveillance. Ann Rheum Dis. 2015;74:2107–16.

129. Zhang J, Delzell E, Xie F, et al. The use, safety, and effectiveness of herpes zoster vaccination in individuals with inflammatory and autoimmune diseases: a longitudinal observational study. Arthritis Res Ther. 2011;13(5):R174.

130. Zhang J, Xie F, Delzell E, et al. Association between vaccination for herpes zoster and risk of herpes zoster infection among older patients with selected immune-mediated diseases. JAMA. 2012;308(1):43–9.

131. Berkowitz EM, Moyle G, Stellbrink HJ, Zoster-015 HZ/su Study Group, et al. Safety and immunogenicity of an adjuvanted herpes zoster subunit candidate vaccine in HIV-infected adults. A phase 1/2a randomized, placebo-controlled study. J Infect Dis. 2015;211(8):1279–87.

132. Stadtmauer EA, Sullivan KM, Marty FM, et al. A phase ½ study of an adjuvanted varicella-zoster virus subunit vaccine in autologous hemopoietic stem cell transplant recipients. Blood. 2014;124(19):2921–9.

133. Jaeger VK, Rüegg R, Steffen R, Hatz C, Bühler S. Travelers with immune-mediated inflammatory diseases: are they different? J Travel Med. 2015;22(3):161–7.

134. Centers for Disease Control and Prevention (CDC). Japanese encephalitis vaccines. Recommendations of the advisory committee on immunization practices (ACIP). MMWR Recomm Rep. 2010;59(RR-1):1–27.

135. Jackson BR, Iqbal S, Mahon B. Updated recommendations for the use of typhoid vaccine – advisory committee on immunization practices, United States, 2015. MMWR Morb Mortal Wkly Rep. 2015;64(11):305–8.

136. Mota LM, Oliveira AC, Lima RA, Santos-Neto LL, Tauil PL. Vaccination against yellow fever among patients on immunosuppressors with diagnoses of rheumatic diseases. Rev Soc Bras Med Trop. 2009;42:23–7.

137. Staples JE, Gershman M, Fischer M, Centers for Disease Control and Prevention (CDC), et al. Yellow fever vaccine. Recommendations of the advisory committee on immunization practices (ACIP). MMMR Recomm Rep. 2010;59(RR-7):1–27.

33 Management of Autoimmune and Inflammatory Disorders in the Setting of Infection or Immunodeficiency

W. Winn Chatham

Abbreviations

ADA	Adenosine deaminase deficiency
AICDA	Activation-induced cytidine deaminase
CVID	Common variable immunodeficiency
DMARD	Disease-modifying antirheumatic drug
GCA	Giant cell arteritis
GPA	Granulomatosis with polyangiitis
IL	Interleukin
IL-6R, IL-17R	Interleukin 6 (17) receptor
IVIG	Intravenous immunoglobulin
MBL	Mannose-binding lectin
MMP	Matrix metalloproteinase
MPA	Microscopic polyangiitis
MTX	Methotrexate
NSAID	Nonsteroidal anti-inflammatory drug
PAN	Polyarteritis nodosa
PID	Primary immunodeficiency
RA	Rheumatoid arthritis
sIgA	Selective IgA deficiency
SLE	Systemic lupus erythematosus
SNSA	Seronegative spondyloarthritis
TACI	Transmembrane activator, calcium-modulator, and cyclophilin ligand interactor
TLR	Toll-like receptor
UNG	Uracil nucleoside glycosylase
WAS	Wiskott-Aldrich syndrome
XLA	X-linked agammaglobulinemia

Managing Autoimmune Disorders in the Setting of Acquired Infection

Rheumatoid Arthritis

Infection risk is increased in rheumatoid arthritis (RA), primarily in the context of high disease activity and intercurrent use of corticosteroids [1, 2]. Risk of joint sepsis is increased due to hypervascular, proliferative synovium permitting easy access of circulating microbial pathogens into affected joints. RA patients with Felty's syndrome may be at even greater risk due to the leucopenia and hypersplenism associated with this RA complication. Traditional disease-modifying antirheumatic drugs (DMARDs) as well as biologic DMARDs targeting inflammatory mediators in RA are highly effective in suppressing synovial inflammation and attendant structural damage due to RA. With the possible exception of anti-TNF antibodies, DMARDs have not been shown to significantly increase overall incident

W. W. Chatham
University of Alabama at Birmingham (UAB), Division of Clinical Immunology and Rheumatology, Birmingham, AL, USA
e-mail: wchatham@uabmc.edu

G. Ragab et al. (eds.), *The Microbiome in Rheumatic Diseases and Infection*,
https://doi.org/10.1007/978-3-319-79026-8_33

infection risk in RA [3–5]. However, traditional DMARDs such as methotrexate and biologic DMARDs may nonetheless impact host responses to acquired infection.

As a general rule, management of RA in the setting of suspected intercurrent infection entails withholding dosing of therapies known to impact phagocytic cell functions, minimizing corticosteroid dosing to the levels required for avoidance of adrenal crisis, assiduous attention to the possibility of joint seeding by bacteria, and prompt institution of antimicrobial therapy with joint drainage as needed. Nonsteroidal anti-inflammatory drugs (NSAIDs) or intra-articular corticosteroids can be used as needed to manage synovitis flares until infection has resolved. If NSAIDs are contraindicated, low-dose prednisone (5–10 mg/day) and/or non-acetylated aspirin (salsalate) which does not inhibit cyclooxygenase activity can be used for managing generalized joint flares. Considerations in this setting with respect to commonly used RA DMARDs and biologics are summarized below (see Chap. 34 for individual drugs and risk of infection).

Methotrexate

The clinical efficacy of methotrexate (MTX), one of the most commonly employed DMARDs in the management of RA, is attributed primarily to the inhibitory effects of intracellular MTX polyglutamates on AICAR transformylase, resulting in increased levels of adenosine which is inhibitory for trafficking of phagocytic cells into joints [6]. As such, it is prudent to hold treatment with methotrexate until intercurrent bacterial infections affecting the lungs, skin, joints, or other tissues have clinically resolved. The presumed effect of MTX on immune cell trafficking has traditionally proscribed MTX use perioperatively with conflicting expert opinion on whether MTX should be held in the context of joint replacement procedures. However, recent studies have shifted expert opinion toward not withholding MTX around the time of elective joint replacement surgery, citing the increased morbidity associated with disease flare in this setting [5].

TNF Inhibitors

TNF promotes a variety of phagocytic cell activation responses including expression of adhesion molecules and activation of the respiratory burst in neutrophils. Although in vitro studies with etanercept showed no direct effect on neutrophil phagocytic cell or microbicidal activity [7], inhibition of TNF locally by etanercept or anti-TNF monoclonal constructs may nonetheless impair phagocytic cell-mediated host defenses to microbial pathogens. Indeed, treatment with TNF inhibitors has been shown to confer increased infection risk in multiple cohorts of patients with disorders in which treatment with these agents is included among the employed therapeutic options [4]. TNF also appears to be an important cytokine in maintaining the integrity of granulomas, and the association of anti-TNF therapies with reactivation of tuberculosis and disseminated fungal infections is also well recognized [8, 9]. Thus, prescribing guidelines include testing for latent tuberculosis in all patients newly started on TNF inhibitors. The risk for non-viral opportunistic infection, including tuberculosis, appears to be higher in patients treated with anti-TNF monoclonal reagents such as infliximab relative to that noted in patients treated with sTNFR:Fc /etanercept [10].

Given the increased risk and morbidity of infection complications observed in patients on TNF inhibitor therapy, it is therefore appropriate to withhold and not initiate anti-TNF therapy in the setting of any active infection. Moreover, patients with RA who have comorbidities such as diabetes have a demonstrated increased risk for bacterial infections as well as increased infection-related morbidity during treatment with TNF inhibitors [11]. An alternative to anti-TNF therapy with less direct impact on phagocytic cell responses might therefore best be considered for managing RA in patients with pre-existing comorbidities associated with increased infection risk.

IL-6 Inhibitors

Due to signaling that can occur through the interleukin (IL)-6 receptor (IL-6R) and trans-signaling through gp130 receptors that recognize IL-6:sIL-6R heterodimer, inhibitors of IL-6 such as tocilizumab have pleomorphic effects on immune as well as nonimmune cells. IL-6 mediates activation of macrophages, terminal proliferation and differentiation of B-cells, differentiation of Th17 cells, and also homeostatic processes including granulopoiesis, induction of some anti-inflammatory cytokines, and mucosal integrity [12, 13]. Given these considerations, it is generally prudent to withhold treatment with IL-6 inhibitors such as tocilizumab (anti-IL6R) or sirukumab (anti-IL6) in the setting of intercurrent infection. Since IL-6 signaling appears to govern homeostasis of the enteric mucosal epithelium, and anti-IL-6 therapy has been associated with increased risk of intestinal perforations [14], treatment with IL-6 inhibitors is not recommended in the setting of inflammatory bowel disease, diverticular disease, or recent colitis in which the integrity of the enteric mucosa may become compromised.

Janus Kinase Inhibitors

Janus kinase inhibitors such as tofacitinib block signal transduction mediating the effects of inflammatory cytokines such as TNF and IL-6, with potent inhibitory effects on the functions of phagocytic cells. Reported rates of infection in patients on treatment with tofacitinib are comparable to those reported in patients on anti-TNF or anti-IL6 therapies [15]. The considerations alluded to above for these respective biologics are therefore equally applicable to tofacitinib, and it is advisable to withhold its use in the setting of intercurrent infection, resuming treatment once the infection is deemed resolved. The experience with other Janus kinase inhibitors is limited, but in the absence of data indicating otherwise, treatment with the newer agents is also advisably withheld in the setting of intercurrent bacterial infection.

Abatacept

Effective in blocking T cell co-stimulation and associated acquired responses to neo-antigens, abatacept does not have direct impacts on phagocytic cell responses. Serious bacterial infection occurs less commonly during treatment of RA with abatacept than with TNF inhibitors [16, 17], and risk of reactivation or acquired infection with tuberculosis is lower among RA patents treated with abatacept relative to those treated with TNF inhibitors [18]. Whether it is necessary to withhold treatment with abatacept in the setting of acute bacterial infection has not been established. Since the occurrence of serious infections does not appear to be increased in RA patients treated with abatacept, this may be a preferred biologic option in patients with RA deemed to have increased risk for bacterial infection.

Rituximab

Depletion of CD20+ lymphocytes impacts primarily B cell-mediated acquired immunity and has little if any impact on the function of phagocytic cells. However, infection risk among RA patients treated with rituximab is nonetheless comparable to that observed among patients treated with TNF inhibitors [17, 19]. This may be due to the not insignificant numbers of patients who develop hypogammaglobulinemia with recurrent dosing of rituximab, with occurrence of serious infection events noted to be higher in such patients [20]. Management of intercurrent infections in patients treated with rituximab or other B cell-depleting reagents (such as obinutuzumab, ofatumumab) is therefore best directed toward ensuring antecedent B cell depletion therapy has not rendered the recipient hypogammaglobulinemic. Should severe infection occur with IgG levels less than 500 mg/dL, consideration should be given to supportive immunoglobulin replacement therapy (usually 0.4 g/kg every 4 weeks as needed). Whether to initiate prophylactic immunoglobulin replacement therapy at lower levels of serum IgG in the absence of infection is subject to debate. Hypogammaglobulinemia in the setting of B cell depletion therapy may be transient, and provided the patient can produce adequate neutralizing antibodies, IgG replacement therapy in such patients may not be required.

Assessment of responses to pneumococcal vaccination may be informative in this setting. With this caveat of needed vigilance for hypogammaglobulinemia, given the absence of its effects on phagocytic cell functions, rituximab may be another preferred option for managing patients with RA who either have comorbidities placing them at increased risk for infections or who have experienced recurring episodes of bacterial infections on anti-TNF biologics.

Seronegative Spondyloarthropathies

Patients with seronegative spondyloarthropathies (SNSA) are at some increased risk for infection due to chronic arthropathy as well as enteric complications due to underlying inflammatory bowel disease (IBD) or subclinical inflammation of the enteric mucosa that may occur in non-IBD-associated SNSA (see Chap. 16). A noted increased occurrence of mannose-binding lectin (MBL) deficiency in patients with SNSA may also confer increased risk for infection [21, 22].

Methotrexate, sulfasalazine, and TNFα inhibitors are commonly employed in the management of SNSA, and the same considerations with regard to the use of these therapies in patients with RA are applicable and relevant to patients with SNSA with intercurrent infection. As discussed below, use of alternative biologics targeting the IL-23/IL-17 pathway that are primarily used in the management of psoriasis and SNSA may also need to be curtailed in the setting of intercurrent infection. *Apremilast*, a phosphodiesterase-4 inhibitor that is used primarily for the management of psoriasis and psoriatic arthropathy, does not have any direct effects on phagocytic cell function and has not been shown in clinical trials to confer increased infection risk [23]. As such, it is usually not necessary to curtail the use of apremilast during episodes of infection. The majority of joint manifestations in SNSA can otherwise be adequately managed with NSAID therapy during episodes of intercurrent infection when anti-TNF biologics or biologics targeting the IL23/IL17 axis need to be appropriately withheld.

Ustekinumab and IL-23 Inhibitors

Ustekinumab is a monoclonal reagent targeting the shared p40 subunit of the IL-12 and IL-23 receptors. Both IL-12 and IL-23 impact primarily T cell lineage development, with minimal if any direct effects on phagocytic cell functions. In clinical trials using ustekinumab in psoriasis as well as ankylosing spondylitis and inflammatory bowel disease, there have been no increased occurrences of serious infections in the ustekinumab treatment arms relative to the placebo treatment arms [24]. While there is no evidence to support holding ustekinumab or IL-23-specific therapies during intercurrent bacterial infection, given the identified role of IL-12 and IL-23 in mediating host defense against mycobacterial, fungal, and *Salmonella* infections, it is prudent to withhold ustekinumab and agents targeting IL-23 (tildrakizumab and guselkumab) in the setting of infection with these pathogens.

Inhibitors of IL-17 and IL-17R

IL-17 is derived from both innate and lymphoid cells, promoting the induction and release of IL-6, TNF, CCL2, CCL3, and matrix metalloproteinase (MMPs) from macrophages as well as the proliferation, maturation, and chemotaxis of neutrophils. In trials with secukinumab and ixekizumab (inhibitors of IL-17A) as well as trials with brodalumab (an inhibitor of the IL-17R), infection rates were increased over those observed in patients randomized to placebo but comparable to what has been observed in similar populations of patients enrolled in trials with TNF inhibitors [25]. Candida infections occurred more frequently in studies with the IL-17 inhibitor brodalumab [26]. It is prudent to withhold therapies targeting IL-17/IL-17R in the setting of active infection with these classes of microbial pathogens. For patients with SNSA who have experienced recurrent serious infections, consideration should be given to use of alternative therapies associated with less infection risk such as apremilast or ustekinumab. Although the therapeutic benefits of ustekinumab in SNSA may be attributable in large part to decreases in the number and survival of Th17 lymphocytes which comprise a significant source of IL-17, there are other (innate) cellular sources of IL-17 and therapies that specifically target IL-17 or its receptor may therefore confer greater infection risk than therapies targeting the Th17 lineage.

Systemic Lupus Erythematosus

For a variety of reasons, patients with systemic lupus erythematosus (SLE) may be at increased risk for infection (see Chap. 21). Defects in innate immunity related to opsonization functions known to also predispose to SLE include deficiencies in early components of the classic complement pathway (C1q, C2, and C4) and mannose-binding lectin [27, 28]. Lymphopenia is a common disease manifestation and a demonstrated risk factor for infectious complications in lupus [29]. Autoreactive T cell clones and/or autoantibodies may potentially target molecules required for appropriate production of granulocytes [30] or the ability of B cells to appropriately mature, proliferate, and secrete high-affinity antibodies capable of neutralizing microbial pathogens [31]. Autoimmunity with SLE features may be the presenting feature of patients with common variable immune deficiency or immunoglobulin IgG subclass deficiency [32]. Although therapies required to suppress autoreactive inflammatory disease are becoming increasingly selective and targeted (one example being belimumab), many of the current therapies required to effectively manage moderate to severe SLE activity result in some degree of nonselective immune suppression impacting innate and/or acquired immune functions.

Due primarily to their direct effects on the function of phagocytic cells as well as the production and survival of T lymphocytes, chronic *corticosteroid therapy* constitutes one of the major risk factors for infection-related morbidity and mortality in SLE patients. For patients who require ongoing treatment with corticosteroids, the dosing of steroids during intercurrent bacterial infection should be the lowest deemed sufficient to avoid SLE-related acute organ damage. In the setting of overwhelming confirmed microbial sepsis deemed life-threatening, it is usually prudent to decrease the dose of steroids to that required to avoid adrenal crisis, even if this entails a risk of SLE-related organ damage. The exception may be in the setting of active lupus-related CNS or pulmonary disease (notably diffuse alveolar hemorrhage) where corticosteroid dosing at high levels may be necessary to avoid imminent demise or brain injury. High-dose intravenous immunoglobulin (IVIG) (2.0 g/kg/day) is often effective in ameliorating acute lupus-related CNS vascular injury [33, 34] or alveolar hemorrhage [35] and should be considered as an alternative to high-dose steroid therapy when these entities require treatment in the setting of serious bacterial infection.

Dosing with *cyclophosphamide* or *azathioprine*, both of which may impact the numbers and production of phagocytic cells, is best withheld in the setting of bacterial infection. Moreover, should lupus patients develop significant granulocytopenia (<500/mcl) during treatment with either of these agents, prophylactic use of levofloxacin (500 mg/day) is recommended to decrease the risk of gram-negative sepsis until the absolute neutrophil count recovers to >500/mcl [36]. Treatment with recombinant granulocyte colony-stimulating factor (rCSF) can be considered if serious intercurrent bacterial infection occurs in this setting, but use of rCSF is otherwise not recommended due to increased risk of lupus flare associated with its use [37]. Since *mycophenolate* and *mycophenolic acid* target primarily the proliferation of lymphoid cells with minimal, if any, impact on the proliferation of phagocytic cells, it may not be necessary to withhold treatment with these agents during episodes of bacterial infection. Antimalarials (*chloroquine*, *hydroxychloroquine*, *quinacrine*), *dapsone*, and *thalidomide* have no significant impact on host responses to microbial pathogens and can be continued as needed to suppress lupus activity during episodes of infection. Since *belimumab* primarily impacts the maturation, proliferation, and survival of autoreactive B cells and has no known effects on phagocytic cell function, it is usually not necessary to withhold scheduled dosing with this biologic during periods of intercurrent infection. Provided patients who may be hypogammaglobulinemic (due to immunosuppression or underlying associated immunodeficiency) are receiving appropriate immunoglobulin replacement treatment in the setting of acute infectious complications, it may also not be necessary to withhold dosing with B cell-depleting agents such as *rituximab* or *obinutuzumab* if needed for managing acute disease complications such as immune thrombocytopenia or hemolytic anemia. However, temporizing measures using a course of high-dose IVIG (2 g/kg) may be a more prudent intervention for treating acute exacerbations of immune cytopenias in lupus patients with intercurrent serious microbial infection [38, 39].

Sjogren's Syndrome

Patients with Sjogren's syndrome may require immunosuppressive therapy for pulmonary complications such as acute interstitial lung disease or organizing pneumonia or neurologic complications such as transverse/longitudinal myelitis. Although corticosteroids and cytotoxic agents are often employed in the initial acute management of these complications, early initiation of steroid-sparing therapy with agents such as mycophenolate with minimal impact on phagocytic cell function may help mitigate infection risk. For patients with intercurrent infection who still have acute myelitis or other central nervous system disease, temporizing measures with use of high-dose IVIG may permit prompt lowering of the employed use of corticosteroids and holding of cytotoxic therapy without increasing the risk of clinical relapse [40]. For patients who develop infection in the setting of active interstitial lung disease or organizing pneumonia, lowering the dose of corticosteroids and use of IVIG with rituximab or mycophenolate may be an effective therapeutic alternative with minimal impact on host defenses required to clear intercurrent infection [41–43].

Systemic Sclerosis

Immunosuppressive therapy is being utilized more frequently in the management of patients with systemic sclerosis who have evidence of alveolitis or who have early active skin disease with dermal edema. Cyclophosphamide is used most commonly for patients with active interstitial lung disease and evidence of active alveolitis on high-resolution CT scan, with concomitant improvements also noted in selected patients with active skin disease. Notably, improvements have also been noted in both lung and skin manifestations among patients treated with mycophenolate [44]. Although not yet assessed in randomized trials, a number of small case series have reported improvements in both lung and skin manifestations following treatment with high-dose (2 g/kg) IVIG [45]. As such, for patients with active lung and skin disease who have ongoing infection complications that would best preclude use of cyclophosphamide, consideration can be given to using IVIG as a suitable alternative for managing acute lung inflammation and/or transitioning to mycophenolate for long-term management of these disease complications.

Polymyositis and Dermatomyositis

The standard management of inflammatory myopathies entails initial use of corticosteroids, most often in divided doses, with early initiation of steroid-sparing immunosuppressive therapy such as mycophenolate, azathioprine, methotrexate, or calcineurin inhibitors. Given the negligible effects of mycophenolate or calcineurin inhibitors on phagocytic cell proliferation and function, it may not be necessary to withhold these medications during treatment for routine bacterial infections. However, withholding mycophenolate and other immune suppressants is advisable in the setting of infection with opportunistic infections, whereby host T cell responses are critical in effecting clearance of the infecting pathogen. IVIG has demonstrated efficacy in both the acute and chronic management of polymyositis as well as dermatomyositis (including associated acute lung inflammation) and would be a preferred option for managing critical weakness and/or pneumonitis in patients with these disorders who have infection complications requiring attenuation of corticosteroid and other immunosuppressive therapy [46].

Vasculitis

Given the intensity of immune suppression often required to induce remission in patients with systemic vasculitis, infectious complications are not uncommon occurrences in patients with these disorders. Moreover, compromise of vascular integrity in patients with disease-involving vessels which supply the dermis and gastrointestinal tract may engender septic complications. Disease management may be further complicated by the propensity of intercurrent infection to trigger flares of disease. These considerations require careful vigilance for infection as well as careful attention to organ-specific disease activity when managing patients with systemic vasculitis.

ANCA-Associated Vasculitis

Infectious complications in patients with granulomatosis and polyangiitis (GPA) or microscopic polyangiitis (MPA) are of particular concern not only from the standpoint of sepsis-associated morbidity but also the possibility of disease flare triggered by neutrophil degranulation of target antigen (proteinase-3 and myeloperoxidase). Flares of ANCA-associated vasculitis and pauci-immune glomerulonephritis occurring in the context of bacteremia are well documented [47–49]. Vigilance for development of bacterial infection as well as antimicrobial prophylaxis is therefore a critical component of disease management strategies in patients with ANCA-associated vasculitis. Daily dosing with trimethoprim-sulfamethoxazole (160–800 mg) has been shown to decrease flares of GPA and is recommended as an adjunct treatment to immune suppression in patients with GPA as well as MPA [50]. Use of trimethoprim-sulfa would be of even greater importance to prevent infection with *Pneumocystis jirovecii* pneumonia in patients who may develop CD4+ T cell counts <300/mm^3 as a consequence of sustained treatment with immune suppression regimens impacting T cells. Leucopenia in association with immunosuppressive therapy is a significant risk factor for sepsis and poor outcomes in ANCA-associated glomerulonephritis [51]. Accordingly, for patients receiving cyclophosphamide as part of their induction treatment or patients managed with azathioprine, prophylactic use of levofloxacin is recommended during periods of severe neutropenia that may occur as a complication of treatment with these immune suppressants [52]. Use of recombinant granulocyte colony-stimulating factor can be considered if intercurrent serious infection occurs but is otherwise best avoided due to potential increased risk of vasculitis flares that may be associated with its use [53].

Since B cell depletion treatments with rituximab, use of cyclophosphamide, or use of azathioprine in the management of ANCA vasculitis may engender hypogammaglobulinemia, it is important to check immunoglobulin levels when patients with ANCA vasculitis develop septic complications. Administration of immunoglobulin replacement therapy (0.4 g/kg) should be considered for patients with bacterial infection and serum IgG levels less than 500 mg/dL. Continuation of immunoglobulin replacement at 3–4-week intervals is recommended until the infection has resolved; longer treatment duration for patients with sustained hypogammaglobulinemia may decrease the likelihood of recurring infection [54].

Giant Cell Arteritis

The primary treatment for giant cell arteritis (GCA) is chronic corticosteroid therapy, placing affected patients at risk for routine as well as opportunistic infection. Optimal disease management of GCA during episodes of infection depends upon when in the course of disease septic complications occur. Should bacterial infection develop within the first month of diagnosis when patients with ophthalmic artery involvement may be at risk for visual loss, it may be necessary to continue prescribed steroid treatment in the setting of bacterial infection. Subsequent to this initial phase of treatment, temporary attenuation of corticosteroid dosing to doses required to avoid adrenal insufficiency can usually safely be undertaken until the infection has resolved.

Similar considerations as were discussed in RA management apply to the more recent use in GCA of anti-IL-6 therapy with tocilizumab, shown to increase the likelihood of GCA remission and lower the cumulative dose of corticosteroid required for management. Should infectious complications occur, treatment with anti-IL-6 therapy is best withheld until infection has resolved, with use of the lowest dose of corticosteroid deemed appropriate to manage the GCA at the time infection occurs. Due to the association of tocilizumab therapy with intestinal perforations and homeostatic role of IL-6 in maintenance of mucosal integrity, tocilizumab or other anti-IL6 therapies are best not resumed in patients with sepsis arising from the gastrointestinal tract [13, 14].

Polyarteritis Nodosa

Optimal management of polyarteritis nodosa (PAN) varies depending upon whether the disease has been demonstrated to develop in the context of infection with viral pathogens such as hepatitis B (HBV), parvovirus B19, or cytomegalovirus. Induction strategies for HBV-associated PAN often entail combinations of a limited (2-week) course of corticosteroids and plasma exchange with antiviral therapy to induce remission [55], and CMV-associated polyarteritis is best managed with corticosteroids, ganciclovir, and either IVIG or anti-CMV immunoglobulin [56]. IVIG alone may be sufficient to effect resolution of parvovirus B19-associated PAN [57]. PAN syndromes in the absence of confirmed viral disease are most often managed with corticosteroids in combination with cyclophosphamide. Should septic complications occur during the prescribed treatment program, use of high-dose IVIG as a temporary alternative to cytotoxic therapy may serve to suppress vasculitis [58, 59]. However, for patients with neurologic or visceral complications of non-viral-associated PAN, the effects of IVIG are often just transient, and it is usually necessary to resume cytotoxic therapy to achieve disease remission.

Cryoglobulinemic Vasculitis

Similar to PAN, optimal management of cryoglobulin syndromes is based upon the disease process that has engendered the development of the cryoprecipitating immunoglobulins. Induction strategies entail combinations of plasma exchange with B cell depletion or alternative cytotoxic therapy for type I cryoglobulins associated with monoclonal gammopathies and type III cryoglobulin-associated autoimmune disease. Use of antiviral therapies with or without a brief course of corticosteroid therapy and plasma exchange constitute the most common strategies for management of severe or life-threatening type II cryoglobulins associated with hepatitis C infection. Rituximab may be added after viral clearance for persistent autoimmune manifestations (see Chap. 26). Should septic complications occur in the course of any of the above cryoglobulin syndromes, high-dose IVIG (2 g/kg) is an effective treatment strategy that can be employed to suppress vasculitis manifestations until intercurrent bacterial infection resolves. Bacterial infections occurring as a complication of plasma exchange may be due in part to associated hypogammaglobulinemia, and IVIG replacement therapy (0.4 g/kg) should be administered to such patients. However, administration of IVIG is not recommended in patients who have cryoglobulins associated with rheumatoid factor activity, as severe disease exacerbations have been reported when IVIG is administered in this setting [60, 61].

Management of Autoimmune Disorders in the Setting of Immune Deficiency

Immune deficiency may occur as a consequence of prescribed immunosuppressive therapy, genetic defects impacting development of mature immune responses, autoimmune responses targeting cells and/or molecules involved in the immune response, or viruses targeting immune effector cells. Since underlying immune deficiency may be an important consideration in the overall management strategy of autoimmune disease, assessment of underlying immune competence should be included in the initial if not ongoing assessment of individuals presenting with autoimmune manifestations.

Immune Deficiency Occurring as a Consequence of Autoimmune Disease Treatment

Although targeted therapies are becoming increasingly available as effective interventions for autoimmune disease, infectious complications due to treatment-related acquired immune deficiency remain a significant cause of disease morbidity and mortality. Accumulated experience with the use of chemotherapeutic agents impacting populations of immune cells has helped define thresholds below which infection complications are likely to occur. When using immune suppressants for treatment of autoimmune disease, periodic surveillance for acquired immune defects known to be associated with their use and employing prophylactic interventions when significant deficiency is recognized may serve to mitigate the risk of infection-related morbidity. Management of autoimmune disease going forward following recognition of treatment-related immune deficiency should include consideration of:

1. Attenuating the dose of prescribed immunosuppressive therapy as disease activity permits
2. Use of prophylactic interventions (Table 33.1)
3. Alternative therapeutic approaches that are least likely to compromise phagocytic cell functions as have been discussed for patients with autoimmune disease and intercurrent infection

Immune Deficiency Occurring as a Consequence of Autoimmunity

Immune deficiency developing as a consequence of autoimmunity poses a significant therapeutic challenge, as the cell line(s) affected may be

Table 33.1 Risk mitigation in the setting of immunosuppressive treatment

Immune defect	Therapeutic agent(s)	Threshold	Intervention options
Neutropenia	Cyclophosphamide Azathioprine 6-mercaptopurine Methotrexate	<500/mm^3	Levofloxacin 500 mg/day
T-lymphopenia	Corticosteroids Cyclophosphamide Azathioprine 6-mercaptopurine Mycophenolic acid	<500/mm^3	Trimethoprim-sulfa 160/800 mg q.o.d. Dapsone 100 mg daily
Hypogammaglobulinemia	Corticosteroids (prolonged use) Cyclophosphamide Azathioprine 6-mercaptopurine Mycophenolic acid Anti-CD20 (rituximab)	<500 mg/dL (<700 mg/dL with infection)	IVIG 0.4 g/kg every 3–4 weeks

further impacted by therapies normally required to manage the underlying autoimmune process. Lymphopenia, neutropenia, and pancytopenia not uncommonly occur in the context of SLE. Autoimmune neutropenia and aplastic anemia occurring in the setting of lupus have been effectively managed with therapies primarily targeting autoreactive T lymphocytes, including cyclosporine, tacrolimus, or anti-thymocyte globulin. Severe peripheral lymphopenia is a hallmark of lupus activity, but the underlying mechanisms giving rise to lymphopenia are not well understood and the extent to which the noted lymphopenia increases infection risk in SLE has not been well defined.

In the presence or absence of lymphopenia, hypogammaglobulinemia may occur in patients with established SLE [62]. For patients in whom low immunoglobulin levels are noted to antedate SLE manifestations, the underlying immunopathology may comprise part of the spectrum of common variable immune deficiency (discussed below). Alternatively, hypogammaglobulinemia may develop in the absence of significant immunosuppressive therapy well into the course of SLE [63, 64]. In such cases, it is hypothesized that autoimmune responses develop that target B cells directly or growth factors or cytokines requisite for B cell maturation and survival. Notably, it has been observed that in patients who develop spontaneous B cell depletion, preceding lupus manifestations may remit [65]. For patients who otherwise continue to have active disease manifestations requiring immune suppression, institution of immunoglobulin replacement therapy may permit proceeding as needed with usual SLE standard of care interventions [62].

Immune Deficiency Occurring as the Primary Disorder Underlying Autoimmunity

Manifestations of autoimmunity are not uncommonly an initial presenting clinical feature in patients with primary immune deficiencies (PID). With the advent of whole genome sequencing, increasing numbers of identified mutations underlying PID have been identified, many of which may be associated with autoimmunity (Table 33.2). The temporal relationships underlying the development of infection-related versus autoimmune complications arising from the underlying immune dysfunction are highly variable, and the mechanisms underlying the development of autoimmunity in these disorders remain incompletely understood. However, there is a developing collection of experience with management of autoimmunity associated with the more common and better characterized primary immune deficiencies (see Chap. 4).

Common variable immune deficiency (*CVID*) is the disorder in which autoimmunity is most commonly linked to immune deficiency. The prevalent immunologic phenotype is hypogammaglobulinemia with low levels of IgG and inability to generate sufficient IgG antibodies in response to pneumococcal or other polysaccharide bacterial antigens. Levels of IgA and/or IgM in CVID may also be attenuated. The mechanisms underlying the immune deficiency are variable; those most well described are failures of immunoglobulin class switch due to mutations in the transmembrane activator, calcium-modulator, and cyclophilin ligand interactor (TACI) receptor, but these account for less than 20% of affected patients [66]. While most patients with CVID have a history of recurring bacterial infections dating to childhood, many patients noted to have clinical and immunologic features consistent with CVID do not develop recurring infections or hypoglobulinemia until the third, fourth, fifth, or even later decades of life [67], begging the question as to whether the immune deficiency in such patients develops as a consequence of autoreactive responses targeting the normal production of mature neutralizing antibodies.

Preventative strategies are employed to minimize infectious complications associated with CVID and to permit management of associated autoimmunity with less infection risk. Milder variants associated with recurring respiratory infections can be successfully managed with rotating antibiotic therapy targeting respiratory pathogens. For patients with more severe levels of hypogammaglobulinemia (less than 500 mg/dL)

Table 33.2 Primary immune deficiencies associated with autoimmunity

Disorder	Mutations	Immune defects	Autoimmune features
CVID	*TACI*, others	Hypogammaglobulinemia	AIHA, ITP, SLE, (multiple)
sIgAD		Low serum IgA	JIA, RA, SLE Celiac disease Hashimoto's thyroiditis Pernicious anemia Myasthenia gravis Dermatomyositis
X-linked agammaglobulinemia	*btk*	Hypogammaglobulinemia FcR, TLR signaling	(rare)
Hyper-IgM [1]	*CD40, CD40 ligand*	Low serum IgG T cell co-stimulation	(rare)
Hyper-IgM [2], hyper-IgM [3]	*AICDA*, *UNG*	Low serum IgG	Autoimmune hepatitis RA, IBD, uveitis Diabetes mellitus
MBL deficiency	*MBL2*	Opsonization	SLE
C1q, C2, C4	*C1q, C2, C4A/C4B*	Opsonization	SLE
Adenosine deaminase deficiency	*ADA*	Th, T reg, variable low IgG	AIHA, ITP
PNP deficiency	*PNP*	Th, T reg, variable low IgG	AIHA, ITP
Wiskot-Aldrich syndrome	*WAS*	Th, T reg	AIHA, ITP, IBD, vasculitis, glomerulonephritis
DiGeorge syndrome	22q11 deletions	Th, T reg	AIHA, ITP, IBD, thyroiditis
LRBA deficiency	*LRBA*	T reg, low serum IgG	AIHA, ITP, enteritis, arthritis, myasthenia gravis, encephalitis, cerebellitis
CHAI	*CTLA4*	Th, T reg, variable low IgG	AIHA, ITP, enteritis, pneumonitis

AICDA activation-induced cytodine deaminase, *AIHA* autoimmune hemolytic anemia, *CHAI* CTLA-4 haploinsufficiency with autoimmune infiltration, *CVID* common variable immune deficiency, *IBD* inflammatory bowel disease, *ITP* immune thrombocytopenia, *JIA* juvenile idiopathic arthritis, *LRBA* lipopolysaccharide (LPS)-responsive beige-like anchor, *MBL* mannose bonding lectin, *PNP* purine nucleoside phosphorylase, *sIgAD* selective IgA deficiency, *TACI* transmembrane activator calcium-modulator and cyclophilin ligand interactor, *TLR* toll-like receptor, *UNG* uracil nucleoside glycosalase

and/or those demonstrating failure to mount sufficient titers of neutralizing antibodies in response to administered vaccine antigens, intravenous (every 3–4 week) or weekly subcutaneous infusions of immunoglobulin replacement therapy are recommended. Although complete selective IgA deficiency is uncommon in CVID, assessment for this is advised to minimize risk of anaphylaxis with IVIG administration. For CVID patients with significant intercurrent infection complications or undergoing major surgery, an additional dose of IVIG (0.4 g/kg) is recommended.

Immune thrombocytopenia, autoimmune hemolytic anemia, neuromyelitis optica, anti-GAD65 dystonias, ANCA vasculitis, or other CVID-associated autoimmune complications associated with defined autoantibodies frequently respond favorably to rituximab in combination with scheduled IVIG replacement therapy [68–71]. A similar therapeutic approach may be effective in managing the granulomatous interstitial lung disease that is not uncommonly associated with CVID [72, 73]. Lupus-related musculoskeletal and cutaneous syndromes that develop on a background of CVID can frequently be managed effectively with antimalarials, weekly methotrexate, and/or dapsone, without requiring significant corticosteroid use. As these drugs do not significantly impact B cell proliferation, the use of background immunoglobulin replacement therapy may not be required in patients who have these lupus-related features in association with milder variants of CVID. The use of immunosuppressive therapies that do impact B cell populations is otherwise best undertaken in CVID patients on a background of immunoglobulin replacement therapy.

Patients with CVID with or without known autoimmunity have been observed to have higher than normal levels of B lymphocyte stimulator (BLyS, BAFF), a known survival factor for autoreactive B cells [74]. Whether and to what extent elevated levels of BLyS/BAFF contribute to autoimmunity in CVID remain an active area of investigation. The noted elevations in BLyS/BAFF in patients with CVID suggest that presently available biologic reagents which neutralize the effects of BLyS/BAFF may be potentially useful in suppressing autoimmune complications in this population of patients.

Selective IgA Deficiency (*sIgAD*) is commonly associated with a variety of autoimmune disorders, and case-control cohort studies have demonstrated greater prevalence of autoantibodies in IgA deficient patients [75, 76]. The immunopathologic mechanisms underlying noted increases in autoimmunity in sIgAD individuals remain poorly understood, but associations with deficiencies in the population of Treg cells and class-switched memory B cells have been observed in sIgAD cohorts with autoimmunity [77]. Since the vast majority of patients with sIgAD in the absence of IgG or IgG subclass deficiency do not have increased prevalence of serious infections, management of autoimmune and rheumatic disease in sIgAD patients can proceed as would be custom for patients who are not IgA deficient.

X-linked agammaglobulinemia (*XLA*), associated with mutations in Bruton's tyrosine kinase (*btk*) resulting in absence of circulating CD19+/CD20+ B cells and hypogammaglobulinemia, is rarely associated with autoimmune disease. In addition to being critical to normal B cell maturation, *btk* also mediates monocyte Fc receptor as well as toll-like receptor (TLR)-associated signal transduction, and in a variety of murine models of autoimmune inflammation, *btk* inhibitors have a profound ameliorative effect on tissue inflammation as well as titers of autoantibodies [78, 79]. The paucity of autoimmune complications in patients with *btk* deficiency is therefore not surprising and selective *btk* inhibitors are now being evaluated in clinical trials of patients with lupus. However, should autoimmune complications occur in a patient with XLA, treatment with indicated immunosuppressive therapy can proceed on a background of immunoglobulin replacement therapy.

Hyper IgM syndromes occur most commonly in the setting of *CD40 or CD40 ligand deficiency*, whereby there are observed failures of Ig class switching, establishment of effective cell memory, and T cell-driven monocyte activation. Laboratory correlates include low levels of IgG and IgA but normal to elevated levels of serum IgM, normal levels of circulating B cells but only expressing IgM or IgD, and absence of circulating memory B cells [80]. Clinical features include frequent respiratory infections and opportunistic infections (histoplasmosis, cryptosporidium, pneumocystis). Given the pivotal role of CD40-CD40 ligand interactions in T cell co-stimulation, it is therefore not surprising that autoimmune complications are seen rarely in patients with deficiency in CD40-mediated signaling and that interruptions in CD40-CD40L signaling can ameliorate autoimmune manifestations in lupus-prone mice.

In a small minority of cases (<5%), hyper IgM syndrome occurs due to deficiencies in either *activation-induced cytidine deaminase* (*AICDA*) or *uracil nucleoside glycosylase* (*UNG*). Both enzymes are required for B cell class switching, and deficiency of either results in low serum levels of IgG and IgA, with normal to high serum levels of IgM and normal levels of circulating B cells expressing IgM [81, 82]. However, unlike CD40/CD40L deficiency, T cell number and functions are essentially intact, and a variety of autoimmune complications have been reported in individuals deficient in AICDA or UNG including autoimmune hepatitis, RA, IBD, uveitis, and diabetes mellitus. Provided they are administered on a background of scheduled immunoglobulin replacement therapy, standard treatments can be employed to manage AICDA- and UNG-associated autoimmune complications.

Complement (*C1q, C2, C4*) and *mannose-binding lectin* (*MBL*) *deficiencies* are associated with increased risk of pyogenic infection with encapsulated organisms. Early complement components as well as MBL also opsonize and facilitate the removal by macrophages of nucleosome products of cellular apoptosis, rather than by plasmacytoid dendritic cells in a manner that renders epitopes in the nucleosomes becoming potentially immunogenic [83]. Deficiencies in C1q, C2, C4, and MBL have all been associated with increased risk of systemic or cutaneous lupus, presumably due to associated impairment in the noninflammatory, non-immunogenic disposal of apoptotic nucleosomes [28, 84]. Management of lupus-related autoimmune disease in patients with early complement or MBL deficiency can proceed with standard lupus therapies. However, it is prudent to monitor for treatment-associated lymphopenia, neutropenia, and hypogammaglobulinemia in affected patients, entertaining a lower threshold for instituting immunoglobulin replacement therapy or prophylactic antibiotic use in patients further immunocompromised (Table 33.1).

Adenosine deaminase deficiency (*ADA*), *Wiskott-Aldrich syndrome* (*WAS*), and *DiGeorge* (*22q11 deletion*) syndromes are combined immune deficiencies associated with defects primarily in T cell function, with variable defects in humoral immunity arising secondarily. Autoimmunity occurs in these syndromes likely due in large part to impairments in the function and/or numbers of T regulatory lymphocytes.

The elevated levels of adenosine and deoxyadenosine associated with ADA are toxic primarily to T lymphocytes, engender feedback inhibition of ribonucleotide reductase with decreased de novo purine synthesis, and inhibit phagocytic cell migration. The primary observed immunologic abnormalities in ADA are very low levels of circulating T cells with variable degrees of hypogammaglobulinemia; immune cytopenias are the most commonly observed autoimmune complications. The noted autoimmunity observed in ADA likely occurs as a consequence of imbalances in the proportions of affected regulatory versus helper/cytotoxic T cells [85].

WAS develops primarily due to loss of function mutations of the *WASp* protein involved in the cytoskeletal functions of hematopoietic cells. The immunodeficiency develops due to loss of formation of lipid rafts required for the formation of the immunologic synapse between T lymphocytes and antigen-presenting cells. This *WASp*-associated cytoskeletal defect also likely accounts for the failure of T regs to form synapses with effector T cells, with attendant failure to suppress effector functions of autoreactive T lymphocytes [86]. As a consequence, autoimmune manifestations including immune cytopenias, vasculitis, IBD, and/or nephritis occur commonly in patients with WAS.

Individuals with DiGeorge syndrome due to deletions of 22q11 have impaired thymic development with low numbers of circulating T lymphocytes. Reported autoimmune complications include immune cytopenias, endocrinopathies, and inflammatory enteropathies [87]. Autoimmunity in DiGeorge syndrome likely occurs as consequence of impaired development of a sufficiently diverse T regulatory cell repertoire [88].

Although management of autoimmune complications in patients with primary immune deficiencies is challenging, the majority of affected patients can be effectively managed with standard therapies employed in the treatment of non-immune deficient individuals. It is nonetheless important to recognize the presence of primary immune deficiency in patients presenting with autoimmunity so as to appropriately choose and minimize the risk of infection that may be heightened as a consequence of employed immunosuppressive therapy. The development of an autoimmune disorder at an unusually early age for that condition, the presence of autoimmunity affecting multiple organ systems, or atypical immune syndromes that cannot be attributed to specific rheumatologic diagnosis should prompt investigation for possible primary immune deficiency. Assessment of immunoglobulin levels, responses to pneumococcal vaccination, and flow cytometry studies to quantify numbers of circulating B cells and T cell subset populations may serve as useful initial screening assessments for many of the immune deficiencies associated with autoimmunity.

References

1. Doran MF, Crowson CS, Pond GR, O'Fallon WM, Gabriel SE. Predictors of infection in rheumatoid arthritis. Arthritis Rheum. 2002;46:2294–300.
2. Curtis JR, Yang S, Patkar NM, Chen L, Singh JA, Cannon GW, et al. Risk of hospitalized bacterial infections associated with biologic treatment among

US veterans with rheumatoid arthritis. Arthritis Care Res. 2014;66(7):990.
3. Aaltonen KJ, Joensuu JT, Virkki L, Sokka T, Aronen P, Relas H, et al. Rates of serious infections and malignancies among patients with rheumatoid arthritis receiving either tumor necrosis factor inhibitor or rituximab therapy. J Rheumatol. 2015;42:372–8.
4. Bongartz T, Sutton AJ, Sweeting MJ, Buchan I, Matteson EL, Montori V. Anti-TNF antibody therapy in rheumatoid arthritis and the risk of serious infections and malignancies: systematic review and meta-analysis of rare harmful effects in randomized controlled trials. JAMA. 2006;295:2275–85.
5. Goodman SM. Rheumatoid arthritis: perioperative management of biologics and DMARDs. Semin Arthritis Rheum. 2015;44:627–32.
6. Chan ES, Cronstein BN. Methotrexate – how does it really work? Nat Rev Rheumatol. 2010;6:175–8.
7. Moreland LW, Bucy RP, Weinblatt ME, Mohler KM, Spencer-Green GT, Chatham WW. Immune function in patients with rheumatoid arthritis treated with etanercept. Clin Immunol. 2002;103:13–21.
8. Xie X, Li F, Chen JW, Wang J. Risk of tuberculosis infection in anti-TNF-alpha biological therapy: from bench to bedside. J Microbiol Immunol Infect. 2014;47:268–74.
9. Dorhoi A, Kaufmann SH. Tumor necrosis factor alpha in mycobacterial infection. Semin Immunol. 2014;26:203–9.
10. Baddley JW, Winthrop KL, Chen L, Liu L, Grijalva CG, Delzell E, et al. Non-viral opportunistic infections in new users of tumour necrosis factor inhibitor therapy: results of the SAfety Assessment of Biologic ThERapy (SABER) study. Ann Rheum Dis. 2014;73:1942–8.
11. Wasson NJ, Varley CD, Schwab P, Fu R, Winthrop KL. Serious skin & soft tissue infections in rheumatoid arthritis patients taking anti-tumor necrosis factor alpha drugs: a nested case-control study. BMC Infect Dis. 2013;13:533.
12. Tilg H, Trehu E, Atkins MB, Dinarello CA, Mier JW. Interleukin-6 (IL-6) as an anti-inflammatory cytokine: induction of circulating IL-1 receptor antagonist and soluble tumor necrosis factor receptor p55. Blood. 1994;83:113–8.
13. Grivennikov S, Karin E, Terzic J, Mucida D, Yu GY, Vallabhapurapu S, et al. IL-6 and Stat3 are required for survival of intestinal epithelial cells and development of colitis-associated cancer. Cancer Cell. 2009;15:103–13.
14. Strangfeld A, Richter A, Siegmund B, Herzer P, Rockwitz K, Demary W, et al. Risk for lower intestinal perforations in patients with rheumatoid arthritis treated with tocilizumab in comparison to treatment with other biologic or conventional synthetic DMARDs. Ann Rheum Dis. 2017;76:504–10.
15. Strand V, Ahadieh S, French J, Geier J, Krishnaswami S, Menon S, et al. Systematic review and meta-analysis of serious infections with tofacitinib and biologic disease-modifying antirheumatic drug treatment in rheumatoid arthritis clinical trials. Arthritis Res Ther. 2015;17:362.
16. Desai RJ, Thaler KJ, Mahlknecht P, Gartlehner G, McDonagh MS, Mesgarpour B, et al. Comparative risk of harm associated with the use of targeted immunomodulators: a systematic review. Arthritis Care Res. 2016;68:1078–88.
17. Yun H, Xie F, Delzell E, Levitan EB, Chen L, Lewis JD, et al. Comparative risk of hospitalized infection associated with biologic agents in rheumatoid arthritis patients enrolled in medicare. Arthritis Rheumatol. 2016;68:56–66.
18. Schiff M, Weinblatt ME, Valente R, van der Heijde D, Citera G, Elegbe A, et al. Head-to-head comparison of subcutaneous abatacept versus adalimumab for rheumatoid arthritis: two-year efficacy and safety findings from AMPLE trial. Ann Rheum Dis. 2014;73:86–94.
19. Silva-Fernandez L, De Cock D, Lunt M, Low AS, Watson KD, Group B-RC, et al. Serious infection risk after 1 year between patients with rheumatoid arthritis treated with rituximab or with a second TNFi after initial TNFi failure: results from the British Society for Rheumatology biologics register for rheumatoid arthritis. Rheumatology. 2017. https://doi.org/10.1093/rheumatology/kex304.
20. van Vollenhoven RF, Emery P, Bingham CO 3rd, Keystone EC, Fleischmann RM, Furst DE, et al. Long-term safety of rituximab in rheumatoid arthritis: 9.5-year follow-up of the global clinical trial programme with a focus on adverse events of interest in RA patients. Ann Rheum Dis. 2013;72:1496–502.
21. Nisihara R, Skare T, Maestri V, Alegretti JS, Campos APB, Messias-Reason I. Mannose-binding lectin (MBL) deficiency and tuberculosis infection in patients with ankylosing spondylitis. Clin Rheumatol. 2017;37(2):555–8.
22. Skare TL, Nisihara R, Cieslinski JZ, Zeni JO, Rasera HN, Messias-Reason I, et al. Mannose-binding lectin deficiency in Brazilian patients with spondyloarthritis. Immunol Investig. 2017;46:183–9.
23. Crowley J, Thaci D, Joly P, Peris K, Papp KA, Goncalves J, et al. Long-term safety and tolerability of apremilast in patients with psoriasis: pooled safety analysis for ≥156 weeks from 2 phase 3, randomized, controlled trials (ESTEEM 1 and 2). J Am Acad Dermatol. 2017;77:310–7e1.
24. Kalb RE, Fiorentino DF, Lebwohl MG, Toole J, Poulin Y, Cohen AD, et al. Risk of serious infection with biologic and systemic treatment of psoriasis: results from the psoriasis longitudinal assessment and registry (PSOLAR). JAMA Dermatol. 2015;151:961–9.
25. Langley RG, Elewski BE, Lebwohl M, Reich K, Griffiths CE, Papp K, et al. Secukinumab in plaque psoriasis – results of two phase 3 trials. N Engl J Med. 2014;371:326–38.
26. Saunte DM, Mrowietz U, Puig L, Zachariae C. Candida infections in patients with psoriasis and psoriatic arthritis treated with interleukin-17 inhibitors and their practical management. Br J Dermatol. 2017;177:47–62.

27. Yang Y, Chung EK, Zhou B, Lhotta K, Hebert LA, Birmingham DJ, et al. The intricate role of complement component C4 in human systemic lupus erythematosus. Curr Dir Autoimmun. 2004;7:98–132.
28. Monticielo OA, Mucenic T, Xavier RM, Brenol JC, Chies JA. The role of mannose-binding lectin in systemic lupus erythematosus. Clin Rheumatol. 2008;27:413–9.
29. Merayo-Chalico J, Gomez-Martin D, Pineirua-Menendez A, Santana-De Anda K, Alcocer-Varela J. Lymphopenia as risk factor for development of severe infections in patients with systemic lupus erythematosus: a case-control study. QJM. 2013;106:451–7.
30. Hartman KR. Anti-neutrophil antibodies of the immunoglobulin M class in autoimmune neutropenia. Am J Med Sci. 1994;308:102–5.
31. Browne SK. Anticytokine autoantibody-associated immunodeficiency. Annu Rev Immunol. 2014;32: 635–57.
32. Perazzio SF, Granados A, Salomao R, Silva NP, Carneiro-Sampaio M, Andrade LE. High frequency of immunodeficiency-like states in systemic lupus erythematosus: a cross-sectional study in 300 consecutive patients. Rheumatology. 2016;55:1647–55.
33. Engel G, van Vollenhoven RF. Treatment of severe CNS lupus with intravenous immunoglobulin. J Clin Rheumatol. 1999;5:228–32.
34. Rodrigues M, Galego O, Costa C, Jesus D, Carvalho P, Santiago M, et al. Central nervous system vasculitis in systemic lupus erythematosus: a case series report in a tertiary referral centre. Lupus. 2017;26:1440–7.
35. Deane KD, West SG. Antiphospholipid antibodies as a cause of pulmonary capillaritis and diffuse alveolar hemorrhage: a case series and literature review. Semin Arthritis Rheum. 2005;35:154–65.
36. Imran H, Tleyjeh IM, Arndt CA, Baddour LM, Erwin PJ, Tsigrelis C, et al. Fluoroquinolone prophylaxis in patients with neutropenia: a meta-analysis of randomized placebo-controlled trials. Eur J Clin Microbiol Infect Dis. 2008;27:53–63.
37. Euler HH, Harten P, Zeuner RA, Schwab UM. Recombinant human granulocyte colony stimulating factor in patients with systemic lupus erythematosus associated neutropenia and refractory infections. J Rheumatol. 1997;24:2153–7.
38. Arnal C, Piette JC, Leone J, Taillan B, Hachulla E, Roudot-Thoraval F, et al. Treatment of severe immune thrombocytopenia associated with systemic lupus erythematosus: 59 cases. J Rheumatol. 2002;29: 75–83.
39. Gomard-Mennesson E, Ruivard M, Koenig M, Woods A, Magy N, Ninet J, et al. Treatment of isolated severe immune hemolytic anaemia associated with systemic lupus erythematosus: 26 cases. Lupus. 2006;15:223–31.
40. Rogers SJ, Williams CS, Roman GC. Myelopathy in Sjogren's syndrome: role of nonsteroidal immunosuppressants. Drugs. 2004;64:123–32.
41. Gueta I, Shoenfeld Y, Orbach H. Intravenous immune globulins (IVIg) treatment for organizing pneumonia in a selective IgG immune deficiency state. Immunol Res. 2014;60:165–9.
42. Kashif M, Arya D, Niazi M, Khaja M. A rare case of necrotizing myopathy and fibrinous and organizing pneumonia with anti-EJ antisynthetase syndrome and SSA antibodies. Am J Case Rep. 2017;18:448–53.
43. Shitenberg D, Fruchter O, Fridel L, Kramer MR. Successful rituximab therapy in steroid-resistant, cryptogenic organizing pneumonia: a case series. Respiration. 2015;90:155–9.
44. Volkmann ER, Tashkin DP, Li N, Roth MD, Khanna D, Hoffmann-Vold AM, et al. Mycophenolate mofetil versus placebo for systemic sclerosis-related interstitial lung disease: an analysis of scleroderma lung studies I and II. Arthritis Rheumatol. 2017;69: 1451–60.
45. Cantarini L, Rigante D, Vitale A, Napodano S, Sakkas LI, Bogdanos DP, et al. Intravenous immunoglobulins (IVIG) in systemic sclerosis: a challenging yet promising future. Immunol Res. 2015;61:326–37.
46. Wang DX, Shu XM, Tian XL, Chen F, Zu N, Ma L, et al. Intravenous immunoglobulin therapy in adult patients with polymyositis/dermatomyositis: a systematic literature review. Clin Rheumatol. 2012;31:801–6.
47. Hellmich B, Ehren M, Lindstaedt M, Meyer M, Pfohl M, Schatz H. Anti-MPO-ANCA-positive microscopic polyangiitis following subacute bacterial endocarditis. Clin Rheumatol. 2001;20:441–3.
48. Kasmani R, Okoli K, Naraharisetty K, Gunning W, Shapiro JI, Ratnam S. Microscopic polyangiitis triggered by recurrent methicillin-resistant Staphylococcus aureus bacteremia. Int Urol Nephrol. 2010;42:821–4.
49. Bell EK, Chugh SS, Cook WJ. A case of infection-associated antiproteinase-3-negative cytoplasmic antineutrophil cytoplasmic antibody pauci-immune focal necrotizing glomerulonephritis. Nephrol Dial Transplant. 2010;25:3119–23.
50. Stegeman CA, Tervaert JW, de Jong PE, Kallenberg CG. Trimethoprim-sulfamethoxazole (co-trimoxazole) for the prevention of relapses of Wegener's granulomatosis. Dutch Co-Trimoxazole Wegener Study Group. N Engl J Med. 1996;335:16–20.
51. Booth AD, Almond MK, Burns A, Ellis P, Gaskin G, Neild GH, et al. Outcome of ANCA-associated renal vasculitis: a 5-year retrospective study. Am J Kidney Dis. 2003;41:776–84.
52. Bucaneve G, Micozzi A, Menichetti F, Martino P, Dionisi MS, Martinelli G, et al. Levofloxacin to prevent bacterial infection in patients with cancer and neutropenia. N Engl J Med. 2005;353:977–87.
53. Freeley SJ, Coughlan AM, Popat RJ, Dunn-Walters DK, Robson MG. Granulocyte colony stimulating factor exacerbates antineutrophil cytoplasmic antibody vasculitis. Ann Rheum Dis. 2013;72:1053–8.
54. Roberts DM, Jones RB, Smith RM, Alberici F, Kumaratne DS, Burns S, et al. Immunoglobulin G replacement for the treatment of infective complications of rituximab-associated hypogammaglobu-

linemia in autoimmune disease: a case series. J Autoimmun. 2015;57:24–9.
55. Guillevin L, Mahr A, Cohen P, Larroche C, Queyrel V, Loustaud-Ratti V, et al. Short-term corticosteroids then lamivudine and plasma exchanges to treat hepatitis B virus-related polyarteritis nodosa. Arthritis Rheum. 2004;51:482–7.
56. Meyer MF, Hellmich B, Kotterba S, Schatz H. Cytomegalovirus infection in systemic necrotizing vasculitis: causative agent or opportunistic infection? Rheumatol Int. 2000;20:35–8.
57. Viguier M, Guillevin L, Laroche L. Treatment of parvovirus B19-associated polyarteritis nodosa with intravenous immune globulin. N Engl J Med. 2001;344:1481–2.
58. Marie I, Miranda S, Girszyn N, Soubrane JC, Vandhuick T, Levesque H. Intravenous immunoglobulins as treatment of severe cutaneous polyarteritis nodosa. Intern Med J. 2012;42:459–62.
59. Balbir-Gurman A, Nahir AM, Braun-Moscovici Y. Intravenous immunoglobulins in polyarteritis nodosa restricted to the limbs: case reports and review of the literature. Clin Exp Rheumatol. 2007;25:S28–30.
60. Barton JC, Herrera GA, Galla JH, Bertoli LF, Work J, Koopman WJ. Acute cryoglobulinemic renal failure after intravenous infusion of gamma globulin. Am J Med. 1987;82:624–9.
61. Yebra M, Barrios Y, Rincon J, Sanjuan I, Diaz-Espada F. Severe cutaneous vasculitis following intravenous infusion of gammaglobulin in a patient with type II mixed cryoglobulinemia. Clin Exp Rheumatol. 2002;20:225–7.
62. Karim MY. Immunodeficiency in the lupus clinic. Lupus. 2006;15:127–31.
63. Stein A, Winkelstein A, Agarwal A. Concurrent systemic lupus erythematosus and common variable hypogammaglobulinemia. Arthritis Rheum. 1985;28:462–5.
64. Baum CG, Chiorazzi N, Frankel S, Shepherd GM. Conversion of systemic lupus erythematosus to common variable hypogammaglobulinemia. Am J Med. 1989;87:449–56.
65. Tarrant TK, Frazer DH, Aya-Ay JP, Patel DD. B cell loss leading to remission in severe systemic lupus erythematosus. J Rheumatol. 2003;30:412–4.
66. Sathkumara HD, De Silva NR, Handunnetti S, De Silva AD. Genetics of common variable immunodeficiency: role of transmembrane activator and calcium modulator and cyclophilin ligand interactor. Int J Immunogenet. 2015;42:239–53.
67. Cunningham-Rundles C, Bodian C. Common variable immunodeficiency: clinical and immunological features of 248 patients. Clin Immunol. 1999;92:34–48.
68. Gobert D, Bussel JB, Cunningham-Rundles C, Galicier L, Dechartres A, Berezne A, et al. Efficacy and safety of rituximab in common variable immunodeficiency-associated immune cytopenias: a retrospective multicentre study on 33 patients. Br J Haematol. 2011;155:498–508.
69. Hill F, Yonkof J, Chaitanya Arudra SK, Thomas J, Altorok N. Successful treatment of ANCA-associated vasculitis in the setting of common variable immunodeficiency using rituximab. Am J Ther. 2016;23:e1239–45.
70. Zephir H, Bernard-Valnet R, Lebrun C, Outteryck O, Audoin B, Bourre B, et al. Rituximab as first-line therapy in neuromyelitis optica: efficiency and tolerability. J Neurol. 2015;262:2329–35.
71. Rizzi M, Knoth R, Hampe CS, Lorenz P, Gougeon ML, Lemercier B, et al. Long-lived plasma cells and memory B cells produce pathogenic anti-GAD65 autoantibodies in Stiff Person Syndrome. PLoS One. 2010;5:e10838.
72. Pathria M, Urbine D, Zumberg MS, Guarderas J. Management of granulomatous lymphocytic interstitial lung disease in a patient with common variable immune deficiency. BMJ Case Rep. 2016;2016. https://doi.org/10.1136/bcr-2016-215624.
73. Jolles S, Carne E, Brouns M, El-Shanawany T, Williams P, Marshall C, et al. FDG PET-CT imaging of therapeutic response in granulomatous lymphocytic interstitial lung disease (GLILD) in common variable immunodeficiency (CVID). Clin Exp Immunol. 2017;187:138–45.
74. Knight AK, Radigan L, Marron T, Langs A, Zhang L, Cunningham-Rundles C. High serum levels of BAFF, APRIL, and TACI in common variable immunodeficiency. Clin Immunol. 2007;124:182–9.
75. Barka N, Shen GQ, Shoenfeld Y, Alosachie IJ, Gershwin ME, Reyes H, et al. Multireactive pattern of serum autoantibodies in asymptomatic individuals with immunoglobulin A deficiency. Clin Diagn Lab Immunol. 1995;2:469–72.
76. Edwards E, Razvi S, Cunningham-Rundles C. IgA deficiency: clinical correlates and responses to pneumococcal vaccine. Clin Immunol. 2004;111:93–7.
77. Abolhassani H, Gharib B, Shahinpour S, Masoom SN, Havaei A, Mirminachi B, et al. Autoimmunity in patients with selective IgA deficiency. J Investig Allergol Clin Immunol. 2015;25:112–9.
78. Ren L, Campbell A, Fang H, Gautam S, Elavazhagan S, Fatehchand K, et al. Analysis of the effects of the Bruton's tyrosine kinase (Btk) inhibitor ibrutinib on monocyte Fc gamma Receptor (FcgammaR) function. J Biol Chem. 2016;291:3043–52.
79. Rankin AL, Seth N, Keegan S, Andreyeva T, Cook TA, Edmonds J, et al. Selective inhibition of BTK prevents murine lupus and antibody-mediated glomerulonephritis. J Immunol. 2013;191:4540–50.
80. Winkelstein JA, Marino MC, Ochs H, Fuleihan R, Scholl PR, Geha R, et al. The X-linked hyper-IgM syndrome: clinical and immunologic features of 79 patients. Medicine. 2003;82:373–84.
81. Quartier P, Bustamante J, Sanal O, Plebani A, Debre M, Deville A, et al. Clinical, immunologic and genetic analysis of 29 patients with autosomal recessive hyper-IgM syndrome due to activation-induced Cytidine Deaminase deficiency. Clin Immunol. 2004;110:22–9.

82. Imai K, Slupphaug G, Lee WI, Revy P, Nonoyama S, Catalan N, et al. Human uracil-DNA glycosylase deficiency associated with profoundly impaired immunoglobulin class-switch recombination. Nat Immunol. 2003;4:1023–8.
83. Gullstrand B, Martensson U, Sturfelt G, Bengtsson AA, Truedsson L. Complement classical pathway components are all important in clearance of apoptotic and secondary necrotic cells. Clin Exp Immunol. 2009;156:303–11.
84. Lood C, Gullstrand B, Truedsson L, Olin AI, Alm GV, Ronnblom L, et al. C1q inhibits immune complex-induced interferon-alpha production in plasmacytoid dendritic cells: a novel link between C1q deficiency and systemic lupus erythematosus pathogenesis. Arthritis Rheum. 2009;60:3081–90.
85. Sauer AV, Brigida I, Carriglio N, Hernandez RJ, Scaramuzza S, Clavenna D, et al. Alterations in the adenosine metabolism and CD39/CD73 adenosinergic machinery cause loss of Treg cell function and autoimmunity in ADA-deficient SCID. Blood. 2012;119:1428–39.
86. Humblet-Baron S, Sather B, Anover S, Becker-Herman S, Kasprowicz DJ, Khim S, et al. Wiskott-Aldrich syndrome protein is required for regulatory T cell homeostasis. J Clin Invest. 2007;117:407–18.
87. Tison BE, Nicholas SK, Abramson SL, Hanson IC, Paul ME, Seeborg FO, et al. Autoimmunity in a cohort of 130 pediatric patients with partial DiGeorge syndrome. J Allergy Clin Immunol. 2011;128:1115–7e1-3.
88. Ferrando-Martinez S, Lorente R, Gurbindo D, De Jose MI, Leal M, Munoz-Fernandez MA, et al. Low thymic output, peripheral homeostasis deregulation, and hastened regulatory T cells differentiation in children with 22q11.2 deletion syndrome. J Pediatr. 2014;164:882–9.

34 Individual Drugs in Rheumatology and the Risk of Infection

Konstantinos Thomas and Dimitrios Vassilopoulos

Abbreviations

AAV	ANCA-associated vasculitis
ABA	Abatacept
ADA	Adalimumab
ANA	Anakinra
ANCA	Antineutrophil cytoplasmic antibody
Anti-HBc	Antibody against hepatitis B core antigen
Anti-HBs	Antibody against hepatitis B surface antigen
AOSD	Adult-onset Still's disease
AS	Ankylosing spondylitis
AZA	Azathioprine
BAFF	B-cell activating factor
BCG	Bacillus Calmette-Guérin
bDMARDs	Biologic disease-modifying antirheumatic drugs
CAPS	Cryopyrin-associated periodic syndromes
CD	Cluster of differentiation
CNS	Central nervous system
CRP	C-reactive protein
CsA	Cyclosporine A
csDMARDs	Conventional synthetic disease-modifying antirheumatic drugs
CYC	Cyclophosphamide
EDTA	European Dialysis and Transplantation Association
EMA	European Medicines Agency
ETN	Etanercept
EULAR	European League Against Rheumatism
FDA	Food and Drug Administration
GCA	Giant-cell arteritis
HBsAg	Hepatitis B surface antigen
HBV	Hepatitis B virus
HZ	Herpes zoster
Ig	Immunoglobulin
IGRA	Interferon-gamma releasing assay
IL	Interleukin
INFL	Infliximab
IV	Intravenous
IVIG	Intravenous immunoglobulin
JAK	Janus kinase
JIA	Juvenile idiopathic arthritis
LEF	Leflunomide
LN	Lupus nephritis
LON	Late-onset neutropenia
LTBI	Latent tuberculosis infection
LTE	Long-term extension
MMF	Mycophenolate mofetil
MTX	Methotrexate
NSAIDs	Nonsteroidal anti-inflammatory drugs
NTM	Nontuberculous mycobacteria

K. Thomas · D. Vassilopoulos (✉)
Joint Rheumatology Program, Clinical Immunology-Rheumatology Unit, 2nd Department of Medicine and Laboratory, National and Kapodistrian University of Athens, School of Medicine, Hippokration General Hospital, Athens, Greece
e-mail: dvassilop@med.uoa.gr

G. Ragab et al. (eds.), *The Microbiome in Rheumatic Diseases and Infection*,
https://doi.org/10.1007/978-3-319-79026-8_34

OIs	Opportunistic infections
PDE4	Phosphodiesterase-4
PJP	Pneumocystis jirovecii pneumonia
PML	Progressive multifocal leukoencephalopathy
PMR	Polymyalgia rheumatica
PsA	Psoriatic arthritis
RA	Rheumatoid arthritis
RCT	Randomized controlled trial
RTX	Rituximab
SC	Subcutaneous
SLE	Systemic lupus erythematosus
TB	Tuberculosis
TCZ	Tocilizumab
TMP/SMX	Trimethoprim/sulfamethoxazole
TNF	Tumor necrosis factor
TNFi	TNF inhibitors
TST	Tuberculin skin test
VZV	Varicella-zoster virus

Introduction

The therapeutic choices for patients with rheumatic diseases have been greatly expanded over the last 20 years. In addition to the traditional treatments such as corticosteroids and conventional synthetic disease-modifying antirheumatic drugs (csDMARDs), biologic DMARDs (bDMARDs) or small molecules have been introduced in daily clinical practice for the treatment of various inflammatory rheumatic diseases (Table 34.1). These novel therapies have been shown to be highly effective in patients with inadequate response to conventional treatments. They provide alternative choices of equal efficacy or function as steroid-sparing agents and have greatly improved patients' ability for work [1].

Despite this progress, infections continue to consist one of the most common comorbidities in patients with rheumatic diseases and to contribute significantly to the morbidity and mortality of this population. Data from the pre-biologic era have shown that patients with inflammatory arthritides, mainly rheumatoid arthritis (RA), have approximately a two-fold higher risk for serious infections in comparison to the general population [2]. This risk is increased for patients with high disease activity and disability scores, indicating that it is partially related to the disease itself and not only to the administered antirheumatic therapy [3].

The infectious diseases' burden remains significantly high also in patients with systemic lupus erythematosus (SLE), in whom the risk for hospitalized infections was 12-fold higher compared to the general population in a recent study [4], with pneumonia being the most frequent infection and bloodstream infection the most common infection-related cause of death (also see Chap. 24) [5]. Similarly, high risk for serious infections and infection-related death has been noticed in patients with systemic vasculitides [6]. Common bacterial and viral infections constitute the majority of infectious complications with the respiratory tract being the most commonly affected, whereas other commonly described infections involve skin, soft tissues and urinary tract [7].

Nevertheless, a number of other bacterial, viral, or fungal pathogens have raised concern in rheumatic patients, given their potential for reactivation especially in those treated with bDMARDs (*Mycobacterium tuberculosis*; hepatitis B virus, HBV; varicella-zoster virus, VZV) or the higher incidence of rare opportunistic infections, such as *Pneumocystis jirovecii*. It should be noted that the risk for developing such infections differs among the several classes of bDMARDs and rheumatologists should be familiar with the safety profile of each specific agent.

In this review the individual risk of different antirheumatic therapies is critically reviewed and presented.

Infection Risk of Individual DMARDs

Non-biological Therapies

Corticosteroids

Despite the well-established risks associated with their use, corticosteroids still remain the most prescribed drug in patients with inflammatory rheumatic diseases. Recent studies have

Table 34.1 Most commonly used biologic agents and small molecules and their targets in the treatment of rheumatic diseases

Target	Agent	Rheumatologic and related disorder indications: Approved	Off-label use
Biologic agents			
TNF-α	Adalimumab	RA, PsA, AS, JIA, psoriasis, hidradenitis suppurativa, Crohn's disease, ulcerative colitis, uveitis	Takayasu arteritis
	Certolizumab pegol		Behcet's disease
	Etanercept		
	Infliximab		
	Golimumab		
IL-1	Anakinra	RA, CAPS	Gout
			Systemic JIA
	Canakinumab	Systemic JIA (>2 years old)	
		AOSD	
		CAPS	
		Gout	
IL-6	Tocilizumab	RA	PMR
		Systemic JIA	
		Polyarticular JIA (>2 years old)	
		GCA	Takayasu arteritis
CD20	Rituximab	RA	SLE
			Cryoglobulinemic syndrome
			Catastrophic antiphospholipid syndrome
		ANCA-associated vasculitides	Inflammatory myopathies
CD80/86	Abatacept	RA	
		JIA (>6 years old)	
		PsA	
BAFF	Belimumab	SLE	
IL-17	Secukinumab	PsA	
		AS	
		Psoriasis	
IL-12/23	Ustekinumab	PsA	
		Psoriasis	
		Crohn's disease	
Small molecules			
PDE4	Apremilast	PsA	Behcet's disease
JAK	Tofacitinib	RA	
	Baricitinib[a]		

[a]Approved by EMA (European Medicines Agency) only

TNF tumor necrosis factor, *RA* rheumatoid arthritis, *PsA* psoriatic arthritis, *AS* ankylosing spondylitis, *IL* interleukin, *JIA* juvenile idiopathic arthritis, *AOSD* adult-onset Still's disease, *CAPS* cryopyrin-associated periodic syndromes, *GCA* giant-cell arteritis, *PMR* polymyalgia rheumatica, *CD* cluster of differentiation, *AAV* ANCA-associated vasculitis, *SLE* systemic lupus erythematosus, *BAFF* B-cell activating factor, *PDE4* phosphodiesterase-4, *JAK* Janus kinase

shown that approximately half of RA patients are treated with corticosteroids [8], whereas almost 90% of patients with SLE have ever taken prednisone [5] and approximately 40% of elderly patients with giant-cell arteritis (GCA) fail to discontinue corticosteroid therapy after 10 years of treatment [9].

Corticosteroids exert their anti-inflammatory and immunosuppressive effects by acting on a variety of immune cells, including macrophages, neutrophils, and B and T lymphocytes, as well as other cells participating in tissue injury including fibroblasts and endothelial cells [10].

In a recent population-based study from the UK, corticosteroid prescription for various indications correlated with an increased risk of infection (hazard ratio (HR) = 2 for cellulitis and 5.8 for lower respiratory tract infections) [11]. Similar data have been derived from observational studies in patients with RA. In these patients, the risk seems to escalate in a dose-dependent manner, although a safe daily dose has not been clearly established. In a large nested-controlled study including more than 16,000 patients with RA, prescription of 5 mg prednisone daily did not result in an increased incidence of nonserious infections, in contrast with doses >20 mg, which were associated with a twofold increase [12]. Other studies have evaluated the role of corticosteroids on the risk for serious infections and have reported a dose-dependent increase [13]. Daily prednisone dose of >10 mg was associated with an up to threefold increase in the risk for serious infection [14]. Other investigators support that even the daily administration of ≤5 mg of prednisone may also pose a risk for hospitalization due to pneumonia [15]. Moreover, the same low dose may be correlated with a significantly increased risk when administered for extended time periods [16]. Interestingly, recent studies derived from the German registry for biologics (RABBIT) showed that the reduction in infection risk observed after 24 months of therapy with biologics may be partly attributed to decreases in the daily prednisone dose [17].

In patients with SLE, corticosteroids have been suggested to increase the risk for both serious and nonserious infections in a dose-dependent manner. In a study from Spain, a 12% increase in the odds for serious infection for each mg increase in daily prednisone was noticed. Mean daily prednisone dose was significantly higher in those SLE patients that experienced a serious infection compared with those without such history (7.5 vs. 2.5 mg) [18]. Another study showed that a daily prednisone dose of >20 mg, combined with ever use of cyclophosphamide, was independently associated with infection [19]. Recently, investigators from the Spanish Rheumatology Society Lupus Registry (RELESSER) reported that any use of ≥10 mg prednisone was associated with 27% increase in the risk of severe infection [5].

Regarding patients with vasculitides, corticosteroid use seems to predispose patients with ANCA-associated vasculitis (AAV) to infections, and alternative regimens containing lower cumulative dose of corticosteroids are being investigated [20]. Similarly, patients with giant-cell arteritis (GCA) are at increased risk for serious infection [21], especially during the first 12 months after treatment initiation, with an incidence reaching 11 cases/100 patient-years and almost 30% of deaths attributed to infectious causes. Daily prednisone dose of >10 mg after 12 months was associated with a 4.6-fold increase in the risk of infection-related death [22].

There is a satisfactory amount of evidence for the role of corticosteroids and the development of opportunistic infections (OIs), although the dose that increases the risk differs for each disease. Thus, daily prednisone doses of 7.5–10 mg correlate with an increased risk for herpes zoster (HZ), whereas the threshold for *Pneumocystis jirovecii* pneumonia (PJP) and tuberculosis (TB) seems to be higher (15 and 30 mg, respectively).

HBV reactivation is still a concern in patients with chronic HBV infection (who do not receive antiviral therapy) treated with corticosteroids for >4 weeks (at daily prednisone doses >10 mg). Although there is a paucity of data regarding rheumatic patients with past HBV infection, this risk is believed to be very low (<1%) [23].

csDMARDs

In contrast to corticosteroids, a risk for infection in csDMARD-treated patients has not been established. Methotrexate (MTX) is the most widely used and best studied csDMARD. Most studies do not show an increased risk for infections in MTX-treated patients. Older studies have shown no correlation between MTX and increased infection incidence or surgical infections after elective orthopedic surgery. Wolfe et al. studied a cohort of 16,788 RA patients to assess the incidence and risk factors for pneumonia. Regarding csDMARDs, only leflunomide (LEF) correlated with a slight increase of the risk by 20%, whereas MTX use was not associated with any increased risk for pneumonia [15].

Regarding HZ, most studies have not shown an increased risk with MTX administration. Smitten et al. used two independent cohorts to study the effect of csDMARDs (including cyclosporine (CsA) and cyclophosphamide (CYC)) on the risk for HZ and found a modestly increased risk (OR, 1.27 and 1.37) [24].

MTX and other csDMARDs are not considered to increase the risk of HBV reactivation in patients with chronic or past HBV infection, although MTX hepatotoxicity can rarely result in severe liver disease in HBV-infected patients [23].

In patients with SLE, antimalarials were found to have a protective effect regarding the risk for serious infections [5], whereas other csDMARDs were not associated with increased infection risk [18]. When mycophenolate mofetil (MMF) was compared with azathioprine (AZA) as maintenance therapy, the rate of serious infection during a 36-month period did not differ between the two drugs (9.6% vs. 11.7%) [25].

Overall, these findings suggest a safe profile for csDMARDs regarding serious infection risk in rheumatic patients.

Biologic DMARDs

TNF Inhibitors (TNFi)

TNFi was the first class of bDMARDs introduced in daily practice almost 20 years ago (Table 34.1). These agents have been found to be highly effective in patients with RA, psoriatic arthritis (PsA), juvenile idiopathic arthritis (JIA), and ankylosing spondylitis (AS). Randomized controlled trials (RCTs) as well as longitudinal registries of bDMARD-treated patients have provided valuable data regarding TNFi infection risk.

In RA patients, the serious infection risk in RCTs was 4.9/100 patient-years [26], while a similar risk was found in registry-derived data (2–6.4/100 patient-years) [27–29] compared to csDMARDs that represent an almost 30% increased risk which in absolute values equals to an annual rate of 2.6% compared to 2% with csDMARDs alone [30]. The infectious risk appears to be lower in PsA (0.9–3.3/100 patient-years) and AS (1.3–2.13/100 patient-years) patients (Table 34.2).

In TNFi-treated patients, corticosteroid use and comorbidities significantly affect this risk. Most serious infections are observed during the first 12 months after TNFi initiation and subside subsequently, which could be partly attributed to

Table 34.2 Serious infections in rheumatic patients treated with biologics

bDMARD	Disease	RCT-LTE studies[a]	Real-world evidence studies[b]
TNF inhibitors	RA	4.9 [26]	2–6.4 [27–29]
	PsA	1.16–2.8 [31–33][c]	0.9–3.3 [34, 35]
	AS	1.4–2.13 [33, 36, 37][c]	1.3 [38]
Rituximab	RA	3.9 [39]	2.5–8.2 [40–42]
	AAV	21 [43]	6–17 [44–46]
	SLE	16.6 [47]	6 [48]
Secukinumab	PsA	2.6–2.9 [49, 50]	–
	AS	1.1 [51]	–
Tocilizumab	RA	5.45 [26]	4.1–10.7 [52, 53]
Abatacept	RA	3.04 [26]	4.1 [54]
Anakinra	RA	5.4 [55]	9 [56]
Belimumab	SLE	3.9–8.3 [57, 58]	–
Ustekinumab	PsA	0.7–0.8 [59, 60]	1.1 [61]
Tofacitinib	RA	2.93 [26]	3.7 [62]

[a]Incidence per 100 patient-years, except otherwise indicated
[b]Registry data for PsA included patients with psoriasis of whom 36% had PsA
[c]Data only for adalimumab [33], etanercept [32, 36], and golimumab [31, 37]
TNF tumor necrosis factor, *RA* rheumatoid arthritis, *PsA* psoriatic arthritis, *AS* ankylosing spondylitis, *AAV* ANCA-associated vasculitis, *SLE* systemic lupus erythematosus, *RCT* randomized controlled trial, *LTE* long-term extension

the gradual reduction of corticosteroids [17]. Evidence from some, but not all, registries supports a trend for lower risk for serious infections in patients treated with the soluble TNFi etanercept (ETN) in comparison with the monoclonal antibodies infliximab (INFL) and adalimumab (ADA) (1.66 vs. 3.86 vs. 2.61/100 patient-years, respectively) [28]. The lower respiratory system, skin, and soft tissues are the most commonly affected sites in TNFi-treated patients with serious infection [15, 40, 63, 64].

Only sparse data are available regarding the prognosis of TNFi-treated patients with serious infections. Interestingly, a recent study demonstrated that patients treated with bDMARDs (mostly TNFi) were at decreased risk for developing or dying from sepsis after a serious infection [64], with the authors suggesting a potential role of cytokine blockade in efficient control of immune host response, as previously showed in experimental models [65].

Post-marketing surveillance has provided some early signals for increased rates of infections caused by intracellular pathogens, such as *Legionella*, *Listeria*, or *Salmonella* [66, 67]. Monoclonal antibodies were found to correlate with higher risk compared with soluble TNFi, and the risk was higher during the first 3 months after treatment initiation, although the absolute risk for these infections still remained quite low [66].

Several opportunistic infections have become of particular interest in patients treated with TNFi. Rates of tuberculosis (TB) infections were increased by 5–20 times in the early era of TNFi therapies [68]. The majority of infections occurred during the first 12 months, and the risk of TB reactivation was significantly higher in patients treated with the monoclonal antibodies INFL and ADA versus ETN [69]. Fortunately, universal screening for latent tuberculosis infection (LTBI) before TNFi initiation has proved highly efficient in reducing the rates of TB reactivation up to 83% in patients with RA [70].

Two methods for LTBI diagnosis are widely used, the tuberculin skin test (TST) and the interferon-gamma releasing assays (IGRAs) that include the T-SPOT.TB test and the QuantiFERON-TB test. These methods seem to have similar sensitivity for active TB diagnosis (~80%), while IGRAs appear to have higher specificity (>90%) and are not affected by previous *Bacillus* Calmette-Guérin (BCG) vaccination. Both methods may be negatively affected by immunosuppressive therapy [71]. There is no universal consensus on the optimal algorithm for LTBI screening in rheumatic patients, with some authorities suggesting interchangeable implementation of the two techniques [72], whereas others supporting screening with both methods [73, 74]. Regular annual rescreening may be of benefit in areas of high endemicity or for patients at high risk for exposure (Table 34.3).

Nontuberculous mycobacterial (NTM) infections are not as well studied as TB in rheumatic patients, although there is evidence supporting a higher incidence in RA patients compared with TB infections [68]. Elderly TNFi-treated patients with RA and chronic lung disease comprise a high-risk group for acquiring NTM infection [75].

Another concern regarding TNFi therapy is their potential for HBV reactivation (Table 34.3) [23]. This risk is significantly higher in patients with chronic HBV infection (hepatitis B surface antigen (HBsAg) positive, 29–64%) [76–79] than those with resolved infection (HBsAg negative/anti-hepatitis B core antigen (HBc) positive, 1–2%) [80, 81]. Current guidelines support the administration of prophylactic antiviral therapy in all TNFi-treated patients with chronic HBV infection [82]. Given an up to 70% risk for emergence of resistant HBV strains after long-term treatment with lamivudine [83], newer third-generation oral nucleos(t)ide analogs with high genetic resistance barrier (entecavir or tenofovir) are recommended as prophylactic therapies in this setting (Table 34.3) [23].

There are conflicting data regarding the risk for HZ in patients treated with TNFi, with some studies failing to show any difference in the HZ incidence between patients treated with TNFi and csDMARDs [84] and others demonstrating a modest increase (HR = 1.5–2.2), especially during the first year after TNFi initiation [85]. The risk for HZ does not differ between different types of TNFi or between TNFi and other

Table 34.3 Most commonly used interventions to reduce infection risk in patients with rheumatic diseases treated with antirheumatic therapies

Intervention	Methods	Comments
Screening for latent tuberculosis infection (LTBI)	– TST – IGRAs – Chest X-ray	• Dual screening (TST and IGRAs) at baseline before starting biologic therapy may increase sensitivity for LTBI detection • Retesting (for patients negative at baseline) recommended only for – Recently TB exposed – High risk for TB exposure patients
Screening for hepatitis B virus (HBV) infection before initiation of – bDMARDs – High-dose CS or certain csDMARDs (i.e., MTX, LEF)	– HBsAg – Anti-HBc – Anti-HBs	• All negative: consider vaccination in high-risk patients • HBsAg (+): antiviral prophylaxis (pos) • HBsAg (−)/anti-HBc (+): close monitoring for HBV reactivation
Chemoprophylaxis against *Pneumocystis jirovecii* pneumonia	TMP/SMX administration	• For AAV patients treated with – CYC – RTX
Vaccinations	Various vaccines according to National Guidelines	• Inactivated vaccines safely administered during any type of therapy and not related with disease flares • Live attenuated vaccines not recommended in patients while on – bDMARDs – High-dose CS – --//-- csDMARDs (although they can be administered prior to treatment initiation)
Intravenous immunoglobulin (IVIG) administration	IgG measurement	• Only recommended as secondary prophylaxis in patients with relapsing infections and IgG levels <400 mg/dl

TST tuberculin skin testing, *IGRAs* interferon-gamma release assays, *HBsAg* hepatitis B surface antigen, *Anti-HBc* antibody against hepatitis B core antigen, *Anti-HBs* antibody against hepatitis B surface antigen, *bDMARD* biologic disease-modifying antirheumatic drugs, *MTX* methotrexate, *LEF* leflunomide, *TMP/SMX* trimethoprim/sulfamethoxazole, *CYC* cyclophosphamide, *RTX* rituximab, *CS* corticosteroids, *csDMARDs* conventional synthetic DMARDs, *IgG* immunoglobulin G

bDMARDs [86, 87]. No data are currently available regarding the severity of HZ infection and postherpetic neuralgia in this group of patients.

Rituximab

Rituximab (RTX), a B-cell-depleting monoclonal antibody that targets CD20 surface antigen, is licensed for a variety of hematologic and rheumatic diseases, including RA and, more recently, AAV, while a steadily increasing number of patients with relapsing or refractory SLE are being treated off-label with RTX (Table 34.1).

Infection risk among RTX-treated rheumatic patients depends on the underlying disease and the concomitant immunosuppressives used, corticosteroids in particular (Table 34.2). Regarding RA, a pooled analysis of the safety data from ten studies of >3000 patients showed a serious infection incidence of 3.9/100 patient-years, not different from the cohort that was treated with MTX (3.8/100 patient-years), with this rate being relatively stable during follow-up [39]. As observed in TNFi-treated patients, the majority of infections involved lower respiratory tract. In real-life settings, the incidence of severe infections has been reported to range between 2.5–8.2/100 patient-years [40–42].

B-cell depletion with RTX has been found to be a non-inferior therapeutic alternative to CYC for patients with AAV, although infectious complications did not differ in the randomized controlled trials (RCTs) [88, 89]. Apart from RCTs, a continuously growing body of real-life-derived evidence has been published over the last years.

In a study from the USA, the annual risk for severe infection was calculated at 12/100 person-years for patients treated solely with RTX, while the respective rate was 17/100 person-years for those with prior or concurrent cyclophosphamide administration. More than 50% of these infections were located at the lower respiratory tract [44].

Renal involvement greatly affects the incidence of serious infections of SLE patients treated with RTX. In a German cohort that included SLE patients (37% with lupus nephritis (LN)), the incidence of serious infections was 6/100 patient-years [48]. The infection risk significantly increased in patients with LN. An RCT compared the efficacy and safety of RTX on top of concomitant treatment with mycophenolate mofetil (MMF) and corticosteroids. The incidence of serious infections was increased in comparison to the previous study, but did not differ between RTX and placebo (16.6 and 20/100 patient-years, respectively) [47].

Two potential complications of RTX treatment, that may predispose patients to infections, have been recognized. Late-onset neutropenia (LON) was first described in lymphoma patients treated with RTX-containing regimens. The underlying mechanism still remains unclear, and no factors predictive of this complication have been identified. Most studies report neutrophil count nadir to become more apparent 3–5 months after last RTX infusion [90–92]. Interestingly, LON is much more common in patients with AAV (12–23%) and SLE (20%) [91, 93] than RA (1.3–4.6%) [90–92]. Sepsis from non-opportunistic pathogens and febrile neutropenia are not uncommon sequelae to LON. Re-treatment with RTX should not be precluded in patients who experienced LON after restoration of normal neutrophil counts.

The negative impact of immunosuppressive therapy on immunoglobulin (Ig) levels has been implicated in the infection risk of these patients. Again, the risk for hypogammaglobulinemia depends on the underlying disease. In a cohort of RA patients treated with RTX, 22.4% developed low IgM, while the respective rates for low IgG and IgA were significantly lower (3.5% and 1%). Overall infections did not differ before and during or after low IgG or IgM, although patients who finally developed hypogammaglobulinemia were in significantly higher risk for developing serious infections compared with those that never had this complication. Older age, longer disease duration, lower mean CD19 + count, lower mean IgG levels, and history of more csDMARDs were predictive factors for hypogammaglobulinemia [39].

Regarding AAV, recent studies have reported a variable incidence of hypogammaglobulinemia, ranging between 10% and 56%, although hypogammaglobulinemia is not rare even before RTX initiation and it may involve 26–30% of AAV patients [94, 95]. Rates of drug discontinuation also vary between 5% and 28% [45, 96, 97], as well as the need for intravenous immunoglobulin (IVIG) administration for recurrent infections, which is reported to range between 3% and 18% [46, 95, 96]. A recent retrospective study explored the risk for hypogammaglobulinemia and serious infections in 283 patients with systemic autoimmune diseases treated with RTX (n = 160 with AAV) [95]. The proportion of patients with hypogammaglobulinemia (<6.9 g/l) increased from 26% at the time of RTX initiation to 56% after RTX treatment. There was a weak association between the previous cumulative dose of CYC and nadir IgG after RTX, whereas IgG levels before RTX initiation were well correlated with nadir IgG levels during RTX therapy. Only a small proportion of patients (4.2%) developed recurrent infections necessitating IVIG replacement. The incidence of IgM and IgG hypogammaglobulinemia in SLE patients treated with RTX has recently been found to be 21% and 5%, respectively, whereas none of the 57 patients needed IVIG replacement [98].

RTX administration has been correlated with a substantial risk of HBV reactivation in HBsAg (+) patients with hematologic malignancies, and this risk has been previously estimated between 30% and 60%. Although the respective incidence in rheumatic patients with chronic HBV infection cannot be accurately calculated, this type of biologic therapy is considered a high-risk one [82]. Regarding the much larger category of RTX-treated rheumatic patients with past (resolved) HBV infection (HBsAg−/anti-HBc+), the risk for HBV reactivation probably is less than 1% [99, 100], warranting increased vigilance but not universal antiviral prophylaxis (Table 34.3).

A 2006 FDA alert, regarding two SLE patients that developed progressive multifocal leukoencephalopathy (PML) after RTX therapy, caused concerns for a possible correlation between iatrogenic B-cell depletion and John Cunningham virus (JCV) reactivation. PML has been disproportionately reported in patients with SLE in comparison with other rheumatic diseases, but it still is quite rare in this group of patients [101], and regarding RTX-treated RA patients, this risk has been estimated to be as low as 1/25,000 patients [102].

Concerns regarding increased risk for PJP during B-cell depletion have been based mainly on experimental animal models and the hematologic literature, but the risk appears to be much lower in rheumatic diseases (~1.2% for AAV [103] and <1/10,000 patient-years for RA) [39]. Current evidence does not support prophylaxis in RA patients treated with RTX (Table 34.3) [72].

Recently published EULAR/ERA-EDTA recommendations for the treatment of AAV advocate the initiation of prophylaxis in all patients being treated with CYC, although many experts extend the indications for prophylaxis in AAV patients concurrently treated with RTX, especially if corticosteroids in daily doses ≥10 mg are coadministered [104]. Of note, studies where prophylaxis was compulsory reported no cases of PJP.

Abatacept

Abatacept (ABA) is a fusion protein that binds to the CD80/86 surface protein of antigen-presenting cells (APCs) and inhibits the co-stimulation of T-cells. The medication is currently licensed for RA, PsA, and JIA and is administered either intravenously (IV) or subcutaneously (SC). Data from the clinical development program that included eight clinical trials of IV ABA calculated an incidence rate of 3.7 serious infections/100 patient-years in the short-term period of exposure (compared to 2.6/100 patient-years in the placebo arm), while in the long-term extension studies, the incidence rate fell to 2.9/100 patient-years [105]. Respiratory and skin infections comprised the majority of the infectious complications. In a recent meta-analysis of all published trials, the overall serious infection risk was estimated at 3.04/100 patient-years (Table 34.2) [26].

The incidence rates of opportunistic infections, such as TB and candidiasis, were <0.1/100 patient-years [105]. A project of similar design that pooled the clinical trials of SC ABA reported a lower incidence of serious infections (1.8/100 patient-years) [106].

Regarding real-life data, a recent prospective French study reported data on ABA safety, out of the context of controlled trials. As expected, the study population of 976 patients was older than the one of clinical trials (58 years) and had longer disease duration (17.5 years), 76% were receiving corticosteroids at ABA initiation, and 35% of the registered patients had a history of serious infection [54]. The incidence rate of serious infections was slightly higher than that of clinical trials (4.1/100 patient-years), although opportunistic infections were rare. No case of TB was reported, partly supporting data from chronic TB animal models showing that, in contrast with TNFi, inhibition of co-stimulation with ABA does not lead to exacerbation of the underlying TB infection [107]. Increased age and a history of serious infection, but not concomitant csDMARD use, were associated with serious infections [54].

Tocilizumab

Tocilizumab is a fully humanized monoclonal antibody that targets the IL-6 receptor. Indications for its use in rheumatology include RA, GCA, and JIA (Table 34.1). In RA patients, a meta-analysis of RCTs showed a serious infection risk of 5.45/100 patient-years (Table 34.2) [26]. In post-marketing surveillance of TCZ in Japan which included >5500 RA patients, the serious infection rate was slightly lower at 4.1/100 patient-years (similar to TNFi cohorts) [52]. Of note, almost 60% of patients that experienced a serious infection permanently discontinued TCZ. In a real-world study, the safety profile of TCZ was compared to TNFi in the context of the Japanese real-world registry for biologics (REAL) [53]. Patients treated with TCZ were older and had higher disease activity and more disability than those treated with TNFi. Incidence rates for serious infection were 10.7 and 3/100 patient-years for TCZ and TNFi, respectively. After adjusting for several factors, a trend for higher incidence of serious infections in the TCZ group still remained (HR, 2.2). Respiratory tract and bone and joint infections accounted for approximately 30% and 20% of the total infections. In the contrary, in the German registry for biologic therapies (RABBIT), TCZ and TNFi had similar risks for serious infections [108].

Neutropenia has been found to be more common in TCZ- compared to placebo-treated patients in controlled trials. The underlying mechanism by which IL-6 inhibition reduces neutrophil counts has yet to be elucidated. Both grade 1–2 and 3–4 neutropenia were more common in patients treated with IV TCZ than with placebo, and neither total nor serious infections were found to occur more frequently during periods with low neutrophil counts. Most cases of neutropenia were reversed after temporary discontinuation of TCZ administration [109].

A signal associated with possible increased risk of low intestinal perforation in TCZ-treated patients was identified during the clinical development program of TCZ. A recent study from Germany reported that, although still rare, TCZ-treated patients carry a higher risk for low intestinal perforation than those exposed to csDMARDs, TNFi, or other bDMARDs such as RTX or ABA (2.7, 0.6, 0.5, 0.2, and 0.5 per 1000 patient-years, respectively). In addition to use of TCZ, multivariate analysis detected higher age and use of corticosteroids and NSAIDs as independent factors for intestinal perforation [110]. Clinicians should be vigilant for clinical symptoms and signs of infectious complications in patients treated with TCZ, given the fact that these may occur in the absence of elevated acute phase reactants, such as CRP, especially during the first days after IV TCZ infusion [110, 111]. For the moment, respective data regarding the kinetics of CRP during infection in patients receiving SC TCZ are lacking.

The high morbidity related to corticosteroids of patients with GCA, especially during treatment initiation, raised the need for alternative steroid-sparing agents, and TCZ has gained interest in this field. Open-label studies have showed the efficacy of TCZ in controlling active disease. Nevertheless, serious common and opportunistic infections were not uncommon [112, 113]. In a recent double-blind, placebo-controlled study, 20 patients treated with TCZ and prednisolone were compared to ten patients treated with placebo and prednisolone. Combination treatment was superior in terms of complete remission at week 12 and relapse-free survival and cumulative prednisolone dose at week 52. Although infections were much more common in combination arm, only one of them was considered serious [114].

Recently, FDA approved TCZ for the treatment of GCA, based on the positive results of a phase 3 RCT which included 250 patients and showed higher rates of sustained remission in patients treated with a combination of TCZ and a 6-month corticosteroid regimen than those treated with corticosteroids alone for 6 or 12 months [115]. No differences in the rates of serious infections were noted across treatment arms. Real-world data is much needed in order to clarify the infection risk of this novel treatment in this vulnerable population.

IL-1 Inhibitors

IL-1 inhibitors that are currently used in rheumatology include the recombinant IL-1 receptor antagonist anakinra (ANA) and the monoclonal antibody targeting IL-1β, canakinumab. Approved indications for ANA include RA and cryopyrin-associated periodic syndromes (CAPS), while canakinumab is licensed for use in patients with several periodic fever syndromes, gout, and systemic JIA.

As for infection risk, most available data are derived from cohorts of ANA-treated patients with JIA and RA. A recent study assessed the risk for hospitalized infection in children with JIA treated with bDMARDs or MTX, and the incidence of serious infections in those treated with ANA was estimated at 8.4/100 patient-years, significantly higher than the respective rates in MTX and TNFi users (1.46 and 1.54/100 patient-years, respectively) [116]. These results have to be interpreted cautiously, given the fact that patients in the ANA cohort were more likely to have a history of serious infection, to be concurrently treated with higher doses of corticosteroids, and to have more severe disease. No cases of opportunistic infections were recorded in the ANA cohort, although the short duration of exposure (226 patient-years) precludes from reaching definitive conclusions [116]. With the advance in biologic therapies, IL-1 inhibitors are not widely used in patients with RA; however, they are widely used in SoJIA and rare pediatric autoinflammatory conditions.

With respect to the risk for serious infections, a double-blind study comparing ANA with placebo followed by a 3-year open-label ANA treatment in adult patients with RA, estimated an incidence rate of 5.4/100 patient-years for patients treated with ANA [55]. In the absence of corticosteroid coadministration, this rate was significantly lower than in patients treated with corticosteroids (2.9 vs. 7.1/100 patient-years). A slightly higher rate of 9/100 patient-years was reported in a smaller cohort of 111 patients from the British Society for Rheumatology Biologics Register (BSRBR), not statistically significantly increased compared with the respective rate in csDMARDs-treated patients (HR = 1.58) [56]. A meta-analysis of RA patients treated with ANA revealed an increased infection risk only in patients treated with higher doses of ANA (≥100 mg/day) and coexisting comorbidities [117].

Indications for canakinumab administration include several autoinflammatory diseases, with JIA being the most common [118]. In two randomized trials, canakinumab was not associated with more serious infections than placebo [119].

Belimumab

Belimumab belongs to a novel class of biologic agents that inhibit the B-lymphocyte stimulator (BLyS), a cytokine with pivotal role in B-cell proliferation and differentiation, and it is the only drug approved for the treatment of SLE in the last 50 years [120].

Belimumab has been studied in two RCTs as an add-on to standard of care therapy in patients with clinically and serologically active SLE without nephritis or CNS involvement and has shown modest effect on musculoskeletal and mucocutaneous manifestations [57]. Both studies reported similar rates of serious infections among low and high dose of belimumab and placebo (8%, 4%, and 6% in BLISS-52 and 7%, 7.3%, and 5.8% in BLISS-76, respectively). Given that belimumab mitigates the differentiation of B-cells to plasma cells, decreases in all immunoglobulin classes (IgG, IgM, IgA) were more prevalent in patients treated with belimumab, although almost none of them developed IgG levels of less than 4 g/L. Low immunoglobulin levels were not associated with increased risk for infection [121, 122]. In the long-term extension of one of the aforementioned studies, an incidence rate of serious infections of 3.9–8.3/100 patient-years was estimated [58]. Patients treated with combination of belimumab and MMF had higher rates of serious infections than those treated with belimumab alone (9.4 vs. 6.3/100 patient-years). Corticosteroid use carried a 2.5-fold increased risk for serious infection in patients treated with belimumab [58].

Ustekinumab

Ustekinumab is a human IgG1 monoclonal antibody that targets the p40 subunit of IL-12 and IL-23. Current indications include plaque psoriasis, PsA, and, more recently, Crohn's disease. Although IL-12 and IL-23 are prominent inducers of a Th1 immune response and their role in the cleavage of intra- and extracellular infections has been well established, no specific alarming signals arose during randomized clinical trials. PSUMMIT-1 recruited only bDMARDs-naïve patients, and 5 out of 615 participants (0.8%) developed serious infection, with all of them occurring in ustekinumab-treated patients [59]. In a subsequent study that included both bDMARDs-naïve and bDMARDs-experienced PsA patients, the incidence rate was estimated at 0.74/100 patient-years [60]. No cases of TB were noted throughout both studies [59, 60].

Most real-world evidence derive from post-marketing surveillance registries that include mainly patients with psoriasis. In the Psoriasis Longitudinal Assessment and Registry (PSOLAR), 36% of patients had also PsA. Incidence rates for serious infection were 0.83, 1.47, 1.97, and 2.49/100 patient-years in patients treated with ustekinumab, ETN, ADA, and INFL [123]. Prescription of INFL and ADA, but not ustekinumab, was associated with increased infection risk [123]. In a small recent cohort of 58 patients with PsA treated with ustekinumab, 22 (38%) discontinued the drug but none due to infectious complications [124].

Patients with chronic HBV infection carry a non-negligible risk for HBV reactivation after ustekinumab initiation and therefore should be handled as described for patients treated with TNFi [23, 125].

IL-17 Inhibitors

Monoclonal antibodies that target IL-17A constitute a novel therapeutic choice for patients with psoriasis, PsA, and AS. The risk for infection in patients treated with these agents seems to be similar with or lower than the respective risk in patients treated with other classes of bDMARDs. In RCTs, serious infections were noted in 2.6–2.9% [49] and 0.7–2.8% [50] of patients during 52-week follow-up. In a large pooled analysis of ten clinical trials of patients with psoriasis, one fifth of whom had psoriatic arthritis, serious infections in secukinumab arms were recorded in 1–1.5% of patients after 52 weeks of follow-up, similar with the proportion of patients treated with ETN [126].

Cytokines implicated in the Th17 pathway are considered to contribute substantially in the protection from fungal infections by several mechanisms (promotion of Th1 response, neutrophil recruitment, and defensins production, among others). Indeed, single nucleotide polymorphisms or genetic defects that lead to impaired Th17 immune response have been recognized and associated with chronic mucocutaneous candidiasis [127]. RCTs of secukinumab in patients with PsA have reported frequencies of *Candida* infections up to 5% during a 52-week follow-up [49, 50]. These rates were observed in patients treated with the 150 and 300 mg doses. The majority of these infections were of mild or moderate severity and affected mainly the oral or genital mucosa and did not lead to drug discontinuation. Esophageal involvement was rare.

Ixekizumab, a monoclonal antibody that also targets IL-17A, is approved for the treatment of plaque psoriasis and PsA. A recently published randomized study reported similar rates of serious infections between ixekizumab and ADA, involving 2% of patients during a 24-week period [128]. The incidence of *Candida* infections was 1% in patients treated with ixekizumab. A higher proportion of patients were reported to develop candidiasis in recent trials involving patients with psoriasis (3.4%) [129]. More data from real-world cohorts are expected to specify the safety profile of these novel agents during the following years.

Small Molecules

Janus Kinase (JAK) Inhibitors

JAK inhibitors comprise the most recent advancement in the field of rheumatic disease therapeutics and have been approved in certain countries for the treatment of moderate to severe RA (Table 34.1). This class includes two oral agents, tofacitinib (approved by FDA and EMA for RA) and baricitinib (approved by EMA for RA). JAK inhibitors act by blocking JAK enzymes that are located intracellularly and are responsible for signal transmission after membrane cytokine receptor activation, resulting in a variety of anti-inflammatory and immunosuppressive effects [130].

The majority of safety data stem from the tofacitinib global development program. The serious infection incidence rate was 2.93/100 patient-years, comparable with respective rates in cohorts with bDMARDs [26]. This rate was stable during 3 years of follow-up, and the majority of those were pneumonias. Age ≥65 years, corticosteroid daily use ≥7.5 mg, presence of diabetes, and high tofacitinib dose were independently correlated with increased infection risk [131].

Data from the same program have raised concern regarding the risk for HZ infection in tofacitinib-treated patients. Incidence risk was calculated at 4.4 cases/100 patient-years, with elderly patients and those from Asia having a significantly higher risk. Tofacitinib-treated patients trended to have a higher incidence when compared with ADA- and placebo-treated patients (2.8 and 1.5/100 patient-years, respectively). Tofacitinib dose affected HZ incidence only during the first 3 months [132]. A more recent study confirmed that tofacitinib carries an almost two-fold increased risk compared with bDMARDs [86].

TB incidence was 0.21/100 patient-years, with notable variability across countries with low, medium, or high background TB incidence and extrapulmonary involvement being more common than pulmonary disease. It has to be noted that 77% of TB cases were diagnosed on the basis of positive acid-fast smear and were not culture confirmed [133].

Strategies to Reduce the Infection Risk in Rheumatic Patients

Although the breakthrough advances in therapeutics have led to a substantially improved control of rheumatic diseases, infections still contribute substantially to the morbidity and mortality of these patients, even in recent cohorts [4, 134, 135]. Measures that assist in preventing infectious complications should be embedded in the daily practice of rheumatologists (see Table 34.3).

Vaccinations (in This Chapter)

As mentioned above, respiratory infections are the most common serious infections in patients with rheumatic diseases, and physicians should bear in mind that a significant proportion of those can be prevented by vaccination against influenza and *Streptococcus pneumoniae*. Other vaccines of special interest for rheumatic patients are those against HZ or against hepatitis A and B virus, especially in high-risk patients for acquiring these diseases. Adherence to vaccination schedules is far from optimal in rheumatic patients [136], although several interventions have been evaluated and found to assist in increasing the vaccination coverage. Concerns regarding potential flares of underlying rheumatic disease after vaccine administration have been discarded by several studies [137–139]. Although disease-modifying therapies may attenuate the immunogenicity of vaccines, all eligible patients should be vaccinated according to recommendations, with the exception of live attenuated vaccines that carry a mostly theoretical risk for disseminating the disease [140].

Chemoprophylaxis

Current evidence supports its use only in patients with AAV during the induction of remission phase of treatment, in order to prevent PJP (see above for details, Table 34.3) [141]. Nevertheless, experts have suggested a more liberal use of antimicrobial prophylaxis that concerns mainly two categories of patients. The first includes TNFi-treated patients for the prevention of bacterial infections and PJP with the administration of co-trimoxazole [142]. Studies deriving mainly from Japan have shown an increased prevalence of colonization with *Pneumocystis jirovecii* in patients treated with INFL [143], although the clinical significance remains unknown, given the fact that some, but not all, studies have shown similar findings in the general population [144, 145]. Regarding the risk for PJP in TNFi-treated patients, the risk remains <0.5/100 patient-years in most series [146]. Identification of additional risk factors, such as increased age, chronic pulmonary disease, and corticosteroid coadministration, may assist in a better selection of candidate patients for PJP prophylaxis [147].

The second category includes rheumatic patients treated with relatively high corticosteroid doses (≥20 mg of prednisone) for at least 2–4 weeks, as those with vasculitis or inflammatory myositis [148]. A retrospective study from Southeastern Asia that included 132 patients treated with such doses for >2 months (~90% with SLE) showed an incidence of PJP in 8% (6/73) in those not taking co-trimoxazole, whereas none occurred in those on prophylaxis (0/59) [149].

Universal consensus on the corticosteroid dose and duration that should prompt physicians to institute prophylaxis against PJP is absent, not only in rheumatic but also in other patient populations [150]. The American Thoracic Society suggests initiating prophylaxis in patients starting prednisone at ≥20 mg/day for >4 weeks, especially in the presence of a coexisting predisposing factors, such as T-cell defects, cytotoxic agents, or TNFi, but this statement is more an expert opinion and not based on solid evidence [151].

At the moment, our opinion is that all patients with AAV treated with CYC or RTX should receive PJP prophylaxis with TMP/SMX for the duration of their treatment. For other patient categories, there is no strong evidence to suggest universal prophylaxis. Nevertheless, in individual high-risk cases, this should be discussed with an infectious disease specialist.

IVIG

Hypogammaglobulinemia, low IgG levels in particular, has been described as a sequela of treatment with RTX, mainly in patients with AAV and to a much lesser extent in patients with RA. In agreement with the findings from hematologic literature, a recent study reported a twofold increased risk for serious infection in AAV patients with IgG levels below 400 mg/dl [152]. Most infections in patients with hypogammaglobulinemia affect the upper and lower respiratory tract and manifest as sinusitis or pulmonary infections with or without bronchiectasis. Patients with recurrent infections and IgG levels near or below 400 mg/dl could benefit from IVIG infusion.

Conclusions

The newer biologic and non-biological therapies have transformed the therapeutic landscape in inflammatory rheumatic diseases offering great hope for a better and longer life for affected rheumatic patients. The long-term clinical experience has shown that overall these agents appear to be safe when appropriate precautions before and during their administration are taken. Infections still represent the most common serious side effect of older and newer antirheumatic therapies, occurring with variable frequency in different rheumatic diseases. Knowledge of the infection risk of each agent and the necessary preventive and monitoring measures for decreasing the infectious risk is necessary for the practicing rheumatologist today worldwide.

References

1. Olofsson T, Petersson IF, Eriksson JK, et al. Predictors of work disability after start of anti-TNF therapy in a national cohort of Swedish patients with rheumatoid arthritis: does early anti-TNF therapy bring patients back to work? Ann Rheum Dis. 2017;76(7):1245–52.
2. Mikuls TR, Saag KG, Criswell LA, et al. Mortality risk associated with rheumatoid arthritis in a prospective cohort of older women: results from the Iowa women's health study. Ann Rheum Dis. 2002;61:994–9.
3. Weaver A, Troum O, Hooper M, et al. Rheumatoid arthritis disease activity and disability affect the risk of serious infection events in RADIUS 1. J Rheumatol. 2013;40:1275–81.
4. Tektonidou MG, Wang Z, Dasgupta A, et al. Burden of serious infections in adults with systemic lupus erythematosus: a national population-based study, 1996–2011. Arthritis Care Res (Hoboken). 2015;67:1078–85.
5. Rua-Figueroa I, Lopez-Longo J, Galindo-Izquierdo M, et al. Incidence, associated factors and clinical

impact of severe infections in a large, multicentric cohort of patients with systemic lupus erythematosus. Semin Arthritis Rheum. 2017;47(1):38–45.
6. Flossmann O, Berden A, de Groot K, et al. Long-term patient survival in ANCA-associated vasculitis. Ann Rheum Dis. 2011;70:488–94.
7. Doran MF, Crowson CS, Pond GR, et al. Frequency of infection in patients with rheumatoid arthritis compared with controls: a population-based study. Arthritis Rheum. 2002;46:2287–93.
8. Dougados M, Soubrier M, Antunez A, et al. Prevalence of comorbidities in rheumatoid arthritis and evaluation of their monitoring: results of an international, cross-sectional study (COMORA). Ann Rheum Dis. 2014;73:62–8.
9. Labarca C, Koster MJ, Crowson CS, et al. Predictors of relapse and treatment outcomes in biopsy-proven giant cell arteritis: a retrospective cohort study. Rheumatology (Oxford). 2016;55:347–56.
10. Youssef J, Novosad SA, Winthrop KL. Infection risk and safety of corticosteroid use. Rheum Dis Clin North Am. 2016;42:157.
11. Fardet L, Petersen I, Nazareth I. Common infections in patients prescribed systemic glucocorticoids in primary care: a population-based cohort study. PLoS Med. 2016;13:e1002024.
12. Dixon WG, Kezouh A, Bernatsky S, et al. The influence of systemic glucocorticoid therapy upon the risk of non-serious infection in older patients with rheumatoid arthritis: a nested case-control study. Ann Rheum Dis. 2011;70:956–60.
13. Grijalva CG, Chen L, Delzell E, et al. Initiation of tumor necrosis factor-alpha antagonists and the risk of hospitalization for infection in patients with autoimmune diseases. JAMA. 2011;306:2331–9.
14. Smitten AL, Choi HK, Hochberg MC, et al. The risk of hospitalized infection in patients with rheumatoid arthritis. J Rheumatol. 2008;35:387–93.
15. Wolfe F, Caplan L, Michaud K. Treatment for rheumatoid arthritis and the risk of hospitalization for pneumonia: associations with prednisone, disease-modifying antirheumatic drugs, and anti-tumor necrosis factor therapy. Arthritis Rheum. 2006;54:628–34.
16. Dixon WG, Abrahamowicz M, Beauchamp ME, et al. Immediate and delayed impact of oral glucocorticoid therapy on risk of serious infection in older patients with rheumatoid arthritis: a nested case-control analysis. Ann Rheum Dis. 2012;71:1128–33.
17. Strangfeld A, Eveslage M, Schneider M, et al. Treatment benefit or survival of the fittest: what drives the time-dependent decrease in serious infection rates under TNF inhibition and what does this imply for the individual patient? Ann Rheum Dis. 2011;70:1914–20.
18. Ruiz-Irastorza G, Olivares N, Ruiz-Arruza I, et al. Predictors of major infections in systemic lupus erythematosus. Arthritis Res Ther. 2009;11:R109.
19. Bosch X, Guilabert A, Pallares L, et al. Infections in systemic lupus erythematosus: a prospective and controlled study of 110 patients. Lupus. 2006;15(9):584.
20. Pagnoux C, Quemeneur T, Ninet J, et al. Treatment of systemic necrotizing vasculitides in patients aged sixty-five years or older: results of a multicenter, open-label, randomized controlled trial of corticosteroid and cyclophosphamide-based induction therapy. Arthritis Rheumatol. 2015;67:1117–27.
21. Petri H, Nevitt A, Sarsour K, et al. Incidence of giant cell arteritis and characteristics of patients: data-driven analysis of comorbidities. Arthritis Care Res (Hoboken). 2015;67:390–5.
22. Schmidt J, Smail A, Roche B, et al. Incidence of severe infections and infection-related mortality during the course of giant cell arteritis: a multicenter, prospective, double-cohort study. Arthritis Rheumatol. 2016;68:1477–82.
23. Koutsianas C, Thomas K, Vassilopoulos D. Hepatitis B reactivation in rheumatic diseases: screening and prevention. Rheum Dis Clin North Am. 2017;43:133–49.
24. Smitten AL, Choi HK, Hochberg MC, et al. The risk of herpes zoster in patients with rheumatoid arthritis in the United States and the United Kingdom. Arthritis Rheum. 2007;57(8):1431.
25. Dooley MA, Jayne D, Ginzler EM, et al. Mycophenolate versus azathioprine as maintenance therapy for lupus nephritis. N Engl J Med. 2011;365:1886–95.
26. Strand V, Ahadieh S, French J, et al. Systematic review and meta-analysis of serious infections with tofacitinib and biologic disease-modifying antirheumatic drug treatment in rheumatoid arthritis clinical trials. Arthritis Res Ther. 2015;17:362.
27. Galloway JB, Hyrich KL, Mercer LK, et al. Anti-TNF therapy is associated with an increased risk of serious infections in patients with rheumatoid arthritis especially in the first 6 months of treatment: updated results from the British Society for Rheumatology biologics register with special emphasis on risks in the elderly. Rheumatology (Oxford). 2011;50:124–31.
28. van Dartel SA, Fransen J, Kievit W, et al. Difference in the risk of serious infections in patients with rheumatoid arthritis treated with adalimumab, infliximab and etanercept: results from the Dutch rheumatoid arthritis monitoring (DREAM) registry. Ann Rheum Dis. 2013;72:895–900.
29. Dixon WG, Watson K, Lunt M, et al. Rates of serious infection, including site-specific and bacterial intracellular infection, in rheumatoid arthritis patients receiving anti-tumor necrosis factor therapy: results from the British Society for Rheumatology biologics register. Arthritis Rheum. 2006;54:2368–76.
30. Singh JA, Cameron C, Noorbaloochi S, et al. Risk of serious infection in biological treatment of patients with rheumatoid arthritis: a systematic review and meta-analysis. Lancet. 2015;386:258–65.
31. Kavanaugh A, McInnes IB, Mease P, et al. Clinical efficacy, radiographic and safety findings through 5 years of subcutaneous golimumab treatment in patients with active psoriatic arthritis: results from a long-term extension of a randomised, placebo-

controlled trial (the GO-REVEAL study). Ann Rheum Dis. 2014;73:1689–94.
32. Gottlieb AB, Gordon K, Giannini EH, et al. Clinical trial safety and mortality analyses in patients receiving etanercept across approved indications. J Drugs Dermatol. 2011;10:289–300.
33. Burmester GR, Panaccione R, Gordon KB, et al. Adalimumab: long-term safety in 23 458 patients from global clinical trials in rheumatoid arthritis, juvenile idiopathic arthritis, ankylosing spondylitis, psoriatic arthritis, psoriasis and Crohn's disease. Ann Rheum Dis. 2013;72:517–24.
34. Kristensen LE, Gulfe A, Saxne T, et al. Efficacy and tolerability of anti-tumour necrosis factor therapy in psoriatic arthritis patients: results from the South Swedish arthritis treatment group register. Ann Rheum Dis. 2008;67:364–9.
35. Saad AA, Ashcroft DM, Watson KD, et al. Efficacy and safety of anti-TNF therapies in psoriatic arthritis: an observational study from the British Society for Rheumatology biologics register. Rheumatology (Oxford). 2010;49:697–705.
36. van der Heijde D, Zack D, Wajdula J, et al. Rates of serious infections, opportunistic infections, inflammatory bowel disease, and malignancies in subjects receiving etanercept vs. controls from clinical trials in ankylosing spondylitis: a pooled analysis. Scand J Rheumatol. 2014;43:49–53.
37. Deodhar A, Braun J, Inman RD, et al. Golimumab administered subcutaneously every 4 weeks in ankylosing spondylitis: 5-year results of the GO-RAISE study. Ann Rheum Dis. 2015;74:757–61.
38. Wallis D, Thavaneswaran A, Haroon N, et al. Tumour necrosis factor inhibitor therapy and infection risk in axial spondyloarthritis: results from a longitudinal observational cohort. Rheumatology (Oxford). 2015;54:152–6.
39. van Vollenhoven RF, Emery P, Bingham CO III, et al. Long-term safety of rituximab in rheumatoid arthritis: 9.5-year follow-up of the global clinical trial programme with a focus on adverse events of interest in RA patients. Ann Rheum Dis. 2013;72:1496–502.
40. Curtis JR, Yang S, Patkar NM, et al. Risk of hospitalized bacterial infections associated with biologic treatment among US veterans with rheumatoid arthritis. Arthritis Care Res (Hoboken). 2014;66:990–7.
41. Vassilopoulos D, Delicha EM, Settas L, et al. Safety profile of repeated rituximab cycles in unselected rheumatoid arthritis patients: a long-term, prospective real-life study. Clin Exp Rheumatol. 2016;34:893–900.
42. Johnston SS, Turpcu A, Shi N, et al. Risk of infections in rheumatoid arthritis patients switching from anti-TNF agents to rituximab, abatacept, or another anti-TNF agent, a retrospective administrative claims analysis. Semin Arthritis Rheum. 2013;43:39–47.
43. Jones RB, Tervaert JW, Hauser T, et al. Rituximab versus cyclophosphamide in ANCA-associated renal vasculitis. N Engl J Med. 2010;363:211–20.
44. McGregor JG, Hogan SL, Kotzen ES, et al. Rituximab as an immunosuppressant in antineutrophil cytoplasmic antibody-associated vasculitis. Nephrol Dial Transplant. 2015;30(Suppl 1):i123–31.
45. Pendergraft WF III, Cortazar FB, Wenger J, et al. Long-term maintenance therapy using rituximab-induced continuous B-cell depletion in patients with ANCA vasculitis. Clin J Am Soc Nephrol. 2014;9:736–44.
46. Alberici F, Smith RM, Jones RB, et al. Long-term follow-up of patients who received repeat-dose rituximab as maintenance therapy for ANCA-associated vasculitis. Rheumatology (Oxford). 2015;54:1153–60.
47. Rovin BH, Furie R, Latinis K, et al. Efficacy and safety of rituximab in patients with active proliferative lupus nephritis: the lupus nephritis assessment with rituximab study. Arthritis Rheum. 2012;64:1215–26.
48. Witt M, Grunke M, Proft F, et al. Clinical outcomes and safety of rituximab treatment for patients with systemic lupus erythematosus (SLE)–results from a nationwide cohort in Germany (GRAID). Lupus. 2013;22:1142–9.
49. Mease PJ, McInnes IB, Kirkham B, et al. Secukinumab inhibition of interleukin-17A in patients with psoriatic arthritis. N Engl J Med. 2015;373:1329–39.
50. McInnes IB, Mease PJ, Kirkham B, et al. Secukinumab, a human anti-interleukin-17A monoclonal antibody, in patients with psoriatic arthritis (FUTURE 2): a randomised, double-blind, placebo-controlled, phase 3 trial. Lancet. 2015;386:1137–46.
51. Baeten D, Sieper J, Braun J, et al. Secukinumab, an interleukin-17A inhibitor, in ankylosing spondylitis. N Engl J Med. 2015;373:2534–48.
52. Yamamoto K, Goto H, Hirao K, et al. Longterm safety of tocilizumab: results from 3 years of followup postmarketing surveillance of 5573 patients with rheumatoid arthritis in Japan. J Rheumatol. 2015;42:1368–75.
53. Sakai R, Cho SK, Nanki T, et al. Head-to-head comparison of the safety of tocilizumab and tumor necrosis factor inhibitors in rheumatoid arthritis patients (RA) in clinical practice: results from the registry of Japanese RA patients on biologics for long-term safety (REAL) registry. Arthritis Res Ther. 2015;17:74.
54. Salmon JH, Gottenberg JE, Ravaud P, et al. Predictive risk factors of serious infections in patients with rheumatoid arthritis treated with abatacept in common practice: results from the Orencia and rheumatoid arthritis (ORA) registry. Ann Rheum Dis. 2016;75:1108–13.
55. Fleischmann RM, Tesser J, Schiff MH, et al. Safety of extended treatment with anakinra in patients with rheumatoid arthritis. Ann Rheum Dis. 2006;65:1006–12.
56. Galloway JB, Hyrich KL, Mercer LK, et al. The risk of serious infections in patients receiving anakinra for rheumatoid arthritis: results from the British Society for Rheumatology biologics register. Rheumatology (Oxford). 2011;50:1341–2.
57. Manzi S, Sanchez-Guerrero J, Merrill JT, et al. Effects of belimumab, a B lymphocyte stimulator-specific inhibitor, on disease activity across multiple organ domains in patients with systemic lupus erythemato-

sus: combined results from two phase III trials. Ann Rheum Dis. 2012;71:1833–8.
58. Merrill JT, Ginzler EM, Wallace DJ, et al. Long-term safety profile of belimumab plus standard therapy in patients with systemic lupus erythematosus. Arthritis Rheum. 2012;64:3364–73.
59. McInnes IB, Kavanaugh A, Gottlieb AB, et al. Efficacy and safety of ustekinumab in patients with active psoriatic arthritis: 1 year results of the phase 3, multicentre, double-blind, placebo-controlled PSUMMIT 1 trial. Lancet. 2013;382:780–9.
60. Ritchlin C, Rahman P, Kavanaugh A, et al. Efficacy and safety of the anti-IL-12/23 p40 monoclonal antibody, ustekinumab, in patients with active psoriatic arthritis despite conventional non-biological and biological anti-tumour necrosis factor therapy: 6-month and 1-year results of the phase 3, multicentre, double-blind, placebo-controlled, randomised PSUMMIT 2 trial. Ann Rheum Dis. 2014;73:990–9.
61. Ritchlin CT, Gottlieb AB, Menter A, Mease PJ, Kalia S, Kerdel F, et al. Serious infections in psoriasis patients with psoriatic arthritis in the psoriasis longitudinal assessment and registry study. Arthritis Rheumatol. 2015;67(suppl 10):2084–5.
62. Kavanaugh AF, Geier J, Bingham CO III, Chen C, Reed GW, Saunders KC, et al. Real world results from a post-approval safety surveillance of tofacitinib (Xeljanz): over 3 year results from an ongoing US-based rheumatoid arthritis registry. Arthritis Rheumatol. 2016;68(suppl 10):2595.
63. Greenberg JD, Reed G, Kremer JM, et al. Association of methotrexate and tumour necrosis factor antagonists with risk of infectious outcomes including opportunistic infections in the CORRONA registry. Ann Rheum Dis. 2010;69:380–6.
64. Richter A, Listing J, Schneider M, et al. Impact of treatment with biologic DMARDs on the risk of sepsis or mortality after serious infection in patients with rheumatoid arthritis. Ann Rheum Dis. 2016;75:1667–73.
65. Beutler B, Milsark IW, Cerami AC. Passive immunization against cachectin/tumor necrosis factor protects mice from lethal effect of endotoxin. Science. 1985;229:869–71.
66. Lanternier F, Tubach F, Ravaud P, et al. Incidence and risk factors of Legionella pneumophila pneumonia during anti-tumor necrosis factor therapy: a prospective French study. Chest. 2013;144:990–8.
67. Slifman NR, Gershon SK, Lee JH, et al. Listeria monocytogenes infection as a complication of treatment with tumor necrosis factor alpha-neutralizing agents. Arthritis Rheum. 2003;48:319–24.
68. Winthrop KL, Iseman M. Bedfellows: mycobacteria and rheumatoid arthritis in the era of biologic therapy. Nat Rev Rheumatol. 2013;9:524–31.
69. Tubach F, Salmon D, Ravaud P, et al. Risk of tuberculosis is higher with anti-tumor necrosis factor monoclonal antibody therapy than with soluble tumor necrosis factor receptor therapy: the three-year prospective French research axed on tolerance of biotherapies registry. Arthritis Rheum. 2009;60:1884–94.
70. Carmona L, Gomez-Reino JJ, Rodriguez-Valverde V, et al. Effectiveness of recommendations to prevent reactivation of latent tuberculosis infection in patients treated with tumor necrosis factor antagonists. Arthritis Rheum. 2005;52:1766–72.
71. Wong SH, Gao Q, Tsoi KK, et al. Effect of immunosuppressive therapy on interferon gamma release assay for latent tuberculosis screening in patients with autoimmune diseases: a systematic review and meta-analysis. Thorax. 2016;71:64–72.
72. Singh JA, Saag KG, Bridges SL Jr, et al. 2015 American college of rheumatology guideline for the treatment of rheumatoid arthritis. Arthritis Rheumatol. 2016;68:1–26.
73. Kleinert S, Tony HP, Krueger K, et al. Screening for latent tuberculosis infection: performance of tuberculin skin test and interferon-gamma release assays under real-life conditions. Ann Rheum Dis. 2012;71:1791–5.
74. Winthrop KL, Weinblatt ME, Daley CL. You can't always get what you want, but if you try sometimes (with two tests–TST and IGRA–for tuberculosis) you get what you need. Ann Rheum Dis. 2012;71:1757–60.
75. Winthrop KL, Baxter R, Liu L, et al. Mycobacterial diseases and antitumour necrosis factor therapy in USA. Ann Rheum Dis. 2013;72:37–42.
76. Perez-Alvarez R, Diaz-Lagares C, Garcia-Hernandez F, et al. Hepatitis B virus (HBV) reactivation in patients receiving tumor necrosis factor (TNF)-targeted therapy: analysis of 257 cases. Medicine (Baltimore). 2011;90:359–71.
77. Lan JL, Chen YM, Hsieh TY, et al. Kinetics of viral loads and risk of hepatitis B virus reactivation in hepatitis B core antibody-positive rheumatoid arthritis patients undergoing anti-tumour necrosis factor alpha therapy. Ann Rheum Dis. 2011;70:1719–25.
78. Ryu HH, Lee EY, Shin K, et al. Hepatitis B virus reactivation in rheumatoid arthritis and ankylosing spondylitis patients treated with anti-TNFalpha agents: a retrospective analysis of 49 cases. Clin Rheumatol. 2012;31(6):931.
79. Ye H, Zhang XW, Mu R, et al. Anti-TNF therapy in patients with HBV infection–analysis of 87 patients with inflammatory arthritis. Clin Rheumatol. 2014;33:119–23.
80. Lee YH, Bae SC, Song GG. Hepatitis B virus (HBV) reactivation in rheumatic patients with hepatitis core antigen (HBV occult carriers) undergoing anti-tumor necrosis factor therapy. Clin Exp Rheumatol. 2013;31:118–21.
81. Fukuda W, Hanyu T, Katayama M, et al. Incidence of hepatitis B virus reactivation in patients with resolved infection on immunosuppressive therapy for rheumatic disease: a multicentre, prospective, observational study in Japan. Ann Rheum Dis. 2017;76(6):1051.
82. Reddy KR, Beavers KL, Hammond SP, et al. American gastroenterological association institute guideline on the prevention and treatment of hepatitis

B virus reactivation during immunosuppressive drug therapy. Gastroenterology. 2015;148:215–9.
83. Vassilopoulos D, Apostolopoulou A, Hadziyannis E, et al. Long-term safety of anti-TNF treatment in patients with rheumatic diseases and chronic or resolved hepatitis B virus infection. Ann Rheum Dis. 2010;69:1352–5.
84. Winthrop KL, Baddley JW, Chen L, et al. Association between the initiation of anti-tumor necrosis factor therapy and the risk of herpes zoster. JAMA. 2013;309:887–95.
85. Galloway JB, Mercer LK, Moseley A, et al. Risk of skin and soft tissue infections (including shingles) in patients exposed to anti-tumour necrosis factor therapy: results from the British Society for Rheumatology biologics register. Ann Rheum Dis. 2013;72:229–34.
86. Curtis JR, Xie F, Yun H, et al. Real-world comparative risks of herpes virus infections in tofacitinib and biologic-treated patients with rheumatoid arthritis. Ann Rheum Dis. 2016;75:1843–7.
87. Yun H, Xie F, Delzell E, et al. Risks of herpes zoster in patients with rheumatoid arthritis according to biologic disease-modifying therapy. Arthritis Care Res (Hoboken). 2015;67:731–6.
88. Stone JH, Merkel PA, Spiera R, et al. Rituximab versus cyclophosphamide for ANCA-associated vasculitis. N Engl J Med. 2010;363:221–32.
89. Guillevin L, Pagnoux C, Karras A, et al. Rituximab versus azathioprine for maintenance in ANCA-associated vasculitis. N Engl J Med. 2014;371:1771–80.
90. Salmon JH, Cacoub P, Combe B, et al. Late-onset neutropenia after treatment with rituximab for rheumatoid arthritis and other autoimmune diseases: data from the AutoImmunity and rituximab registry. RMD Open. 2015;1:e000034.
91. Tesfa D, Ajeganova S, Hagglund H, et al. Late-onset neutropenia following rituximab therapy in rheumatic diseases: association with B lymphocyte depletion and infections. Arthritis Rheum. 2011;63:2209–14.
92. Abdulkader R, Dharmapalaiah C, Rose G, et al. Late-onset neutropenia in patients with rheumatoid arthritis after treatment with rituximab. J Rheumatol. 2014;41:858–61.
93. Knight A, Sundstrom Y, Borjesson O, et al. Late-onset neutropenia after rituximab in ANCA-associated vasculitis. Scand J Rheumatol. 2016;45:404–7.
94. Besada E, Koldingsnes W, Nossent JC. Serum immunoglobulin levels and risk factors for hypogammaglobulinaemia during long-term maintenance therapy with rituximab in patients with granulomatosis with polyangiitis. Rheumatology (Oxford). 2014;53:1818–24.
95. Roberts DM, Jones RB, Smith RM, et al. Rituximab-associated hypogammaglobulinemia: incidence, predictors and outcomes in patients with multi-system autoimmune disease. J Autoimmun. 2015;57:60–5.
96. Venhoff N, Niessen L, Kreuzaler M, et al. Reconstitution of the peripheral B lymphocyte compartment in patients with ANCA-associated vasculitides treated with rituximab for relapsing or refractory disease. Autoimmunity. 2014;47:401–8.
97. Besada E. Risk factors and adverse events poorly predict infections and hypogammaglobulinemia in granulomatosis with polyangiitis patients receiving rituximab. Autoimmune Dis. 2016;2016:8095695.
98. Reddy V, Martinez L, Isenberg DA, et al. Pragmatic treatment of patients with systemic lupus erythematosus with rituximab: long-term effects on serum immunoglobulins. Arthritis Care Res (Hoboken). 2016;69(6):857–66.
99. Mitroulis I, Hatzara C, Kandili A, et al. Long-term safety of rituximab in patients with rheumatic diseases and chronic or resolved hepatitis B virus infection. Ann Rheum Dis. 2013;72:308–10.
100. Varisco V, Vigano M, Batticciotto A, et al. Low risk of hepatitis B virus reactivation in HBsAg-negative/anti-HBc-positive carriers receiving rituximab for rheumatoid arthritis: a retrospective multicenter Italian study. J Rheumatol. 2016;43:869–74.
101. Molloy ES, Calabrese CM, Calabrese LH. The risk of progressive multifocal leukoencephalopathy in the biologic era: prevention and management. Rheum Dis Clin North Am. 2017;43:95–109.
102. Clifford DB, Ances B, Costello C, et al. Rituximab-associated progressive multifocal leukoencephalopathy in rheumatoid arthritis. Arch Neurol. 2011;68:1156–64.
103. Besada E, Nossent JC. Should Pneumocystis jiroveci prophylaxis be recommended with rituximab treatment in ANCA-associated vasculitis? Clin Rheumatol. 2013;32:1677–81.
104. Kronbichler A, Jayne DR, Mayer G. Frequency, risk factors and prophylaxis of infection in ANCA-associated vasculitis. Eur J Clin Invest. 2015;45:346–68.
105. Weinblatt ME, Moreland LW, Westhovens R, et al. Safety of abatacept administered intravenously in treatment of rheumatoid arthritis: integrated analyses of up to 8 years of treatment from the abatacept clinical trial program. J Rheumatol. 2013;40:787–97.
106. Alten R, Kaine J, Keystone E, et al. Long-term safety of subcutaneous abatacept in rheumatoid arthritis: integrated analysis of clinical trial data representing more than four years of treatment. Arthritis Rheumatol. 2014;66:1987–97.
107. Bigbee CL, Gonchoroff DG, Vratsanos G, et al. Abatacept treatment does not exacerbate chronic Mycobacterium tuberculosis infection in mice. Arthritis Rheum. 2007;56:2557–65.
108. Zink A, Manger B, Kaufmann J, et al. Evaluation of the RABBIT risk score for serious infections. Ann Rheum Dis. 2014;73:1673–6.
109. Moots RJ, Sebba A, Rigby W, et al. Effect of tocilizumab on neutrophils in adult patients with rheumatoid arthritis: pooled analysis of data from phase 3 and 4 clinical trials. Rheumatology (Oxford). 2017;56:541–9.
110. Strangfeld A, Richter A, Siegmund B, et al. Risk for lower intestinal perforations in patients with rheumatoid arthritis treated with tocilizumab in comparison

to treatment with other biologic or conventional synthetic DMARDs. Ann Rheum Dis. 2017;76:504–10.
111. Lang VR, Englbrecht M, Rech J, et al. Risk of infections in rheumatoid arthritis patients treated with tocilizumab. Rheumatology (Oxford). 2012;51:852–7.
112. Loricera J, Blanco R, Hernandez JL, et al. Tocilizumab in giant cell arteritis: multicenter open-label study of 22 patients. Semin Arthritis Rheum. 2015;44:717–23.
113. Regent A, Redeker S, Deroux A, et al. Tocilizumab in giant cell arteritis: a multicenter retrospective study of 34 patients. J Rheumatol. 2016;43:1547–52.
114. Villiger PM, Adler S, Kuchen S, et al. Tocilizumab for induction and maintenance of remission in giant cell arteritis: a phase 2, randomised, double-blind, placebo-controlled trial. Lancet. 2016;387:1921–7.
115. Stone JH, Tuckwell K, Dimonaco S, et al. Trial of tocilizumab in giant-cell arteritis. N Engl J Med. 2017;377:317–28.
116. Beukelman T, Xie F, Baddley JW, et al. The risk of hospitalized infection following initiation of biologic agents versus methotrexate in the treatment of juvenile idiopathic arthritis. Arthritis Res Ther. 2016;18:210.
117. Salliot C, Dougados M, Gossec L. Risk of serious infections during rituximab, abatacept and anakinra treatments for rheumatoid arthritis: meta-analyses of randomised placebo-controlled trials. Ann Rheum Dis. 2009;68:25–32.
118. Orrock JE, Ilowite NT. Canakinumab for the treatment of active systemic juvenile idiopathic arthritis. Expert Rev Clin Pharmacol. 2016;9:1015–24.
119. Ruperto N, Brunner HI, Quartier P, et al. Two randomized trials of canakinumab in systemic juvenile idiopathic arthritis. N Engl J Med. 2012;367:2396–406.
120. Fanouriakis A, Boumpas DT, Bertsias GK. Balancing efficacy and toxicity of novel therapies in systemic lupus erythematosus. Expert Rev Clin Pharmacol. 2011;4:437–51.
121. Navarra SV, Guzman RM, Gallacher AE, et al. Efficacy and safety of belimumab in patients with active systemic lupus erythematosus: a randomised, placebo-controlled, phase 3 trial. Lancet. 2011;377:721–31.
122. Furie R, Petri M, Zamani O, et al. A phase III, randomized, placebo-controlled study of belimumab, a monoclonal antibody that inhibits B lymphocyte stimulator, in patients with systemic lupus erythematosus. Arthritis Rheum. 2011;63:3918–30.
123. Kalb RE, Fiorentino DF, Lebwohl MG, et al. Risk of serious infection with biologic and systemic treatment of psoriasis: results from the Psoriasis Longitudinal Assessment and Registry (PSOLAR). JAMA Dermatol. 2015;151(9):961.
124. Almirall M, Rodriguez J, Mateo L, et al. Treatment with ustekinumab in a Spanish cohort of patients with psoriasis and psoriatic arthritis in daily clinical practice. Clin Rheumatol. 2017;36:439–43.
125. Chiu HY, Chen CH, Wu MS, et al. The safety profile of ustekinumab in the treatment of patients with psoriasis and concurrent hepatitis B or C. Br J Dermatol. 2013;169:1295–303.
126. van de Kerkhof PC, Griffiths CE, Reich K, et al. Secukinumab long-term safety experience: a pooled analysis of 10 phase II and III clinical studies in patients with moderate to severe plaque psoriasis. J Am Acad Dermatol. 2016;75:83–98.
127. Romani L. Immunity to fungal infections. Nat Rev Immunol. 2011;11:275–88.
128. Mease PJ, van der Heijde D, Ritchlin CT, et al. Ixekizumab, an interleukin-17A specific monoclonal antibody, for the treatment of biologic-naive patients with active psoriatic arthritis: results from the 24-week randomised, double-blind, placebo-controlled and active (adalimumab)-controlled period of the phase III trial SPIRIT-P1. Ann Rheum Dis. 2017;76:79–87.
129. Gordon KB, Blauvelt A, Papp KA, et al. Phase 3 trials of ixekizumab in moderate-to-severe plaque psoriasis. N Engl J Med. 2016;375:345–56.
130. Winthrop KL. The emerging safety profile of JAK inhibitors in rheumatic disease. Nat Rev Rheumatol. 2017;13:234–43.
131. Cohen S, Radominski SC, Gomez-Reino JJ, et al. Analysis of infections and all-cause mortality in phase II, phase III, and long-term extension studies of tofacitinib in patients with rheumatoid arthritis. Arthritis Rheumatol. 2014;66:2924–37.
132. Winthrop KL, Yamanaka H, Valdez H, et al. Herpes zoster and tofacitinib therapy in patients with rheumatoid arthritis. Arthritis Rheumatol. 2014;66:2675–84.
133. Winthrop KL, Park SH, Gul A, et al. Tuberculosis and other opportunistic infections in tofacitinib-treated patients with rheumatoid arthritis. Ann Rheum Dis. 2016;75:1133–8.
134. Sokka T, Abelson B, Pincus T. Mortality in rheumatoid arthritis: 2008 update. Clin Exp Rheumatol. 2008;26:S35–61.
135. van den Hoek J, Boshuizen HC, Roorda LD, et al. Mortality in patients with rheumatoid arthritis: a 15-year prospective cohort study. Rheumatol Int. 2017;37:487–93.
136. Hmamouchi I, Winthrop K, Launay O, et al. Low rate of influenza and pneumococcal vaccine coverage in rheumatoid arthritis: data from the international COMORA cohort. Vaccine. 2015;33:1446–52.
137. Fomin I, Caspi D, Levy V, et al. Vaccination against influenza in rheumatoid arthritis: the effect of disease modifying drugs, including TNF alpha blockers. Ann Rheum Dis. 2006;65:191–4.
138. Huang Y, Wang H, Wan L, et al. Is systemic lupus erythematosus associated with a declined immunogenicity and poor safety of influenza vaccination?: a systematic review and meta-analysis. Medicine (Baltimore). 2016;95:e3637.
139. Del PF, Lagana B, Biselli R, et al. Influenza vaccine administration in patients with systemic lupus erythematosus and rheumatoid arthritis. Safety and immunogenicity. Vaccine. 2006;24:3217–23.

140. Thomas K, Vassilopoulos D. Immunization in patients with inflammatory rheumatic diseases. Best Pract Res Clin Rheumatol. 2016;30:946–63.
141. Yates M, Watts RA, Bajema IM, et al. EULAR/ERA-EDTA recommendations for the management of ANCA-associated vasculitis. Ann Rheum Dis. 2016;75:1583–94.
142. Bodro M, Paterson DL. Has the time come for routine trimethoprim-sulfamethoxazole prophylaxis in patients taking biologic therapies? Clin Infect Dis. 2013;56:1621–8.
143. Wissmann G, Morilla R, Martin-Garrido I, et al. *Pneumocystis jirovecii* colonization in patients treated with infliximab. Eur J Clin Invest. 2011;41:343–8.
144. Ponce CA, Gallo M, Bustamante R, et al. Pneumocystis colonization is highly prevalent in the autopsied lungs of the general population. Clin Infect Dis. 2010;50:347–53.
145. Fritzsche C, Riebold D, Munk-Hartig A, et al. High prevalence of *Pneumocystis jirovecii* colonization among patients with autoimmune inflammatory diseases and corticosteroid therapy. Scand J Rheumatol. 2012;41:208–13.
146. Mori S, Sugimoto M. *Pneumocystis jirovecii* infection: an emerging threat to patients with rheumatoid arthritis. Rheumatology (Oxford). 2012;51:2120–30.
147. Katsuyama T, Saito K, Kubo S, et al. Prophylaxis for pneumocystis pneumonia in patients with rheumatoid arthritis treated with biologics, based on risk factors found in a retrospective study. Arthritis Res Ther. 2014;16:R43.
148. Fillatre P, Decaux O, Jouneau S, et al. Incidence of *Pneumocystis jirovecii* pneumonia among groups at risk in HIV-negative patients. Am J Med. 2014;127:1242–7.
149. Vananuvat P, Suwannalai P, Sungkanuparph S, et al. Primary prophylaxis for *Pneumocystis jirovecii* pneumonia in patients with connective tissue diseases. Semin Arthritis Rheum. 2011;41:497–502.
150. Liebling M, Rubio E, Ie S. Prophylaxis for *Pneumocystis jirovecii* pneumonia: is it a necessity in pulmonary patients on high-dose, chronic corticosteroid therapy without AIDS? Expert Rev Respir Med. 2015;9:171–81.
151. Limper AH, Knox KS, Sarosi GA, et al. An official American Thoracic Society statement: treatment of fungal infections in adult pulmonary and critical care patients. Am J Respir Crit Care Med. 2011;183:96–128.
152. Cortazar FB, Pendergraft WF III, Wenger J, et al. Effect of continuous B cell depletion with rituximab on pathogenic autoantibodies and total IgG levels in antineutrophil cytoplasmic antibody-associated vasculitis. Arthritis Rheumatol. 2017;69:1045–53.

35 The Promise of Personalized Medicine

Matthew L. Stoll

List of Abbreviations

AID	Anti-inflammatory diet
CGR	Cardiac glycoside reductase
EEN	Exclusive enteral nutrition
FMT	Fecal microbial transplantation
HMP	Human Microbiome Project
IBD	Inflammatory bowel disease
JIA	Juvenile idiopathic arthritis
RA	Rheumatoid arthritis
ReA	Reactive arthritis
SCFA	Short-chain fatty acids
SpA	Spondyloarthritis

Introduction

The promise of personalized medicine is that in the future, we will be able to take a biospecimen from a patient and use the information contained within to design the patient's therapy. One potential source of information is the human genome. Unfortunately, there are very few situations in which genetic testing can be used to guide therapy; rheumatologists are familiar with testing for thiopurine methyltransferase activity prior to starting azathioprine, as patients with defective gene activity are at increased risk of drug toxicity [1].

It is intuitively apparent that the microbiota, which among the organisms therein have been estimated to contain 100 times as many genes as their human hosts [2], are highly likely to contain genes that can both promote a disease and effect response to therapy. An essential difference between microbial and human genetics is that only the former can easily be modified with today's technology. This ability to modify the microbiota offers both peril and promise to microbiota-based therapy. The peril reflects whether assessment of the microbiota at any particular point in time actually reflects any truth about the patient's microbiota or whether it merely reflects the microbiota on the particular day it is sampled, which could be unrecognizably different by the next day. The promise, of course, is that it can be changed. As rheumatologists, we are familiar with genes that increase the risk of a particular condition, such as the strong association between HLA-B27 and ankylosing spondylitis [3]. Alas, if a patient with AS is HLA-B27+, there is scant that can be done about this polymorphism beyond continuing to work to understand the mechanism underlying its association with the disease. In contrast, if the same patient carried an abundance of microbial genes that contributed to his risk of developing the disease, then there is cause for optimism that microbial gene therapy may provide a therapeutic option.

M. L. Stoll
Department of Pediatrics, Division of Rheumatology, University of Alabama at Birmingham, Birmingham, AL, USA
e-mail: mstoll@peds.uab.edu

G. Ragab et al. (eds.), *The Microbiome in Rheumatic Diseases and Infection*,
https://doi.org/10.1007/978-3-319-79026-8_35

Stability of Microbiota

A detailed discussion of the ontogeny of the microbiota is beyond the scope of this review and has been summarized elsewhere [4]. In brief, in children born vaginally, the initial microbiota is highly similar to that of the genitourinary tract of the mother [5]. It then undergoes successive maturational changes throughout early childhood until it reaches an adult state [4]. Early data from the Human Microbiome Project (HMP) indicated that the adult state is reached around 2–3 years of age [6], although a subsequent study indicated that even older children have distinct microbiota from adults [7]. Even so, it is highly likely that the pace of the changes of the microbiota slows down after age 2–3 years. However, formal assessments of the stability of the microbiota have not been performed in school-age children.

In contrast, several studies performed in adult subjects have queried the stability of the microbiota by evaluating samples taken from adults at two or more points in time. Costello et al. obtained baseline and repeat samples from multiple different habitats (skin, gut, oral cavity, hair, nostril, outer ear) at baseline and after 3 months [8]. With respect to habitats, the variation between habitats (e.g., comparing stool to mouth) was far greater than that within habitats (e.g., comparing the mouth of one subject versus that of another). This was also the situation with individual participants, comparing two samples from the same habitat in different participants versus two samples from the same habitat in the same subject. However, the passage of time did not greatly increase the distance between the samples.

Likewise, Faith et al. followed 37 adults over a period 296 weeks [9]. To quantify the similarity between the samples, they used the Jaccard index, which in this case measures the fraction of shared strains between an individual at baseline and any time in the future—in essence, it measures the extent of overlap in a Venn diagram. The Jaccard index started off at approximately 0.9 in the first post-baseline collection, indicating 90% similarity. This gradually fell over time, but even at the end of the 5+-year study period, the Jaccard index was over 0.6, indicating 60% similarity. In contrast, two unrelated individuals had a Jaccard index of approximately 0.3.

The microbiota is so stable that it is a potential forensic tool. This was assessed by Curtis Huttenhower and colleagues at Harvard, who studied baseline and follow-up samples obtained from healthy adults through the Human Microbiome Project [10]. Their aim in this study was to assess whether an individual's baseline sample could be identified through sequencing of the second. For this study, they evaluated multiple habitats (feces, skin, etc.) as well as multiple informatics tools of querying the contents of the microbiota. It emerged that feces provided more stability than any of the other habitats. In addition, traditional sequencing approaches (e.g., 16S) did not yield as much accuracy as a marker-based approach, which takes into account the bacterial counterparts to genetic polymorphisms to compare baseline and follow-up samples. Using this marker approach from fecal samples, the authors demonstrated that the correct subject could be identified a respectable 80% of the time, with most errors consisting of failure to identify the correct subject (false negative) rather than incorrectly attributing one subject's sample to another (false positive).

Do the Microbiota Cause Illness?

In order for assessment of the microbiota to be useful as a clinical tool, one would likely argue it has to be both associated with and even causal of a disease state and/or predictive of response to therapy. In animal models of the disease, it is relatively easy to prove causality. For example, germ-free arthritis-prone animals do not develop HLA-B27 spondyloarthritis (SpA) [11], rheumatoid arthritis [12], multiple sclerosis [13], or gout [14]. Clearly, in these model systems, gut bacteria are necessary for the development of the disease. However, since a germ-free human system is obviously impossible, a direct pathogenic role for the microbiota cannot be evaluated in humans with the same degree of rigor that it can be studied in laboratory animals. Nevertheless, the body of literature does provide some evidence of a pathogenic role, and that comes from the consistency of findings within a particular disease state. The discussion in section IV of this textbook provided numerous examples of associations of an altered microbiota with a specific disease. For example, several studies in patients with inflammatory bowel disease (IBD; Chap. 15) demonstrated decreases in one particular organism, *Faecalibacterium prausnitzii* [15, 16], which was also found to be present in decreased abundance in children with the related condition of SpA [17]. Another study demonstrated that low *F. prausnitzii* abundance predicted poor response to therapy in children with IBD [18]. In contrast, *Prevotella copri* was found to be overly abundant in two unrelated studies of newly diagnosed RA patients (Chap. 15) [19, 20] yet has not been identified in any other disease models. Abundance of *Bacteroides* species was linked to multiple categories of JIA (Chap. 17) [17, 21], as well as to type I diabetes [22, 23], yet is depleted in adult IBD [24] and adult RA [20]. That the same bacteria often emerge as being associated in the same direction in the same disease using different patient populations is highly suggestive of a pathogenic or protective role for these particular organisms in the specific diseases in question.

Furthermore, it can be argued that the microbiota need not be dysbiotic for therapeutic alterations in such to have a potential benefit. First, as will be discussed below, the microbiota can influence response to drug therapy, by enhancing either effectiveness or toxicity. Thus, an alteration in the microbiota may permit usage of a drug that might otherwise result in dose-limited adverse events. Also, alterations in the overall diversity of the microbiota—the breadth and depth of organisms present in a sample—have been linked to a variety of diseases, including irritable bowel syndrome [25], psoriatic arthritis [26], and IBD [27]. Altered diversity may even have a predictive capacity, such as in the case of patients undergoing bone marrow transplantation, where patients with low diversity were less likely to survive treatment, even after adjustments for multiple confounding factors [28]. Likewise, in children at risk for developing type I diabetes, decreased bacterial diversity preceded the development of diabetes-associated antibodies [22]. Thus, therapeutic alterations in microbial diversity could provide benefit, even if no single organism can be identified as being deficient or overly abundant. Third, to the extent that bacteria differ in their metabolic capacities or effects on the immune system, there might be a family of organisms whose levels are normal in comparison with the general population, but for which it is the case that alterations in their levels can repair a metabolic or immunologic defect caused by some other source such as host genetics or an undefined environmental trigger. For example, certain bacteria are highly capable of producing short-chain fatty acids such as butyrate, which are generally considered to have anti-inflammatory effects (reviewed by [29]). Even if the levels of such bacteria are normal in comparison with the general population, enhancing the production of these metabolites might still be beneficial for the patient: their levels may be too low at an active disease site, or increased levels may be required to counteract an abnormal pro-inflammatory stimulus. Finally, alterations in the microbiota may be able to influence disease states through modulation of immune function. The microbiota has profound influences on multiple arms of the immune system. Some elements of the microbiota influence innate immunity through modulation of innate lymphoid cells as well as through binding to innate receptors such as the toll-like receptors and the nucleotide oligomerization domain among others [30]; *Bacteroides fragilis* can program regulatory T cells [31]; the mouse bacteria segmented filamentous bacteria generate Th17 T cells [32]; and helminths can promote Th2 function [33], a property which has enabled their therapeutic use in IBD [34, 35].

The Microbiota and Drug Metabolism

Many therapeutic compounds are either prodrugs that have to be metabolized to active moieties (e.g., sulfasalazine, mycophenolate mofetil, azathioprine) or are taken as active compounds that are subsequently inactivated by enzymes within the liver (e.g., nonsteroidal anti-inflammatory drugs, cyclosporine, tacrolimus). As many of the microbial genes have metabolic functions, the human intestinal microbiota constitutes a reservoir of metabolic enzymes that puts our livers to shame. In-depth reviews about the role of the microbiota in drug metabolism are available [36, 37]. Briefly, the microbiota appears to influence the absorption or metabolism of a variety of medications, including several such as nonsteroidal anti-inflammatory drugs, methotrexate, and sulfasalazine, which are widely used in rheumatology [36]. The microbiota may influence the tolerability of one of the most widely used medicines in rheumatology, methotrexate. Folic acid supplementation has long been recognized to reduce AEs associated with this therapy [38]. The microbiome of young children is far more efficient than that of adults at producing endogenous folic acid [4]; one can only speculate as to whether this might in part be responsible for the observation that methotrexate tends to be better tolerated in children with JIA as compared to adults with RA [39]. Data presented at the 2016 American College of Rheumatology conference showed that 2 of 25 bacterial species tested were able to metabolize oral methotrexate into polyglutamated methotrexate [40], the active moiety of the drug.

However, it is a non-rheumatic medicine, digoxin, that may best illustrate how the microbiota might impact drug delivery. Digoxin has long been used to treat congestive heart failure and arrhythmias. Digoxin can be metabolized to the inactive form dihydrodigoxin through reduction of the lactone ring [41]. Pronounced interindividual variability in absorption of the active form has been recognized for over 40 years [42], and a role of the intestinal microbiota in the inactivation of digoxin was initially recognized in 1981 [43]. In 1983, it was hypothesized that a specific organism, *Eubacterium lentum* (now called *Eggerthella lenta*), may be responsible for interindividual variations in digoxin pharmacokinetics in vivo due to its in vitro ability to inactivate this medicine [44]. However, the authors of that study were not able to confirm that this organism was responsible for digoxin inactivation in vivo, due to their observations that many subjects unable to reduce digoxin also had high *E. lentum* abundance. Using technology not available in 1983, Haiser et al. identified a genetic element that they termed the cardiac glycoside reductase (cgr) operon that was present only in *E. lenta* strains capable of inactivating digoxin [45]. This study also revealed that in vitro supplementation of the amino acid arginine resulted in decreased expression of the cgr operon and thus decreased digoxin inactivation. These in vitro observations also translated to decreased in vivo digoxin inactivation in mice fed a high-protein diet, as evidenced by higher active digoxin levels in high-protein- versus low-protein-fed mice. Thus, not only can a specific strain of a single organism predict response to a cardiac drug, but diet may also influence drug levels.

Therapeutic Alterations of the Microbiota

There are several potential ways to alter the microbiota: antibiotics, probiotics, diet, and fecal transplantation are the most widely discussed.

Antibiotics

Certain antibiotics have long been used in the treatment of IBD, particularly the postsurgical complication of pouchitis [46]. Otherwise, their role in the management of chronic inflammatory diseases appears to be limited. There are compelling reasons to limit use of antibiotics for autoimmune diseases, including induction of bacterial resistance, risks of development of *C. difficile* colitis, and availability of safer and more effective alternatives in the current era, but it is certainly worth exploring the data to see what can be learned from the previous era. Along those lines, the effectiveness of antibiotics in patients with SpA has been disappointing. The vast majority of the studies of antibiotics in SpA patients specifically included those with reactive arthritis (ReA), which by definition has a known or strongly suspected infectious trigger [47]. Despite this, a meta-analysis published in 2013 showed that antibiotics as a whole were ineffective in the management of ReA [48]. Likewise, a single randomized trial of doxycycline in patients with other forms of SpA also yielded negative findings [49]. In contrast, as discussed in this textbook (Chap. 15), studies in adults with RA have often shown multiple classes of antibiotics to be of benefit, although the mechanism of benefit remains unknown.

Probiotics

There may be a place for probiotics in the management of ulcerative colitis, although as recently reviewed, the data are not compelling [50]. Overall, this line of therapy has shown the least promise as a therapeutic tool. For example, two studies conducted in adult SpA, one a randomized placebo-controlled study [51] and the other a study conducted over the Internet that used only patient-reported outcomes but was nevertheless a randomized controlled trial [52], both yielded negative findings. Likewise, a RCT performed in children with juvenile SpA demonstrated improvement in both arms, possibly attributable to therapeutic nonsteroidal anti-inflammatory drug usage, with no differences between the groups among a panel of clinical and immunologic outcomes [53]. The studies of probiotics in RA showed minimal improvement, discussed in (Chap. 15).

One very plausible reason for their failure to alter the disease course is that they do not necessarily succeed in altering the contents of the microbiota, as summarized by a meta-analysis [54]. Work performed in Gary Wu's lab in mice showed that pretreatment with polyethylene glycol (the standard washout used for colonoscopies) and antibiotics permitted uptake of an engineered microbiota, while mice exposed to the same organisms without any pretreatment did not demonstrate any changes in their microbiota [55]. Thus, future studies involving probiotics may need to deplete the existing microbiota prior to adding new organisms. However, even this step does not guarantee success. Even if the probiotics did alter the microbiota, it does not necessarily follow that the changes would be beneficial. Prior to any large-scale probiotic study, proof-of-concept studies need to be performed to evaluate the effects of the intervention on the community structure (e.g., diversity), as well as abundances of specific organisms that may be relevant to the disease state. So far this has not been done.

Diet

There is an abundance of data indicating that dietary therapies can rapidly alter the microbiota [56, 57] as well as specific data on the effects of individual nutrients on the fecal microbiome or metabolome. Examples include increased production of fecal short-chain fatty acids following exposure to poorly digestible carbohydrates [58], decreased abundance of *Prevotella* following exposure to a high-fat diet [59], and increased *Bifidobacteria* with whey as compared with casein protein [60]. These measures have demonstrated benefit in animal models of inflammatory diseases [59, 61, 62], although there are mixed data in human conditions. As discussed elsewhere, studies of dietary therapy have not shown much promise. In IBD, the studies have been small and somewhat contradictory. There are some proponents of excluding complex carbohydrates from the diet of IBD patients on the grounds that the enzymes required for breaking down disaccharides may be impaired in patients with IBD [63] and thus the specific carbohydrate diet and the low fermentable oligo-, di-, and monosaccharide and polyol (commonly known as FODMAP) diet have gained some attention, although controlled studies with objective endpoints are lacking [64]. On the other hand, nondigestible carbohydrates are fermented in the colon to make short-chain fatty acids (SCFAs) [65], and organisms responsible for the production of SCFAs are generally depleted in patients with IBD [66], indicating a potential role for consumption of complex carbohydrates in patients with IBD. Indeed, high-fiber diets have also resulted in symptomatic improvement in patients with IBD, although, again, rigorous studies are lacking [67]. There has recently been success with an "anti-inflammatory diet (AID)" in the management of IBD. Olendzki1 et al. introduced 40 adult patients with IBD to an AID enriched for lean meats, omega-3 fatty acids, fibers, fruits, and vegetables, also encouraging foods with soft textures [68]. In this retrospective study, the 11 subjects who completed the diet for 1 month reported decreased symptom severity scales for Crohn disease (CD) and ulcerative colitis, as appropriate, based upon their IBD diagnosis. Likewise, Sigall-Boneh et al. treated 34 pediatric and 13 adult patients with CD with a combination of enteral nutrition and their version of an AID for 12 weeks [69]. This diet excluded gluten, dairy, animal fat, processed meats, emulsifiers, canned goods, and packaged products containing an expiration date. They reported remission in 33 (70%) of the subjects, including 6 of 7 subjects who followed the AID without supplemental enteral nutrition.

One form of dietary intervention that has had some consistent success is exclusive enteral nutrition (EEN), which consists of administration of a liquid diet, typically a polymeric formula, which is typically administered via a nasogastric or gastrotomy tube due to poor taste [70]. Randomized controlled studies in children with IBD have shown EEN to be equally effective as compared to corticosteroids in the induction of remission [71], while it appears to be less effective in adults [64]. There is also a case series of EEN use in children with JIA, demonstrating effectiveness among the 7 (of 13) children who maintained the therapy for more than 2 weeks [72]. The same group has also reported changes in the fecal microbiome and metabolome in association with EEN use [73].

A recent study indicated that a subject's baseline microbiota may influence response to dietary interventions. Kang et al. obtained baseline and follow-up fecal specimens from 12 healthy adults administered controlled diets containing varying doses of capsaicin in order to assess its effects on a variety of metabolic functions [74]. Consistent with the work of Wu et al. [56], they found that the baseline microbiota could be clustered into one of two enterotypes: one driven by *Bacteroides* and the other by *Prevotella*. Overall, subjects with the *Bacteroides* enterotype were far more sensitive to the metabolic effects of capsaicin as compared to those with the *Prevotella* enterotype. They also demonstrated more pronounced effects on the fecal microbiota and metabolome.

Another study that evaluated baseline patient factors and response to dietary intervention used baseline IgG4 antibodies against 16 nutrients, the rationale being that IgG4 antibodies reflect chronic antigenic exposure [75] and thus might reflect specific intolerance. A total of 98 subjects with CD were randomized to exclude either the nutrients against which they had the four highest IgG4 antibodies (intervention group) or the four lowest (control). The intervention group demonstrated statistically significant improvements in the short IBD quality of life score as well as in the Crohn's Disease Activity Index.

Finally, it bears mentioning that effects of diet on inflammatory diseases need not be limited to the microbiota. Certain foods may have a direct pro- or anti-inflammatory potential [76]. Additionally, proper nutrition may affect the nutritional status or weight of a subject, factors which themselves may have salutary effects on the disease state.

In summary, the following conclusions may be reached about dietary interventions on inflammatory diseases:

- Diet has the potential to alter the microbiota, which itself may alter the disease state.
- Diets that otherwise may be considered unhealthy may nevertheless have a beneficial effect on arthritis. An illustration is the ability of a high-fat diet to prevent development of a mouse model of auto-inflammatory bone disease [59]. Conversely, simply changing to a more healthful diet does not automatically translate to clinical benefits for a specific disease.
- As inflammatory diseases are chronic, potentially lifelong processes, dietary therapy will have to be acceptable to the patient and family for it to be sustained long term.
- Dietary therapy may need to be tailored to individual subjects based upon their disease state, baseline microbiota, and potentially other factors.

Fecal Microbial Transplant

Originally designed for treatment of recurrent *C. difficile* infection, fecal microbial transplant (FMT) is an effort to alter the fecal microbiota in a patient by replacing with one from a healthy individual. Feces are administered by gavage or rectally, although efforts are also in progress to introduce a defined consortium of bacteria that can act as a functional microbiota, thus avoiding the need for human donors and permitting use of capsules as the delivery vehicle. Although there are websites providing instructions on at-home FMT, comprehensive screening of potential donors is performed at medical centers. Following anecdotal reports of improvement in IBD [77, 78], randomized trials were conducted, showing mixed benefit [79, 80]. These studies have generally shown this procedure to be safe, although bacteremia caused by the introduced bacteria has been reported [81].

Targeting Individual Bacteria

All of the above approaches use broad strokes to alter the microbiota. Although this might be appropriate in some situations, such as in patients with recurrent *C. difficile* infection or in patients with a highly dysfunctional microbiota due to a combination of genetics, inflammation, and antibiotics, a directed approach may provide a safer and more effective means of providing microbial-based therapy. Some potential mechanisms of doing so were suggested in a recent review [82]. For example, Guo et al. tested a peptide with an antimicrobial moiety attached to a targeting moiety that was specific to the oral pathogen *Streptococcus mutans* [83]. A second potential approach would be use of bacteriophages targeting specific bacteria. As reviewed [84], this concept has been around for nearly one century, although it has yet to find widespread use in medicine. One limitation to both these approaches is that depleting one organism may have downstream effects on the abundances of multiple organisms, which either fill the niche of the depleted organism or were dependent upon the depleted organism and subsequently decrease in abundance [83]. Finally, Kuntz and Gilbert also proposed designing therapeutics to target specific microbial enzymes, an approach that has the advantage that it would not result in community-wide changes to the microbiota [82]. To the extent that by-products of bacterial metabolism may be involved in the inflammatory process, as recently suggested by Stoll et al. with respect to the tryptophan pathway in juvenile SpA [85], blocking bacterial enzymes not otherwise present in humans may have the potential to ameliorate disease.

Peek into the Future

So what might microbiota-based personalized medicine look like? In some cases, the microbiota might assist with diagnosis. In others, at time of diagnosis, the microbiota could be sampled and subjected to amplicon (16S) sequencing or perhaps shotgun sequencing. Based upon this, a unique treatment plan might be designed, in which the goal would be to generate a microbiota that might be more healthful for that particular disease state. This might involve introduction of organisms that affect the metabolism of drugs used to treat the disorder; using dietary, probiotic, or even bacteriophage therapy to increase or decrease the abundance of specific organisms that are associated with the disease state; or simply increasing the fecal microbial diversity. Drug therapy targeting bacterial enzymes predisposing to an unfavorable metabolic milieu might also be contemplated. Situations with more severe dysbiosis might require more drastic measures, such as EEN or FMT.

One final consideration is cost. Monitoring the fecal microbiota may sound interesting, but is it feasible from an economic standpoint? Here at UAB, the cost of performing 16S sequence analysis inclusive of all steps from DNA preparation to bioinformatics analysis is approximately $50/sample. This is equivalent to a complete blood count and metabolic panel, labs routinely ordered in medical practice. At approximately $1000/sample, shotgun sequencing is substantially more expensive, although it will likely fall in price in the future. Even at its current price, it is in line with numerous types of advanced testing, and to the extent that such testing could aid in the management of chronic diseases, it may well be worth its cost.

References

1. Clunie GP, Lennard L. Relevance of thiopurine methyltransferase status in rheumatology patients receiving azathioprine. Rheumatology (Oxford). 2004;43(1):13–8.
2. Qin J, Li R, Raes J, Arumugam M, Burgdorf KS, Manichanh C, et al. A human gut microbial gene catalogue established by metagenomic sequencing. Nature. 2010;464(7285):59–65.
3. Brewerton DA, Hart FD, Nicholls A, Caffrey M, James DC, Sturrock RD. Ankylosing spondylitis and HL-A 27. Lancet. 1973;1(7809):904–7.
4. Backhed F, Roswall J, Peng Y, Feng Q, Jia H, Kovatcheva-Datchary P, et al. Dynamics and stabilization of the human gut Microbiome during the first year of life. Cell Host Microbe. 2015;17(6):852.
5. Dominguez-Bello MG, Costello EK, Contreras M, Magris M, Hidalgo G, Fierer N, et al. Delivery mode shapes the acquisition and structure of the initial microbiota across multiple body habitats in newborns. Proc Natl Acad Sci U S A. 2010;107(26):11971–5.
6. Yatsunenko T, Rey FE, Manary MJ, Trehan I, Dominguez-Bello MG, Contreras M, et al. Human gut microbiome viewed across age and geography. Nature. 2012;486(7402):222–7.
7. Hollister EB, Riehle K, Luna RA, Weidler EM, Rubio-Gonzales M, Mistretta TA, et al. Structure and function of the healthy pre-adolescent pediatric gut microbiome. Microbiome. 2015;3:36.
8. Costello EK, Lauber CL, Hamady M, Fierer N, Gordon JI, Knight R. Bacterial community variation in human body habitats across space and time. Science. 2009;326(5960):1694–7.
9. Faith JJ, Guruge JL, Charbonneau M, Subramanian S, Seedorf H, Goodman AL, et al. The long-term stability of the human gut microbiota. Science. 2013;341(6141):1237439.
10. Franzosa EA, Huang K, Meadow JF, Gevers D, Lemon KP, Bohannan BJ, et al. Identifying personal microbiomes using metagenomic codes. Proc Natl Acad Sci U S A. 2015;112(22):E2930–8.
11. Taurog JD, Richardson JA, Croft JT, Simmons WA, Zhou M, Fernandez-Sueiro JL, et al. The germfree state prevents development of gut and joint inflammatory disease in HLA-B27 transgenic rats. J Exp Med. 1994;180(6):2359–64.
12. Wu HJ, Ivanov II, Darce J, Hattori K, Shima T, Umesaki Y, et al. Gut-residing segmented filamentous bacteria drive autoimmune arthritis via T helper 17 cells. Immunity. 2010;32(6):815–27.
13. Berer K, Mues M, Koutrolos M, Rasbi ZA, Boziki M, Johner C, et al. Commensal microbiota and myelin autoantigen cooperate to trigger autoimmune demyelination. Nature. 2011;479(7374):538–41.
14. Vieira AT, Macia L, Galvao I, Martins FS, Canesso MC, Amaral FA, et al. A role for gut Microbiota and the metabolite-sensing receptor GPR43 in a murine model of gout. Arthritis Rheumatol. 2015;67(6):1646–56.
15. Sokol H, Seksik P, Furet JP, Firmesse O, Nion-Larmurier I, Beaugerie L, et al. Low counts of Faecalibacterium prausnitzii in colitis microbiota. Inflamm Bowel Dis. 2009;15(8):1183–9.
16. Machiels K, Joossens M, Sabino J, De Preter V, Arijs I, Eeckhaut V, et al. A decrease of the butyrate-producing species Roseburia hominis and Faecalibacterium prausnitzii defines dysbiosis in patients with ulcerative colitis. Gut. 2013;63(8):1275–83.
17. Stoll ML, Kumar R, Morrow CD, Lefkowitz EJ, Cui X, Genin A, et al. Altered microbiota associated with abnormal humoral immune responses to commensal organisms in enthesitis-related arthritis. Arthritis Res Ther. 2014;16(6):486.
18. Shaw KA, Bertha M, Hofmekler T, Chopra P, Vatanen T, Srivatsa A, et al. Dysbiosis, inflammation, and response to treatment: a longitudinal study of pediatric subjects with newly diagnosed inflammatory bowel disease. Genome Med. 2016;8(1):75.
19. Maeda Y, Kurakawa T, Umemoto E, Motooka D, Ito Y, Gotoh K, et al. Dysbiosis contributes to arthritis development via activation of autoreactive T cells in the intestine. Arthritis Rheumatol. 2016;68(11):2646–61.
20. Scher JU, Sczesnak A, Longman RS, Segata N, Ubeda C, Bielski C, et al. Expansion of intestinal Prevotella copri correlates with enhanced susceptibility to arthritis. Elife. 2013;2:e01202.
21. Tejesvi MV, Arvonen M, Kangas SM, Keskitalo PL, Pirttila AM, Karttunen TJ, et al. Faecal microbiome in new-onset juvenile idiopathic arthritis. Eur J Clin Microbiol Infect Dis. 2015;35(3):363–70.
22. Giongo A, Gano KA, Crabb DB, Mukherjee N, Novelo LL, Casella G, et al. Toward defining the autoimmune microbiome for type 1 diabetes. ISME J. 2011;5(1):82–91.
23. Murri M, Leiva I, Gomez-Zumaquero JM, Tinahones FJ, Cardona F, Soriguer F, et al. Gut microbiota in children with type 1 diabetes differs from that in healthy children: a case-control study. BMC Med. 2013;11:46.
24. Zhou Y, Zhi F. Lower level of Bacteroides in the gut Microbiota is associated with inflammatory bowel disease: a meta-analysis. Biomed Res Int. 2016;2016:5828959.
25. Durban A, Abellan JJ, Jimenez-Hernandez N, Salgado P, Ponce M, Ponce J, et al. Structural alterations of faecal and mucosa-associated bacterial communities in irritable bowel syndrome. Environ Microbiol Rep. 2012;4(2):242–7.

26. Scher JU, Ubeda C, Artacho A, Attur M, Isaac S, Reddy SM, et al. Decreased bacterial diversity characterizes the altered gut microbiota in patients with psoriatic arthritis, resembling dysbiosis in inflammatory bowel disease. Arthritis Rheumatol. 2015;67(1):128–39.
27. Michail S, Durbin M, Turner D, Griffiths AM, Mack DR, Hyams J, et al. Alterations in the gut microbiome of children with severe ulcerative colitis. Inflamm Bowel Dis. 2012;18(10):1799–808.
28. Taur Y, Jenq RR, Perales MA, Littmann ER, Morjaria S, Ling L, et al. The effects of intestinal tract bacterial diversity on mortality following allogeneic hematopoietic stem cell transplantation. Blood. 2014;124(7):1174–82.
29. Stoll ML. Gut microbes, immunity, and spondyloarthritis. Clin Immunol. 2015;159(2):134–42.
30. Thaiss CA, Zmora N, Levy M, Elinav E. The microbiome and innate immunity. Nature. 2016;535(7610):65–74.
31. Round JL, Lee SM, Li J, Tran G, Jabri B, Chatila TA, et al. The toll-like receptor 2 pathway establishes colonization by a commensal of the human microbiota. Science. 2011;332(6032):974–7.
32. Farkas AM, Panea C, Goto Y, Nakato G, Galan-Diez M, Narushima S, et al. Induction of Th17 cells by segmented filamentous bacteria in the murine intestine. J Immunol Methods. 2015;421:104–11.
33. Hussaarts L, Yazdanbakhsh M, Guigas B. Priming dendritic cells for th2 polarization: lessons learned from helminths and implications for metabolic disorders. Front Immunol. 2014;5:499.
34. Summers RW, Elliott DE, Urban JF Jr, Thompson R, Weinstock JV. Trichuris suis therapy in Crohn's disease. Gut. 2005;54(1):87–90.
35. Summers RW, Elliott DE, Urban JF Jr, Thompson RA, Weinstock JV. Trichuris suis therapy for active ulcerative colitis: a randomized controlled trial. Gastroenterology. 2005;128(4):825–32.
36. Spanogiannopoulos P, Bess EN, Carmody RN, Turnbaugh PJ. The microbial pharmacists within us: a metagenomic view of xenobiotic metabolism. Nat Rev Microbiol. 2016;14(5):273–87.
37. Jourova L, Anzenbacher P, Anzenbacherova E. Human gut microbiota plays a role in the metabolism of drugs. Biomed Pap Med Fac Univ Palacky Olomouc Czech Repub. 2016;160(3):317–26.
38. Morgan SL, Baggott JE, Vaughn WH, Austin JS, Veitch TA, Lee JY, et al. Supplementation with folic acid during methotrexate therapy for rheumatoid arthritis. A double-blind, placebo-controlled trial. Ann Intern Med. 1994;121(11):833–41.
39. Graham LD, Myones BL, Rivas-Chacon RF, Pachman LM. Morbidity associated with long-term methotrexate therapy in juvenile rheumatoid arthritis. J Pediatr. 1992;120(3):468–73.
40. Nayak RR, O'Loughlin C, Fischbach M, Turnbaugh PJ. Methotrexate is an antibacterial drug metabolized by human gut Bacteria [abstract]. Arthritis Rheum. 2016;68(suppl 10).
41. Robertson LW, Chandrasekaran A, Reuning RH, Hui J, Rawal BD. Reduction of digoxin to 20R-dihydrodigoxin by cultures of Eubacterium lentum. Appl Environ Microbiol. 1986;51(6):1300–3.
42. Greenblatt DJ, Smith TW, Koch-Weser J. Bioavailability of drugs: the digoxin dilemma. Clin Pharmacokinet. 1976;1(1):36–51.
43. Lindenbaum J, Rund DG, Butler VP Jr, Tse-Eng D, Saha JR. Inactivation of digoxin by the gut flora: reversal by antibiotic therapy. N Engl J Med. 1981;305(14):789–94.
44. Saha JR, Butler VP Jr, Neu HC, Lindenbaum J. Digoxin-inactivating bacteria: identification in human gut flora. Science. 1983;220(4594):325–7.
45. Haiser HJ, Gootenberg DB, Chatman K, Sirasani G, Balskus EP, Turnbaugh PJ. Predicting and manipulating cardiac drug inactivation by the human gut bacterium Eggerthella lenta. Science. 2013;341(6143):295–8.
46. Sokol H. Probiotics and antibiotics in IBD. Dig Dis. 2014;32(Suppl 1):10–7.
47. Carter JD. Reactive arthritis: defined etiologies, emerging pathophysiology, and unresolved treatment. Infect Dis Clin N Am. 2006;20(4):827–47.
48. Barber CE, Kim J, Inman RD, Esdaile JM, James MT. Antibiotics for treatment of reactive arthritis: a systematic review and metaanalysis. J Rheumatol. 2013;40(6):916–28.
49. Smieja M, MacPherson DW, Kean W, Schmuck ML, Goldsmith CH, Buchanan W, et al. Randomised, blinded, placebo controlled trial of doxycycline for chronic seronegative arthritis. Ann Rheum Dis. 2001;60(12):1088–94.
50. Derikx LA, Dieleman LA, Hoentjen F. Probiotics and prebiotics in ulcerative colitis. Best Pract Res Clin Gastroenterol. 2016;30(1):55–71.
51. Jenks K, Stebbings S, Burton J, Schultz M, Herbison P, Highton J. Probiotic therapy for the treatment of spondyloarthritis: a randomized controlled trial. J Rheumatol. 2010;37(10):2118–25.
52. Brophy S, Burrows CL, Brooks C, Gravenor MB, Siebert S, Allen SJ. Internet-based randomised controlled trials for the evaluation of complementary and alternative medicines: probiotics in spondyloarthropathy. BMC Musculoskelet Disord. 2008;9:4.
53. Shukla A, Gaur P, Aggarwal A. Effect of probiotics on clinical and immune parameters in enthesitis-related arthritis category of juvenile idiopathic arthritis. Clin Exp Immunol. 2016;185(3):301–8.
54. Kristensen NB, Bryrup T, Allin KH, Nielsen T, Hansen TH, Pedersen O. Alterations in fecal microbiota composition by probiotic supplementation in healthy adults: a systematic review of randomized controlled trials. Genome Med. 2016;8(1):52.
55. Shen TC, Albenberg L, Bittinger K, Chehoud C, Chen YY, Judge CA, et al. Engineering the gut microbiota to treat hyperammonemia. J Clin Invest. 2015;125(7):2841–50.
56. Wu GD, Chen J, Hoffmann C, Bittinger K, Chen YY, Keilbaugh SA, et al. Linking long-term dietary patterns with gut microbial enterotypes. Science. 2011;334(6052):105–8.

57. David LA, Maurice CF, Carmody RN, Gootenberg DB, Button JE, Wolfe BE, et al. Diet rapidly and reproducibly alters the human gut microbiome. Nature. 2014;505(7484):559–63.
58. Bindels LB, Neyrinck AM, Salazar N, Taminiau B, Druart C, Muccioli GG, et al. Non digestible oligosaccharides modulate the gut Microbiota to control the development of Leukemia and associated Cachexia in mice. PLoS One. 2015;10(6):e0131009.
59. Lukens JR, Gurung P, Vogel P, Johnson GR, Carter RA, McGoldrick DJ, et al. Dietary modulation of the microbiome affects autoinflammatory disease. Nature. 2014;516(7530):246–9.
60. McAllan L, Skuse P, Cotter PD, O'Connor P, Cryan JF, Ross RP, et al. Protein quality and the protein to carbohydrate ratio within a high fat diet influences energy balance and the gut microbiota in C57BL/6J mice. PLoS One. 2014;9(2):e88904.
61. Le Leu RK, Young GP, Hu Y, Winter J, Conlon MA, et al. Dig Dis Sci. 2013;58(12):3475–82.
62. Sprong RC, Schonewille AJ, van der Meer R. Dietary cheese whey protein protects rats against mild dextran sulfate sodium-induced colitis: role of mucin and microbiota. J Dairy Sci. 2010;93(4):1364–71.
63. Kakodkar S, Farooqui AJ, Mikolaitis SL, Mutlu EA. The specific carbohydrate diet for inflammatory bowel disease: a case series. J Acad Nutr Diet. 2015;115(8):1226–32.
64. Ruemmele FM. Role of diet in inflammatory bowel disease. Ann Nutr Metab. 2016;68(Suppl 1):33–41.
65. Arpaia N, Campbell C, Fan X, Dikiy S, van der Veeken J, de Roos P, et al. Metabolites produced by commensal bacteria promote peripheral regulatory T-cell generation. Nature. 2013;504(7480):451–5.
66. Cao Y, Shen J, Ran ZH. Association between Faecalibacterium prausnitzii reduction and inflammatory bowel disease: a meta-analysis and systematic review of the literature. Gastroenterol Res Pract. 2014;2014:872725.
67. Brotherton CS, Taylor AG, Bourguignon C, Anderson JG. A high-fiber diet may improve bowel function and health-related quality of life in patients with Crohn disease. Gastroenterol Nurs. 2014;37(3):206–16.
68. Olendzki BC, Silverstein TD, Persuitte GM, Ma Y, Baldwin KR, Cave D. An anti-inflammatory diet as treatment for inflammatory bowel disease: a case series report. Nutr J. 2014;13:5.
69. Sigall-Boneh R, Pfeffer-Gik T, Segal I, Zangen T, Boaz M, Levine A. Partial enteral nutrition with a Crohn's disease exclusion diet is effective for induction of remission in children and young adults with Crohn's disease. Inflamm Bowel Dis. 2014;20(8):1353–60.
70. Whitten KE, Rogers P, Ooi CY, Day AS. International survey of enteral nutrition protocols used in children with Crohn's disease. J Dig Dis. 2012;13(2):107–12.
71. Heuschkel RB, Menache CC, Megerian JT, Baird AE. Enteral nutrition and corticosteroids in the treatment of acute Crohn's disease in children. J Pediatr Gastroenterol Nutr. 2000;31(1):8–15.
72. Berntson L, Hedlund-Treutiger I, Alving K. Anti-inflammatory effect of exclusive enteral nutrition in patients with juvenile idiopathic arthritis. Clin Exp Rheumatol. 2016;34(5):941–5.
73. Berntson L, Agback P, Dicksved J. Changes in fecal microbiota and metabolomics in a child with juvenile idiopathic arthritis (JIA) responding to two treatment periods with exclusive enteral nutrition (EEN). Clin Rheumatol. 2016;35(6):1501–6.
74. Kang C, Zhang Y, Zhu X, Liu K, Wang X, Chen M, et al. Healthy subjects differentially respond to dietary capsaicin correlating with the specific gut enterotypes. J Clin Endocrinol Metab. 2016;101(12):4681–9. jc20162786.
75. Stapel SO, Asero R, Ballmer-Weber BK, Knol EF, Strobel S, Vieths S, et al. Testing for IgG4 against foods is not recommended as a diagnostic tool: EAACI task force report. Allergy. 2008;63(7):793–6.
76. Shivappa N, Steck SE, Hurley TG, Hussey JR, Hebert JR. Designing and developing a literature-derived, population-based dietary inflammatory index. Public Health Nutr. 2014;17(8):1689–96.
77. Russell GH, Kaplan JL, Youngster I, Baril-Dore M, Schindelar L, Hohmann E, et al. Fecal transplant for recurrent Clostridium difficile infection in children with and without inflammatory bowel disease. J Pediatr Gastroenterol Nutr. 2014;58(5):588–92.
78. Zhang FM, Wang HG, Wang M, Cui BT, Fan ZN, Ji GZ. Fecal microbiota transplantation for severe enterocolonic fistulizing Crohn's disease. World J Gastroenterol. 2013;19(41):7213–6.
79. Suskind DL, Brittnacher MJ, Wahbeh G, Shaffer ML, Hayden HS, Qin X, et al. Fecal microbial transplant effect on clinical outcomes and fecal microbiome in active Crohn's disease. Inflamm Bowel Dis. 2015;21(3):556–63.
80. Suskind DL, Singh N, Nielson H, Wahbeh G. Fecal microbial transplant via nasogastric tube for active pediatric ulcerative colitis. J Pediatr Gastroenterol Nutr. 2015;60(1):27–9.
81. Quera R, Espinoza R, Estay C, Rivera D. Bacteremia as an adverse event of fecal microbiota transplantation in a patient with Crohn's disease and recurrent Clostridium difficile infection. J Crohns Colitis. 2014;8(3):252–3.
82. Kuntz TM, Gilbert JA. Introducing the Microbiome into precision medicine. Trends Pharmacol Sci. 2016;38(1):81–91.
83. Guo L, McLean JS, Yang Y, Eckert R, Kaplan CW, Kyme P, et al. Precision-guided antimicrobial peptide as a targeted modulator of human microbial ecology. Proc Natl Acad Sci USA. 2015;112(24):7569–74.
84. Kutter E, De Vos D, Gvasalia G, Alavidze Z, Gogokhia L, Kuhl S, et al. Phage therapy in clinical practice: treatment of human infections. Curr Pharm Biotechnol. 2010;11(1):69–86.
85. Stoll ML, Kumar R, Lefkowitz EJ, Cron RQ, Morrow CD, Barnes S. Fecal metabolomics in pediatric spondyloarthritis implicate decreased metabolic diversity and altered tryptophan metabolism as pathogenic factors. Genes Immun. 2016;17(7):400–5.

Index

G. Ragab et al. (eds.), *The Microbiome in Rheumatic Diseases and Infection*,
https://doi.org/10.1007/978-3-319-79026-8

D

P

Q

R

MIX
Papier aus verantwortungsvollen Quellen
Paper from responsible sources
FSC® C105338

If you have any concerns about our products,
you can contact us on
ProductSafety@springernature.com

In case Publisher is established outside the EU,
the EU authorized representative is:
Springer Nature Customer Service Center GmbH
Europaplatz 3, 69115 Heidelberg, Germany

Printed by Libri Plureos GmbH
in Hamburg, Germany